Physical Diagnosis in Neonatology

Physical Diagnosis in Neonatology

Mary Ann Fletcher, M.D.
Clinical Professor of Pediatrics and of Obstetrics and Gynecology
George Washington University
Attending Physician
The George Washington University Medical Center
Children's National Medical Center
Washington, D.C.

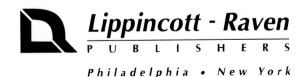

Lippincott - Raven
P U B L I S H E R S
Philadelphia • New York

Acquisitions Editor: Paula Callaghan
Developmental Editor: Julia Benson
Manufacturing Manager: Dennis Teston
Production Manager: Larry Bernstein
Production Editor: Linda B. Bass
Cover Designer: Betty Booker
Indexer: Linda Fetters
Compositor: Maryland Composition
Printer: Phoenix Offset

Printed and bound in China

9 8 7 6 5 4 3 2 1

Library of Congress Cataloging-in-Publication Data
Fletcher, Mary Ann.
    Physical diagnosis in neonatology / Mary Ann Fletcher.
        p.   cm.
    Includes bibliographical references and index.
    ISBN 0-397-51386-0
    1. Infants (Newborn)—Medical examinations.   2. Infants (Newborn)—
Diseases—Diagnosis.   I. Title.
    [DNLM: 1. Physical Examination—in infancy & childhood.
2. Diagnosis—in infancy & childhood.   3. Infant, Newborn.   WS 141
F613p 1997]
RJ255.5.F54   1997
618.92′01—dc21
DNLM/DLC
for Library of Congress

Care has been taken to confirm the accuracy of the information presented and to describe generally accepted practices. However, the authors, editors, and publisher are not responsible for errors or omissions or for any consequences from application of the information in this book and make no warranty, express or implied, with respect to the contents of the publication.

The authors, editors, and publisher have exerted every effort to ensure that drug selection and dosage set forth in this text are in accordance with current recommendations and practice at the time of publication. However, in view of ongoing research, changes in government regulations, and the constant flow of information relating to drug therapy and drug reactions, the reader is urged to check the package insert for each drug for any change in indications and dosage and for added warnings and precautions. This is particularly important when the recommended agent is a new or infrequently employed drug.

Some drugs and medical devices presented in this publication have Food and Drug Administration (FDA) clearance for limited use in restricted research settings. It is the responsibility of the health care provider to ascertain the FDA status of each drug or device planned for use in their clinical practice.

*To Maureen Edwards, my partner in neonatology for 17 years.
Her clinical skills, unselfish work ethic, and friendship
have always made a difference.*

*In loving memory of my son,
Declan J. Hurley,
April 25, 1974 to July 26, 1997.*

Contents

SECTION A: GENERAL

Purpose of Examination • First Neonatal Examination • Assessment of
Transition • Newborn Examination • Discharge Examination • First
Outpatient, Well-Baby Examination • Sick-Baby Examination •
Evaluation of the Dysmorphic Infant • *Interpreting Findings Based on
Time of Examination* • *Environment* • *Equipment Needed* • *History* •
Elements of Neonatal History • Techniques for Taking the History •
General Principles in Physical Examination • Tools of Physical
Examination • Descriptions of Alternation in Anatomic Structure •
Areas for Potential Error • Order of Examination • *Documentation* •
General Examination • General Observations • *References*

Indications for Measuring Growth Parameters • Morbidity and Mortality
Statistics for Outcome • Identification of Infant at Risk for Problems
Associated with Aberrant Growth Pattern • Providing a Quantitative
Value to Qualitative Assessment • Determine Pathophysiology
Contributing to a Disproportion • Monitor Efficacy of Nutritional
Interventions • Monitor Complications of Disease Processes • *Define
Aberrant Growth* • *Standard Curves* • *Equipment for Measuring* •
What Should be Measured • *Specific Measurement Techniques* •
General Measurement • Measurement of Head • Measurement of Ears •

Hearing by Behavior Response • *Clinical Examples* • Aural Atresia •
Auricular Sinus • Auricular Appendage • Microtia • Lop Ear • Cup
Ear • *Glossary* • *References*

SECTION C: THE TRUNK REGION

Steps in Examination of the Trunk • *I. THE UPPER TRUNK* •
Technique of Examination of the Chest • Pertinent History for
Pulmonary Assessment • Inspection and Palpation of the Chest •
Auscultation • Percussion of Chest • Transillumination of the Chest •
Causes of Respiratory Distress • Breasts • *Techniques of Examination
of the Cardiovascular System* • Pertinent History for Cardiovascular
Assessment • Cardiac Transition • Inspection • Palpation • Measure
Blood Pressure • Auscultation • Select Appropriate Laboratory
Information • Lymph Nodes • *II. THE LOWER TRUNK AND BACK* •
The Abdomen • Steps in Examination • Pertinent History for Abdominal
Conditions • Inspection • Palpation and Percussion of the Abdomen •
Auscultate the Abdomen • Transillumination of the Abdomen • *The
Perineum and Genitalia* • Pertinent History for Perineum and
Genitourinary System • Examination of the Female Genitalia •
Examination of Male Genitalia • Ambiguous Genitalia • Anus •
Inguinal Region • *The Back* • Steps in Examining the Back • *Glossary*
• *References*

SECTION D: NEUROSKELETAL EVALUATION

Embryology • *Anatomy* • *Techniques of Examination of the Extremities*
• Upper Extremities • Lower Extremities • Special Clinical
Assessment: Examination of the Hips • Special Clinical Assessment:
Examination of the Clavicles • Special Clinical Assessment: Defining
Direction and Range of Motion in Major Joints • *Clinical Examples* •
Clinical Example: Preaxial Duplication • Clinical example: Abnormal
Limb Length in Achondroplasia • Clinical example: Abnormal Range of
Motion in Arthrogryposis • *Glossary* • *References*

Purpose of Neonatal Neurologic Examination • Assessing Behavior •
Infant State • *The General Neuromotor Examination* • *Sequence of
Examination* • *Muscle Tone* • *Specific Examination Techniques* •
Cranial Nerves • Deep Tendon Reflexes • Skin Reflexes • Primitive
Reflexes • *Indicators of Behavior* • Irritability • Cuddliness • Self-
Quieting Activity • Visual and Auditory Response Decrement • Visual
and Auditory Orientation Responses • Defensive Reaction • *General
Reflexes* • Posture Supine and Prone (Resting Posture) • Spontaneous
Motor Activity • Spontaneous Movements of the Head in the Prone
Position • Spontaneous Crawling or Bauer's Response • Moro Reflex •
Startle Reflex • Asymmetrical Tonic Neck Reflex • *Upper Segmental
Reflexes: Passive Tone* • Square Window • *Upper Segmental* Reflexes:
Active Tone • Palmar Grasp (Upper Extremity Grasp, Tonic Reflex of
the Finger Flexors, Hand Grasp) • *Axial Reflexes* • Active Tone •

Upper Segmental Reflexes: Passive Tone • Lower Segmental Reflexes: Passive Tone • Lower Segmental Reflexes: Active Tone • Other Lower Segmental Reflexes • Maturation and Reflexes of Early Infancy • Symmetrical Tonic Neck Reflex STNR (Cat Reflex) • Tonic Labyrinthine Reflexes in Supine and Prone • Landau Reflex • Derotative Body • Downward Thrust • Upper Extremity Placing • Glossary • References

General Growth Measurements • Head and Neck Region • The Trunk Region • The Extremities • Periods of Critical Human Development • Blood Pressure • References

Preface

The eye of the master will do more work than both his hands.
—Benjamin Franklin

Physical diagnosis represents *old* medicine. Advanced technology involving detailed imaging and microanalysis that refines diagnoses to a subcellular level has come to define *new* medicine. In many cases, this exciting technology leads to early and precise diagnoses and improves the level of care, widening the options for both medical and surgical intervention. As both availability and demand for technology-assisted diagnosis have increased, dependence on traditional physical diagnosis has decreased, contributing to deteriorating levels of skill in this vital component of our discipline. Additionally, the expanding volume of information presented during the years of formal medical education shorten the time available for the basics of anatomy, embryology, and physical examination. Less emphasis by educators makes the process of physical diagnosis seem unimportant to students. For resident trainees, far less time is likely to be devoted to physical examination than is spent discussing use of advanced technological diagnostic and therapeutic tools. Further, intensive care practices appropriately discourage touching fragile infants, but that does not mean careful examination is inappropriate.

Physical diagnosis lacks the glamour of advanced technology. This aspect of our practice is more the true art than the strict science of medicine. It may seem old-fashioned because it relies on clinical experience and acumen. Yet, it is a process that keeps the physician-patient relationship personal. A balance between the new and old means that technology supplements, rather than replaces, the traditional tools of physical diagnosis. The history and physical examination direct how, if at all, we can use modern technology to augment or refine our findings.

This book is intended to remind us of the irreplaceable value of looking at, listening to, and touching infants during their many changes in the newborn period. The book's preparation has relied both on available literature and on my own clinical experience, supplemented with greatly appreciated advice from other master clinicians. Unfortunately, many of our traditionally accepted standards are based on few cases with questionable or absent statistical testing. Others have evolved into accepted "facts" from incorrect or over-zealous interpretations of published or unpublished findings. There has been a sincere effort to identify these issues, but the readers are encouraged to help with this process. This book will not discuss diagnosis of syndromes (except as isolated findings) because there are already seminal reference books detailing these conditions. The intention has been, rather, to identify when specific findings are likely to be abnormal and related so that one can then investigate a possible syndromic relationship.

Technological capabilities aside, the approach to each patient should always begin with the patient's history and a physical examination. After all, good beginnings are what both the art and the science of neonatology are all about.

Mary Ann Fletcher, M.D.

Acknowledgments

As always, a project such as this results from the contributions of many helpful teachers, coworkers, and students. Maureen Edwards and Anne B. Fletcher willingly opened up their own photography collections to provide many of the unusual case illustrations. Howland Hartley cheerfully reviewed all the dermatology illustrations. Ayman El Mohandes helped by lending important reference materials and by capturing some cases on film. The staff nurses and physicians at The George Washington University Medical Center remembered to tell me about unusual findings. This project was really a group effort from which we all learned.

I would like to thank Benjamin M. Manalasay, Jr. for photographs and assistance in helping to organize files; and our office staff of Mary Reed and Saundra Moore for their cheerful support. Sincere appreciation goes to the audio-visual department at The George Washington University School of Medicine. Fine drawings by Judy Guenther and patient advice on photography by Jim Kendrick were truly special contributions.

Thanks to the editors and assistants at Lippincott-Raven Publishers, especially to Richard Winters, who started me off with solid suggestions; Paula Callaghan for her guidance as an editor; and Julia Benson for her assistance and gentle reminders.

And finally, a great measure of appreciation goes to my husband and children, John, Declan, Ryan, and Jennifer Hurley, for doing what only families can do. They are the source of my strength. I would especially like to thank our daughter Jen for doing everything that we asked during her summers of work.

Physical Diagnosis in Neonatology

General

1

General Information

PURPOSE OF EXAMINATION

In the clinical practice of pediatrics there are two fundamental types of physical examinations: a periodic, comprehensive physical assessment and a sporadic, problem-specific evaluation. The purpose of the first type of assessment is preventive health maintenance but the purpose of the second is evaluation of a specific complaint in order to establish a diagnosis and determine therapy. The first examination covers all regions and systems and the second focuses on either regional or single systems unless physical findings indicate otherwise.

In neonatology, there are probably at least seven fundamental reasons for physical examinations; the details sought in each vary according to the purpose as well as to the patient's tolerance and accessibleness. Clearly, the tolerance of a healthy term infant will be much greater than that of a sick premature infant, but even the healthy infant will be more tolerant at 2 weeks of age than at 2 hours. Sick infants may be relatively inaccessible because of both their fragility and impeding equipment (Fig. 1). The various examinations include the first examination at birth; the assessment as the infant completes transition, which is the procedure commonly referred to as the newborn examination; the general health assessment at 24 to 72 hours after transition, or the discharge examination; well-baby examinations in the office visits; evaluation because of illness; a determination of gestational age; and an evaluation of a dysmorphic infant. There are many overlaps in each of these examinations, but each has slightly different purposes and requirements. Not all of these examinations will necessarily be conducted by physicians, and it is usually someone other than the primary physician who is the first to detect major anomalies at the time of birth or that the infant is premature or ill. Because of shortened postpartum hospital stays, most infants undergo a single complete newborn examination by their physician rather than one on admission and another on discharge.

A prospective study by Moss et al. assessed the value of more than one complete newborn examination by determining how many abnormalities were detected on a second examination that were not found on the first (1). This study found that some type of abnormality of variable significance was found in 8.8% of newborn infants on a first examination. On a second complete examination, only 0.5% had findings considered important that were not detected on the first examination. These findings primarily were hip instabilities. Two complete examinations of healthy newborn infants, particularly when done within a short interval, are unlikely to be fully time and effort productive. Of course,

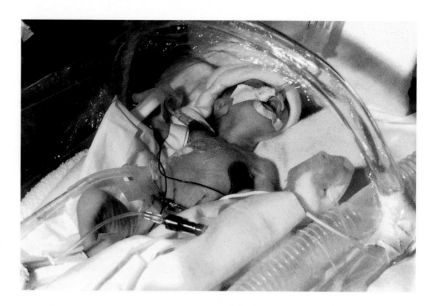

Figure 1. The neonatal patient may be quite inaccessible and intolerant for physical examination because of size, illness, and environmental barriers.

the prerequisites for relying on a single newborn assessment are that there is a thorough examination at some point after a successful transition and that there are no dynamic conditions present in the infant. A second evaluation is probably sufficient for apparently healthy infants when it is directed at areas most likely to be informative such as the hips and the cardiovascular system (1,2).

First Neonatal Examination

The truly first examination on any infant may be a prenatal sonogram. With improved technology and experience, increased access to fetal detail has allowed far more description of many physical characteristics, including sex, detection of major anomalies, and evaluation of internal structures. Nevertheless, there are likely few clinicians who have not been surprised to find an opposite sex or an unexpected malformation despite thorough sonographic examination. One must remember that not only do many things change in the fetus during development and birth transition, but no matter how refined any technique or experience may be, there are always difficulties in making complete and fully accurate fetal diagnoses and predictions about successful transition. Prenatal sonography surely augments but cannot replace physical examination.

Assign Apgar Score

The first explicit neonatal assessment occurs immediately after birth in the assigning of Apgar scores (Table 1). As originally developed, the score was to be assigned at 1 minute (3). Current guidelines suggest scoring at 1 and 5 minutes for all infants, and if the score is less than 7, at every 5 minutes until 20 minutes have passed or until two successive scores of 7 or greater are obtained (4). The scores, which are cursory assessments of the cardiopulmonary and neurologic systems, give an immediate estimation of the infant's status and need for resuscitation. They provide a shorthand for documenting the state of an infant and assessing the effectiveness of a resuscitation, but except for the heart rate, they are still subjective descriptions and are impacted by a variety of neonatal conditions, especially gestational age (5). For example, muscle tone and reflex irritability are at least partially dependent on the physiologic maturity of an infant. Also at issue and dependent on individual practice is whether to factor in whatever assistance the infant is receiving at the time. For instance, when an infant is receiving oxygen but is fully pink at 5 minutes, should he or she receive full, partial, or no score for color? Similarly, if an infant is intubated and receiving sufficient artificial ventilation but does not give a good, strong cry, how should he

Table 1. *Apgar score*

Sign	0	1	2
Heart rate	Absent	Slow (<100 beats/min)	100 beats/min
Respirations	Absent	Weak cry; hypoventilation	Good, strong cry
Muscle tone	Limp	Some flexion	Active motion
Reflex irritability (response to brisk slap on soles of feet)	No response	Grimace	Cough or sneeze
Color	Blue or pale	Body pink; extremities blue	Completely pink

From AAP Committee, ref. 4, with permission.

or she be scored? Finally, the Apgar scores may be the least accurate in the most severely depressed infant who is being resuscitated because they are usually assigned either retrospectively or by someone busy with other tasks as well. It may be ideal but unrealistic to have someone whose sole responsibility is noting the time and assigning the Apgar score when all hands are needed to resuscitate the infant. Evaluating the efficacy of the resuscitation steps is more important than determining the score at exact time intervals. Nonetheless, using these observations does help in quantifying the response and condition of the infant so they need to be as accurate as possible. Taking the potential variables into account, one should not try to make more of the Apgar score than what it is.

There have been a few attempts to improve on the original Apgar score, including weighting the various components, but this makes scoring more cumbersome (6). Another proposal is to eliminate the color value to give a maximum score of 8, thus taking away the most subjective measure and any possible confusion because of skin pigmentation (7,8). Of all the components, color correlates the least with umbilical pH, arterial carbon dioxide tension, and base excess (7). Another factor is that the reproducibility between observers is so low that valid research studies would not accept this system as reliable. One study found only a 68% interobserver correlation (9).

In and of themselves, low Apgar scores are not diagnostic of asphyxia. The American Academy of Pediatrics reminds us that to equate the presence of a low Apgar score solely with asphyxia represents a misuse of the score (10). The 1-minute score does not correlate with future outcome, although it does indicate an infant who requires resuscitation. An Apgar score of 0 to 3 at 5 minutes is associated with a risk of cerebral palsy that is increased from the general 0.3% to 1%. Scores of 4, 5, and 6 are not markers of later neurologic dysfunction. Later scores at 10, 15, and 20 minutes that are as low as 0 to 3 have a higher correlation but are still not specific in the absence of other clinical correlation such as evidence of neuroencephalopathy. Long-term assessments have failed to confirm a correlation between performance and the 1- and 5-minute scores (11).

Evaluate the Completion of Early Transition

As the circulation changes from fetal to neonatal routes, there may be a brief period when the oxygen saturation in the blood going to the head, upper body, and right arm is sufficiently higher than that going to the lower body that there will be a visible line of demarcation across the chest. The upper body and face appear pink, and the lower body and legs appear pale or blue. This visual phenomenon reflects a persistence of a fetal pathway of unsaturated blood across a still patent ductus arteriosus with little mixing of saturated blood from the left ventricle. In order to have a demarcation, there has to be a marked difference in the saturation of the blood. The disappearance of demarcation as the ductal flow decreases serves as a sign of beginning transition from fetal to neonatal circulation pathways but does not exclude all ductal shunting.

Evaluating early transition includes auscultating the chest to assure that there is sufficient air entry, listening to the cry to evaluate for obstruction or narrowing of the airway and overall infant vigor, appraising perfusion and oxygenation, and judging appropriateness of state. The breath sounds may not yet be clear but should be present and equal.

Other Components of a First Examination

The delivery room examination includes designation of sex and inspection for major anomalies and for the presence of three umbilical vessels. If the appearance of the external genitalia are such that there may be some question about the sex of the baby, delay pronouncing the sex until accurate assessment of the ambiguity can be completed. It is best to inform the parents gently that the appearance of the genitalia is unclear enough that you will need to examine the infant further before declaring definitely the sex of the infant. Be sure to show them what you are talking about and tell them what will be done.

Routine procedures in the delivery room include passing a catheter through both nostrils and into the stomach. Besides establishing patency of the upper airway and esophagus, passing a catheter allows removal and description of the stomach contents. A term fetus swallows approximately 450 ml of amniotic fluid each day (12) and has a gastric emptying time of approximately 20 ml/hour. An aspirated volume of greater than 15 ml is increased. More than 25 ml is always abnormal and suggests an obstruction at the pylorus or duodenum. The gastric contents may be green–brown, indicating old swallowed meconium or blood, or an obstruction below the outlet of the bile duct into the duodenum (13). If bloody, the source may be fetal or maternal; an Apt test will distinguish the two.

Look at the Back

Any obvious abnormality in this first assessment merits more immediate evaluation, but the definitive examination in seemingly healthy infants should be finished after the infant completes transition and spends time with his parents. Similarly, in infants who are ill and require diagnostic and therapeutic intervention, the complete examination should be deferred until they are initially stabilized. All infants should undergo a cursory inspection of all external areas before leaving the delivery suite. It is especially important to develop a habit of looking at the back of every infant because it is easy to forget to look when an infant has required intubation and other procedures.

Do Not Forget the Placenta

Finally, in the delivery suite, there should be a general examination of the placenta to detect any gross abnormalities that could influence early neonatal care or resuscitation (see Chapter 4).

Assessment of Transition

An interpretation of physical findings in infants in the first day of life is affected by how completely the infant has made the transition from fetal to neonatal life. Transition requires significant adjustments to tolerate change from a relatively stable, fluid filled environment with nutrition and respiration provided through the placenta and amniotic fluid to one in which the newborn must be far more physiologically independent. Healthy term infants should complete the essential parts of the process within a few hours, whereas preterm infants take much longer and require more external assistance to complete the process. The evaluation of transition includes noting all the vital signs and observing for general alertness, color, signs of respiratory distress, cardiac rate and rhythm, ability to suck and swallow, and handling of secretions.

Three particular observations during transition are reassuring indications of a healthy baby: normal variations in behavior state, comfortable respiratory effort with an intermittent, vigorous cry, and a transitional blush or erythema neonatorum. The neurobehavioral stages are discussed in more detail below (14).

Changes in Behavior State

Immediately after birth, healthy term infants are awake for 30 to 60 minutes in a comfortably flexed posture with intermittent gross body movements such as stretching or sucking on a fist. During this period, infants may breast feed, cry periodically, or lie rather quietly. They appear to be aware, with eyes open but not staring. After initial wakefulness, infants sleep for several hours. If aroused, they go back to sleep when left alone. By the end of this first nap, healthy infants are ready to tolerate a bath and feeding. Term infants who fail to have a period of wakefulness before sleep may be abnormally lethargic. Infants who remain alert, stare, do not have some semipurposeful body movements, or fail to go into a quiet sleep are likely demonstrating neurologic irritability. Premature infants, even those that are well, may not demonstrate a definite period of alert, quiet awareness and the same sleep cycling.

Resolution of Tachypnea

The respiratory rate during early transition ranges from 60 to 100 breaths per minute and then slows to 50 to 60. During the first hours of transition, infants who have been delivered by elective section or after a precipitous labor tend to grunt and to breathe faster than those who have been born after several hours of labor. Although healthy infants may continue to breathe well above 60 breaths per minute, they do not appear distressed and can slow their rate enough to nipple feed successfully. Infants with tachypnea and hyperventilation to compensate for a metabolic acidosis, to increase their oxygen intake, or to eliminate excess carbon dioxide are unlikely to slow their respiratory rate enough to nipple feed well. They are less active and have accompanying nasal flaring and retractions. Infants hyperventilating because of neurologic irritability have other signs of abnormal state or consciousness.

The respiratory rate may be inappropriately low, reflecting an inability to respond to hypoxemia or hypercarbia. If an infant is cyanotic, has poor air movement on auscultation, or elevation of carbon dioxide tension, he should be tachypneic. An absence of tachypnea indicates inadequate respiratory drive and suggests depression from maternal drugs including magnesium sulfate, analgesics, anesthetics, or illicit drugs, or from other causes of perinatal depression, hypoglycemia, extreme hypothermia, or complete respiratory failure.

Transitional Blush (Erythema Neonatorum)

An interesting finding that occurs most commonly several hours into transition, often at the time of the first bath when an infant is vigorously stimulated, is the appearance of an overall blush to a brilliant red, the *erythema neonatorum*. The blush lasts from 30 minutes to several hours. After the first episode it does not return with the same intensity if at all and is not repeated after the first day. The occurrence of this phenomenon probably indicates normal cardiovascular pathways and a healthy baby but this relationship has not been scientifically studied.

Newborn Examination

The comprehensive newborn examination is best performed after the infant has completed transition because its purpose is an evaluation of the overall well-being and physical normality of the infant. This procedure is the series of steps described in most discussions of newborn examination and has its main purpose of determining the physical normality of

Table 2. *Examination sequence in relation to infant's state*

Area to assess	Required state	Arousing maneuvers	Equipment
Observe general appearance			
Observe color			
Observe resting posture	Quiet		
Observe spontaneous activity	Active		
Count respiratory rate	Quiet		Clock
Count heart rate	Quiet		Clock
Inspect facies at rest	Quiet		
Auscult heart sounds	Quiet		Stethoscope
Auscult breath sounds	Quiet		Stethoscope
Measure blood pressure	Quiet		BP cuff
Inspect head and neck region			
Stimulate response to sound	Quiet		Calibrated noise maker
Inspect trunk anteriorly			
Palpate abdomen, cardiac impulse	Quiet		
Feel pulses			
Examine genitalia			Lubricant for rectal
Inspect trunk posteriorly			
Inspect arms and hands			
Inspect legs and feet			
Assess passive tone			
Assess active tone	Active	x	
Elicit primitive reflexes	Active	x	
Assess muscle strength	Active	x	
Assess gestational age			
Test range in major joints		x	
Manipulate hips	Quiet	x	
Measure temperature			Thermometer
Examine ears with otoscope		x	Otoscope
Determine pupil response to light			Bright light
Examine fundi	Quiet	x	
Elicit tendon reflexes		x	Percussion hammer
Simulate response to pain		x	
Weigh infant	Quiet	x	Scales, growth chart
Measure head circumference			Tape measure, growth chart
Measure chest and abdominal circumference		x	Tape measure
Measure length			Tape measure, growth chart
Transilluminate head		x	High intensity light
Percuss abdomen	Quiet		
Percuss lungs	Quiet		

an infant. A schema for this examination is included in Table 2. If the infant is quiet at the beginning of the examination, the examination proceeds from the least invasive and noxious of stimuli to those most likely to irritate the infant but the sequence has to be modified according to the infant's condition and response.

Discharge Examination

The discharge examination specifically assesses an infant's ability to be outside a hospital environment where tools for resuscitation and direct medical evaluation are available. When an infant is to be discharged within the first two days of life, this assessment may be part of a single newborn examination for the physician, obligating other personnel and the parents to take more responsibility in detecting any significant changes in the infant.

The details of examination for discharge depend in part on how long the infant has been in the hospital. Clearly, if the infant is less than 24 hours old, there needs to be emphasis on his or her ability to survive by being able to maintain temperature and take sufficient nutrition as well as no evidence of dynamic or life-threatening conditions. If the infant has been in the hospital for an extended period, the assessment needs to include evaluation for complications of care or illness and of neurodevelopment. Part of the evaluation in preparation for discharge is assessment of maternal competence in caring and observing for changes in her infant. The plan for follow-up for the mother and infant comes at the conclusion of the discharge examination.

Some of the factors to consider in the discharge examination (when done as a supplement to the comprehensive newborn examination):

Vital signs
Temperature stability in a normal, ambient environment
Ability and success of feeding
    Weight change since birth
    Amount or duration and frequency of feeding
    State of hydration and urine output
    Bowel movements
Normal color (absence of cyanosis, pallor, plethora, significant jaundice)
Cardiovascular system
    Absence of murmur unless cause is determined
    Normal pulses
    Splitting of second sound
    Good perfusion
Pulmonary system (resolution of tachypnea or respiratory distress)
Drying of the umbilical cord
Hip stability
Normal state and behavior
Assess whatever might not have been accessible at earlier examination (eyes, hearing)

First Outpatient, Well-Baby Examination

After discharge the office or home visits may require that more time be spent on discussing care issues and the adequacy of breast feeding, but several areas require careful examination. These include any areas that might have been relatively inaccessible during the first examinations, such as the eyes, ear canals, and eardrums, as well as an assessment of overall well-being as suggested by the neuromotor evaluation and feeding and sleep patterns. Repeated assessment for hip stability, clavicular fractures, or murmurs and equality of pulses is appropriate with each examination opportunity (1,15).

Sick-Baby Examination

At any time during the neonatal period, there may be a need for examination because of signs and symptoms suggesting illness or because historical factors put an infant at risk for certain problems. Older patients are likely to present with more specific complaints, but the neonate rarely demonstrates explicit signs. For example, fever is not a reliable sign of infection. It is sometimes present in an overheated but healthy infant and absent in a septic one. The only symptoms that may suggest illness might be a change in the feeding/sleeping pattern or demonstrated hunger or irritability. The younger the infant in both chronologic and gestational age, the more subtle and general are clues to illness. Because signs are vague, there might be a tendency for caregivers to rely primarily on laboratory tests rather than to use the physical examination to determine a cause. Laboratory assessment is essential for many evaluations, but careful examination narrows the approach and is a valuable tool in assessing response to therapy.

Scoring Severity of Illness

There have been many attempts to quantitate certain factors in neonates to provide information about their current condition or their potential for survival and long-term morbidity. Scoring systems have been devised to measure the level of illness for each infant within larger groups to allow for interinstitutional comparison of care or to assist in predicting overall morbidity and mortality (16–18). One scoring system is based on what types of intervention are needed in order to quantitate the neonatal therapeutic intensity (19). Although such scores have been validated for groups of babies, they have not been validated for predicting the survival of individual infants or for decisions regarding discontinuation of life support. Additionally, each system is relatively cumbersome to apply. As the predictability increases, so does the number of parameters measured or scored.

One of the earliest scoring systems that assesses the degree of respiratory distress in an infant still has some merit because it forces the observation of several respiratory signs and it is extremely simple (20). For someone not used to caring for sick neonates, this score or similar ones assists in recognizing respiratory distress. Like the Apgar score, the Silverman-Anderson score uses five observations of synchrony in the chest and abdomen, retractions of the lower ribs, retractions of the sternum, nasal flaring, and presence and intensity of grunt on expiration, and assigns scores of 0, 1, or 2 to each factor (20). A total score of 0 means no respiratory disease and 10 means severe respiratory disease. A total of more than 7 indicates impending respiratory failure. When this is the only means available to determine how much respiratory disease is present, it holds some merit in that it allows comparison of an infant over time. Having staff personnel use such a score during the early transition of infants who are not likely to worsen does allow some standardization of observation. Besides oversimplifying the evaluation of illness, one problem with this system is that, as an infant tires with respiratory failure and makes less vigorous effort, the score would probably decrease and falsely suggest improvement. More modern interventions and monitoring devices have largely supplanted this system, but its original value still holds in that it encourages a close look at the breathing pattern.

Determining Presence of Illness

Besides applying scoring systems to predict morbidity and mortality or to compare care outcomes, some observations help the clinician and parent decide if an infant is ill and to estimate if he or she requires admission to a hospital or a higher level of neonatal care. Determining whether an infant is sick as well as the extent of illness, particularly when he or she does not present with definite indications for intervention, is one of the more challenging aspects of caring for newborn infants. In this respect it is relatively easy to decide to intervene and start therapy for infants who have met criteria for admission to an intensive care nursery based on their prematurity, the presence of obvious anomalies, or a clearly defined perinatal event requiring intervention. It is more difficult to determine whether an infant without these factors but with some signs is sick or not. Here the clinician is faced with judgment decisions that carry one risk if initiation of therapy is delayed too long and another if therapy is begun unnecessarily.

Morley et al. have devised and tested a scoring system based on what signs and symptoms are seen and reported in infants less than 6 months of age (21). The findings were correlated with severity of illness being well or mildly, moderately, or seriously ill. Most symptoms were associated with all levels of illness, with only four symptoms not present in some of the well infants. These four symptoms were a fluid intake less than a third of normal, convulsions, frank blood in stools, and bile-stained vomit. Specific signs were more helpful than symptoms in that they were present only in infants who were ill. These included marked retractions of the lower ribs, high-pitched or moaning cry, expiratory grunt, loss of alertness, central cyanosis, and severe hypotonia. Some signs were so common in both well and sick infants that they were not helpful in determining if an infant was ill; in particular, they noted that congested breathing and respiratory rate were poor predictors of illness.

Morley et al. have pointed out the need to relate symptoms and signs to grades of illness rather than to specific diagnoses for three reasons: "(1) When infants become ill, their symptoms and signs are often nonspecific and it is not easy to make a firm diagnosis. (2) The severity of illness in specific diagnostic categories (e.g., gastroenteritis or viral respiratory infections) can vary so much that the diagnosis alone does not help decide how ill an infant is. (3) Parents and doctors need to know whether an infant's symptoms indicate a serious illness that needs further attention even though the diagnosis may not be obvious" (21). Although their study included more than just neonates, their findings are helpful for neonates if environmental conditions and factors affected more by maturation are also considered. The types of symptoms and signs are described in Tables 3 and 4 and the definitions of symptoms are included in Table 5.

Evaluation of the Dysmorphic Infant

Another type of physical examination that may be needed during the newborn period is one determining if certain findings represent malformations or deformations and if their presence constitutes a definable syndrome or consequence. This type of examination is the cornerstone of clinical genetics. When malformations are obvious, the examination defines the full extent of each malformation as well as all other associated findings. It requires care-

Table 3. *Proportion of infants in each illness category with each symptom*

Symptom	Well (n = 290)	Mildly ill (n = 305)	Moderately ill (n = 247)	Seriously ill (n = 165)
Increased irritability	8	43	61	78
Cough (>5 episodes/day)	6	28	39	34
Runny nose	6	21	30	26
Not himself/herself	5	43	59	79
Not feeding normally	5	30	51	71
Noisy breathing	5	29	36	43
Feels hot	5	22	47	53
An abnormal cry	4	27	47	69
Vomiting (not possetting)	3	21	32	41
Diarrhea	3	15	25	27
Cold hands and feet	3	13	27	39
Pallor	3	13	29	56
Sweating	2	16	19	33
Fluids intake, approximately half normal	1	15	29	36
Drowsiness occasionally	1	6	25	53
Decreased activity	1	6	15	46
Breathing difficulty	<1	15	28	34
Vomiting more than half the feed after the last three feeds	<1	7	12	10
Projectile vomiting	<1	5	9	10
Less urine	<1	5	17	34
Cyanotic episodes	<1	3	5	12
Apneic episodes	<1	3	5	4
Jaundice	<1	1	0	<1
Drowsy most of the time	<1	<1	7	35
Fluids less than ⅓ normal intake	0	1	3	19
Convulsions	0	1	<1	4
Blood in stools (not streaks)	0	<1	<1	5
Bile-stained vomiting	0	0	<1	3

For the definition of each symptom, see Table 5. Values are given in percentages.
From Morley et al., ref. 21, with permission.

Table 4. *Proportion of infants in each illness category with each sign*

Sign	Well (n = 290)	Mildly ill (n = 305)	Moderately ill (n = 247)	Seriously ill (n = 165)
Respiratory rate >50/min	76	69	70	62
Pulse rate >140/min	72	69	81	76
Not smiling at examiner	32	42	54	82
Intermittent cry during examination	24	33	50	62
Mild retraction of lower ribs	7	20	44	43
Rash (moderate or severe)	3	14	17	12
Big toe squeeze; color return takes >3 seconds	3	12	23	31
Mild hypotonia	3	11	22	36
Persistent cry during examination	3	2	5	10
Soft tissue mass (>2 cm diameter)	3	2	2	6
Nasal discharge	2	9	8	5
Peripheral cyanosis	2	2	6	15
Hyperinflation of the chest	2	1	7	19
Stridor	2	1	3	3
Pale arms and legs	1	8	16	29
Wheeze	<1	4	14	17
Calves feel cold	<1	0	3	11
Bleeding into skin (any cause)	<1	0	2	2
Inflamed tympanic membranes	0	6	15	11
Pallor of whole body	0	5	9	36
Partially extended posture	0	3	3	25
Distended and tense abdomen	0	2	2	6
Transient loss of eye contact with examiner	0	1	2	31
Transient loss of awareness of surroundings	0	1	2	33
Rectal temperature >100.8°F[a]	0	1	13	29
Crepitations (on auscultation)	0	<1	6	13
Cry; weak or whimpering	0	<1	5	23
Reduced hydration	0	<1	2	12
Obvious sweating	0	<1	2	3
Inguinal hernia	0	<1	1	5
Palpable mass in abdomen	0	<1	1	6
Tender abdomen on palpation	0	<1	<1	17
Obvious retraction of lower ribs	0	0	3	6
Cry; high pitched or moaning	0	0	<1	67
Expiratory grunt; audible	0	0	<1	7
No eye fixation with examiner	0	0	0	5
Central cyanosis	0	0	0	5
No awareness of surroundings	0	0	0	3
Completely extended posture	0	0	0	2

Values are given in percentages.
[a] >38.2°C.
From Morley et al., ref. 20, with permission.

Table 5. *Definition of symptoms used to assess infant illness*

Symptom	Definition
Cold hands and feet	Hands, feet, or limbs have felt cold.
Noisy breathing	Persistent noises, including mucusy sounds, snuffles, stridor, grunt, or wheeze.
Runny nose	Mucus seen over philtrum (not just a blocked nose).
Sweating	Beads of sweat on forehead, or obviously wet hair when at rest or feeding.
Increased irritability	More fractious and difficult to settle than usual.
Cough	More than five episodes of coughing per day.
Feels hot	Feeling hotter than normal.
Pallor	Looking generally pale.
Not feeding normally	Taking less fluids or solids, or feeding more slowly than usual. The amount of fluid taken was scored in thirds of normal intake.
Vomiting	Forceful regurgitation of significant quantity of fluid. The number of vomiting episodes of more than half the feed was recorded.
Not himself/herself	Baby has not been his or her usual self.
Diarrhea	Excessively fluid motions. If present the number of stools in the last 24 hours was recorded.
Abnormal cry	Any unusual characteristics to the cry.
Less urine	Fewer wet diapers than usual, or drier diapers than usual. If fewer, the number of wet ones was recorded.
Breathing difficulty	Working harder to breathe, or heaving chest.
Decreased activity	Moving arms and legs less than usual.
Drowsy	Less alert than usual. A score was then used that allowed a more objective assessment of drowsiness: "When the baby is awake is he or she (a) always alert, (b) occasionally drowsy, (c) occasionally alert, (d) never alert?"
Jaundice	Yellow skin or sclera.
Projectile vomiting	Vomit that travels more than 45 cm.
Cyanotic episodes	Periods of obvious blueness of the tongue and lips.
Apneic episodes	Cessation of breathing for 20 seconds or more.
Bile-stained vomiting	Episodes of green vomiting.
Blood in stools	Frank blood mixed with the stool (not streaks).
Convulsion	Shaking movements with decreased awareness.

Symptoms were recorded as present only if they had been present within the previous 24 hours.

From Morley et al., ref. 21, with permission.

ful attention to the entire infant so that less obvious abnormalities are not overlooked. Unfortunately many of the findings described as typical of most syndromes are not apparent or fully developed in newborn infants, so no matter how thorough and careful the examination may be, many will be missed.

A major component of evaluating an infant with an unusual or dysmorphic appearance is being able to measure various body parts and to compare them to standards from a similar population as well as to determine proportionality within the same infant. Details on how to take these measurements are discussed in the next chapter on growth as well as in chapters on individual regions. Selected standards for measurements are included in these chapters or in the appendix.

INTERPRETING FINDINGS BASED ON TIME OF EXAMINATION

The timing of examinations on neonates affects how one should interpret findings: some may be normal if present during transition but not if they first appear thereafter. An example is the presence of a single heart sound that is normal for only a few hours after birth and thereafter represents definite cardiac pathology. Tachypnea is normal during transition but abnormal afterward. Jaundice on the first day of life is abnormal and requires investigation, whereas jaundice on the third day may be only physiologic and require little further evaluation. If an infant is premature, one has to understand the expected course of these transitional changes as it relates to gestational age and be able to distinguish that impact on the physical findings.

Findings may be interpreted as normal or abnormal depending not only on day of life but also on the phase of an infant's sleep–feeding cycle. For instance, infants who have just had a satisfactory feeding may be so deeply asleep that it is difficult to arouse them. During the first 1 to 3 days after delivery, many infants spend most of their time sleeping. Because the ability to demonstrate a normal, alert, and hungry state is one of the satisfying findings that generally indicates a healthy baby, further assessment is necessary if sleeping is the only state observed during examination. If any suspicious finding is present at one examination, a later reevaluation should lessen the impact of state and age.

ENVIRONMENT

A routine neonatal examination, normally taking 5 to 10 minutes, should be conducted in a quiet, warm environment. The room should be light enough to detect skin markings and color but not so bright that it discourages the infant from keeping his eyes open. If the area is too cold or drafty, the infant may resort to crying to keep warm. Even healthy infants do not tolerate extended handling, and the sicker or more immature they are, the less they tolerate it.

The environment in which the examination of a newborn infant takes place impacts significantly on the response of that neonate and must be taken into account while interpreting findings. For example, there needs to be as little extraneous noise as possible to provide not only a quiet milieu for auscultation or assessing the infant's hearing but also not to overwhelm an immature infant. Because of an inability to filter sensory input selectively, the newborn, particularly when premature, habituates very quickly to all types of sensory input. When overwhelmed, he may become flaccid with little response to directed input (22). If the environment includes noisy support equipment such as ventilators, continuous suction drainage, incubator fans, monitor alerts, telephones, or people, there should be as much modification of that environment as possible to decrease noise interference. In the physician's office, the neonatal examinations deserve the same considerations regarding warmth, light, and noise.

Parental Presence

In routine care situations, having one or both parents present during the process allows discussion about physical findings and offers the opportunity for pointing out infant behaviors and responses that can help the parent better understand their child. When appropriate in the hospital, a newborn examination can take place in the mother's room at her bedside. Having parents present facilitates assessment of their competence in caregiving as well as uncovering some of their anxieties. Some topics in the history or the examination require privacy for discussion, so there should be consideration for confidentiality. One would certainly not want to point out to a parent and discuss a major anomaly and syndrome in the presence of either roommates, relatives, visitors, or other parents. Even if parents are not present, it may not be prudent to discuss abnormal or suspect physical findings in the presence of other personnel.

Inhibited Environment

For most newborn examinations, the infant will be either on an open warmer or in a bassinet. Most healthy term infants can tolerate being completely undressed in a reasonably warm room for a period of 5 to 10 minutes. If the infant is ill, premature, or undergrown, or if the ambiance is cool or drafty, an external heat source should be provided. The heat lamps approved for use in nurseries have protection against shattering of hot glass and a recommended distance from the infant's skin, but there should be further consideration on the potential effects of prolonged exposure of the infant's eyes to the bright light in the heat lamp. If a warming lamp is used, shield the infant's eyes.

Infants are not fully accessible in an incubator or when restrained and attached to equipment on an open bed, and they cannot be assessed as completely as infants who are free to be turned, put into a sitting position, or lifted into ventral and vertical suspension (Fig. 1). The portions of the examination requiring this kind of mobility have to be modified or delayed but not forgotten. Infants who are so sick that they need full resuscitation at birth should undergo a full examination as soon as possible in the early treatment period. If complete examination is delayed because of patient condition, a thorough examination is needed as soon as it can be tolerated.

EQUIPMENT NEEDED

The equipment needed for the physical examination is limited but should be specific for use in neonates in whom size is a factor, especially for items such as blood pressure cuffs and stethoscope heads. Essential equipment includes a bright pen light with a pinpoint beam, pneumatic otoscope with small head, ophthalmoscope, standardized sound source, tongue blade, tape measure, and a clear, flexible ruler. In order to effect a seal, the bell on the stethoscope needs to have a soft contact surface for use on thin walled chests. One piece of equipment that is not essential but is extremely helpful is a good camera used with as much natural light as possible. If not of the single-use variety, equipment must be cleaned between patients. Nosocomial infections have been linked to multi-use examination equipment, including blood pressure cuffs and stethoscopes (23).

There is no documented benefit to wearing cover gowns or masks to prevent infant colonization, although many physicians prefer to wear gowns to protect their own clothes (24,25). For the earliest examinations before an infant is first bathed and until the risk of sexually transmitted diseases is determined, it is prudent to wear gloves throughout the examination. An examiner with a skin infection should wear gloves. Even after the infant has been bathed, portions of the examination require gloved hands.

HISTORY

Elements of Neonatal History

The elements of a neonatal medical history are essentially the same as those that comprise a history for an adult or older child so will include some information about past medical history, present condition, and the family. The neonatal history clearly emphasizes the relationship of maternal medical conditions and includes more than merely the events of the interval since birth. Even though an infant will not have a work or education history, the parents will and theirs may be particularly important factors either as causes of problems or for setting reasonable care plans for the neonate.

Just as there are several types of neonatal examinations, so too are there different degrees of detail needed. These range from a brief review after a normal pregnancy in a healthy mother and father already known to the physician to a complete family tree if the infant appears dysmorphic. When a newborn represents the first member of a family to enter a practice, there will need to be a more comprehensive review of family history than when siblings join an already known family. With more pregnancies resulting from donated eggs or sperm, it is rarely necessary to know exactly who the donor is, but it is always helpful to know if it is someone other than a parent.

Much of the information that constitutes the basics of a neonatal history should be available through the maternal records if they are complete and accessible at the time of delivery. Many of the items requested in the antepartum record, such as the one suggested by the American College of Obstetrics, provide information about the mother and the pregnancy, although more information will be needed in specialized cases. Suggested information for a complete newborn history is shown in Table 6.

Table 6. *Components of complete newborn history*

Maternal general history	Newborn patient	Paternal general history	Sibling history
Age	Age in hours or days	Age	Ages of infant's siblings
Race/ethnic group		Race/ethnic group	Identify father
Occupation		Occupation	Levels in school
Highest level of school completed		Highest level of school completed	School difficulties
Type of medical insurance for infant		Consanguinity	Known inherited diseases
Living accommodations		Living in home or not	Where they are living; if not with mother, why not.
Access to transportation			
Plans for care of infant		Availability to assist in care	Identity of care givers and any problems with that
Time for return to work			
Primary caregiver and the immune and tuberculosis status, particularly if recent immigrant			
Feeding plans	Ability to latch and suckle	Food allergies	Success with breast feeding
Previous breast surgery	Demonstration of hunger		Feeding intolerances
Breast or bottle feeding of previous children	Movement of bowels, urine		Allergies
Food allergies			
Use of	Presence of symptoms consistent with withdrawal	Use of	
Illicit drugs		Illicit drugs	
Alcohol		Alcohol	
Smoking		Smoking	
Prescribed or non-prescribed drugs			
Presence of any congenital conditions: deafness, visual impairment, or malformation	Reported reactions to light and sound	Presence of any congenital conditions: deafness, visual, or malformation impairment	Presence of any congenital conditions
Blood type	If mother is rh negative or type O	Blood type	
Sensitization status if rh negative			
Previous pregnancies (gravida)	If multiple gestations, order of birth and type of placentation	Is father the same for previous pregnancies?	Early infancy problems of
Number liveborn, born at term, abortions			Significant jaundice
Dates of each delivery			Feeding difficulties
Birth weights			Allergies
Problems encountered			Sudden infant death
Immune status	Receipt of immunization or immune globulin to date		
Rubella	Results of neonatal tests as indicated		
Hepatitis			
HIV			
Syphilis			
Current pregnancy	Results of any prenatal sonograms or other diagnostic tests	If father is the donor, in an artificial insemination pregnancy	
Fertilization history			
Due date	Placental examination		
Number of prenatal visits	Documentation of type of medical and environmental support required since birth (particularly when other than healthy term newborn)		
Prescription and nonprescription drugs taken just before conception and during pregnancy including prenatal vitamins			
Nutrition: excessive or inadequate weight gain			
Hydrorrhea			
Vaginal bleeding			
Fetal activity			

continued

Table 6. *Continued.*

Maternal general history	Newborn patient	Paternal general history	Sibling history

Physical activity
  Care of animals
  Exercise
  Travel
  Exposure to potential
    teratogens
	Physical activity
	  Sleep/wake pattern
	  Alertness
	  Crying activity		

Infectious exposure
  particularly risky for infant
  Tuberculosis
  Hepatitis
  Sexually transmitted
    diseases including
    herpes, syphilis,
    gonococcus, chlamydia,
    HIV
	Vital signs	Presence of any current
		  infections
			Presence of any current
			  infections, particularly
			  recent contagious
			  infections

Diabetes: type of treatment,
  adequacy of control
  throughout pregnancy,
  and especially in 48 hours
  before delivery
Hypertension: chronic or
  pregnancy induced
Heart disease: type and
  severity
Kidney disease: urinary
  infections, congenital
  anomalies
Mental illness
Neuromotor conditions,
  particularly seizure
  disorders
Hepatitis or other liver
  diseases
Thyroid dysfunction
Allergies
Blood dyscrasia
Hemoglobinopathy
Congenital hearing disability
	Ability to maintain blood
	  glucose
	Documentation of blood
	  draw for state-mandated
	  neonatal screening:
	  congenital endocrine/
	  metabolic diseases and
	  hemoglobinopathies
			Presence of any chronic or
			  acute medical conditions,
			  including congenital heart
			  disease, cystic fibrosis,
			  allergies, neuromotor
			  disorders,
			  hemoglobinopathy,
			  neonatal illness

Current labor and delivery
  Duration
  Fetal monitoring
    abnormalities
  Anesthesia
  Delivery route
	Presenting part
	Apgar scores
	Requirement for
	  resuscitation, time to
	  spontaneous breathing
	Ease of transition		

Techniques for Taking the History

In a hospital setting it is often more practical to conduct the physical examination before speaking to the parents, but basic information about the pregnancy and delivery history as well as the information since birth should be present in the infant's and mother's charts. Consideration for privacy must be taken, including the potential need for separate histories from mother and father. Even other relatives may be helpful in providing essential information, particularly when parents are not available to talk, but the privacy of the parent remains important.

The best way to get a complete history is to be an active listener and direct the questioning only as needed to encourage pertinent but complete answers. Taking the time and effort to allow the parent to say what is needed not only allows the physician to get the most information but also helps establish rapport. One needs to be aware of the many cultural differences that parents may present in order to be effective in communicating and listening. When English is not the primary language, finding a medically literate interpreter who can demonstrate the same sentiment as you may yield far more information. The reader is referred to an excellent and easy-to-read reference on improving communication skills by Platt (26).

GENERAL PRINCIPLES IN PHYSICAL EXAMINATION

Tools of Physical Examination

Inspection

Inspection is the most valuable tool in the physical assessment of neonates. An immediate assessment of wellness comes just from noting the state, color, respiratory effort, posture, and spontaneous activity of the infant. Inspection suggests if the appearance of an infant is aberrant or merely that of a newborn baby temporarily deformed by intrauterine environment; confirming or changing this impression requires further inspection of the infant as well as of both parents. The visual impression one gets from careful inspection forms the basis for assessing changes that occur during illness. It provides the fastest tool to detect changes in the physical examination, but it requires thoughtful inspection rather than merely looking.

Inspection begins before making any physical contact and from enough of a distance to encompass the infant as a whole. When infants are undressed on an open warmer or in an incubator, partial inspection is possible without disturbing them. If infants are clothed, undressing them for full inspection affects some of the observations that should be made before they are touched. Inspection continues throughout the entire physical examination and should not stop at the end of the formal assessment but continue as long as an infant is in the nursery or in an office.

Palpation

Palpation is used to sense temperature, moisture, turgor, texture, consistency, tension, tenderness, pulsation, vibration, and amplitude, as well as depth, size, shape, and location of concealed structures. As in older patients, palpation must be gentle and performed with the flat of the finger pads rather than with the tips. It is important not to apply too much pressure to sensitive organs such as the liver, spleen, or skin, which are at greater risk for disruption and bleeding in neonates, particularly those who are premature or have hepatosplenomegaly. The small size of neonates makes it possible to palpate the entire infant in a matter of seconds.

Percussion

Of all the traditional tools of physical diagnosis, percussion is used the least in neonatology but nonetheless should not be overlooked for its value in determining the size of abdominal viscera and the presence of abnormal tympanicity or dullness in the head, chest, or abdomen. An effective variation of the finger-to-finger percussion technique in detecting liver size or the height of the diaphragm is to listen with the diaphragm of the stethoscope applied over the solid organ and then map that area by lightly scratching on the skin until there is a change in the pitch.

Auscultation

Auscultation is done first by just listening to whatever sounds an infant may be making spontaneously before and after physical contact and stimulation. Listening includes assessing all utterances, including grunts, whines, and whimpers, and the cry for its intensity, pitch, quality, and duration, as well as any extraneous sounds at rest or during feeding and other activities. The open bell of a stethoscope can augment these sounds and help localize their origin. Auscultation of the heart, lungs, abdomen, neck, and head with a stethoscope is an important tool but requires a quiet subject to be effective. It is best to take whatever time is needed to console the infant before applying a stethoscope. Many sounds are relatively louder on auscultation because of the closeness of the structure through a thinner wall, but the presence of extraneous noises and the rapid rate of the heart and breathing makes distinguishing the characteristics more challenging than in older patients. Because there will be no patient cooperation in breathing on cue or remaining quiet, effective auscultation requires filtering the many extraneous sounds that envelop the neonate.

Descriptions of Alteration in Anatomic Structure

Physical diagnosis involves making careful observations and then interpreting their meaning in the context of the particular patient. It requires training and experience to make valid observations rather than just to look at something. Observations involve both scientific and systematic descriptions, whereas looking is merely using the eyes to see. In training ourselves to be careful observers and to be able to communicate what it is we are seeing, we should use a consistent set of descriptions in the possible alterations in anatomic structure as well as the possible alteration in physiologic variables for each body system or area. Athreya and Silverman have suggested consistently using seven variables to describe potential alterations in anatomic structure: size, number, shape, position, color, texture or consistency, continuity, and alignment (Table 7) (27). Unfortunately, these words do not suggest an easy mnemonic, but the descriptions are fully applicable to the newborn examination. To describe the potential changes in the physiologic variables, Athreya and Silverman have further suggested considering the presence or absence of a function and then, if present, considering if it is present in full capacity or with a variation in degree or pattern. Because neonates cannot directly describe sensations even though they are capable of experiencing them, the descriptions of physiologic function require modification for application to the newborn. The questions asked about each physiologic function being assessed on examination are its presence or absence and how much or how fast it is and in what way it is functioning (Table 8).

Areas for Potential Error

There are several categories of potential errors in physical diagnosis, including poor technique, omission of areas in the examination, failure to recognize signs, and incomplete or poor recording of what is present or absent on the examination as well as improper interpretation of what the findings mean (28). Most physical diagnosis is taught on adult patients with more limited time devoted to gaining experience in pediatrics and even less or none in neonatology. Modification of standard techniques applicable to adults is necessary in approaching the smallest and most fragile of all patients who are unable to cooperate actively, have limited tolerance for handling, and present with different physiologic norms, variations, and disease conditions than other age groups. These factors make errors in physical diagnosis quite possible even though the establishment of a normal physical examination is one of the most important events in the newborn period.

To avoid making errors in neonatal physical diagnosis, one should first learn the specialized techniques and use them methodically to prevent omissions and errors in reporting. Avoiding errors in interpretation comes with experience and careful application of scientific principles to everyday practice. Athreya and Silverman have pointed out that all findings must be interpreted within the context of the whole patient to avoid accepting the findings that confirm a clinical suspicion while ignoring those that contradict that diagnosis (27). One should consider the true likelihood of a patient having a particular condition before interpreting whether or not a finding is diagnostic, coincidental, or insignificant. For example, some problems commonly encountered in premature infants are far less likely in term infants and vice versa. Respiratory distress due to hyaline membrane disease occur-

Table 7. *Possible alterations in anatomic structures*

Descriptors	Size	Number	Shape	Position	Color	Texture/ consistency	Continuity	Alignment
Normal	Normal	Normal	Normal	Normal	Normal	Normal	Normal	Normal
Variables	Abnormal (large or small in relation to itself and in relation to other structures) Rate of growth	Fewer (fused, absent) More (split, extra)	Uniformity (defines entire organ) Concave Convex	Right/left Anterior/posterior Superior/inferior In relation to other structures: Far off Elevated Depressed Moved in Moved out Rotated In relation to itself (pushed or twisted): Forward Backward Inward Outward Multiple (combinations)	Less of normal color More of normal color Abnormal color Black Green Dark Red Blue Yellow Cherry red Milky white Brown Pink	Soft Firm Hard Fluctuant Uniform Variable	Abnormal (a) Extra growth (not normally present) including skin rash, swellings, and projections Location Size Shape Rate of growth Flat or elevated Margin-regulated/irregular Surface-smooth/rough Consistency (as listed) Color (as listed) Temperature (hot, cold) Tenderness Pulsation Attachment to skin and to surrounding structures (b) Loss of continuity such as ulcers and fractures	Abnormal In relation to itself In relation to other structures

From Athreya and Silverman, ref. 27, with permission.

Table 8. *Description of possible aberration in physiologic function*

Question	Descriptions			
Presence	Absent	Partially absent		
	Present	Present but painful	Present but difficult	Present but abnormal
Quantity (how often)				
Rate	Normal	Fast	Slow	
Rhythm	Regular	Irregular	Regularly irregular	Irregularly irregular
Quantity (how much)				
Volume	Normal	Increased	Decreased	Variable, changing
Size	Normal	Increased	Decreased	
Depth	Normal	Increased	Shallow	
Amplitude	Normal	Widened	Narrowed	
Force	Normal	Strong	Weak	
Duration	Normal	Short	Prolonged	Continuous
Quality	Smooth, rough, jerking, writhing, tremulous, harsh, coarse, clear, vibratory, moist, dry			

Modified from Athreya and Silverman, ref. 27, with permission.

ring in premature infants is unlikely in term infants. Respiratory distress as a sign of meconium aspiration is far more likely in term infants and is unlikely in premature infants.

Order of Examination

The order in which an examination progresses depends on its purpose as well as on the current state of the infant. It is not possible to follow an exact routine with each infant, but it is essential to keep an organized routine in mind so that all regions and systems are included at some point. In general, one starts with the least invasive observations and leaves the most disturbing aspects to the end. The small size of the newborn infant lends itself to a regional approach, but a lot of crossover is dependent on the infant's state and on specific findings. Clearly, observations of the skin and neurobehavior continue throughout the examination, with more directed assessment toward the end. Items that require a specific state or a higher degree of cooperation from the infant are done whenever the opportunity arises. Considering the impact of each step in the process in either calming or upsetting the infant is key to completing a thorough examination. Here is a suggested order for examination of the infant:

General observation
Head and neck region
  Facies
  Nose
  Mouth
  Ears
Trunk
  Cardiorespiratory systems
  Abdomen
  Back
  Genitalia and rectum
Extremities
Neurologic examination
Head circumference and length
Eye examination

DOCUMENTATION

A written report is the formal description of an examination. Using standard terms that are clear and familiar as well as descriptive, such as those suggested in Tables 7 and 8, makes each report more reliable and makes observations by different examiners more comparable. Using specific measurements, growth charts for percentile relationships, drawings, or photographs result in more precise documentation than do general descriptors.

For many practices, standard forms are used for the newborn examination. When the only descriptors are either normal or abnormal, one must be clear in understanding what both terms mean for each infant. Providing a quantity or a specific description is far more meaningful although more time consuming. When a finding is not clearly normal, there should be further description of that variation. Obviously, a prerequisite here is that each examiner understand what is truly normal for each type of examination situation and how the findings relate to day of life, race, gestational age, intrauterine positioning, or familial traits.

GENERAL EXAMINATION

General Observations

State

Important indicators of infant well-being are the states or levels of arousal the infant achieves throughout the examination and throughout the day as described by the parent or nursing staff. Several investigators have described the states from their clinical observations (29–31) or from electroencephalographic studies, but for practical purposes, the states originally categorized by Prechtl and Beintema are still relevant (14):

Deep sleep
Light sleep
Awake, light peripheral movements
Awake, large movements, not crying
Awake, crying

During examination, a healthy infant should demonstrate several levels of arousal. The most useful states for assessing an infant are those of light sleep and quiet awake so irritating maneuvers are held until the conclusion. What it takes to assist an infant to move from one state to another, or how well he or she does it spontaneously, is noteworthy. Because the deep sleep that follows a recent feeding may give an appearance of lethargy on arousal, knowing the feeding history and pattern is paramount to determining appropriateness of state.

Quieting an infant may require anything from simply stopping the handling to holding and talking to him or her. The amount of time spent in unstimulated crying is normally limited in the first 24 hours. Excessive crying, requiring more than routine consoling, particularly when there are no intervals of quiet alert states, indicates abnormal irritability. Similarly, a complete absence of crying is abnormal.

Color

Color assessment includes noting perfusion and skin color for the presence of cyanosis, jaundice, pallor, plethora, or any unusual cast and evaluating the distribution and types of pigmentation.

Respiratory Effort

The degree of respiratory effort is a primary indicator of how distressed or comfortable a newborn infant is, even when the cause of distress is not pulmonary. The physician can observe the respiratory rate, depth of excursions, use of accessory muscles with retractions or nasal flare, and any emitted sounds such as grunting or whining. Understanding the infant's pattern of respiratory effort can suggest a specific illness and guide a more directed examination. As the severity of a condition increases, these distinctions among the patterns may be lost.

Posture

One of the more important clues to physical status is the resting posture assumed by an unrestrained infant. This posture reflects intrauterine positioning and general body tone, and it varies with gestational age. At term, the healthy infant lies with thighs partially abducted and the hips, knees, ankles, elbows, and shoulders comfortably flexed. Premature infants lie in a less flexed posture than term infants as might also any infants who are not well. While observing neck position, the examiner looks for symmetry between the sides and compares upper and lower extremities. If there is lateral asymmetry and the head is turned to one side, there may be an asymmetric tonic neck reflex with the extremities on the mental side in extension and on the occipital side in flexion. In that case, the head should be turned to the opposite side to verify that the asymmetry reverses.

When the fetal presentation is not vertex or known or there is asymmetry or deformation, it is helpful to assist the infant in assuming a position reflecting his or her intrauterine attitude. The physician can fold the extremities into the fetal position by applying moderate pressure to a relaxed infant's feet while gently shaking the legs and by directing the arms toward the thorax through gentle pressure on the elbows.

Spontaneous Activity

The examiner should observe what the infant does in states of light sleep and awake. Does the infant stretch, move all extremities equally, open and close the hands, root and start sucking when something touches his or her face, and yawn with great facial expression, or does the infant lie quietly and move only in response to noxious stimulation?

Premature infants spend more time sleeping but should have spontaneous activity and resting postures commensurate with their gestational age. Because upon handling they quickly habituate and become disorganized, inspection before contact is even more important.

Vital signs

Temperature

The environment exerts a great effect on the temperature of a newborn infant who is poorly equipped to control his own body response. Maternal temperature is the most frequent cause of elevated temperature in a newborn immediately after birth, but the infant's temperature subsides to normal within an hour. Bundling or excess heat from an incubator, heated and humidified air, or warming lamps are frequent causes of temperature elevations in the first few days of life (32,33). Grover et al. studied the effect of bundling in an infant population 2 weeks to 3 months of age and determined that it would cause an elevation in skin temperature but did not significantly alter the rectal temperature. They cautioned that elevated rectal temperature should not be attributed to bundling in that age group (34). In general, if the infant's temperature remains elevated after the environment is returned to normal, or if the infant is more than 3 days of age, evaluation for infectious or neurologic causes is indicated to determine the cause of fever (32,33,35,36). From a meta-analysis of all studies addressing outcome has come a recommendation that all febrile infants less than 28 days of age should be hospitalized for parenteral antibiotic therapy because of the risk of serious infection in infants with little immunogenic reserve (37).

When infants are in a controlled environment the ambient temperature of which is determined by electronic biofeedback, their own body temperature may not increase in a typical fever but the ambient temperature they require may decrease. In such cases, one then has to interpret the measured body temperature compared with the energy output of the heat in the unit to determine if there are changes that would have the same significance as a true fever. For each major birth weight group and age there are different environmental temperatures that are expected to maintain a body temperature. When an infant develops a fever equivalent, the ambient temperature in a feedback system falls to or below the lowest limits for that expected temperature range.

Infants easily become hypothermic, again usually in response to the environment but also in clinical situations in which fever would be an expected response in older children. This is especially true if the infant generally remains quiet and does not cry vigorously. Infants who are either premature or underweight for length or for their gestational age are at greatest risk for hypothermia. Their environment should be controlled, especially during examination to prevent both hypo- and hyperthermia. Persistent hypothermia despite a controlled environment with an ambient temperature appropriate for the infant suggests infection but for the smallest and most immature infant, particularly in the first few days of life, temperature instability more likely reflects difficulty with environment. Later onset temperature instability is more likely to indicate a new onset infection.

Term infants will sweat, albeit poorly, in response to thermal stress. Preterm infants develop a measurable response by 2 weeks of age (38). Visible sweating at rest or on feeding in an afebrile infant is abnormal and may indicate distress, typically from cardiac disease.

Respiratory Rate and Heart Rate

As soon as an infant is touched, the respiratory rate and depth change. The rate is slightly faster when obtained by listening with a stethoscope than when obtained by observation and counting (39). The normal respiratory rate is 30 to 60 inspirations per minute in a term infant, with lower rates occurring after cardiopulmonary transition but continuing to decrease for several weeks. There is a much wider range of normal for respiratory rates in the neonatal period than in older infants (39). When awake, some normal infants breathe shallowly and rapidly but are able to slow sufficiently to feed well. Deep sleep is characterized by a more regular breathing pattern, whereas the awake state is characterized by more bursts of rapid breathing.

The heart rate is 110 to 160 beats per minute in healthy term infants but may vary significantly during deep sleep or active awake states. Preterm infants have resting heart rates at the higher end of the normal range. Tachycardia, with a rate persistently greater than 160, is a sign of many conditions, including central nervous system irritability, congestive heart failure, sepsis, anemia, fever, and hyperthyroidism.

Blood Pressure

The range of normal for blood pressure in neonates depends on the method used for assessment and gestational age (see Appendix Fig. 35 and Appendix Tables 1–3). The values obtained by the blanching and flush method are mean pressures and are lower than those registered by direct intravascular or Doppler monitoring. The flush method for mean pressure is easier to obtain in an active infant and requires only a sphygmomanometer so should remain as a clinical screening tool in the outpatient setting. The Doppler methods, although providing both diastolic and systolic pressures, require electronic equipment and a quieter patient. Two important elements for obtaining accurate blood pressures are a quiet infant and a properly sized cuff. The cuff should have a width approaching 50% to 67% of the length of the arm or leg. The inflatable bladder should encircle the entire limb (40,41).

For the flush method, the hand or foot is wrapped or squeezed firmly enough to blanch the skin (42). The cuff is inflated, the wrapping removed, and the pressure slowly lowered until there is a flush of color, at which point the pressure is read.

Diaper Colors and Abnormal Odors

Young infants provide frequent opportunities for us to observe the appearance of their bowel and bladder contents. The appearance and odor of the waste should not be ignored as part of the general examination. Unless the amnionic fluid is also notably foul smelling, bowel contents are odorless until colonized with gas forming organisms. Not only is the odor of the infant and his excreta worthy of noting, but the breath and general odor of the mother and amnionic fluid may give clues as well.

The appearance and frequency of stool is dependent on the what type of feeding has been taken as well as on how well it is absorbed and on what medications are being administered, particularly iron. The first stool is thick, green, tenaceous meconium. As air and fluids reach the meconium, there is a period of transition in the stools with bubbling and more watery content. As milk feedings are excreted, the stools become more seedy, pasty, or mushy in character (Fig. 2) Stools are rarely hard or firm after feedings are started but tend to be either mushy or watery. The exception to this is the greater incidence of firm or hard stool in infants fed a soy formula compared with breast, cow's milk formula, with and without iron, or a modified cow's milk formula with casein hydrolysate (Nutramigen) (43). Yellow stools are more common in breast-fed infants and brown stools more common in cow's milk formula without iron. Green stools are more frequent in iron-fortified formula, soy, and the casein hydrolysate (43). In breast-fed infants, brown or green stools are infrequent but there is more range of color in non–breast-fed infants.

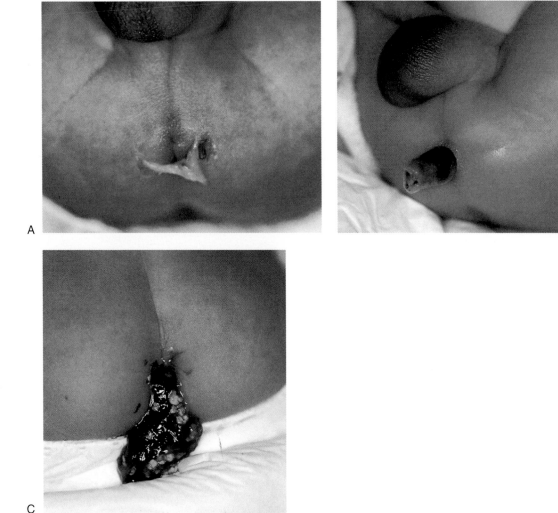

Figure 2. **A:** Initial mucus without color. The earliest elimination is not colored because it represents secretions of the bowel below the level of the bile duct. After the first small amount of rectal mucus, the stool should be colored. **B:** Initial meconium plug. The lower bowel contents can be dehydrated enough to be firm and shaped as illustrated. When too dry and extensive, the difficulty in passing the plug leads to the meconium plug syndrome of lower bowel obstruction. **C:** An early transitional stool. The stool shown is a combination of meconium (the dark green material) and a formula feed (the yellow seedy matter).

Table 9. *Causes of abnormally colored diapers*

Color	Disorder
Black	Homogentisic aciduria
Blue	Tryptophan malabsorption
Pink	Disorders with hematuria, stone formation
Port wine	Porphyrias
Yellow–orange	Disorders with increased uric acid

A historical fact of some importance in the physical assessment is the timing of the first void and stool. Term infants pass meconium before or shortly after birth, with 98.5% having passed their first stool in 24 hours and 100% by 48 hours (44,45). Premature infants are more delayed in their first passage so that 20.4% of infants weighing less than 1,500 g at birth do not stool until after 48 hours (46). Infants weighing less than 1,000 g at birth are the most delayed, with a median day for first passage of 3 days and 90% by 12 days (47). As in term infants, initiation of feeding was not prerequisite to stooling with 77% of the smallest infants having stooled before feeding (47).

The time to the first voiding is dependent on the infant's state of hydration and therefore indicates adequacy of intake as much as renal function. An early void at the time of delivery or shortly thereafter generally reflects fetal hydration state and perfusion. Spontaneous output after a delivery room void is often delayed until after the first stool, although a bladder catheter would indicate some urine formation. Premature infants may void even earlier than term infants unless they are not well. In the first 8 hours, 51%, and by 16 hours of age, 91% of term infants have voided (45). Urine color reflects excreted pigments with the intensity related in part to the concentration of any particular pigment. The various causes of abnormally colored diapers are noted in Table 9.

The overall odor of a person comes from the body's secretions and excretions, with most of the body odor coming from apocrine gland secretion. The general odor of infants is mild and pleasant, with little activity from their apocrine glands. Changes in fragrance most often indicate change in skin, oral, or bowel flora, but they may be due to metabolic or bio-

Table 10. *Causes of unusual urine odor*

General category of odor	Disease or offending substance
Acrid	Glutaric acidemia II
Ammoniacal	Urinary infection with urea-splitting bacteria (e.g., *Proteus* species)
Cabbage	Tyrosinemia
Fishy (rancid butter; boiled cabbage)	Hypermethioninemia
Fishy (rancid butter; musty)	Tyrosinosis, tyrosinemia
Fishy (rotting fish)	Trimethylaminuria
Medicinal	Penicillin and its derivatives
Musty (mouselike; barny; horselike; stale, sweaty locker room towels)	Phenylketonuria
Sweaty feet	Isovaleric acidemia glutaric acidemia (type II)
Sweet	Maple syrup urine disease (branched chain ketonuria)
Maple syrup (caramel-like; malty; burnt sugar)	
Sweet (Dried malt, celery, or hops; burnt sugar; yeastlike; brewerylike)	Oasthouse syndrome (methionine malabsorption)
Sweet (violets)	Turpentine
Swimming pool	Hawkinsinuria
Tomcat urine	3-Methylcrotonoyl-CoA carboxylase deficiency

Data from Hayden (48), Mace et al. (49), and Liddell (50).

Table 11. *Causes of unusual odors in parent or infant*

Source of odor	General category of odor	Disease or offending substance
Breath	Fruity; acetonelike; like decomposing apples	Ketoacidosis (diabetes or starvation)
	Fruity; alcoholic	Alcohol, phenol
	Fruity; pearlike; penetrating	Chloral hydrate, paraldehyde
	Fishy or ammoniacal	Uremia (trimethylamine, ammonia)
	Feculent; foul	Intestinal obstruction
	Bitter almond	Cyanide
	Burned rope	Marijuana
Pus	Nauseatingly sweet; like rotting apples	Gas gangrene
	Fecal; like overripe Camembert cheese	Proteolytic bacteria
Skin[a]	Foul; putrid	Skin disease with protein breakdown (infection, pemphigus)
Stool	Vile; foul	Malabsorption (e.g., cystic fibrosis, enzyme deficiency)
	Rancid	Shigellosis
	Garlic	Arsenic
Vaginal discharge	Foul	Vaginitis, foreign body
Vomitus	Fecal	Intestinal obstruction, peritonitis
	Garlic	Arsenic, phosphorus
	Violets	Turpentine

[a] Any odors affecting the urine will make the skin appear to smell the same in the incontinent neonate.
Data from Hayden (48), Mace et al. (49), and Liddell (50).

chemical abnormalities in either the infant or mother. Careful assessment would include considering abnormal maternal odor as well. Conditions causing remarkable odors are noted in Tables 10 and 11.

References

1. Moss GD, Cartlidge PHT, Speidel BD, Chambers TL. Routine examination in the neonatal period. *Br Med J* 1991;302:878–879.
2. Hughes AP, Stoker AJ, Milligan DWA. One or two routine neonatal examinations? *Br Med J* 1991;302:1209.
3. Apgar VA. A proposal for a new method of evaluation of the newborn infant. *Curr Res Anesth Analg* 1953;32:260.
4. AAP Committee on Fetus and Newborn and ACOG Committee on Obstetrics: *Maternal and Fetal Medicine. Guidelines for Perinatal Care.* 3rd ed. Elk Grove Village, IL, and Washington, DC: American Academy of Pediatrics and American College of Obstetricians and Gynecologists; 1992.
5. Catlin EA, Carpernter MW, Brann BW. The Apgar score revisited: influence of gestational age. *J Pediatr* 1986;109:865–868.
6. Apgar V, Holaday DA, James LS, Weisbrot IM. Evaluation of the newborn infant—a second report. *JAMA* 1958;168:843–848.
7. Crawford JS, Davies P, Pearson JF. Significance of the individual components of the Apgar score. *Br J Anaesth* 1973;45:148–158.
8. Yama AZ, Marx GF. Race and Apgar scores [Letter]. *Anaesthesia* 1991;46:330–331.
9. Clark DA, Hakanson DO. The inaccuracy of Apgar scoring. *J Perinatol* 1988;8:203–205.
10. American Academy of Pediatrics CoFaN. Use and abuse of the Apgar score. *Pediatrics* 1986;78:1148–1149.
11. Seidman DS, Paz I, Laor A, Gale R, Stevenson DK, Danon Y. Apgar scores and cognitive performance at 17 years of age. *Obstet Gynecol* 1991;77:875–878.
12. Pritchard JA. Fetal swallowing and amniotic fluid volume. *Obstet Gynecol* 1966;28:606–610.
13. Lilien LD, Srinivasan G, Pyati SP, Yeh TF, Pildes RS. Green vomiting in the first 24 hours in normal infants. *Am J Dis Child* 1986;140:662–664.
14. Prechtl H, Beintema D. The neurologic examination of the full-term newborn infant. In: *Clinics in developmental medicine.* Vol. 12. London: SIMP Heinemann; 1964.
15. Joseph PR, Rosenfeld W. Clavicular fractures in neonates. *Am J Dis Child* 1990;144:165–167.
16. Richardson DK, Phibbs CS, Gray JE, McCormick MC, Workman-Daniels K, A GD. Birth weight and illness severity: independent predictors of neonatal mortality. *Pediatrics* 1993;91:969.
17. Richardson DK, Gray JE, McCormick MC, Workman K, A GD. Score for neonatal acute physiology: a physiologic severity index for neonatal intensive care. *Pediatrics* 1993;91:617–623.
18. The International Neonatal Network. The CRIB (clinical risk index for babies) score: a tool for assessing initial neonatal risk and comparing performance of neonatal intensive care units. *Lancet* 1993;342:193–198.

19. Gray JE, Richardson DK, McCormick MC, Workman-Daniels K, Goldmann DA. Neonatal therapeutic intervention scoring system: a therapy-based severity-of-illness index. *Pediatrics* 1992;90:561–567.
20. Silverman WE, Andersen DH. Controlled clinical trial of effects of water mist on obstructive respiratory signs, death rate and necropsy findings among premature infants. *Pediatrics* 1956;17:1.
21. Morley CJ, Thornton AJ, Cole TJ, Fowler MA, Hewson PH. Symptoms and signs in infants younger than 6 months of age correlated with the severity of their illness. *Pediatrics* 1991;88:1119–1124.
22. Brazelton TB. Neonatal behavioral assessment scale. In: *Clinics in developmental medicine.* 2nd ed. Vol. 88. Philadelphia: JB Lippincott; 1984.
23. Myers MG. Longitudinal evaluation of neonatal nosocomial infections: association of infection with a blood pressure cuff. *Pediatrics* 1978;61:42–45.
24. Cloney DL, Donowitz LG. Overgown use for infection control in nurseries and neonatal intensive care units. *Am J Dis Child* 1986;140:680–683.
25. Birenbaum HJ, Glorioso L, Rosenberger C, Ashad C, Edwards K. Gowning on a postpartum ward fails to decrease colonization in the newborn infant. *Am J Dis Child* 1990;144:1031–1033.
26. Platt FW. Conversation repair: case studies in doctor-patient communication. Boston: Little, Brown; 1995.
27. Athreya BH, Silverman BK. *Pediatric physical diagnosis.* Norwalk: Appleton-Century-Crofts; 1985. [Revised ed. of *Clinical methods on pediatric diagnosis,* 1980].
28. Weiner S, Nathanson M. Physical examination: frequently observed errors. *JAMA* 1976;236:852–855.
29. Brazelton TB. Neonatal behavioral assessment scale. In: *Clinics in developmental medicine.* 1st ed. Vol. 50. Philadelphia: Spastics International Medical Publications with JB Lippincott; 1973.
30. Michaelis R, Parmelee AH, Stern E, Haber A. Activity states in premature and term infants. *Dev Psychobiol* 1973;6:209–215.
31. Parmelee AH Jr, Wenner WH, Akiyama Y, Schultz M, Stern E. Sleep states in premature infants. *Dev Med Child Neurol* 1967;9:70–77.
32. Voora S, Srinivasan G, Lilien LD, Yeh TF, Pildes RS. Fever in full-term newborns in the first four days of life. *Pediatrics* 1982;69:40–44.
33. Cheng TL, Partridge JC. Effect of bundling and high environmental temperature on neonatal body temperature. *Pediatrics* 1993;92:238–240.
34. Grover G, Berkowitz CD, Lewis RJ, Thompson M, Berry L, Seidel J. The effects of bundling on infant temperature. *Pediatrics* 1994;94:669–673.
35. Bonadio WA, Romine K, Gyuro J. Relationship of fever magnitude to rate of serious bacterial infections in neonates. *J Pediatr* 1990;116:733–735.
36. Jaskiewicz JA, McCarthy CA, Richardson AC, et al. Febrile infants at low risk for serious bacterial infection—an appraisal of the Rochester criteria and implications for management. *Pediatrics* 1994;94:390–396.
37. Baraff LJ, Bass JW, Fleisher GR, et al. Practice guideline for the management of infants and children 0 to 36 months of age with fever without source. Agency for Health Care Policy and Research. *Ann Emerg Med* 1993; 22:1198–1210 [erratum *Ann Emerg Med* 1993;22:1490].
38. Harpin VA, Rutter N. Sweating in preterm babies. *J Pediatr* 1982;100:614–618.
39. Rusconi F, Castagneto M, Gagliardi L, et al. Reference values for respiratory rate in the first 3 years of life. *Pediatrics* 1994;94:350–355.
40. Moss AJ. Indirect methods of blood pressure measurement. *Pediatr Clin North Am* 1978;25:3–14.
41. Blumenthal S, Epps RP, Heavenrich R, et al. Report of the task force on blood pressure control in children. *Pediatrics* 1977;59(Suppl):797–820.
42. Goldring D, Wohltmann HJ. "Flush" method for blood pressure determinations in newborn infants. *J Pediatr* 1952;40:285.
43. Hyams JS, Treem WR, Etienne NL, et al. Effect of infant formula on stool characteristics of young infants. *Pediatrics* 1995;95:50–54.
44. Sherry SN, Kramer I. The time of passage of the first stool and first urine by the newborn infant. *J Pediatr* 1955;46:158–159.
45. Clark D. Times of the first void and stool in 500 newborns. *Pediatrics* 1977;60:457.
46. Jhaveri MK, Kumar SP. Passage of the first stool in very low birth weight infants. *Pediatrics* 1987;79: 1005–1007.
47. Verma A, Dhanireddy R. Time of first stool in extremely low birth weight (≤1000 grams) infants. *J Pediatr* 1993;122:626–629.
48. Hayden GF. Olfactory diagnosis in medicine. *Postgrad Med* 1980;67:110–118.
49. Mace JW, Goodman SI, Centerwall WR, Chinnock RF. The child with an unusual odor. *Clin Pediatr* 1976;January:57–62.
50. Liddell K. Smell as a diagnostic marker. *Postgrad Med J* 1976;52:136–138.

2

Assessment of Size and Growth

One of the general indicators of well-being in the fetal and neonatal periods is a normal growth pattern. When all the parameters that we use to assess growth in any infant follow a consistent trend and fall within expected ranges, there is some reassurance of general health in that infant. Weight is an objective measurement that can be plotted against day of life to establish a weight-for-age curve or a growth curve. When we see an infant increasing in weight on a daily, weekly, or monthly basis, we assume that that infant is growing and, therefore, must be thriving. But can we make that assumption just because there is weight gain? No, there has to be some pattern of weight gain that is appropriate, that is neither too little nor too much, and that correlates with nutritional and fluid intake. Additionally, growth represents increase in size as well as increase in weight, so there must be appropriate change in the dimensions as well as in total mass.

From the time of conception through the neonatal period and beyond, growth follows a predictable path that is influenced by genetic and environmental factors. Disturbances in the normal pattern of growth may be proportionate or disproportionate in their effect. For instance, in fetuses whose weight is disproportionately lower than the length or head circumference, we say that there is head sparing or that there is asymmetric growth retardation. In syndromes with a specific phenotype, many of the dysmorphic features are manifestations of disproportionate growth of more localized areas. This explains why facies described as typical of some dysmorphic syndromes change depending on the age and, therefore, the duration of abnormal growth at the time of the description.

We assess growth in the fetus and neonate by measuring parameters that are accessible and reproducible. For the fetus, measurements by ultrasonography include the biparietal diameter, chest or abdominal circumference, crown–rump length, and femur length. Putting these dimensions on standard graphs allows extrapolation of fetal weight. For the normal neonate, standard measurements include weight, length, and head circumference. For an assessment of nutrition, we could measure skin-fold thickness or mid-arm circumference or calculate the ponderal index. For specific conditions or where abnormal development is suspected, any external body part can be measured and compared with values derived from similar patients.

We can measure different parameters at one time or over a period of time and can express the results as a number, as a comparison, or as a statistical relationship to an expected normal value. We compare an individual infant to him- or herself over time by looking at a rate of growth or we compare that infant to what would be an expected pattern based on measurements from many other infants with the same sex, race, genetic potential, or nutritional/environmental factors. When the measurements of one infant are compared with standard curves, we assess on what percentile curve the measurements lie. We can also calculate the deviations from the mean of any parameter. The most common practice is to plot an infant's measurements on standard growth curves with several sets of measurements over time to determine the curve, representing rate of growth, and to determine for each parameter the percentile group to which the infant may be assigned. It is easy to determine the weight for length ratio or to calculate the ponderal index from the two basic measurements to evaluate general proportionality, obesity, or leanness.

INDICATIONS FOR MEASURING GROWTH PARAMETERS
Morbidity and Mortality Statistics for Outcome

Because the weight of a newly born infant is an objective measurement, it provides a means of classifying infants in outcome data that are more accurate than classifying infants by gestational age, even though morbidity and mortality may be more greatly affected by gestational age than by weight. Standard reporting of reproductive health statistics rely on classification of all infants by birth weight (1). Unfortunately, for the lowest weight groups in which there is the highest mortality and morbidity, there is no consistent grouping of infants among studies. Some reports on outcome that are based on birth weight alone group infants by 250-g partitions, whereas others, particularly those emphasizing infants weighing less than 1,000 grams at birth, divide the population into 100-g partitions or use less than or greater than 800 g as a division.

Infants weighing less than 2,500 g are low birth weight infants regardless of gestational age. Very low birth weight refers to a weight of less than 1,500 g, and extremely low birth weight refers to a weight of less than 1,000 g. Classification by these weight groups helps establish level of risk for neonatal and long-term morbidity and mortality (2).

Identification of Infant at Risk for Problems Associated with Aberrant Growth Pattern

If an infant's measurements fall between the 10th and 90th percentiles for a given gestational age on a standard growth curve that matches the infant's sex, race, and environment,

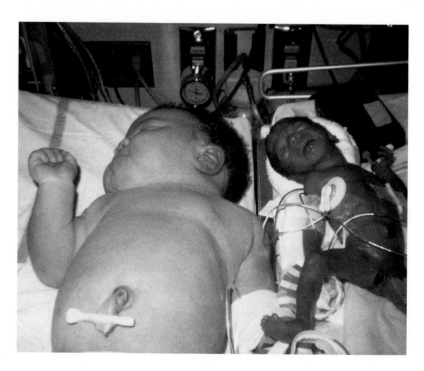

Figure 1. Clinical examples of the extremes of large for gestational age and SGA. Both infants are of the same gestational age, but one weighed 5,500 g and the other 770 g at birth.

the infant is said to have growth within a normal range for that population. He or she is considered appropriate for gestational age (AGA). There is no concurrence if the outer limit for percentile range should be at the 10th (90th) or 3rd (97th) percentile curve. Published studies use either limit, but for clinical application the narrower range of 10 to 90 is the more appropriate one to use. If the weight is at less than the 10th percentile, the infant is small for gestational age (SGA); if above the 90th percentile, the infant is large for gestational age (LGA) (Fig. 1). Clearly, accuracy in gestational age assessment is a critical variable in determining if a weight is appropriate. Infants born prematurely should be plotted at their corrected gestational age until 2 years of age. AGA infants born at term are at lowest risk for problems associated with neonatal mortality and morbidity (2). Infants who are both premature and also SGA are at highest risk (3,4).

If the three parameters of weight, length, and head circumference fall on the same curve, the infant is symmetric, even though he or she may still be AGA, LGA, or SGA. The infant is asymmetric if the parameters are on different curves, most often with the weight lower. This distinction may occur in either prenatal or postnatal growth and is helpful in defining pathologic processes. If the process occurs prenatally, particularly when there is a slowing of intrauterine growth rate documented by serial fetal sonography or a presumed slowing by low weight for length measurements at birth, the infant is classified as having intrauterine growth retardation (IUGR). An infant can have IUGR without being SGA (Fig. 2). Using only the outer limit of the 10th or 90th percentile to define abnormally grown fetuses would miss some otherwise abnormal infants whose weight and length may be well below the normal expected for that individual. Other comparisons are necessary to pick up these infants.

Infants that are SGA or LGA or have IUGR are at risk for perinatal and long-term problems. The risks for LGA infants are primarily maximum in the perinatal period. The risks for SGA infants are both perinatal and long term, and morbidity and mortality for SGA infants depend on the etiology (Fig. 3). Infants who are premature and SGA have been thought to be at less risk for some of the problems of prematurity than are those premature infants who are of the same weight and AGA. Better determination of gestational age as well as use of more appropriate growth charts has suggested that this impression is not correct. SGA infants appear to have an increased risk for hyaline membrane disease and death or poor outcome when compared with other infants of the same gestational age, as compared with infants of the same weight (3,4). The changes that lead to fetal and neonatal problems encountered by SGA infants are found in Table 1. Problems encountered by LGA infants are listed in Table 2.

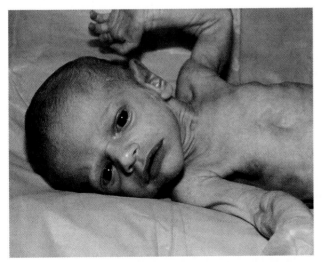

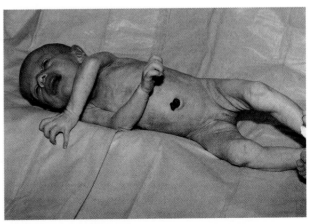

A

B

Figure 2. Clinical example of an extremely IUGR infant who was thyrotoxic from maternal hyperthyroidism. This infant was not SGA but has many of the physical findings of severe undernutrition and would score between 10 and 15 on a CANS score.

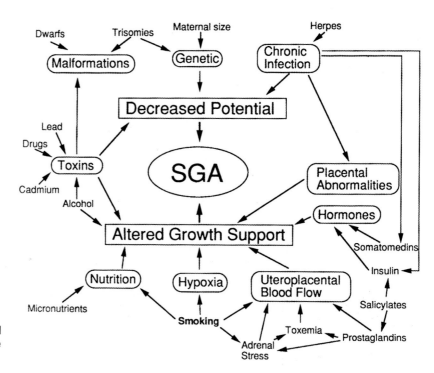

Figure 3. Selected risk factors associated with impaired growth. Reprinted from Crouse and Cassady (61) with permission.

When an infant is LGA because of maternal diabetes, he or she is more likely to have problems relating to abnormal glucose metabolism after birth if the intrauterine growth pattern is disproportionate and leads to a relatively heavy weight for length; in other words, if the weight is on a higher percentile curve than the length, the infant has a greater risk for the problems characteristic of infants of poorly controlled diabetic mothers (5). This risk appears to be greater even when the mother's diabetes is well controlled if the weight for length ratio is excessive (5).

The definitions of aberrant growth based solely on weight for gestational age using 10th and 90th percentiles as limits for normal are recognized as too imprecise to detect all infants at risk or those with intrauterine malnutrition. Fetal malnutrition is not synonymous with SGA or IUGR, although many of these infants are malnourished. It may be present at almost any birth weight and indicates an effect on body composition and, potentially, brain growth. As such, fetal malnutrition may carry a separate, higher risk for infant outcome. Other parameters that have been suggested include Ponderal index, weight/length ratio, skin-fold thickness measurements, and actual weight/estimated weight ratios. The techniques for these calculations are detailed below or in the glossary. An interesting use of physical diagnosis to assess fetal nutritional status in newborn infants is the Clinical Assessment of Nutritional Status (CANS), which is based on physical findings described by McLean and Usher that suggest weight loss or poor nutrition (6). Metcoff looked for these physical signs in 1,382 term infants, applying a weighted observation system, the CANSCORE (Fig. 4), and suggested that fetal malnutrition was present in 10.9% of these infants (7). Without applying these criteria, he suggested that 5.5% of 1,229 AGA infants would not have been classified as malnourished. Fifty-four percent of 153 SGA infants had physical findings suggesting malnutrition, but the rest did not. Whether or not a score is applied to each infant during initial assessments, recognizing the physical signs is helpful as part of a complete evaluation.

Some physical signs manifest when specific nutrients are insufficient or absent (Table 3) (8). These signs are unlikely to be present within the true neonatal period but could develop in infants who remain in hospital nurseries for prolonged times because of neonatal conditions.

Providing a Quantitative Value to Qualitative Assessment

When we look at a patient as part of our physical assessment, we form an impression as to whether the appearance is normal. Much of this impression derives from observing pro-

Table 1. *Biochemical and metabolic changes in infants small for gestational age*

Proteins and collagen	Carbohydrate and fat metabolism
Increased ammonia	Fetal or neonatal hypoglycemia
Increased urea; increased uric acid	No change or increased glucose K_t
Decreased OH-proline turnover early; increased later	Decreased, increased, or no change in insulin
Increased uronic acid turnover	Low urinary adrenaline after hypoglycemia
Decreased or no change in total protein	Decreased or no change in β-hydroxybutyrate
Decreased or no change in prealbumin	No change or increased ketone bodies
Decreased IgG	Decreased, increased, or no change in FFA and glycerol
Increased IgM in some	Decreased hepatic gluconeogenesis
Immunocompetence	Increased lactate and pyruvate
Decreased humoral or cellular bactericidal capacity	Increased alanine
Decreased phagocytic index	Increased glucagon
Decreased lysozyme	Other
Decreased humoral and cellular immunocompetence	Decreased serum Ca^{2+}
Hematology	Decreased, increased, or no change in amniotic fluid L/S ratio
Increased hematocrit; increased RBC volume; increased fetal hemoglobin; increased erythropoietin	Transient diabetes
Increased viscosity	Increased cortisol or 11-OH corticosteroids
Decreased platelets	No change or increased HGH
Increased PT, PTT	Decreased, increased, or no change in O_2 consumption
No change in retic count (% or absolute), but increased reticulocyte index	

FFA, free fatty acids; K_t, rate constant for glucose metabolism; PT, prothrombin time; PTT, partial thromboplastin time; RBC, erythrocyte.
From Crouse and Cassady, ref. 61, with permission.

portionality of the individual parts; either they go together or they do not. When there is disproportion, we use terms like long or short, broad or narrow, flattened or prominent, to describe the findings. These are qualitative descriptors that are highly subjective and certainly depend on the experience of the observer to understand the differences inherent in individuals due to race, sex, gestational age, or day of life. Measuring the features allows quantitative comparison against normal values from population studies or against other fea-

Table 2. *Problems encountered by LGA infants*

Iatrogenic prematurity due to overestimation of fetal gestational age
Increased requirement for delivery by cesarean section
Shoulder dystocia with increased risk for trauma or asphyxia
Birth injuries
    Ecchymoses
    Local fat necrosis associated with forceps applications
    Cephalohematoma
    Intracranial hemorrhage
    Brachial plexus injuries
    Paralysis of diaphragm
    Fracture of clavicle or humerus
Polycythemia
    Jaundice
    Hyperviscosity syndrome
    Hypoglycemia
    Seizures
    Renal vein thrombosis
    Increased total blood volume
Pulmonary hypertension
Poor feeding
Hyperinsulinemia

Table 3. *Clinical findings of nutritional deficiency in neonates*

Clinical findings	Deficiency
Lethargy	Protein, calorie
Pallor	Iron, copper, folate, vitamin B12
Muscle wasting	Protein, calorie
Edema	Protein, zinc
Craniotabes, frontal bossing	Vitamin D
Hair depigmentation	Protein, zinc
Keratomalacia (eyes)	Vitamin A
Angular stomatitis	Vitamin B2
Glossitis	Niacin
Goiter	Iodine
Follicular hyperkeratosis	Vitamin A
Dry skin, scaly dermatitis	Essential fatty acids
Acrodermatitis	Zinc
Petechia, ecchymosis	Vitamin C
Rachitic rosary, bone thickening	Vitamin D
Osteopenia	Calcium, phosphorus

From Pereira and Georgieff, ref. 8, with permission.

tures in the same infant. The first impression of proportionality comes from observation and qualitative description; the confirmation comes from quantitative measurements.

Many of the syndromes that have characteristic facies in childhood represent disproportionate growth of individual features. At birth the growth may not be as disproportionate as it is later in infancy and childhood, making diagnosis based on these physical differences alone more difficult or impossible. When an infant with such a syndrome is born prematurely, the facies may be even less remarkable. Most fetuses in pregnancies that are terminated in mid-trimester because of known trisomy 21 do not have features that are characteristic enough to make that diagnosis on physical examination. Until the fetus and infant have had enough time to grow and develop the disproportional features that distinguish some of the syndromes, the outward appearance may not be typical.

Determine Pathophysiology Contributing to a Disproportion

Aberrant or asymmetric patterns of total growth may suggest their etiology. Similarly, asymmetries of the face or body parts suggest timing and etiology. The abnormal shape the head assumes in craniosynostosis is typical: growth is prevented in one area and uninhibited in the other areas (see Chapter 6, Figs. 14 and 16).

Monitor Efficacy of Nutritional Interventions

Growth requires assimilation of nutrition so it is outward evidence of the adequacy of caloric intake. Regaining birth weight by 1 week of age in a breast-feeding infant is a reassurance that lactation, intake, and digestion are probably normal and that the presence of significant, active pathology is unlikely. Similarly, rate of growth is an important parameter in recovery for infants in intensive care or after premature birth. Some specific measurements for nutritional status include weight and length, plotted on growth curves or velocity curves, or calculated as a ponderal index (9,10), mid-arm circumference compared with head circumference and weight (10,11), and skin-fold thickness (11,12).

Monitor Complications of Disease Processes

The pattern of growth of individual parts or of the infant as a whole helps to monitor disease processes or complications. For instance, the rate of change of the head circumference

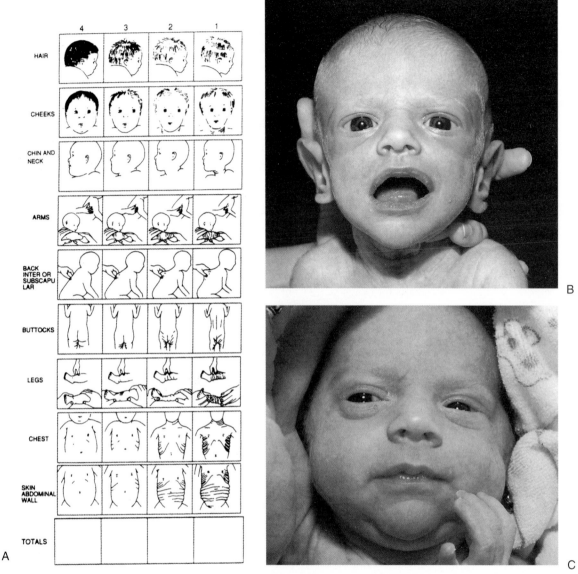

Figure 4. A: CANS. Nine signs for assessing nutritional status in newborn term infants. Each of the signs is rated from 4 (best) to 1 (worst). The CANSCORE is the sum of the nine CANS signs. Hair: large amount, smooth, silky, easily groomed (4 points); thinner, some straight "staring" hair (3 points); still thinner, more straight, with depigmented hair that does not respond to brushing (2 points); and straight staring hair with depigmented stripe (flag sign). Cheeks: Progression from full buccal pads and round face (4 points); to significantly reduced buccal fat with narrow, flat face (1 point). Neck and chin: Double or triple chin fat folds, neck not evident (4 points); to thin chin, no fat folds, neck with loose, wrinkled skin very evident (1 point). Arms: Full, round, cannot elicit "accordion" folds or lift folds of skin from elbow or triceps area (4 points); to striking accordion folding of lower arm elicited when examiner's thumb and fingers of the left hand grasp the arm just below the elbow of the baby and thumb and fingers of the examiner's right hand circling the wrist of the baby are moved toward each other; skin is loose and easily grasped and pulled away from the elbow (1 point). Back: Difficult to grasp and lift skin in the interscapular area (4 points); to skin loose, easily lifted in a thin fold from the interscapular area (1 point). Buttocks: Full, round gluteal fat pads (4 points); to virtually no evident gluteal fat and skin of the buttocks and upper, posterior thigh loose and deeply wrinkled (1 point). Legs: Like arms. Chest: Full; round ribs not seen (4 points), to progressive prominence of the ribs with obvious loss of intercostal tissue (1 point). Abdomen: Full, round, no loose skin (4 points) to distended or scaphoid, but with very loose skin, easily lifted, wrinkled, and accordion folds demonstrable (1 point). Reprinted with permission from Metcoff (7). **B:** Intrauterine growth-retarded infant at term with sparse hair, reduced buccal fat, and thin, wrinkled neck. Full view of same infant is shown in Fig. 2A and B. **C:** Premature infant in growth spurt at term corrected gestational age. Note his extra chin, fat cheeks and neck, and plump fingers.

correlates with the rate of brain growth. When that rate falls below expected levels, particularly when other parameters do not decrease as much, there is a strong suggestion of poor brain growth and atrophy (13). In contrast, excessive head growth beyond other parameters might suggest hydrocephalus. The notable exception to this is the acceleration of brain growth after a reversal of disease or poor intrauterine nutrition. In this situation, weight gain is first, head growth second, and length follows within 10 days.

Infants who have required intensive care are at risk for impaired growth either because of continuing disease process or localized complications. Disproportionate growth of an extremity suggests vascular insufficiency if it is undergrown or a vascular malformation if it is hypertrophied.

DEFINE ABERRANT GROWTH

In order to determine if a patient's measurements fall within normal ranges, one has to apply an appropriate standard against which the measurements can be compared. If the comparison is to population-based growth curves, the population has to represent the patient in gender, race, gestational age, genetic potential, and geographic regions of the world for altitude and other environmental variances. For example, the growth pattern for head circumference in an infant with Down's syndrome should be compared with the growth charts for Down's infants of the same sex (14). Twin or higher multiple gestations infants require specific intrauterine growth charts (15–17) (see Tables 4 and 5).

Aberrant growth also can be detected by a change in the rate of growth of an individual infant for either all or individual parameters. A notable example of this is with a rapid increase in head growth indicating progressive hydrocephalus. Unfortunately, there may be significant hydrocephalus before aberrant head growth is detectable.

Not only must measurements be compared with those from similar population backgrounds and potential, but there also must be some agreement as to the limits for definition of abnormal. Some studies use less than 10th percentile or greater than 90th percentile for the limits, whereas others use less than 3rd percentile or greater than 97th percentile. Still

Table 4. *Percentiles of birth weight for live singleton births in 1986 by sex and gestational age*

Gestational age (wk)	Boys				Girls			
	Total no.	Percentile[a]			Total no.	Percentile[a]		
		10	50	90		10	50	90
25	100	651	810	950	73	604	750	924
26	113	714	950	1,170	109	700	880	1,130
27	138	827	1,010	1,331	105	738	1,000	1,300
28	219	900	1,190	1,550	140	833	1,100	1,517
29	179	990	1,320	1,610	127	942	1,280	1,624
30	257	1,156	1,530	2,214	216	1,040	1,485	2,001
31	294	1,230	1,680	2,105	244	1,220	1,605	2,205
32	578	1,459	1,915	2,400	428	1,359	1,800	2,430
33	648	1,610	2,100	2,601	472	1,543	2,040	2,571
34	1,181	1,880	2,350	2,940	894	1,750	2,235	2,830
35	1,840	2,060	2,570	3,140	1,454	1,950	2,460	3,040
36	4,654	2,280	2,820	3,490	3,870	2,210	2,740	3,370
37	8,576	2,530	3,050	3,640	7,504	2,410	2,940	3,520
38	22,898	2,740	3,280	3,850	20,814	2,630	3,140	3,710
39	35,909	2,900	3,430	4,000	33,931	2,780	3,290	3,850
40	68,102	3,020	3,570	4,160	67,149	2,900	3,430	4,000
41	25,048	3,140	3,700	4,300	25,294	3,000	3,540	4,120
42	10,309	3,200	3,770	4,390	9,636	3,060	3,610	4,190

[a] Values are birth weights in grams.
From Arbuckle and Sherman, ref. 17, with permission.

Philtrum Length

With the infant at rest, without crying or sucking, measure the distance from the base of the collumella to the top of the vermillion border in the midline (48).

Mouth Width (Intercommissural Distance)

With the infant at rest, without crying or sucking, measure the distance between the corners of the mouth. Mean width at term is approximately 20 mm (48).

Measurement of Trunk

Chest Circumference

Measure horizontally around the upper body at the level of the nipples or just below the scapular angles. If the level of the nipples is abnormal, measure at the fourth intercostal space in the mid-clavicular line (see Appendix Fig. 21).

Thoracic Index

Measure the anteroposterior diameter from the sternum at the level of the nipples to the vertebrae. Measure the lateral diameter between the mid-axillary lines at the level of the nipples. If calipers are not available, the lateral margins with the infant lying supine and the anterior margins with the infant in lateral recline may be marked on a pad and measured. At term birth the index should be between 0.87 and 1.04 (47). It decreases progressively after birth unless there are conditions causing an increase in thoracic volume (air trapping, diaphragmatic hernia).

Internipple Distance

Measure between the center of both nipples (51,52). The internipple index stays more constant during gestation and allows another means of assessing abnormal spacing (see glossary and Appendix Fig. 22).

Sternal Length

Measure from the top of the manubrium to the lower edge of the sternum but not including the xiphoid (see Appendix Fig. 23).

Torso Length

Measure the distance from the manubrial notch to the superior aspect of the symphysis pubis (see Appendix Fig. 24).

Measurement of Perineum

Anal Placement

Measure the distance between the posterior aspect of the introitus of the vagina (fourchette) in the female (AF), or the end of scrotal skin in the male, and the anterior border of the anal opening (53). A ratio of AF to anus-clitoris (AC) or fourchette-clitoris to AC has less variability dependent on size or gestational age (see glossary and Appendix Fig. 26).

Penile Length

Gently stretch the penis and measure from the base of the penis (pubis ramus) to the tip of the glans (54–56) (see Appendix Fig. 25).

Testicular Volume

The length and width of the testis can be measured along a vertical axis between the upper and lower pole of the testis and at the broadest width: $0.71 \times \text{length}^2 \times \text{width}$ (volume of an ellipsoid) (57).

Measurement of Extremities

Angle of Thumb Attachment

With the hand at rest and the palm facing up, draw an imaginary line through the main axis of the index finger and another imaginary line through the main axis of the thumb. Measure the angle made at the point of intersection of the two imaginary lines. Normal angle is between 75° and 90° in the resting position (29). The technique for determining the thumb placement index is shown in Fig. 11.

Carrying Angle

With the elbow extended and the forearm supinated, extend an imaginary line along the axis of the humerus to the level of the hand. Establish a second line through the axis of the forearm and the hand. Measure the angle between the two lines at the elbow. The angle increases with age, so the measurement at birth may be within normal range in syndromes characteristically associated with abnormal carrying angles.

Limb Length and Circumference

Techniques for measuring lengths of parts of the extremities are illustrated in Figures 12–18. Measure at the widest or largest diameter of the limb or from a fixed bony point. In the upper arm the widest point is at the middle of the biceps just below the insertion of the deltoid. The widest point of the thigh is usually just below the gluteal crease. The widest point in the calf is in the mid-upper calf muscle (12,33,58–60) (Figs. 11–18).

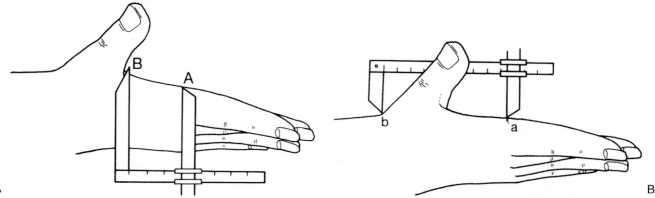

Figure 11. Thumb placement index. This is the ratio of the distance between the distance between the proximal flexion crease at the base of the index finger on the distal insertion of the thumb and the distance between the proximal crease at the base of the index finger and distal flexion crease at the wrist. **A:** Measure on the lateral aspect of the index finger from the proximal crease at the base of the index finger to the basal crease of the thumb insertion. **B:** Measure from the proximal crease at the base of the index finger, on the palmar aspect, to the distal flexion crease at the wrist. Maintain the thumb at 90° in abduction. The ratio is measurement (a)/measurement (b) = 0.51 ± 0.4. Reprinted from Hall et al. (29) with permission from Oxford University Press.

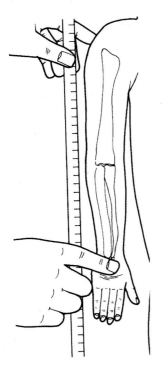

Figure 12. Total upper limb length. Measure between the acromion and the tip of the middle finger. Reprinted from Hall et al. (29) with permission from Oxford University Press.

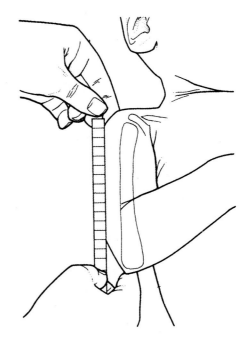

Figure 13. Upper arm length. Measure from the acromion along the posterior lateral aspect of the arm until reaching the distal medial border of the olecranon. Reprinted from Hall et al. (29) with permission from Oxford University Press.

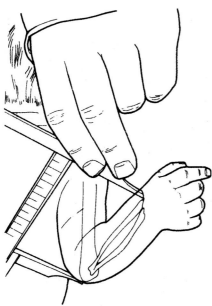

Figure 14. Forearm length. With the forearm pronated, measure from the most prominent point of the olecranon to the distal lateral process of the radius along the lateral surface of the forearm. Reprinted from Hall et al. (29) with permission from Oxford University Press.

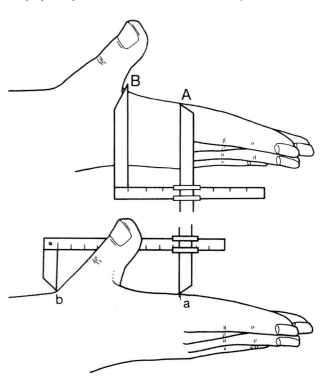

Figure 15. Hand length. Measure from the distal crease at the wrist to the tip of the middle finger. If the hand cannot be held opened fully, walk a tape measure along the palmar surface. **A:** Middle finger length. Measure from the proximal flexion creases at the base of the middle finger to the tip of the middle finger on the palmar surface. Because the crease does not overlie the joint, this measurement does not reflect the lengths of the finger bones. **B:** Palm length. With the wrist in neutral position and the hand held open, measure the distance between the distal flexion crease at the wrist and the proximal flexion crease of the middle finger. Palm width. With the wrist in neutral position and the hand held open, measure the distance across the palm between the edges of the hand at the level of the metacarpophalangeal joints. Reprinted from Feingold et al. (63) with permission.

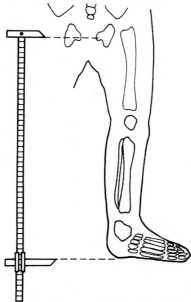

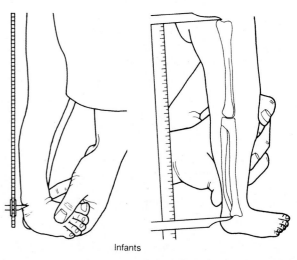

Figure 16. Lower segment. Measure from the top of the middle part of the pubic bone to the sole of the foot. By convention, this does not equal the sum of the lengths of the upper and lower legs or the total lower limb length. Reprinted from Hall et al. (29) with permission from Oxford University Press.

Infants

Figure 17. Total lower limb length. Measure from the greater trochanter of the femur to the lateral malleolus of the ankle along the lateral aspect of the leg. Lower limbs account for approximately one third total length at birth and somewhat less than 20% of weight. Leg length is not equivalent to the lower segment in infants. Reprinted from Hall et al. (29) with permission from Oxford University Press.

Figure 18. Foot length. Foot length is the longest axis of the foot. Measure from an imaginary vertical line drawn from the posterior prominence of the heel, to the tip of the longest toe, on the plantar aspect of the foot with the ankle perpendicular to the foot. Foot length correlates well enough with other anthropometrics in gestations less than 37 weeks to allow estimation of weight and length for calculations of medication doses when infants are too ill to tolerate the handling required in other measurements (64). Reprinted from Hall et al. (29) with permission from Oxford University Press.

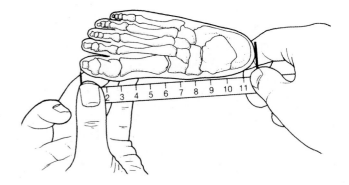

GLOSSARY

Anogenital ratio   Anus to fourchette/anus to base of the clitoris. The anogenital ratio follows a normal distribution and does not correlate with weight, length, or age. The mean ($\pm$SD) value was 0.37 ± 0.07 in infants and 0.36 ± 0.07 in adults. An anogenital ratio of >0.50 falls outside the 95% confidence limits, suggesting labioscrotal fusion (53).

Anthropometrics   The study of comparative measurements of the human body.

Bi-iliac distance   Distance between the most prominent lateral points of the iliac crest.

Bigonial distance   Distance between the lateral aspect of the angle of the jaw on the right and the same point on the left (mandible width).

Bizygomatic distance   Maximal distance between the most lateral points on the zygomatic arches (zygion). This measurement represents facial width.

Bone age   Radiologic assessment of physiologic age relating growth and skeletal maturation; stage of development of the skeleton as judged by radiography and compared with chronologic age.

Bony interorbital distance   The distance between the medial margins of the bony orbit, measured cephalometrically on radiography.

Caliper   Instrument used for measuring distance or thickness.

Canthal distance, inner   Distance between the inner canthi (inner corners) of the two eyes.

Canthal distance, outer   Distance between the outer canthi (outer corners) of the two eyes.

Carpal angle   Angle made by the carpal bones at the wrist.

Carrying angle   Angle subtended by the forearm on the humerus; the deviation of the forearm relative to the humerus; the angle at the elbow joint.

Cephalic index   The ratio of the head width expressed as a percentage of head length. CI = Head width $\times$ 100/head length. Normal head CI is 76–80.9%. Dolichocephaly: CI < 75.9%. Brachycephaly: CI > 81%.

Cephalometrics   The science of precise measurement of bones of the cranium and face, using fixed reproducible positions.

Chest circumference   Circumference of the chest at the level of the nipple.

Cornea, transverse diameter   Distance between the medial and lateral border of the iris.

Corrected gestational age (CGA)   An adjustment in assigned age that allows for prematurity. CGA = chronologic age in weeks $-$ (40 minus gestational age). The term "post-conceptional age" is not synonymous and would be 2 weeks-less because gestational age is calculated the time of the last menstrual period, not from the date of conception.

Crown–rump length   Distance from the top of the head to the bottom of the buttock, with hips in flexion.

Crown–rump/total length ratio   Crown–rump length/total length. The mean value is 0.653 at 27 weeks to 0.673 at 40 weeks. See Table 7.

Dental age   Physiologic age of the teeth as determined by the number and type of teeth that have erupted or been shed.

Ear length   Maximum distance from the superior aspect to the inferior aspect of the external ear (pinna).

Ear position   Location of the superior attachment of the pinna. The size and rotation of the external ear are not relevant.

Ear protrusion   Protrusion of each ear measured by the angle subtended from the posterior aspect of the pinna to the mastoid plane of the skull.

Ear rotation   Rotation of the longitudinal axis of the external ear (pinna).

Ear width   Width of the external ear (pinna), from just anterior to the tragus to the lateral margin of the helix.

Facial height   Distance from the root of the nose (nasion) to the lowest median landmark on the lower border of the mandible (menton of gnathion); lower two thirds of adult craniofacies. In neonates this is the lower half of the craniofacies.

Facial height, lower   Distance from the base of the nose (subnasion) to the lowest median landmark on the lower border of the mandible (menton or gnathion); length of the lower one third of adult craniofacies. In neonates this is the approximate one fourth of the craniofacies.

Facial height, upper   Distance from the root of the nose (nasion) to the base of the nose (subnasion); middle one third of adult craniofacies. In neonates this is the approximate third quarter of the craniofacies.

Facial index   Ratio of the facial height (nasion to menton) to facial width (bizygomatic distance) used to assess a long, narrow face as compared with a short, wide face.

Facial width   See *Bizygomatic distance.*

Finger-to-hand ratio   Middle finger length/total hand length = 0.43 ± 0.02 (1SD) or ± 0.055 (2SD) at term birth (47).

Forehead height   See *Skull height.*

Frankfurt plane (FP)   Eye–ear plane, which is standard horizontal cephalometric reference. The Frankfurt plane or Frankfurt horizontal is established when the head is held erect, with the eyes forward, so that the lowest margin of the lower bony orbit (orbitale) and the upper margin of the external auditory meatus (porion) are in the same horizontal plane (Frankfurt plane).

Goniometer   A hinged device that allows measurement of angles of joints.

Head circumference   Synonym *Occipitofrontal circumference.* Distance around the head at its largest part.

Head circumference ratio   100% × patient head circumference/mean head circumference for age ≈ 100. A decrease of >3.1% between birth and 4 months is strongly predictive of subsequent microcephaly at 18 months in term infants who experienced severe birth asphyxia (13).

Head length   Maximum dimension of the sagittal axis of the skull.

Head width   Maximal biparietal diameter.

Imperial system   System of measuring, using pounds and inches, used by Anglo-American countries.

Individualized birth weight ratio   The actual birth weight divided by the birth weight predicted for a given gestation (24,65,66).

Interalar distance (nasal width)   Distance between the most lateral aspects of the alae nasi.

Intercommissural distance   Mouth width at rest; the distance between the two outer corners of the mouth (cheilion).

Internipple distance   Distance between the centers of both nipples.

Internipple index   Index = internipple distance (cm) × 100/chest circumference (cm). The index stays constant during various gestational ages. An internipple index of >28% (>2SD) at any gestational age or during immediate postnatal period suggests widely spaced nipples (52).

Interpupillary distance   Distance between the centers of the pupils of the two eyes.

Knemometer   Hand-held electronic device, resembling a pair of callipers, used for measuring knee–heel length in small infant. The measuring system, based on a magnetic encoder automatically records the knee–heel length when the pressure applied on the heel reaches a preset value. It is sensitive in detecting small increments in length (67).

Length   Distance between the top of the head and the sole of the foot when the individual is lying down.

Lower segment   Distance from the pubic bone to the sole of the foot.

Mandible width   See *Bigonial distance.*

Mandibular length, effective   Effective length and prominence of the mandible on cephalometry.

Maxillomandibular differential   Measurements determined on cephalometry subtracting the effective midfacial length from the effective mandibular length.

Metric system   A measuring system based on the use of the meter as a unit; used by most of Europe.

Mid-parental height   Sum of the parents' heights divided by two.

Midfacial length, effective   Size and prominence of the maxilla on cephalometry.

Mouth width   See *Intercommissural distance.*

Nasal length   The distance from the nasal root (nasion) to base (subnasion).

Nasal width   See *Interalar distance.*

Obliquity (slant) of the palpebral fissure   Slant of the palpebral fissure from the horizontal.

Occipitofrontal circumference (OFC)   Distance around the head, the largest obtainable measurement (head circumference).

Orchidometer   Measuring device for quantifying testicular size.

Palm width–to–palm length ratio   Palm width/palm length $\times$ 100 = 0.97 $\pm$ 0.085 (2SD) (68).

Palpebral fissure length   Distance between the inner and outer canthus of one eye.

Ponderal index   Birth weight (kg) $\times$ 100/length^3 (cm) (10,69–72). For calculation of fetal ponderal index, the length used may be the femur length (73). All variations on ponderal index use the length to the third power.

Prader beads   A series of standardized ellipsoid models used to estimate testicular volume.

Sitting height   Distance from the top of the head to the buttocks when in sitting position.

Skin-fold thickness   Thickness of skin in designated area (triceps, subscapular, suprailiac), used to assess subcutaneous fat and nutrition.

Skull height (forehead height)   Distance from the root of the nose (nasion) to the highest point of the head (vertex).

Span   Distance between the tips of the middle fingers of each hand when the arms are stretched out horizontally from the body.

Sternal length   Length of the sternum from the top of the manubrium to the inferior border of the xiphisternum.

Testicular volume   Volume of the testis established by an orchidometer, or calculated from measurement or ultrasound.

Thoracic index   Ratio of the anteroposterior diameter of the chest to the lateral diameter (chest width) multiplied by 100. The ratio approaches 1 in term neonates (47).

Torso length   Distance from the top of the sternum to the symphysis pubis.

Umbilical cord length   Length of the umbilical cord from the insertion at the placenta to the abdominal wall of the neonate.

Upper segment   Distance from the top of the head to the pubic bone.

Upper-to-lower segment ratio   Upper segment/lower segment = (crown heel length $-$ lower segment)/lower segment.

Weight velocity   The rate of weight gain or loss over a period of time representing the slope of weight curve. The intrauterine and postnatal weight velocity is greater than at any other time. Immediately after birth the normal weight loss is maximal by the third day and normally equals 7% of birth weight. Greater than 10% is considered excessive in term infants (74,75).

Weight/length ratio   The ratio obtained by dividing the metric weight by the length. It will be abnormally low in infants with low total body fat and high in obese infants (76)

References
1. AAP Committee on Fetus and Newborn and ACOG Committee on Obstetrics: Maternal and Fetal Medicine. *Guidelines for perinatal care.* 3rd ed. Elk Grove Village, IL, and Washington, DC: American Academy of Pediatrics and American College of Obstetricians and Gynecologists; 1992.
2. Wilcox AJ, Russell IT. Birthweight and perinatal mortality: II. On weight-specific mortality. *Int J Epidemiol* 1983;12:319–325.
3. Tyson JE, Kennedy K, Broyles S, Rosenfeld CR. The small for gestational age infant: accelerated or delayed pulmonary maturation? Increased or decreased survival? *Pediatrics* 1995;95:534–538.
4. Kramer MS, Olivier M, McLean FH, Willis DM, Usher RH. Impact of intrauterine growth retardation and body proportionality on fetal and neonatal outcome. *Pediatrics* 1990;86:707–713.
5. Ballard JL, Rosenn B, Khoury JC, Miodovnik M. Diabetic fetal macrosomia: significance of disproportionate growth. *J Pediatr* 1993;122:115–119.
6. McLean F, Usher R. Measurements of liveborn fetal malnutrition infants compared with similar gestation and with similar birth weight normal controls. *Biol Neonate* 1970;16:215–221.
7. Metcoff J. Clinical assessment of nutritional status at birth. *Pediatr Clin North Am* 1994;41:875–891.
8. Pereira G, Georgieff MK. Nutritional Assessment. In: Polin RA, Fox WW, eds. *Fetal and neonatal physiology.* 1st ed. Vol. 1. Philadelphia: WB Saunders; 1992:277–285.
9. Walther FJ, Ramaekers LH. The ponderal index as a measure of the nutritional status at birth and its relation to some aspects of neonatal morbidity. *J Perinatol Med* 1982;10:42–47.

10. Fay RA, Dey PL, Saadie CM, Buhl JA, Gebski VJ. Ponderal index: a better definition of the "at risk" group with intrauterine growth problems than birth-weight for gestational age in term infants. *Aust N Z J Obstet Gynaecol* 1991;31:17–19.

11. Demarini S, Pickens WL, Hoath SB. Changes in static and dynamic skin fold measurements in the first 60 hours of life: higher values following cesarean delivery. *Biol Neonate* 1993;64:209–214.

12. Golebiowska M, Ligenza I, Kobierska I, et al. [Use of mid-arm and head circumference to estimate gestational age and nutritional status of newborns]. *Ginekol Pol* 1992;63:221–226.

13. Cordes I, Roland EH, Lupton BA, Hill A. Early prediction of the development of microcephaly after hypoxic-ischemic encephalopathy in the full-term newborn. *Pediatrics* 1994;93:703–707.

14. Palmer CG, Cronk C, Pueschel SM, et al. Head circumference of children with Down syndrome (0–36 months). *Am J Med Genet* 1992;42:61–67.

15. Gruenwald P. Growth of the human fetus. II. Abnormal growth in twins and infants of mothers with diabetes, hypertension, or isoimmunization. *Am J Obstet Gynecol* 1966;94:1120–1132.

16. Secher NJ, Kaern J, Hansen PK. Intrauterine growth in twin pregnancies: prediction of fetal growth retardation. *Obstet Gynecol* 1985;66:63–68.

17. Arbuckle TE, Sherman GJ. An analysis of birth weight by gestational age in Canada. *Can Med Assoc J* 1989;140:157–160,165.

18. Lubchenco LO, Hansman C, Boyd E. Intrauterine growth in length and head circumference as estimated from live births at gestational ages from 26 to 42 weeks. *Pediatrics* 1966;37:403–408.

19. Usher R, McLean F. Intrauterine growth of live-born Caucasian infants at sea level: standards obtained from measurements in 7 dimensions of infants born between 25 and 44 weeks of gestation. *J Pediatr* 1969;74:901–910.

20. Nellhaus G. Head circumference from birth to eighteen years. Practical composite international and interracial graphs. *Pediatrics* 1968;41:106–114.

21. Gruenwald P. Growth of the human fetus. I. Normal growth and its variation. *Am J Obstet Gynecol* 1966;94:1112–1119.

22. Babson SG, Behrman RE, Lessel R. Fetal growth. Liveborn birth weights for gestational age of white middle class infants. *Pediatrics* 1970;45:937–944.

23. Britton JR, Britton HL, Jennett R, Gaines J, Daily WJ. Weight, length, head and chest circumference at birth in Phoenix, Arizona. *J Reprod Med* 1993;38:215–222.

24. Wilcox MA, Johnson IR, Maynard PV, Smith SJ, Chilvers CE. The individualised birthweight ratio: a more logical outcome measure of pregnancy than birthweight alone. *Br J Obstet Gynaecol* 1993;100:342–347.

25. Weaver DD, Chritian JC. Familial variation of head size and adjustment for parental head circumference. *J Pediatr* 1980;96:990–994.

26. Sivan Y, Merlob P, Reisner SH. Upper limb standards in newborns. *Am J Dis Child* 1983;137:829–832.

27. Merlob P, Sivan Y, Reisner SH. Lower limb standard in newborns. *Am J Dis Child* 1984;138:140–142.

28. Williams J, Hirsch NJ, Corbet AJ, Rudolph AJ. Postnatal head shrinkage in small infants. *Pediatrics* 1977;59:619–622.

29. Hall JG, Froster-Iskenius UG, Allanson JE. *Handbook of normal physical measurements.* Oxford: Oxford University Press; 1989.

30. Hurgoiu V, Mihetiu M. The skinfold thickness in preterm infants. *Early Hum Dev* 1993;33:177–181.

31. Schluter K, Funfack W, Weber B. Longitudinal studies on changes of skinfold diameters during infancy. In: Laron Z, Dickerson Z, eds. *The adipose child.* Basel, Switzerland: Karger; 1976:70–77.

32. Copper RL, Goldenberg RL, Cliver SP, DuBard MB, Hoffman HJ, Davis RO. Anthropometric assessment of body size differences of full-term male and female infants. *Obstet Gynecol* 1993;81:161–164.

33. Peters J, Ulijaszek SJ. Population and sex differences in arm circumference and skinfold thicknesses among Indo-Pakistani children living in the East Midlands of Britain. *Ann Hum Biol* 1992;19:17–22.

34. Verma M, Singh D, Chhatwal J, Jayaharan S. Measurement of neonatal skinfold thickness—is it of any clinical relevance? *Ind Pediatr* 1991;28:1291–1297.

35. Swain S, Bhatia BD, Pandey S, Pandey LK, Agrawal A. Birthweight: its relationship with maternal and newborn skinfold thickness. *Ind Pediatr* 1991;28:259–264.

36. Sheng HP, Muthappa PB, Wong WW, Schanler RJ. Pitfalls of body fat assessments in premature infants by anthropometry. *Biol Neonate* 1993;64:279–286.

37. Sumners JE, Findley GM, Ferguson KA. Evaluation methods for intrauterine growth using neonatal fat stores instead of birth weight as outcome measures: fetal and neonatal measurements correlated with neonatal skinfold thicknesses. *J Clin Ultrasound* 1990;18:9–14.

38. Bray PF, Shields WD, Wolcott GJ, Madsen JA. Occipitofrontal head circumference—an accurate measure of intracranial volume. *J Pediatr* 1969;75:303–305.

39. Bhushan V, Paneth N. The reliability of neonatal head circumference measurement. *J Clin Epidemiol* 1991;44:1027–1035.

40. Gross SJ, Eckerman CO. Normative early head growth in very-low-birth-weight infants. *J Pediatr* 1983;103:946–949.

41. Guo S, Roche AF, Moore WM. Reference data for head circumference and 1-month increments from 1 to 12 months of age. *J Pediatr* 1988;113:490–494.

42. Illingworth RS, Eid EE. The head circumference in infants and other measurements to which it may be related. *Acta Paediatr Scand* 1971;60:333–337.

43. Popich GA, Smith DW. Fontanels: range of normal size. *J Pediatr* 1972;80:749–752.

44. Davies DP, Ansari BM, Cooke TJH. Anterior fontanelle size in the neonate. *Arch Dis Child* 1975;50:81–83.

45. Duc G, Largo RH. Anterior fontanel: size and closure in term and preterm infants. *Pediatrics* 1986;78:904–908.

46. Faix RG. Fontanelle size in black and white term newborn infants. *J Pediatr* 1982;100:304–306.

47. Feingold M, Bossert WH. Normal values for selected physical parameters: an aid to syndrome delineation. *Birth Defects* 1974;10:1–16.

48. Merlob P, Sivan Y, Reisner SH. Anthropomorphic measurements of the newborn infant. In: Paul NW, ed.

Birth defects. Original article series. Vol. 20. White Plains, NY: March of Dimes Birth Defects Foundation, 1984.

49. Jones KL, Hanson JW, Smith DW. Palpebral fissure size in newborn infants. *J Pediatr* 1978;92:787–788.
50. Thomas IT. Palpebral fissure length from 29 weeks gestation to 14 years. *J Pediatr* 1987;111:267–268.
51. Sivan Y, Merlob P, Reisner SH. Sternum length, torso length, and internipple distance in newborn infants. *Pediatrics* 1983;72:523–525.
52. Hassan A, Karna P, Dolanski EA. Intermamillary indices in premature infants. *Am J Perinatol* 1988;5:54–56.
53. Callegari C, Everett S, Ross M, Brasel JA. Anogenital ratio: measure of fetal virilization in premature and full-term newborn infants. *J Pediatr* 1987;111:240–243.
54. Flatau E, Josefsberg Z, Reisner SH, Bialik O, Laron Z. Penile size in the newborn infant. *J Pediatr* 1975;87: 663–664.
55. Lee PA, Mazur T, Danish R, et al. Micropenis. I. Criteria, etiologies and classification. *Johns Hopkins Med J* 1980;146:156–163.
56. Bergeson PS, Hopkin RJ, Bailey RB, McGill LC, Piatt JP. The inconspicuous penis. *Pediatrics* 1993;92: 794–799.
57. Cassoria FG, Golden SM, Johnsonbaugh RE, Heroman WM, Lariaux L, Sherins RJ. Testicular volume during early infancy. *J Pediatr* 1981;99:742–743.
58. Ball TM, Pust RE. Arm circumference v. arm circumference/head circumference ratio in the assessment of malnutrition in rural Malawian children. *J Trop Pediatr* 1993;39:298–303.
59. Chang TC, Robson SC, Spencer JA. Neonatal morphometric indices of fetal growth: analysis of observer variability. *Early Hum Dev* 1993;35:37–43.
60. Georgieff MK, Sasanow SR, Chockalingam UM, Pereira GR. A comparison of the mid-arm circumference/head circumference ratio and ponderal index for the evaluation of newborn infants after abnormal intrauterine growth. *Acta Paediatr Scand* 1988;77:214–219.
61. Crouse DR, Cassady G. The small-for-gestational-age infant. In: Avery GB, Fletcher MA, MacDonald MG, eds. *Neonatology. Pathophysiology and management of the newborn.* 4th ed. Vol. 1. Philadelphia: JB Lippincott; 1994:369–398.
62. Yip R, Li A, Chong W-H. Race and birth weight: the Chinese example. *Pediatrics* 1991;87:688–689.
63. Feingold M. Congenital malformations. In: Avery GB, Fletcher MA, MacDonald MG, eds. *Neonatology: pathophysiology and management of the newborn.* 4th ed. Philadelphia: JB Lippincott; 1994:744–763.
64. James DK, Dryburgh EH, Chiswick ML. Footlength: a new and potentially useful measurement in the neonate. *Arch Dis Child* 1979;54:226–230.
65. Sanderson DA, Wilcox MA, Johnson IR. The individualised birthweight ratio: a new method of identifying intrauterine growth retardation. *Br J Obstet Gynaecol* 1994;101:310–314.
66. Sanderson DA, Wilcox MA, Johnson IR. Relative macrosomia identified by the individualised birthweight ratio (IBR). A better method of identifying the at risk fetus. *Acta Obstet Gynecol Scand* 1994;73:246–249.
67. Michaelsen KF, Skov L, Badsberg JH, Jorgensen M. Short-term measurement of linear growth in preterm infants: validation of a hand-held knemometer. *Pediatr Res* 1991;30:464–468.
68. Snyder RG, Spencer ML, Owings CL, Schneider LW. Hand measurements. In: Roche AF, Malina RM, eds. *Manual of physical status and perforance in childhood.* New York: Plenum; 1975.
69. Rohrer F. Eine neue formel fur bestimmung der korperfulle. *Gesellschaft Anthrophol* 1908;39(Korr.-B1):5.
70. Khoury MJ, Berg CJ, Calle EE. The ponderal index in term newborn siblings. *Am J Epidemiol* 1990;132: 576—583.
71. Colley NV, Tremble JM, Henson GL, Cole TJ. Head circumference/abdominal circumference ratio, ponderal index and fetal malnutrition. Should head circumference/abdominal circumference ratio be abandoned? *Br J Obstet Gynaecol* 1991;98:524–527.
72. Guaschino S, Spinillo A, Stola E, Pesando PC, Gancia GP, Rondini G. The significance of ponderal index as a prognostic factor in a low-birth-weight population. *Biol Res Pregnancy Perinatol* 1986;7:121–127.
73. Yagel S, Zacut D, Igelstein S, Palti Z, Hurwitz A, Rosenn B. In utero ponderal index as a prognostic factor in the evaluation of intrauterine growth retardation. *Am J Obstet Gynecol* 1987;157:415–419.
74. Brandt I. Growth dynamics of low-birth-weight infants with emphasis on the prenatal period. In: Falkner F, Tanner JM, eds. *Human growth. A comprehensive treatise.* Vol. I. New York: Plenum; 1986:415–475.
75. Guihard-Costa AM, Larroche JC. Growth velocity of some fetal parameters. II. Body weight, body length and head circumference. *Biol Neonate* 1992;62:317–324.
76. Yau KI, Chang MH. Weight to length ratio—a good parameter for determining nutritional status in preterm and full-term newborns. *Acta Paediatr* 1993;82:427–429.
77. Goldenberg. RL, Cliver SP, Cutter GR, Hoffman HJ, Cassady G, Davis RO, Nelson KG. Black–white differences in newborn anthropometric measurements. *Obstet Gynecol* 1991;78:785.
78. Merlob P, Sivan Y, Reisner SH. Ratio of crown–rump distance to total length in preterm and term infants. *J Med Genet* 1986;23:339.

3

Assessment of Gestational Age

INDICATIONS FOR CLASSIFICATION BY GESTATIONAL AGE

All infants should be classified by both gestational age and birth weight for standard reporting of reproductive health statistics (1). Estimation of gestational age by physical examination is possible because there is a predictable pattern in physical changes throughout gestation. Assessment of gestational age is part of all first neonatal examinations, but the detail of information needed depends on the clinical situation. The first and most common reason to assess gestational age is simply to verify the term status for that infant after a routine gestation with known obstetric dates. This verification of maturity can provide some assurance that there is decreased risk for problems that are more likely to develop with either prematurity or postmaturity. A second reason for establishing a gestational age exists if there has been no prenatal care, there is a discrepancy in weight for presumed gestational age, or the dates and the screening examination do not agree. Estimating gestational age as closely as possible is important so that interpretation of physical findings, diagnostic procedures, and therapy can be appropriately aided based on the determination. A third need for assessing maturation is to follow progression of the development of an infant as part of routine or high-risk follow-up care.

Definition of Preterm, Term, Postterm, and Corrected Gestational Age

Assessment of gestational age includes assigning a group designation based on obstetric dates of term, preterm, or postterm. Obstetric dating is based on weeks since the last menstrual period with an average cycle length of 28 days (Fig. 1). A term infant is any infant whose birth occurs from the beginning of the first day of week 37 through the end of the last day of week 42 after the onset of the last menstrual period (i.e., 260–294 days' gestation) (Fig. 1). A preterm infant is one born before the end of the last day of the 37th week (i.e., before 259 days), and a postterm infant is one whose birth occurs from the beginning of the first day of the 43rd week (i.e., after 294 days). Classifying infants born at term, preterm, or postterm helps to establish the level of risk for neonatal morbidity and long-term developmental problems. Further definition of gestational age

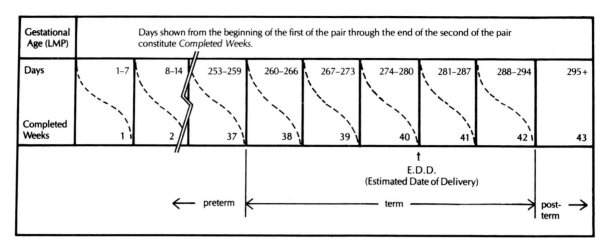

Gestational Age (LMP)	Days shown from the beginning of the first of the pair through the end of the second of the pair constitute *Completed Weeks.*							
Days	1–7	8–14	253–259	260–266	267–273	274–280	281–287	288–294	295+
Completed Weeks	1	2	37	38	39	40	41	42	43

E.D.D.
(Estimated Date of Delivery)

← preterm   ←————————— term —————————→   post-term →

Figure 1. Definition of gestational age. Reprinted with permission (1).

means to assign as closely as possible the estimated weeks in prematurity. Corrected gestational age is the adjustment in chronologic age taken to account for prematurity and applied generally until 2 years of age. By convention, the corrected gestational age is chronologic age less (40 minus the number of weeks of gestation) so that an infant born during the 28th week of gestation, who is now 12 months old would be $52 - (40 - 28) = 9$ months corrected gestational age. Corrected gestational age and corrected conceptional age are not synonymous because a conceptional age would be approximately 2 weeks less than one based on the standard definition of gestational age, which uses last menstrual period as week zero. Strictly speaking, conceptional age would be a more precise dating for embryologic and fetal development given the variability of menstrual cycles, but the true date of conception is not often known, so a corrected conceptional age is no more accurate.

Confirmation of Term Status

In the most common clinical situation of confirming a term status, the assessment is brief when certain physical attributes characteristic after term gestation are found: true plantar creases over at least two-thirds of the foot, stiff ear cartilage, full areola with a breast bud of 5 to 10 mm, and a resting posture of full flexion. The four external characteristics of skin color, texture, ear firmness, and breast development suggested by Parkin are sufficient and rapid for normal term pregnancies (2). When the need is for more specific estimation, as in the last two clinical situations, or when the basic external characteristics suggest a discrepancy in dates, the examination should be as accurate as possible. To that end there needs to be an understanding of how to do the evaluation as well as what individual factors might influence the findings and which findings are likely to be most reliable even in the presence of illness.

METHODS FOR ASSESSING GESTATIONAL AGE

There have been a variety of methods devised for assessing gestational age in the newly born infant. These systems range in complexity from simple visualization of as few as four physical findings to a more highly technical and cumbersome assessment of nerve conduction velocities. When put to careful study of reproducibility and accuracy, using either known dates of conception or early ultrasound dating, no examination on the infant is com-

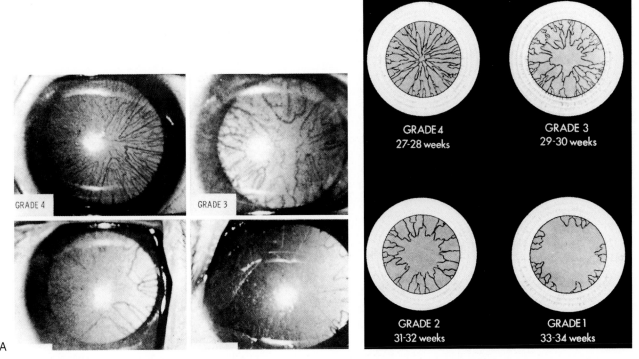

Figure 2. Assessment of maturity by examination of anterior vascular capsule of the lens. Reprinted from Hittner et al. (6) with permission.

pletely accurate with at least 2-week variances in many of the tested systems. This should not be surprising because not only do infants differ, but each gestation also has factors that can impact on fetal maturation and physical examination. Additionally, a number of the earlier studies were conducted on relatively small numbers of racially homogeneous patients and no patients at less than 28 weeks gestation. The gestational age was based on last menstrual period, and it is likely that infants were included who were small for gestational age. **A list of the systems for determining gestational age of an infant is provided, and reference citations reflect the studies that are mentioned most frequently in textbooks or other studies:**

Neurologic characteristics
Robinson. Five neurologic findings: pupillary reflex, glabellar tap, neck-righting reflex, arm traction, head turning to light (3)
Amiel-Tison. Neck-righting reflex, arm traction, scarf sign, square window, ankle flexion, heel to ear (4)
Physical characteristics
Farr. Twelve external characteristics (5)
Hittner eye examination. Anterior vascular capsule of lens (6) (Fig. 2)
Parkin. Four external characteristics: skin color, skin texture, ear firmness, breast development (2)
Narayan. Eye plus three external characteristics: anterior vascular capsule of the lens, plantar creases, ear firmness, and breast nodule (7)
Eregie. Anthropomorphic measurements: relationship of circumference of arm and head (8)
Combination of physical and neurologic characteristics
Dubowitz Score (9). Ten neurologic characteristics from Robinson, Amiel-Tison, and

Konigsberger and 11 external characteristics of Farr (eliminated skull firmness) (3–5,10)

Ballard Maturational Score (revised Dubowitz). Six neurologic and six external characteristics from original Dubowitz: posture, square window, arm recoil, popliteal angle, scarf sign, heel to ear, skin appearance, lanugo, plantar creases, breast development, eyelids/ear firmness, appearance of genitalia (11)

New Ballard Score. Same number of characteristics but with scores for extremely immature and postmature characteristics (12) (Fig. 3)

Capurro Score. Four external and two neurologic signs: skin texture, ear form, nipple formation, breast size, plantar creases, scarf sign, head lag (13)

Laboratory assessment

Alpha-fetoprotein and albumen (14)

Fetal hemoglobin level (15)

Nerve conduction velocity (16–18)

Radiologic examination of ossification centers (19)

Assessment Techniques

The scoring systems that have been studied and reported the most extensively are those devised by Dubowitz and Ballard (4,9,11,20). Compared with reliable ultrasound dates, the earlier Ballard system tended to overestimate the age of premature infants and underestimate the age of postterm infants (21,22). It was particularly inaccurate in very low birth weight infants with a deviation of over 2 weeks (23). However great the inaccuracies, many

Neuromuscular Maturity

	-1	0	1	2	3	4	5
Posture							
Square Window (wrist)	>90°	90°	60°	45°	30°	0°	
Arm Recoil		180°	140°–180°	110°–140°	90°–110°	<90°	
Popliteal Angle	180°	160°	140°	120°	100°	90°	<90°
Scarf Sign							
Heel to Ear							

Physical Maturity

Skin	sticky friable transparent	gelatinous red, translucent	smooth pink, visible veins	superficial peeling &/or rash, few veins	cracking pale areas rare veins	parchment deep cracking no vessels	leathery cracked wrinkled
Lanugo	none	sparse	abundant	thinning	bald areas	mostly bald	
Plantar Surface	heel-toe 40-50 mm:-1 <40 mm:-2	>50mm no crease	faint red marks	anterior transverse crease only	creases ant. 2/3	creases over entire sole	
Breast	imperceptible	barely perceptible	flat areola no bud	stippled areola 1-2mm bud	raised areola 3-4mm bud	full areola 5-10mm bud	
Eye/Ear	lids fused loosely:-1 tightly:-2	lids open pinna flat stays folded	sl. curved pinna; soft; slow recoil	well-curved pinna; soft but ready recoil	formed &firm instant recoil	thick cartilage ear stiff	
Genitals male	scrotum flat, smooth	scrotum empty faint rugae	testes in upper canal rare rugae	testes descending few rugae	testes down good rugae	testes pendulous deep rugae	
Genitals female	clitoris prominent labia flat	prominent clitoris small labia minora	prominent clitoris enlarging minora	majora & minora equally prominent	majora large minora small	majora cover clitoris & minora	

Maturity Rating

score	weeks
-10	20
-5	22
0	24
5	26
10	28
15	30
20	32
25	34
30	36
35	38
40	40
45	42
50	44

Figure 3. New Ballard score sheet for assessment of gestational age. Reprinted from Ballard et al. (12) with permission.

studies on developmental outcome were based on either the Dubowitz or original Ballard maturational assessments.

Further modifications of the original Ballard score and comparison with dates by ultrasonography produced the New Ballard Score (NBS), which extended the range and accuracy of age assessment to within 1 week, diminishing many of the earlier problems (12) (Fig. 3). Precision requires experience and consideration of the infant's history and condition in scoring. Examination as soon as possible after initial stabilization or by 12 hours increases the accuracy in gestations of less than 28 weeks. The use of the NBS is particularly attractive for infants who are both very immature and instrumented because it does not require lifting the infant. Although described separately from other components of the examination, the steps for assessing gestational age are done as part of the general physical examination (Figs. 4–12 and Table 1).

Influences on Age Assessment Results

If there is a discrepancy between expected and achieved scores, factors that influence the demonstrated findings should be sought before assigning gestational age. Included in the factors that determine the score is timing of the examination after birth and conditions that influence joint mobility and active and passive tone. Important is the unpredictable factor of experience in the observer and interpretation of findings. There is variation even when two experienced and independent observers examine the same infant. At best, assessment of gestational age is a confirmation of dates if the obstetric dating is secure. When the assessment and these dates do not agree, the discrepancy can help suggest historical factors or pathologic conditions that would not otherwise be considered. The dating by the examination may not be more accurate than the obstetric dating by ultrasound or known specific dates of conception, but it still will provide important information toward the physical diagnosis.

Table 1. *Technique and interpretation of New Ballard Score*

Item	Technique	Maturation progression	Factors affecting finding
Neuromuscular maturity: Resting posture	Observe infant in unrestrained position on his back and estimate the degree of flexion or extension of the extremities.	Increase in flexion, arms before legs	
Square window (Fig. 4)	Flex the wrist and measure the minimum angle between the hypothenar eminence and the ventral surface of the forearm.	Decrease in angle	
Arm recoil (Fig. 5)	With the infant supine and head midline, first flex the elbow and hold the arm against the forearm for 5 seconds. Then fully extend the elbow and release. Note the time it takes for the infant to resume a flexed posture.	Increase in angle and rapidity of recoil	
Popliteal angle (Fig. 6)	Flex the hips with the thighs held in knee chest position on the abdomen. Without lifting the hips from the bed surface, extend the knee as far as possible. Estimate the popliteal angle.	Decrease in angle	

continued

Table 1. *Continued.*

Item	Technique	Maturation progression	Factors affecting finding
Scarf sign (Fig. 7)	Pull the hand across the chest to encircle the neck as a scarf; observe the position of the elbow in relationship to the midline. Keep the head in midline.	Increase in resistance to crossing midline.	
Heel to ear (Fig. 8)	Press the feet as far as possible toward the head while keeping the pelvis on the table. The knees may be positioned alongside the abdomen. Measure the angle made by an arc from the back of the heel to the table.	Decrease in angle	
Physical maturity: Skin texture	Look for translucency of skin over the abdominal wall.	The skin gets thicker, more keratinized, and opaque with cracking and dryness. Increase of pigmentation progresses.	Hours after birth: skin becomes dryer. Pigmentation increases under effect of phototherapy or sunlight.
Lanugo	Assess presence and length of hair over the back. (It helps to shine a light over the area.)	Lanugo first emerges at 19 to 20 weeks but is not readily apparent for a few weeks. At its peak, it covers all the back and then disappears in areas of baldness from the lower back first and then from at least one-half of the back.	The pigmentation and quantity of body hair correlate to race, sex, and nutritional status.
Plantar surface (Fig. 9)	Measure foot length. Determine presence and distribution of deep creases, not wrinkles.	Foot length correlates with fetal growth in early gestation. Creases develop from the toes toward the heel.	Intrauterine fetal activity: increase in creasing with constriction; decrease in creasing with lack of fetal activity. Suggested racial difference (26).
Breast (Fig. 10)	Assess color, stippling of areola. Estimate diameter of breast bud.	Increase in definition and stippling around areola with pigmentation appearing near term. Bud size increasing in response to maternal hormone and deposition of fat.	Decrease in breast tissue from poor intrauterine growth but no affect on areolar development.
Ear cartilage	Fold top of external ear down and observe vigor and recoil.	Increasing firmness and rapidity of recoil.	Compression decreases firmness. Absence or dysfunction of auricular muscles decreases firmness.
Eyelid opening	Evaluate unfusing of eyelids but without attempting to separate them.	Opening starts by 22 weeks and complete unfusing is evident by 28 weeks (27).	Decrease. In anophthalmia, may have a fused lid at term.
External genitalia, male (Fig. 11)	Feel for level of descent of testes into scrotum. Observe rugation and suspension of scrotum.	There is a fairly reliable timed descent in the third trimester of the testes through the canal into the scrotum.	Decrease in conditions associated with cryptordism. Edema decreases rugae.
External genitalia, female (Fig. 12)	Assess progression of growth of the minora and majora.	Labia minora increases in size before the majora, which eventually fully covers the minora and clitoris.	Decreased covering with poor nutrition. Increase in covering with edema, bruising. The clitoris assumes its full size relatively early in response to maternal androgens, so may appear hypertrophied in otherwise normal premature females.

Factors that Influence Neurologic Evaluation of Maturation

Fetal/neonatal conditions
Obesity
   Hydrops
   Infant of diabetic mother
Hydrops with massive chest wall edema
Intrauterine growth retardation
Presence of orthopedic anomalies
   Arthrogryposis
   Hip dislocation
   Amputation or phocomelia
Neuropathology affecting tone
   Postasphyxial depression
   State: deep sleep, coma
   Anomaly
Intrauterine compression
   Twin
   Oligohydramnios
Fetal or neonatal illness likely to be associated with hypotonia
   Congestive heart failure
   Severe anemia
   Hypoglycemia
   Marked hypoxia
   Marked acidosis
Genetic aberrations associated with tonal deviations: e.g., Trisomy 21
Restraining devices or arm boards
Race: acceleration seen in infants of color[a] (24)
Delivery conditions
Fetal presentation: frank breech
Birth injury
   Brachial plexus injury
   Fracture of clavicle, humerus, or femur
Route of delivery[b]
Maternal conditions
Maternal medications
   Chronic intrauterine sedation: narcoleptics, beta-blockers
   Magnesium sulfate for premature labor or hypertension
   Sedation for labor or delivery
Uterine malformation
Bicornuate, septate
Uterine tumor
   Myoma

---

[a] Other studies do not confirm this. Individual findings vary, but when both physical and neurologic factors are used there is little or no difference (26–28).

[b] Cesarean section decreases neurologic maturity score (25).

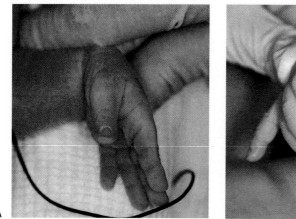
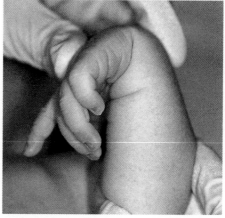

Figure 4. Comparison of square window tests. **A:** At 28 weeks the wrist would not flex beyond 90° (NBS score = 1). **B:** At 36 weeks the wrist flexed to 30° (NBS score = 3).

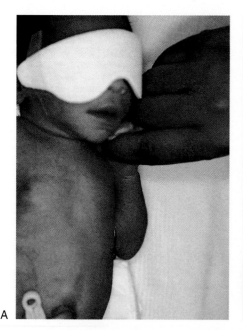
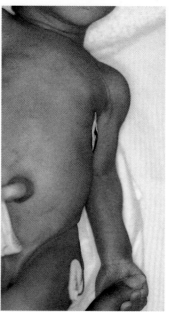
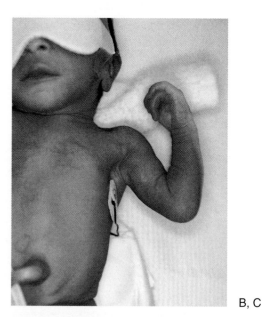

Figure 5. Testing arm recoil. **A:** Hold the forearms flexed against the arms for 5 seconds. **B:** Extend the elbow. **C:** Release the forearms and observe the recoil upon release (NBS score = 4).

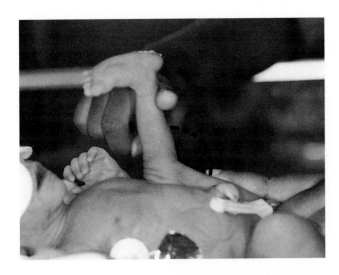

Figure 6. Measuring popliteal angle. Keeping the fully flexed hips on the bed surface with the thighs on the abdomen, extend the knee by gentle pressure at the ankle. Measure the angle from the back of the leg to the thigh (angle measures 130°; NBS score = 1—2).

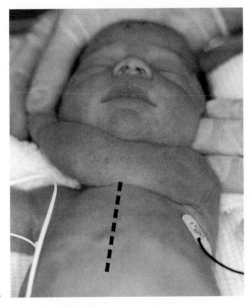

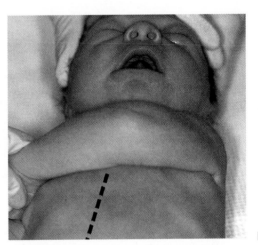

A   B

Figure 7. Comparison of scarf sign test. **A:** At 28 weeks the arm wraps to the border of the opposite chest wall (NBS score = 1). There is abundant lanugo apparent on the upper body, and the veins are easily seen over the abdomen (NBS score = 1 for lanugo, 1 for skin). **B:** At 36 weeks the arm wraps just to the midline (NBS score = 2). Note how the head is being kept in the midline.

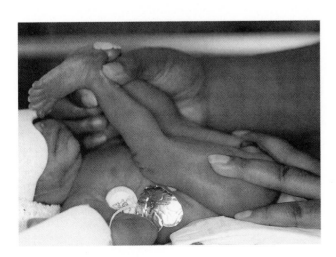

Figure 8. Heel to ear maneuver. The leg should be placed alongside the abdomen with the pelvis kept flat on the matress, and the distance judged as soon as possible. The longer the leg is held in position, the more likely there will be relaxation at the joint. (NBS score = 1).

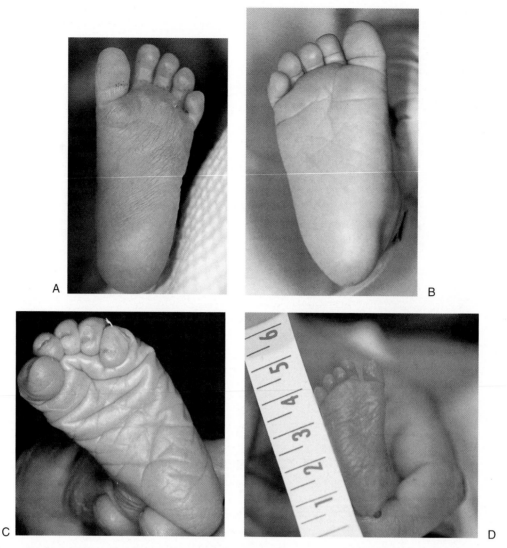

Figure 9. Comparison of sole creases. **A:** At 28 weeks there are wrinkles apparent over much of the foot, but true creases are only faint red marks (NBS score = 1). **B:** There is only anterior transverse creasing, although wrinkles are apparent to the ball of the foot (NBS score = 2). **C:** At 42 weeks the wrinkles are true creases on the entire sole (NBS score = 4 for creases, 5 for leathery skin). **D:** Measurement of this foot is 45 mm for an NBS score of −1. Note that the extent of wrinkles and true creases is not consistent, scoring a 2. This infant was extremely small for gestational age, so her foot measurements were discordant with her gestational age.

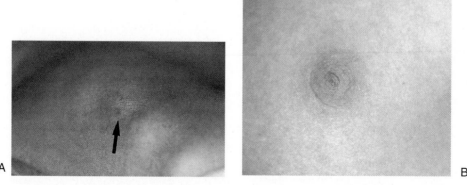

Figure 10. Comparison of breast formations. **A:** At 28 weeks the areola is flat with no bud (NBS score = 1). **B:** At 36 weeks the areola is well stippled, slightly raised, and the bud is 3 mm (NBS score = 3).

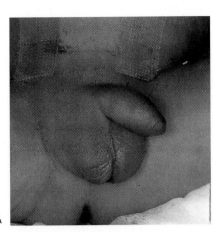
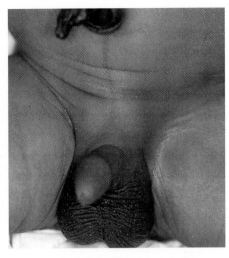

Figure 11. Comparison of mature and immature male genitalia. **A:** At 28 weeks the testes are still in the canal or high in the scrotum. There is begining formation of rugae (NBS score = 1). **B:** At term the testes are in a pendulous scrotum with well defined rugae. After 36 weeks in both male and female infants of color a line from the umbilicus to the genitalia starts to darken into a linea nigra in response to maternal hormones. The genitalia show pigmentation before 36 weeks (NBS score = 4).

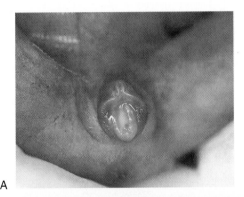
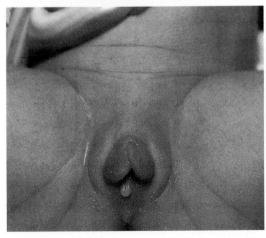
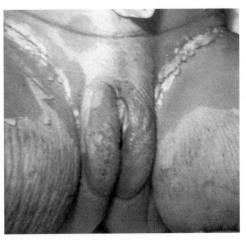

Figure 12. Comparison of mature and immature female genitalia. **A:** At 25 weeks the labia majora are flat and the minor prominent (NBS score = −1 for genitalia, 0 for skin.). **B:** At 28 weeks the labia minora are significantly more prominent than the majora and pigmentation is developing there first. A hymenal tag is evident (NBS score = 1 for genitalia, 1 for skin). **C:** At 42 weeks the skin is starting to wrinkle and peel, the vernix is coming off in dry plaques and is meconium stained. The labia majora cover the minora completely and there is pigmentation in the skin folds and linea nigra as well (NBS score = 4 for genitalia, 5 for skin).

References

1. AAP Committee on Fetus and Newborn and ACOG Committee on Obstetrics: Maternal and Fetal Medicine. *Guidelines for perinatal care.* 3rd ed. Elk Grove Village, IL, and Washington, DC: American Academy of Pediatrics and American College of Obstetricians and Gynecologists; 1992.
2. Parkin JM, Hey EN, Clowes JS. Rapid assessment of gestational age at birth. *Arch Dis Child* 1976;51: 259–263.
3. Robinson RJ. Assessment of gestational age by neurological examination. *Arch Dis Child* 1966;41:437.
4. Amiel-Tison C. Neurological evaluation of the maturity of newborn infants. *Arch Dis Child* 1968;43:89–93.
5. Farr V, Mitchell RG, Neligan GA, Parkin JM. The definition of some external charactristics used in the assessment of gestational age in the newborn infant. *Dev Med Child Neurol* 1966;8:507.
6. Hittner HM, Hirsch NJ, Rudolph AJ. Assessment of gestational age by examination of the anterior vascular capsule of the lens. *J Pediatr* 1977;91:455.
7. Narayanan I, Dua K, Gujral VV, Mehta DK, Mathew M, Prabhakar AK. A simple method of assessment of gestational age in newborn infants. *Pediatrics* 1982;69:27–32.
8. Eregie CO. Determination of maturity at birth: further observations on a maturity scoring system for head circumference and mid-arm circumference. *East Afr Med J* 1993;70:48–50.
9. Dubowitz LM, Dubowitz V, Goldberg C. Clinical assessment of gestational age in the newborn infant. *J Pediatr* 1970;77:1–10.
10. Koenigsberger MR. Judgment of fetal age. I. Neurologic evaluation. *Pediatr Clin North Am* 1966;13: 823–833.
11. Ballard JL, Kazmaier Novak K, Driver M. A simplified score for assessment of fetal maturation of newly born infants. *J Pediatr* 1979;95:769.
12. Ballard JL, Khoury JC, Wedig K, Wang L, Eilers-Walsman BL, Lipp R. New Ballard Score, expanded to include extremely premature infants. *J Pediatr* 1991;119:417–423.
13. Capurro H, Konichezky S, Fonseca D, Caldeyro-Barcia RA. A simplified method for diagnosis of gestational age in the newborn infant. *J Pediatr* 1978;93:120.
14. Finnstrom O, Karlsson B, Zetterlund B. Studies on maturity in newborn infants. VIII. Alpha-foetoprotein and albumin. *Acta Paediatr Scand* 1975;64:409–412.
15. Finnstrom O, Gothefors L, Zetterlund B. Studies on maturity in newborn infants. VII. Foetal haemoglobin. *Acta Paediatr Scand* 1975;64:404–408.
16. Finnstrom O. Studies on maturity in newborn infants. VI. Comparison between different methods for maturity estimation. *Acta Paediatr Scand* 1972;61:33–41.
17. Miller G, Heckmatt JZ, Dubowitz LMS, Dubowitz V. Use of nerve conduction velocity to determine gestational age in infants at risk and in very-low-birth-weight infants. *J Pediatr* 1983;103:109–112.
18. Blom S, Finnstrom O. Maturity estimation in newborn infants motor and sensory nerve conduction velocities. *Acta Paediatr Scand Suppl* 1970;206(Suppl):24.
19. Finnstrom O. Studies on maturity in newborn infants. IV. Postnatal radiological examination of epiphyseal centers. *Neuropadiatrie* 1971;3:119–128.
20. Saint-Anne Dargassies S. *Neurological development in the full-term and premature neonate.* 1st ed. Amsterdam: Elsevier; 1977.
21. Alexander GR, Hulsey TC, Smeriglio VL, Comfort M, Levkoff A. Factors influencing the relationship between a newborn assessment of gestational maturity and the gestational age interval. *Paediatr Perinatol Epidemiol* 1990;4:133–146.
22. Alexander GR, de Caunes F, Hulsey TC, Tompkins ME, Allen M. Validity of postnatal assessments of gestational age: a comparison of the method of Ballard et al. and early ultrasonography. *Am J Obstet Gynecol* 1992;166:891–895.
23. Sanders M, Allen M, Alexander GR, et al. Gestational age assessment in preterm neonates weighing less than 1500 grams. *Pediatrics* 1991;88:542–546.
24. Alexander GR, de Caunes F, Hulsey TC, Tompkins ME, Allen M. Ethnic variation in postnatal assessments of gestational age: a reappraisal. *Paediatr Perinatol Epidemiol* 1992;6:423–433.
25. Gagliardi L, Scimone F, DelPrete A, et al. Precision of gestational age assessment in the neonate. *Acta Paediatr* 1992;81:95–9.
26. Damoulaki-Sfakianaki E, Robertson A, Cordero L. Skin creases on the foot and the physical index of maturity: comparison between caucasian and negro infants. *Pediatrics* 1972;50:483–485.
27. Constantine NA, Kraemer HC, Kendall-Tackett KA, Bennett FC, Tyson JE, Gross RT. Use of physical and neurologic observations in assessment of gestational age in low birth weight infants. *J Pediatr* 1987;110: 921–928.
28. Stevens-Simon C, Cullinan J, Stinson S, McAnarney ER. Effects of race on the validity of clinical estimates of gestational age. *J Pediatr* 1989;115:1000–1002.

4

Gross Examination
of the Placenta

When a clinician is seeking a diagnosis in a newborn infant, he may ignore the placenta because gross placental examination is not a comfortable routine for many clinicians. Even when it is examined at delivery, there is generally very little documentation other than a cursory mention of the placenta as being intact and complete. In many clinical practices, unless one suspects that there might be something abnormal in the placenta, it is not routinely sent for pathologic evaluation. If the placenta is sent to pathology, a final report is certain to be more detailed and to include a microscopic examination but unlikely to be available until well after a healthy neonate is discharged or treatment decisions have been made for sick infants. Because helpful information is neither timely nor expected, there is little reliance on placental examination in most clinical management or diagnosis. Unfortunately, in many respects completely ignoring the placenta may be comparable with attempting a physical examination on the cardiovascular system by only listening to the precordium. Because the majority of maternal–fetal units have normal placentation, most of the time it is possible to make reasonable diagnoses and care plans without examining the placenta. However, if one is not in the habit of including it as part of a complete examination, it is too easy to forget about that source of information when it would be either helpful or diagnostic. For medicolegal reasons, having a written description as part of the medical record and maintaining section blocks or slides that can document normalcy and the absence of any evidence of microscopic or gross pathology may become part of the normal procedure (1–5). Many conditions that are apparent only some months after birth seem to come from normal pregnancies, so having information about each placenta available in retrospect is still potentially useful.

Clearly, the first examination of the placenta should be conducted in the delivery room. For the vast majority of normal pregnancies and healthy newborn infants, a general examination in the delivery room by someone knowledgeable in gross placental pathology is probably sufficient as long as there is documentation of the information. Unless the pediatrician is present at the delivery and remembers to look at it himself, he or she relies on the obstetric staff for information. Even when the pediatrician is present, the placenta will not be available until he or she is otherwise occupied in resuscitating the infant. Nonetheless,

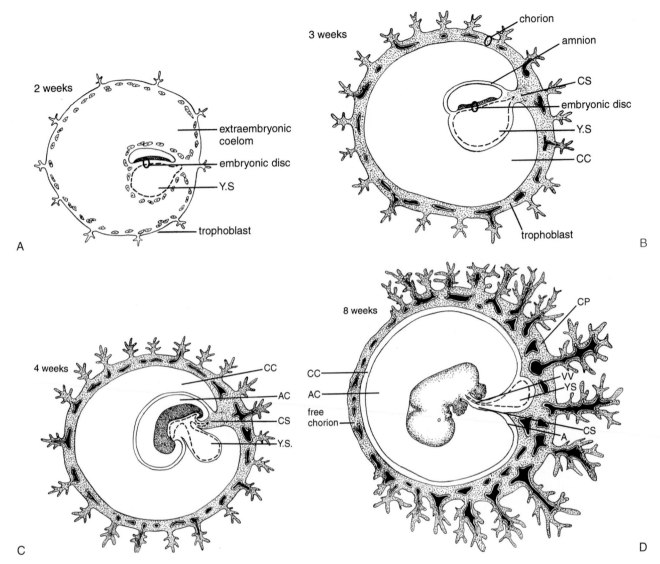

Figure 1. Schematic drawing depicting development of placenta, membranes, and cord from 3 weeks postconception to Eight weeks. **A:** Two weeks. **B:** Three weeks. **C:** Four weeks. **D:** Eight weeks. The amnionic cavity (AC) enlarges to fill the chorionic cavity (CC) and becomes tightly adherent by 12 weeks' gestation. Before that time, there remains a potential space between the membranes. As the amnion (A) enlarges, it encloses the vitelline vessels (VV), which connect the fetus to the yolk sac (YS), and the connecting stalk (CS), forming the umbilical cord (UC). The cord most often connects to the portion of the chorion (C) that forms the chorionic plate (CP). Initially, functioning chorionic villi completely cover the sphere of the conceptus, but then degenerate to form the free chorion. The remaining functioning villous tissue forms the placental disk (PD). (Drawing by Judy Guenther.)

situations requiring resuscitation usually are those for which the placenta is most likely to yield helpful information to guide that resuscitation and care plan. One example would be the resuscitation of a pale, hypotensive infant whose pale placenta clearly showed ruptured fetal vessels. A second would be the difficult resuscitation of an infant whose placenta shows amnion nodosum, a finding commonly associated with fatal pulmonary hypoplasia.

The examination described in this chapter is directed at giving the clinician helpful information to complement the rest of the physical examination. The findings described are both the most common and a few of the uncommon, but revealing, examples. The appropriate examination of the placenta by the clinician in the delivery suite should be brief but should include the cord, membranes, fetal surface, and maternal surface. In my experience, cutting into the placenta to look at the villous structure is only rarely helpful unless there are external signs, and then the cutting might best be done during a complete pathologic examination. Using a simple form for recording observations facilitates the examination. An example is included at the end of the chapter in the placenta gross examination worksheet (see Fig. 30).

If it is not routine to submit all placentas for examination, there are clinical situations in which gross and microscopic examination by a pathologist is likely to contribute important information (See Tables 6 and 7 on pages 99–101.).

Indications for placental microscopy are listed as follows (3):

Fetal–neonatal conditions
　　Stillbirth
　　Possible infection
　　Congenital anomalies
　　Multiple gestation
　　Preterm birth before 37 weeks
　　Postterm birth after 42 weeks
　　Intrauterine growth retardation
　　Small for gestational age
　　Large for gestational age
　　Anemia
　　Hydrops with and without anemia
　　Meconium staining
　　Fetal bradycardia or tachycardia
　　Admission to neonatal intensive care
　　Apgar score less than 3 at 5 minutes
　　Any infant requiring more than minimal resuscitation
Gross placental findings
　　Abnormal fetal/placental weight ratio
　　Single umbilical artery
　　Foul odor
　　Cloudy membranes
　　Unusual color
　　Retroplacental hemorrhages
　　Extensive infarction
　　Excessive fibrin deposition
　　Villous atrophy
　　Chorangioma
　　Any gross finding that is confusing
Maternal conditions
　　Oligohydramnios
　　Maternal disorders (hypertension, diabetes, drug abuse)
　　Possible infection
　　Poor reproductive history
　　Abruption placenta
　　Repetitive bleeding or spotting during pregnancy
　　Leaking membranes
　　Premature or prolonged rupture of membranes
　　Premature labor (even without premature delivery)

The embryology of the placenta and umbilical cord are illustrated in Figs. 1 and 2. The anatomy of the placenta is illustrated in Fig. 3.

retinal pigment   umbilical cord   amnion   amnionic membrane   chorion

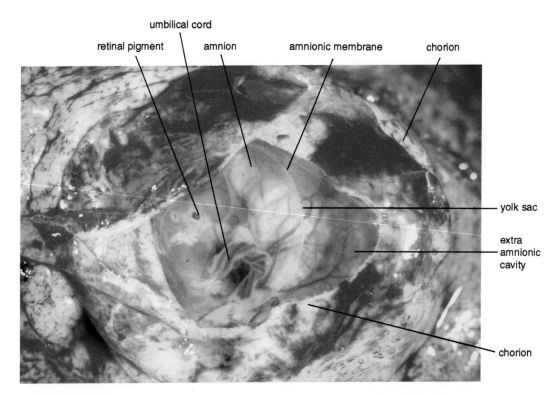

yolk sac

extra
amnionic
cavity

chorion

Figure 2. Eight-week postimplantation conceptus with space between the amnion (clear membrane) and chorion (opaque covering with remnants of villous tissue). The vitelline vessels leading from the yolk sac (arrow at 2 o'clock position) to the umbilical cord is evident at this early gestation. The space between the amnion and the chorion is filled with a gelatinous material that will disappear by 12 weeks of gestation. Note how relatively thick and opaque the chorionic membrane is in comparison to the amnion.

TECHNIQUE OF GROSS PLACENTAL EXAMINATION

Always wear gloves, observe universal precautions, and wash carefully after handling a placenta. Examine the placenta in the delivery suite in an area that is reserved for contaminated specimens.

Weighing the placenta has always been a standard part of the examination, but weights obtained on fresh specimens in the delivery room compared with those in the pathology laboratory differ enough to make delivery room weights not clinically useful. Similarly, weights of placentas preserved in formalin are greater than those refrigerated without preservative (6). Studies of placental weights in relation to gestational age or to fetal weights have been conducted by pathologists, so their techniques should be followed for comparisons. The range of sizes at gestational ages in the last part of pregnancy when pediatric clinicians are likely to become involved are presented in Table 1. If the placenta appears to fall well outside the expected weight range, pathologic examination should be conducted. Low placental weight has been associated with low maternal pregravid body weight, low pregnancy weight gain, high maternal hemoglobin levels during pregnancy, gestational hypertension, paid employment outside the home during pregnancy, and low parity (7). Causes for exceptionally large placentas of greater than 600 g at term are listed in Table 2.

What to look for in gross placental examination (5):
Length
Diameter
Color
Consistency
Vessel number (single artery)
True knots
Insertion (central, marginal, velamentous)
Any unusual markings or masses
Angioma, allantoic, and omphalomesenteric remnants

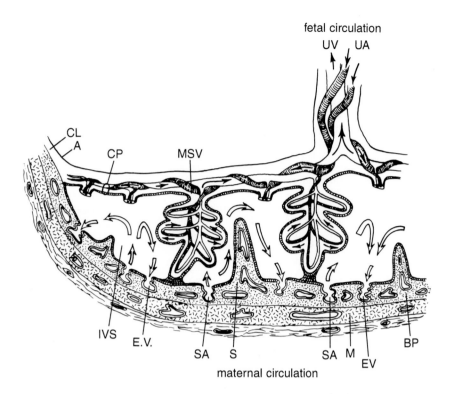

Figure 3. Schematic drawing of mature placenta to indicate the relationship of fetal parts of the placenta (villous chorion) to the maternal parts (decidua basalis) and the relationship between the two circulations. The blood flows from the fetus by way of the two umbilical arteries (UA), which split either just before or on the surface of the placenta into three to five branches each. Each fetal arteriole dives into a mainstem villous (MSV), where the blood can exchange with maternal blood that is flowing around the intervillous space (IVS) in a fountain directed toward the chorionic plate (CP). Blood returns to the fetus by way of a single umbilical vein (UV). The maternal blood enters the intevillous space (IVS) at the base of each mainstem villus through spiral arteries (SA) in the basal plate (BP) attached to the myometrium (M). The pressure from the arterial flow into the area pushes the maternal blood out of the villi into endometrial veins (EV) scattered throughout the basal plate. There are 10 to 40 cotyledons in normal placentation, separated by grooves that contain the placental septa (S), with each cotyledon containing two or more stem villi. The portion of the chorion in the free membrane is the chorion laeve (CL) internally lined by amnion (A). The solid arrows indicate the direction of fetal blood flow. The open arrows indicate the direction of maternal blood flow. Drawings by Judy Guenther.

Table 1. *Placental measurements latter half of gestation*

Gestational age (wk)	Thickness (mm)[a]	Diameter (mm)[a]	Placental weight (g)[b]	Fetoplacental ratio[b]
24	18	120	160 ± 5 (3)	3.7 ± 0.1
28	20	145	215 ± 25 (11)	5.3 ± 0.7
32	22	170	305 ± 20 (13)	5.4 ± 0.6
36	24	195	385 ± 10 (59)	6.9 ± 0.3
40	25	220	435 ± 5 (598)	7.7 ± 0.1
42			465 ± 10 (68)	7.4 ± 0.2

[a] Data from Kaufmann (90).

[b] Placentas were trimmed of cord, membranes, and excess blood. Weight was rounded to nearest 5 g; values are means ± SEM. Values in parentheses are number of cases. Fetoplacental ratio is of appropriate weight for gestational-aged infants using local (Denver, Colorado) criteria, rounded to nearest 0.1, mean ± 95% confidence limits. Data from Molteni et al. (89).

Table 2. *Causes of placentomegaly and placental hydrops*

Immune hemolytic anemia	Placental tumors (primary and metastatic)
Rhesus isoimmunization	Vena caval, portal, or umbilical vein
Fetal–maternal ABO blood group	obstruction
incompatibility	Sacrococcygeal teratoma (also
Kell Ag isoimmunization	intratumoral hemorrhage)
Nonimmune chronic fetal anemia	Diaphragmatic hernia
Intrauterine infection (syphilis,	Congenital cystic adenomatoid
toxoplasmosis, CMV, etc.)	malformation (type III)
Fetomaternal hemorrhage	Thrombosis
Hemoglobinopathy (alpha-thalassemia)	Congenital cirrhosis/hepatic fibrosis
Red cell membrane defect	Cystic kidneys/ovarian cysts
(spherocytosis)	Neuroblastoma
Red cell enzyme defect (glucose-6-	Miscellaneous fetal conditions
phosphate dehydrogenase deficiency)	Chromosomal errors/partial molar
Microangiopathic hemolytic anemia	change
(giant hemangioendothelioma)	Open neural tube defects
Twin transfusion syndrome	Beckwith-Wiedermann syndrome
Fetal cardiac failure	Osteochondrodystrophy
Premature closure of foramen ovale	Metabolic storage disease (Gaucher's
Endocardial fibroelastosis	sialidosis)
Myocarditis (Coxsackie virus B_3)	Small bowel volvulus
Hypoplastic left heart syndrome	Arterial calcification of infancy
Cardiac myxoma	Maternal factors
Large AV malformation	Diabetes mellitus (gestational; without
Intrauterine heart block (maternal SLE)	vasculopathy)
or tachyarrhythmia	Severe anemia
Fetal hypoproteinemia	Heavy cigarette smoking
Congenital nephrosis (Finnish type)	High altitude pregnancy
Renal vein thrombosis	Decompensated cyanotic heart disease
Congenital cirrhosis/hepatitis	
Noonan's syndrome (lymphangiectasia)	

Ag, antigen; AV, arteriovenous; CMV, cytomegalovirus; SLE, systemic lupus erythematosus.
From Heifetz, ref. 91, with permission.

Umbilical Cord

Measure the length and diameter of the cord including the portion attached to the fetus. Look for any irregularity of shape of the umbilical cord along its length. Feel the consistency of the cord, particularly in any area of unusual appearance or swelling. Determine the insertion site on the placenta and the continuity of the vessels and the supporting tissue. Look at the cut surface of the cord and count the vessels. Note any extravascular markings or abnormalities in the color or surface texture. Note the spiral direction of the vessels by holding the cord upright. Look for absent or excessive twisting.

Umbilical Cord Length

Throughout gestation the length of the cord should approximate the length of the fetus; the average length at term is about 60 cm when measured in the delivery room. Lengths longer than 86 cm or shorter than 35 cm are more than two standard deviations (2SD) from the means established by Naeye in the National Collaborative Perinatal Study of the National Institute of Neurologic and Communicative Disorders and Stroke (8). In another study, only 6% of cords were shorter than 40 cm at term (9). The cord increases in length throughout gestation but at a slowed rate in the last weeks of pregnancy (Fig. 4). Thirty-two centimeters is suggested as the minimum length of cord needed for vaginal delivery (10).

Umbilical cord length probably relates to fetal activity because pregnancies associated with decreased fetal movement before the last trimester have shorter cords. Miller et al. found short cords in infants for whom there was evidence of intrauterine constraint or of

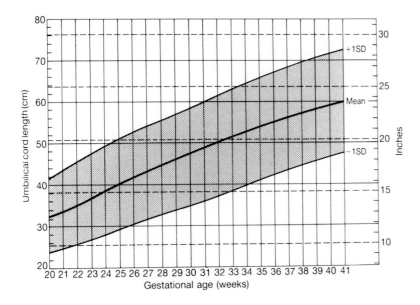

Figure 4. Length of the umbilical cord in relation to gestational age as measured in 35,779 placentas. Data from Naeye (8). Reprinted from Hall (88) with permission.

structural or functional defects that limited movement in early gestation. These patients included infants with intrauterine compression due to amnion rupture, oligohydramnios, or structural uterine anomalies, as well as infants with decreased limb movement because of amelia, acardia, arthrogryposis, or spinal muscular atrophy (11,12). The theory that constraint and fetal activity influence the umbilical length is confirmed in animal studies where oligohydramnios or induced paralysis with curare resulted in shorter cords (13). Analyzing a subset of the same patient population as Naeye, Moessinger reported shorter cords in infants with Down's syndrome as compared with normal infants with cords generally 1SD below the mean expected for gestational age (14). Short cords have also been noted after long-term maternal therapy with medication (atenolol) that is likely to decrease fetal movements (15). Further clinical confirmation of the relationship of fetal activity to umbilical cord length is found in the presence of shorter cords in association with breech presentation and twin gestations (16,17). Fetal sex also affects cord length, with boys having slightly longer cords than girls (9).

The extreme clinical example of a short cord is essentially complete absence of the umbilical cord (Fig. 5). This rare and fatal malformation represents failure of the caudal folding to form the body stalk so it includes absence of variable portions of the anterior abdominal wall and externalization of abdominal contents onto which the placenta is implanted (18–20).

Cords that are especially long are associated with several types of fetal injuries and physical findings when there is cord entanglement and strangulation. When the cord encircles the neck multiple times, not only is there difficulty with delivery and a potential for blood volume shifts away from the fetus, but there is also the potential for compression of the fetal neck vessels and trachea. Such compression may lead to intracranial hemorrhage or transient neonatal stridor. Most commonly, there will be a finding of plentiful petechiae immediately after birth but limited to the head and face and not associated with thrombocytopenia (see Chapter 5 Fig. 29). Tight entanglement of an extremity leads to a grooving and deformation of that extremity.

Umbilical Cord Knot

When the cord is long enough and the fetus is active in utero, there is ample opportunity for knots to form. They may be simple or complicated. Knots occur in 0.1% to 0.35% of deliveries and account for fetal mortality of around 10% (21,22). If a knot is of long standing, the curve in the cord tends to remain when the knot is untied (Fig. 6B). Knots are of no consequence unless there is extreme compression, tension, or both on the cord. Tightening

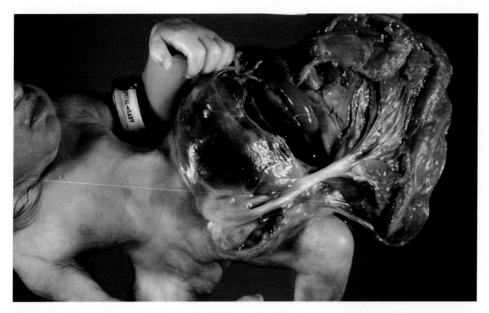

Figure 5. Failure of formation of umbilical cord. This lethal malformation reflects failure of the amnion to enclose the vitelline and body stalk vessels to form a normal umbilical cord. Placental tissue is implanted on abdominal organs. The body stalk defect includes absence of part of the abdominal wall and torsional deformation of the spine. This is one type of ADAM complex (18–20).

of a knot may occur only at the time of delivery as tension is put on the cord. If a knot is tight enough to cause a decrease in blood flow, there should be histologic evidence of venous stasis thrombosis. Grossly, there should be overdistension of the vein between the placenta and the knot (differential congestion), and there may be a proximal hematoma or leakage of blood into the surrounding cord tissue. When knots are found in stillbirths or infants with unexplained fetal stress, it is easy to assume the knot to be causative. In general, there must be correlating gross or histologic evidence of stasis before a knot can be blamed; approximately 90% of knots are not associated with fetal compromise.

Umbilical Coiling

Early in gestation the cord develops a spiral that is most often counterclockwise (Fig. 2). When viewed in profile, the direction of a counterclockwise twist will appear as the left arm

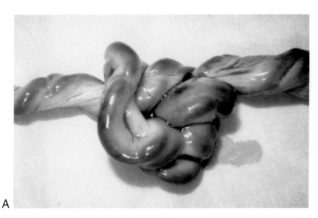

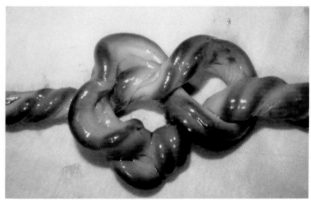

A   B

Figure 6. Umbilical knot. **A:** Complicated knot in umbilical cord. The amount of Wharton's jelly is decreased so there is not as much protection against vascular compression. Evidence of stasis thrombosis should be present before diagnosing obstruction to umbilical blood flow by a knot. **B:** The shape of the knot was maintained after loosening, indicating a tie of long standing. A false knot is visible at the bottom of the true knot and has no significance. The counterclockwise (left) twist of the cord is apparent.

of a V. Left twisting is seven times more common than right twisting but does not relate to handedness or other demonstrable factors (23). The same cord may have both left and right coiling along its course. Noncoiling occurs in 3.7% to 5% of pregnancies (23,24). The absence of spiraling is associated with increased fetal demise, anomalies, and twinning; there is a higher than normal incidence of no twist or right twist in cords with a single umbilical artery (23,24). Pregnancies associated with an abnormally low number of coils may have a higher incidence of fetal heart rate disturbances and interventional delivery, whereas those that have hypercoiled cords appear to involve a greater likelihood of premature delivery or maternal cocaine use (25).

Stricture or Torsion of the Cord

A short segment of the cord that is extremely narrowed, lacking Wharton's jelly and allowing vessel compression, is a cord stricture or coarctation. Exceptionally tight twisting of the cord in localized or diffuse areas of the cord is torsion. A stricture occurs most often at the fetal end of the cord and is generally associated with torsion and obliteration of the umbilical vessels. Both torsion and stricture can occur in isolation but are most commonly found together and so for clinical purposes may be considered part of the same phenomenon (2). Torsion without complete obstruction may cause cardiac failure and nonimmune hydrops (26). Stricture and torsion may develop only after fetal demise from another cause, so that in the absence of vascular changes that indicate obstruction, this may be a sequela of maceration rather than cause of the demise. If torsion is sufficient to impede blood flow, the blood vessels will dilate and develop edema and thrombosis. Stricture with fetal demise has been reported after amniocentesis, suggesting that loss of Wharton's jelly contributed to a coarctation of the umbilical vessels (27).

Umbilical Vessel Number

There are normally two arteries and one vein running the course of the umbilical cord, but there may be bridges between the arteries close to the placental surface and areas of merging and dividing along the course. The number of vessels should be determined by looking at a cut section of the cord closest to the fetal end or at the mid-point. If only two vessels are identified, look at other sections. If three vessels are not clearly discernible, a section of cord should be sent for microscopic evaluation. The arteries tend to have a smaller diameter and thicker wall than the vein but immediately after cutting may appear very similar. As the Wharton's jelly dries, the vein retracts but the arteries extend beyond the cut end. Remnants of the urachus or allantoic ducts may mimic a small artery but are identifiable on microscopic examination.

Single Umbilical Artery

Jones et al. found a single umbilical artery (SUA) in 0.2% of 17,777 singleton births, but the diagnosis was missed in 24% and 16% of cases by the obstetrician and pediatrician, respectively (28). In examining 35,000 placentas, Bourke found an SUA in 0.32% (29). The incidence of SUAs increases with multiple gestations, velamentous insertion, and spontaneous abortions, and was prevalent at autopsy in cases of infants with multiple anomalies (6). In spontaneous abortions the incidence has been reported to be at least twice as high as in other fetuses. In discordant twins it is almost always the smaller twin who has a single artery.

Infants with SUA have a higher incidence of poor intrauterine fetal growth, prematurity, associated congenital abnormalities, and perinatal mortality, even in the absence of prematurity or anomalies (30,31). Several studies have suggested that prenatal ultrasonography is sensitive enough to detect the presence of concurrent anomalies, making neonatal studies unnecessary (32,33). In the absence of other detectable anomalies, there is still an association with poor intrauterine growth and prematurity. Others suggest a strong correlation with renal defects (most of which can be detected on prenatal ultrasound), including absent kidney(s), pelvic kidney, and reflux. These investigators advocate renal ultrasonography on all cases of SUA (29,34). In Bourke's renal sonography study of 112 infants with an SUA, 7.1% had abnormal renal images, with vesicoureteric reflux in 4.5%. Other investigators have argued that there is not enough difference from the general incidence to warrant study in all infants in the absence of other findings (35). Anorectal and esophageal atresias are other common major malformations associated with renal anomalies (31). Most cases of SUA associated with cytogenetic abnormalities have other major malformations (36). There is no increased incidence of SUA with Down's syndrome without other major anomalies (37).

Funisitis

Also visible on cut section may be perivascular bands that resemble the zones of identity on Ouchterlony gel plates. These bands indicate funisitis and suggest the need for evaluation for intrauterine infection or other causes of fetal inflammatory reaction. If marked enough, the reaction is necrotizing funisitis (synonym *chronic funisitis, sclerosing funisitis*). This is an unusual but important finding because it indicates a prolonged inflammatory reaction. Perivascular white bands or arcs give a barber pole appearance to the umbilical cord because of exceptional prominence of the vessels. A white–yellow band may appear to parallel the vessels and become more prominent nearer the fetal surface. The cord feels exceptionally firm if the condition is of long enough duration or appears discolored, edematous, or fibrotic. On cross section, the area around each vessel has a visible white band of inflammatory debris that calcifies and may have neovascularization of the arterial walls or into the adjacent cord substance. The bands may circumscribe the vessels only partially, surround one, two, or all vessels, or have central necrosis. The width of the band, degree of necrosis, band patterns, calcification, and neovascularization suggest a continuum of severity that reflects the intensity and duration of the lesion. There is variable recovery of organisms from these lesions and no predominance of isolate type; almost all the associated placentas show chorioamnionitis, although not necessarily as chronic in appearance as that of the cord. There is no direct relationship to duration of rupture of membranes.

Necrotizing funisitis is found in slightly less than 0.1% of all placentas (38), and discordance between twins occurs. Compared with infants with acute funisitis, there is a higher incidence of stillbirth, prematurity, infection, and other postnatal complications. The mothers have more clinical evidence of acute chorioamnionitis, and histories of oligohydramnios or of prolonged rupture of membranes. Additionally, the incidence of small size for gestational age is significantly higher than expected. Necrotizing funisitis has been described as strongly suggestive of congenital syphilis, but it is not unique to this infection (39,40). Infants with apparent funisitis should be fully evaluated for infection.

Sclerosing funisitis is likely a more chronic form of necrotizing funisitis that has undergone calcification of necrotic inflammatory debris. The finding of firmness and prominent vessel stripes is clearly of significance only in a cord that has not yet started to dry out. Cords with true sclerosing funisitis may be difficult to clamp because of their firmness. They will not shrink in the same manner as normal cords because there is such a calcified supporting exoskeleton.

Candida Funisitis

In another pattern of necrotizing funisitis easily seen on gross examination, the umbilical cord is studded with 1- to 3-mm yellow–white plaques that are embedded in the surface (Fig. 7). The plaques may be present with other changes typical of chorioamnionitis on the surface of the placenta as well but are most distinct on the cord. In histologic examination, the plaques are seen to lie just under the surface of the cord and may contain necrotic de-

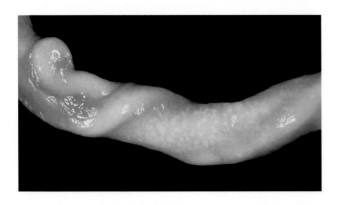

Figure 7. *Candida* funisitis. The white–yellow plaques along the cord contain hyphae and yeast cells visible on an India ink preparation.

bris or inflammatory cells and typical pseudohyphae and fungal elements (38,41). The gross finding is virtually pathognomonic of *Candida* infection (42). The appearance of the plaques in *Candida* funisitis may suggest amnion nodosum, but amnion nodosum does not develop on the cord (see examination of membranes below). The nodules of amnion nodosum can be removed from the amnionic surface, whereas *Candida* plaques cannot.

UMBILICAL CORD DIAMETER

Umbilical cord diameter varies with gestational age but has an average diameter of 1.5 to 2 cm. Umbilical cord diameter less than 1.6 cm after 41 weeks' gestation is associated with significant cord compression patterns on fetal monitoring, particularly when accompanied by oligohydramnios (43). Areas of exceptional narrowness may be associated with torsion and stricture of the cord and are most likely to be significant when at the base of the umbilicus on the fetal abdomen. Areas of swelling may represent varices, aneurysm, thrombosis, hematoma, cysts, or angiomas. When the swelling is near the fetal insertion, there needs to be a strong consideration of possible small omphalocele or umbilical hernia with herniation of abdominal contents (Fig. 8). If the swelling is particularly edematous, it may represent fetal urine leakage from a patent urachus. Edema of the cord with pseudocysts are one of the more frequently found abnormalities of the umbilical cord found on prenatal sonograms and do not appear to relate to any fetal pathology (44).

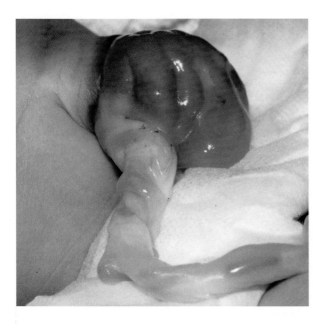

Figure 8. Small herniation of bowel through a defect that measured only 3 cm in diameter in a well-formed umbilical stump. This omphalocele represents failure of intestines to return to the abdomen during the 10th week of fetal development.

Wharton's jelly normally gives a white and generally semi-opaque appearance to the cord. In the presence of cord edema, the cord may be more transparent in contrast to the increase in opacity and firmness that occurs with chronic inflammation. The cord may be stained with meconium, old blood, or bilirubin pigments. The depth of the staining correlates with the duration of the exposure. Dyes injected into the amnionic fluid to detect rupture of membranes will stain the cord as well.

Marginal Insertion of Cord

Instead of the more common slightly eccentric insertion site, the cord inserts at the margin of the placental disk. The configuration resembles a badminton racket, hence, the name "battledore," which was a flat wooden paddle used in an early form of badminton. The general incidence of marginal insertions is higher in stillbirths, spontaneous abortions, malformed infants, and multiple gestations (6,45). Robinson et al. evaluated 4,677 consecutive placentas, including multiple gestations, and found marginal insertions in 8.5%. In contrast to other investigators, they did not find an increased association with malformations beyond the expected occurrence rate in the general population (46).

Velamentous Insertion of Umbilical Cord

Velamentous insertion (synonym *membranous insertion*) is insertion of the cord into the free membranes (Fig. 9). The cord may insert fairly close to the placental surface (most commonly) or, in the extreme, at the apex of the membranous sac. There are fewer fetal surface vessels in this type of insertion, perhaps accounting for the association with intrauterine growth retardation. Velamentous insertion occurs in about 1% of deliveries (47). It is associated with intrauterine growth retardation, multiple gestation, single umbilical artery, and vasa previa. Some studies have suggested an increased incidence in malformed infants, but others suggest that there is an association with deformation syndromes but no increase in major malformations (46). In monochorionic–diamnionic twins, velamentous cord insertion is significantly more prevalent in those with twin-to-twin transfusion syndrome than in those without it (63.6% vs. 18.5%) (48). Both groups have a higher prevalence of velamentous insertions than does the general population.

Because there is no protection to the vessels, they are especially prone toward compression and thrombosis or to rupture, causing a pure fetal hemorrhage and potentially rapid exsanguination (Benckiser's hemorrhage) (49). Uterine contractions causing compression

Figure 9. Marginal and velamentous insertions. This is a monochorionic diamnionic placenta in which the twin on the left (twin B) has a velamentous insertion into a bilobed placenta. Twin A has a marginal insertion. A prenatal sonogram was mistakenly interpreted as dichorionic because of the seemingly separate placentas. The occurrence of marginal and velamentous insertions increases with increasing numbers of fetuses (6). The risk for twin-to-twin transfusions is more than three times higher when a monochorionic placenta has a velamentous insertion (48).

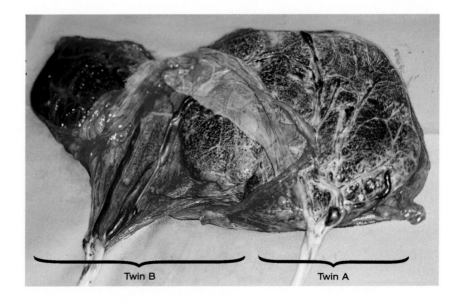

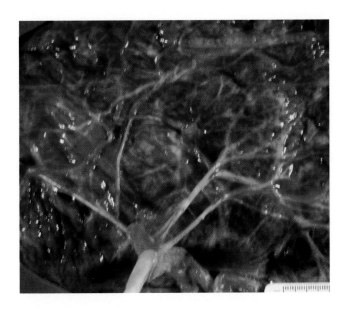

Figure 10. Furcate cord insertion. When the vessels of the umbilical cord divide before entering the placenta the insertion resembles a fork. Having lost protection from Wharton's jelly, the vessels are subject to rupture and compression.

of velamentous vessels may be associated with variable decelerations on fetal heart rate monitoring. An estimated one in 50 instances of velamentous insertion ruptures, although many of these occur in small vessels that do not cause significant blood loss, or they occur after delivery of the fetus (47). The Apt test on bloody vaginal or amnionic fluid would indicate predominantly fetal hemoglobin.

The same intrauterine forces that shape the placenta and influence cord insertion affect the fetus and make it subject to deformation syndromes. It is no wonder that both deformation and velamentous insertions occur with increasing frequency when there are increasing numbers of fetuses in the same uterus.

In furcate cord insertion the cord divides and loses the protection of the Wharton's jelly before reaching the placental disk (Fig. 10). The name comes from the forklike appearance to the placental end of the cord. Without the surrounding protective buffering of the Wharton's jelly, these vessels are at the same risk for compression, thrombosis, and rupture that velamentous vessels are (6,45),

Cord hematoma develops as a swelling of the umbilical cord anywhere along its length in single or multiple segments with a typical appearance of a collection of blood in a firm, round or sausage shape (Fig. 11). Hematomas appear most typically closer to the fetal end of the umbilical cord and vary considerably in size from 1 cm up to 40 cm in length. About 20% may rupture into the amnionic cavity.

In most cases the extravasation into the cord comes from rupture of the umbilical vein, often in association with short cord, trauma, or entanglement (6). With the increased use of prenatal umbilical cord blood sampling, there is likely to be an increase in the number of cases of iatrogenic hematoma after vessel perforation; cord hematoma has been observed after general amniocentesis (50,51). When seen after an intra-amnionic procedure, there tends to be a need for rapid delivery because of fetal exsanguination into the amnionic fluid.

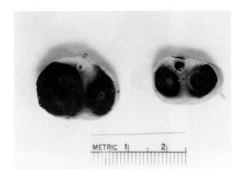

Figure 11. Umbilical hematoma in cross section. Most hematomas occur after rupture of the umbilical vein so appear as collections surrounding that vessel. The vein is the thin-walled structure on the left containing a thrombus and surrounded by blood. An umbilical artery has also been surrounded. The second artery is seen at the 12 o-clock position.

Before the use of intra-amnionic procedures, the reported incidence of cord hematoma ranged from one in 5,500 to one in 10,000 livebirths (6). The hematoma can cause a number of problems for the fetus, including loss of blood volume and compression of the other cord vessels. We reported an infant who experienced myocardial and cerebral infarctions from embolization associated with stasis thrombosis and a cord hematoma (52).

Membranes

Reconstruct the intrauterine configuration of the placenta and membranes. Determine if the volume of the gestational sac seems appropriate to the size of the fetus. Assess the transparency of the membranes. Note if there are any areas of thickening or masses present on the membranes. Inspect the insertion of the membranes on the placenta to find evidence of marginal, circummarginate, or circumvallate placentation. Look for adherent blood clot or old blood at the sites of insertion.

Determine the chorionicity in fused placentas. In same sex, multiple gestations with fused placentas, determine the number of layers in the dividing membranes. Blot off any blood and hold up and look through the dividing membranes to detect any remnants of vessels or chorionic tissue remnants. Separate the membranes with tissue forceps and count the layers. When only two layers of amnion are present, without intervening chorion or when there is no dividing membrane, look for the vascular communications. If none are apparent grossly, inject major vessels from one twin to detect flow to the other.

The membranes regularly invert with vaginal delivery, so it is usually necessary to return them to their anatomic relationship. Because they tear easily, they require careful handling. When the membranes have ruptured before delivery, one can assume that the point of rupture is over the cervical os. If there is at least 2 cm of membrane between the point of rupture and the placental disk, the placenta is unlikely to have been lying next to or over the cervical os in placenta previa. The free membranes should originate from the margins

A

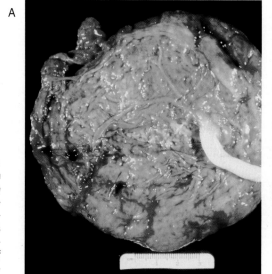

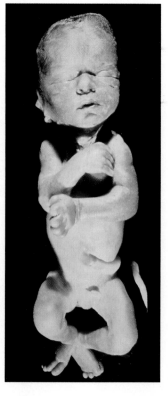

Figure 12. Extra-amnionic pregnancy. **A:** The amnionic cavity, measuring 3 cm in width, was too small to have contained the fetus that developed in the chorionic cavity. The extreme cloudiness and discoloration indicates chronic chorioamnionitis but not from infection. **B:** The fetus, delivered at 24 weeks, had physical findings of severe prolonged compression with normal kidneys.

B

of the placenta so that there is no extramembranous placenta suggesting circumvallate or circummarginate placentation.

The size of the gestational sac should be appropriate to the size of the fetus. If it is obviously too small, the fetus may have developed in the chorionic cavity outside the amnion (extra-amnionic fetus) or in a chronically low amnionic fluid volume (oligohydramnios) (Fig. 12). See Fig. 2 for illustration of early gestation with a chorionic cavity still present outside the amnion. An extramembranous fetus is one that develops free in the uterine cavity outside both the amnion and chorion. In these rare situations, there is always severe fetal compression and chronic leakage of amnionic fluid.

Placenta Color

The membranes are normally colorless and transmit the color of the underlying structures, primarily the blue–purple of lowly saturated hemoglobin in the placental mass. With increasing prematurity the color is more slate blue. With marked anemia the transmitted color is pink. The free membranes may have areas of tan–brown fibrinous material from degenerated chorionic villous tissue but are generally translucent without intrinsic color. Ghosts of chorionic vessels course through the chorion, but there should not be any fetal vessels leading to the umbilical cord. Other masses that may be present in the membranes are succenturiate lobes in various stages of atrophy or even a fetus papyraceus. Like the umbilical cord, the membranes will stain with whatever pigments are present in the amnionic fluid.

Meconium staining of the placenta occurs in 10% to 30% of placentas examined (Fig. 13). In examinations of 12,951 placentas in consecutive deliveries at all gestations, Benirschke found true meconium present in 17.81%. Usher found it to double when the gestational age went past term, with 31.5% occurrence when the pregnancy went past 42 weeks compared with 15.3% 1 week before term (53). Meconium staining is positively correlated with fetal distress as variously described in the different studies but clearly occurs almost as often in the absence of any evidence of fetal distress (53). Because meconium itself may cause placental and umbilical vasoconstriction, its passage may have a role in causing fetal distress (1). The finding of meconium staining in preterm gestations of less than 34 weeks is unusual enough in the absence of major malformations that one should first consider that the dates are inaccurate or that the staining is by hemolyzed blood pigments from an earlier bleeding episode.

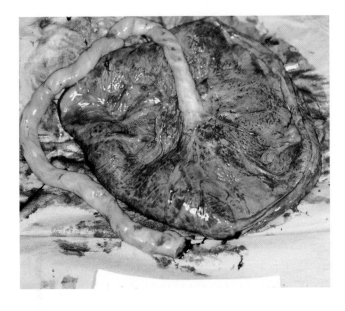

Figure 13. Fetal surface with meconium staining of long enough duration to discolor the full diameter of the umbilical cord and to cause chorioamnionitis in this term placenta.

The bile pigments of meconium undergo changes from a dark blue green to muddy brown and then a lighter, almost chartreuse color. Its endpoint color transition is the same as bilirubin or metabolized hemoglobin. When discharged just before birth, particulate meconium can be wiped or rinsed off without leaving any stain on the amnion. Meconium-containing macrophages may be found in the amnion within 1 hour; the chorion will be stained within 3 hours (54). An earlier literature review suggested that it takes 4 to 6 hours for the meconium to stain the chorion (55). Cord staining with bile pigments to the center of the cord is a later finding, as is degeneration of the amnionic epithelium and the presence of meconium-stained macrophages within the decidua.

Amnion nodosum is the presence of yellow–white nodules 1 to 5 mm in diameter on the fetal surface of the membranes and placenta but not on the umbilical cord (Fig. 14). The nodules can be easily picked off the surface and represent material such as hair, squames, and sebum that is normally floating in the amnionic fluid but has been ground into the membrane surface by the fetus in close and constant contact. These nodules are signs of prolonged, severe oligohydramnios and signify the probable presence of pulmonary hypoplasia.

Amnion nodosum is found most commonly in cases of renal agenesis or leakage of amnionic fluid from at least the mid-trimester with clinically absent amnionic fluid. Nodules also may be seen in the placenta of a chronic donor twin in twin-to-twin transfusion syndrome, as well as in diamnionic acardiac twinning, sirenomelia, or in other fetal conditions that lead to profound, prolonged oligohydramnios (2,6,45,56). Besides the nodules on the amnion, the infant has features typical of prolonged compression, the oligohydramnios sequence: creasing advanced for age, up-slanting creases under the eyes, flattened nose, limb positioning defects, particularly of the hands and feet, and growth deficiency with decreased subcutaneous fat (Fig. 15).

Because of the association of amnion nodosum with pulmonary hypoplasia in fetal compression syndromes, recognition of this entity is essential to assist in resuscitation decisions. Not all fetal compression syndromes are associated with amnion nodosum, but the presence of amnion nodosum in the placenta of an infant who is extraordinarily difficult to ventilate would clarify the probable etiology for the ventilation failure as fatal pulmonary hypoplasia.

It is important to distinguish amnion nodosum, a sign of severe oligohydramnios and fetal compression, from squamous metaplasia, a sign of normal placental maturation, as well as from normal vernix deposits which are few in number, larger, and wipe off easily.

Squamous metaplasia is the name applied to the gray or white plaques 0.5 to 3 mm in largest diameter that are generally flat or only slightly elevated (2,6). These tend to be localized near the base of the umbilical cord on the fetal surface, and they appear dull compared with the surrounding amnion. The plaques are tightly adherent and cannot be removed without disturbing the underlying amnion. Found in about 25% to 60% of term placentas, the lesions represent focal keratinization of the normal squamous epithelium that makes up the amnion. There is no clinical significance for these lesions except as a sign of pregnancy maturation but they should not be confused with amnion nodosum. They do not increase in syndromes of hyperkeratinization of the fetal skin. The name squamous metaplasia is really a misnomer because there is no change in the cell type.

Amnionic Band Syndrome

This entity is also known as the ADAM sequence or complex (*Amnionic Deformities, Adhesions, Mutilation*), amnionic band disruption complex, early amnion rupture sequence, amniochorionic mesoblastic strings, and congenital annular constricting bands syndrome. Strangulation of a body part by a portion of amnion may lead to amputation of the developing part (Fig. 16). The areas affected in decreasing order of frequency are the fingers, toes, limbs, cranium, and abdominal wall. Strangulation of the umbilical cord leads to fetal demise (57). In severe cases there are unpredictable combinations of complex craniofacial malformations that include clefting of the face, palate, eye lids, and eye deformities, as well as absence of portions of the skull and brain. Failure of formation of the umbilical cord may represent one type of ADAM sequence because the cord develops as normal amnion surrounds it (Fig. 5).

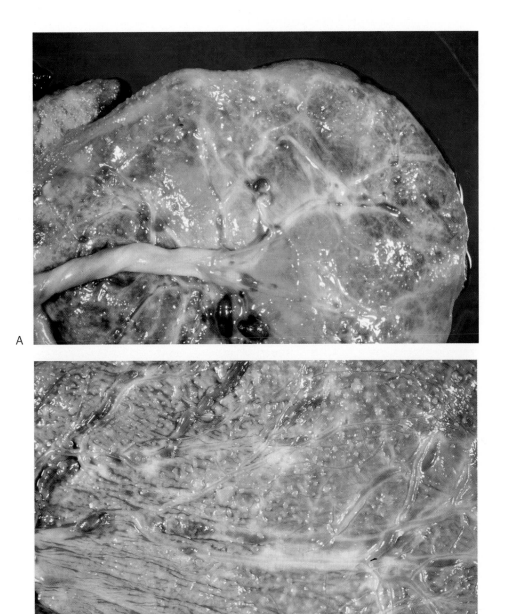

Figure 14. Amnion nodosum indicating severe, chronic oligohydramnios from at least the mid-trimester. **A:** Yellow–orange nodules stud the fetal surface but not the umbilical cord. **B:** A close-up view of amnion nodosum shows how superficial and variably sized the nodules are. Any infant born with this finding would have marked compression facies and probably severe pulmonary hypoplasia (see Figs. 12 and 15). Renal agenesis is the most common reason for severe oligohydramnios.

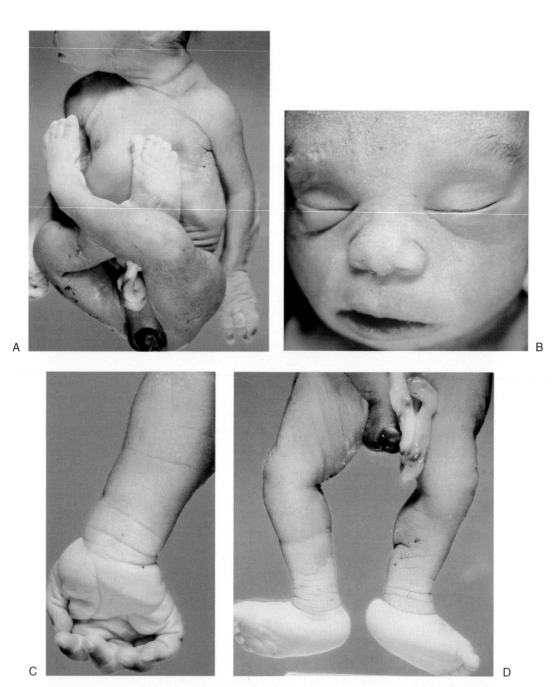

Figure 15. Findings of severe fetal compression (Potter's facies). **A:** The fetal position shows one foot compressing the anterior chest wall. There is an ecchymotic region around the neck where the umbilical cord was tightly wrapped. **B:** The face shows inferior epicanthal folds from flattening of the mid-facies. On the skin, nodules of vernix and amnionic debris are evident. **C:** The hands have deep folds consistent with positioning in a fixed flexion. **D:** The feet have deep vertical creases and rocker bottoms consistent with lack of free movement. A single umbilical artery and renal agenesis were present.

In the absence of amputation, amnionic bands may cause constrictions that result in grooves of varying deepness with underlying dermal necrosis or linear erosions (58).

There is controversy over the cause, particularly when the syndrome includes a range of abnormalities, but the majority of evidence suggests that there is an abnormal attachment of the amnion to the fetus, either because the amnion has lost its integrity or has ruptured and become tightly adherent to the body part. In some cases there appears to be an association with maternal trauma, but in the majority of instances there is nothing remarkable about the history. The possible association with early chorionic villous sampling and amniocentesis is controversial (59–61). Amnionic bands are identified via ultrasound early in gestation and suggest that some of the most severe conditions that involve disruption and internal anomalies occur in the first month after conception because the anomalies may be explicable in terms of interference with neuropore closure, mal migration of cephalic neural crest tissue, and damage to the mesonephros, resulting in local defects (62–64). Others argue that the limb–body wall complex syndromes are a phenomenon separate from amnionic bands (65). Some amnionic bands diagnosed on sonography are benign. When a band is diagnosed on ultrasound in the absence of other major anomalies, there is little increased risk for that pregnancy except for a higher occurrence of delivery at less than 37 weeks and birth weight less than 2,500 g (65,66).

This syndrome is relatively rare, but unlike some of the neural tube defects or malformations of the extremities that it mimics, there is little probability for repetition in future pregnancies, although familial recurrence has been reported (67–69). In an Australian study that included all types of limb defects and limb–body wall defects, the annual prevalence rate was 2.03 per 10,000 births, with males and females being equally affected. In another study of over a million liveborn infants that included only limb amputations, the incidence was 0.19 per 10,000 livebirths (70). The full incidence is likely higher than these reports because most of the cases that represent the earliest fetal effects end in spontaneous early abortion or stillbirth.

The finding of asymmetric, nonuniform amputation suggests amnionic band syndrome rather than either a vascular accident or an intrinsic defect such as split hand, split foot syndrome, which shows more bilateral involvement and an inheritance pattern. The ADAM sequence is diagnosed by examining the placenta. It will be possible to see an absence of amnionic epithelium on the fetal surface of the placenta and, often, a small, fibrotic amnionic band remnant attaching to the umbilical cord at the placental end (Fig. 17). This is one example of the need to make placental examination a habit because the flurry of anxiety and

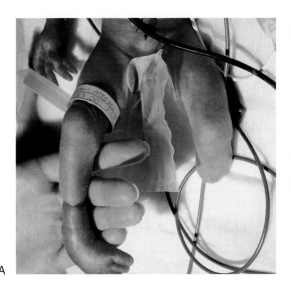
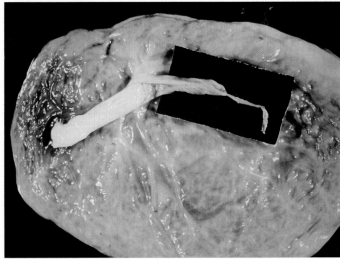

A
B

Figure 16. Amnionic band syndrome in 28-week gestation infant. **A:** A stricture on the right leg did not require therapy. The amputated left leg had a small tag attached. The amputated lower leg and foot were found in the amnionic cavity of the placenta after delivery and measured at a length compatible with 19 weeks. **B:** A placenta with a typical band remnant at the base of the umbilical cord had marked chorioamnionitis without maternal evidence of infection.

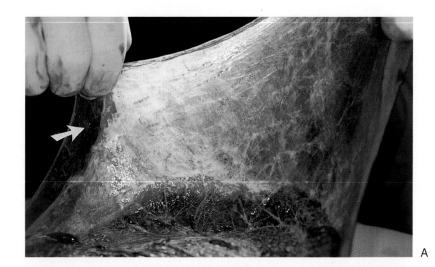

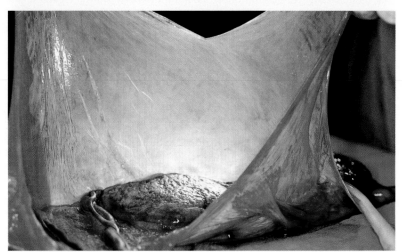

A

B

Figure 17. Dividing membranes. **A:** Membrane with chorionic remnants visible. A single layer of amnion (*arrow*) that has torn away is completely transparent. When there are visible remnants in a dividing membrane, the placenta is dichorionic. **B:** Transparent dividing membrane in a monochorionic diamnionic placenta. There are no remnants of chorionic tissue.

Table 3. *Forms of twin placentation*

Type	%	No. of placental disks	Dividing septum			Zygosity
			Present	No. of amnions	No. of chorions	
DCDA, separate	35	2	In utero only	—	—	DZ or MZA[a]
DCDA, fused	40	1	Yes	2	2	DZ or MZA[a]
MCDA	25	1	Yes	2	0	MZ
MCMA	<1	1	No	—	—	MZ

DCDA, dichorionic—diamnionic; DZ, dizygotic; MCDA, monochorionic—diamniotic; MCMA, monochorionic—monoamnionic; MZ, monozygotic.
[a] Ten percent to 15% of DC placentas, mostly fused, are MZ; 20% to 40% of MZ twins are DC.
From Heifetz, ref. 91, with permission.

activity that accompanies the birth of a malformed infant may distract the clinician and cause him to miss the answer about the diagnosis immediately available to him.

Determining Chorionicity in Fused Placentas

The types of placentation in twin pregnancies are described in Table 3. The information that one gets from knowing that placentas are fused is little more than that they were adjacent within the uterus. Fused placentas may be from more than one zygote and appear tightly joined. If the twins are the same sex, the number of layers in the dividing membrane should be determined to suggest zygosity.

A dividing membrane that is dichorionic with two layers of chorion inside the two layers of amnion appears more opaque with minute but visible remnants of vessels and villi in the layers (Fig. 18). If the membranes are completely transparent, there is less likelihood that chorion is present, but the layers should be divided and counted.

One of the important reasons to determine if there is monochorionicity is to diagnose the probability of interfetal vascular communications. The easiest way to determine if vessels in monochorionic placentas communicate is to inject a contrast substance into an umbilical or fetal surface vessel and to observe if there is filling of vessels leading to the other umbilical cord. The most readily available contrast material for clinicians is air, but any injection should be noted if a histologic examination is to follow (Fig. 19). An injection will detect major communications but will not detect the many more microscopic communications that are likely to be present. Vessels from one twin that dive into a shared region from which a vessel from the other twin emerges may not necessarily be in communication. When vascular communications are balanced between the twins, there is little demonstrable effect unless one twin experiences a catastrophic event. If the communications are unbalanced, one twin may become a chronic donor to the other in a twin-to-twin transfusion syndrome (TTTS) (Figs. 20 and 21). The findings of a unidirectional TTTS are shown in Table 4. The

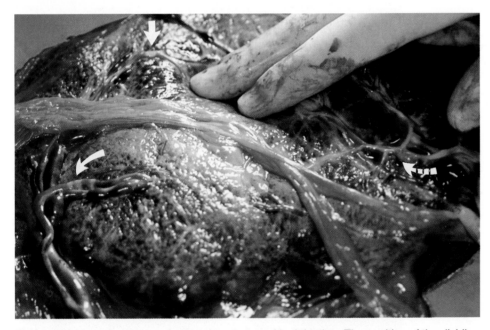

Figure 18. Vascular communication demonstrated by injection. The position of the dividing membrane does not necessarily indicate the location of a vascular equator, the dividing point for the circulation, between twins. There were many apparent vascular communications, including one that stretched across the membrane between the two lobes (see Fig. 9). Air has been injected into an artery at the base of the cord of twin A on the right (*broken arrow*). Bubbles are apparent in arteries of twin A (*straight arrow*) and the arteries and veins of twin B (*curved arrow*). The communications were in both directions and balanced so there was almost identical growth and blood volumes between the twins at birth.

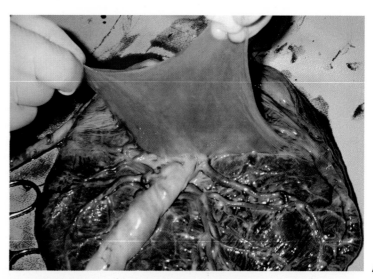

A

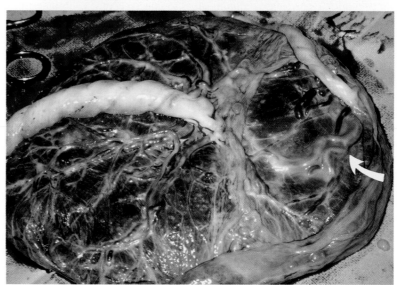

B

Figure 19. Placenta with twin-to-twin transfusion. **A:** Dividing membrane in monochorionic placenta that shows no chorionic remnants, indicating only amnion. These twins were diagnosed with a unidirectional twin-to-twin transfusion syndrome prenatally. **B:** The donor twin's cord and placental mass on the right is smaller than the recipient twin's on the left. Their growth rates were correspondingly asymmetric. After a decompressing amniocentesis from the cavity on the left 3 weeks before delivery, the TTTS abated, and the donor twin started growing better. A recent thrombosis (*arrow*) in a dilated communicating surface vessel is visible, suggesting a reason for the apparent clinical improvement in the donor.

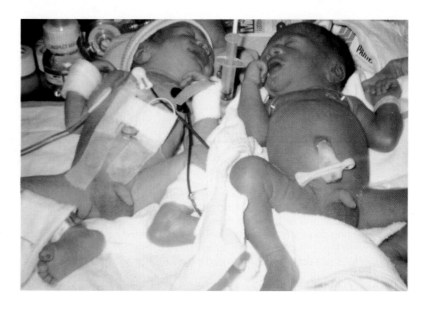

Figure 20. Twins after an acute intrauterine twin-to-twin transfusion. The recipient (right) is more plethoric and donor (left) paler but the weights were similar. The majority of vascular communications in monochorionic twins are probably balanced and dependent on differences in placental or fetal vascular resistance and pressure. When not unidirectional or long standing, acute changes in pressures can cause hypovolemic shock in one and hypervolemia in another without affecting weights and hemoglobin levels at birth. Photo from M.C. Edwards.

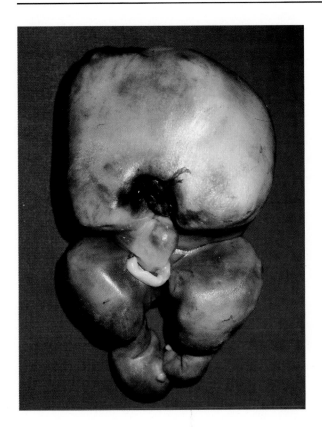

Figure 21. Acardiac twin. The ultimate example of TTTS is the complete support of one fetus's circulation by the other. This twin, measuring 30 cm long, weighed almost twice as much as her supporting twin and caused her severe cardiovascular stress. As is typical, there is no formation of structures above the upper thorax. Rudimentary ectopia cordis is present above the umbilical stump.

Table 4. *Twin transfusion syndrome*

Parameter	Donor	Recipient
Appearance	Small, pale, hydrops; cutaneous erythroblastosis	Large, plethoric, hydrops
Viscera	Asymmetric growth retardation; osteosclerosis; increased hematopoiesis	Congestive cardio- and hepatosplenomegaly; enlarged thymus and adrenal cortex; osteopenia; increased medial smooth muscle in systemic and pulmonary arteries 2° hypertension; more mature and enlarged glomeruli with increased urinary output
Cord blood	Anemia; erythroblastosis	Polycythemia
Placenta	Pale, but bulky	Deep red, firm
Chorionic vessels	Small	Congested
Umbilical cord	Thin	Edematous
Villi	Large, edematous	Normal, but congested
Hofbauer cells	Increased	Normal
Syncytial knots	Decreased	Normal
Nucleated RBCs	Increased	Slightly increased
Amnion	Amnion nodosum (rare; hypotension, hypovolemia, decreased fetal urination)	Hydramnios (excessive fetal urination)

RBC, red blood cell.
From Heifetz, ref. 91, with permission.

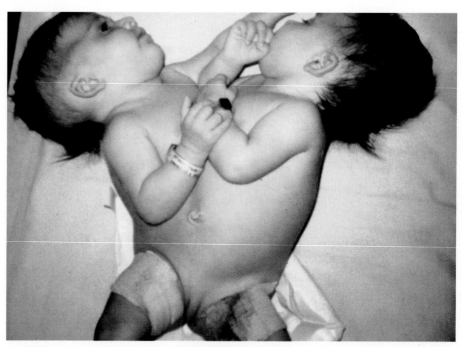

Figure 22. Conjoined twins (thoracoabdominopagus). Twins whose single zygote divides relatively late (day 13) can be joined at almost any site from the head to the pelvis. The broader the area of joining, the more likely there is sharing of common vital organs. Photo from A.B. Fletcher.

ultimate in shared circulation is a situation in which the circulation of one fetus fully supports the other acardiac twin with usually devastating stress on the donor twin (Fig. 22).

The number of dividing membranes depends on how early the zygote divides into twins, with the earliest divisions resulting in dichorionic placentas and the latest in conjoined twinning (Fig. 23). The types of placentation in higher than twin monozygotic multiples are any of several mathematically possible combinations. Because of crowding and, therefore,

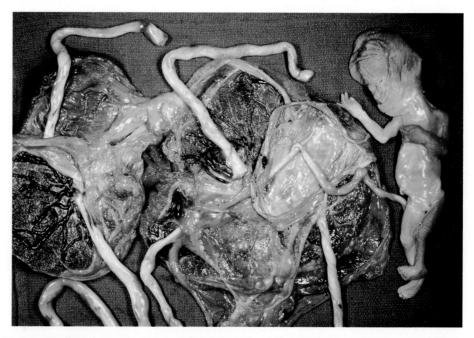

Figure 23. Sextuplet pregnancy delivered at 34 weeks with a fetus papyraceous. All placentas were dichorionic. The membranes and chorionic plate of the dead fetus are cloudy as is typical after fetal demise of long duration.

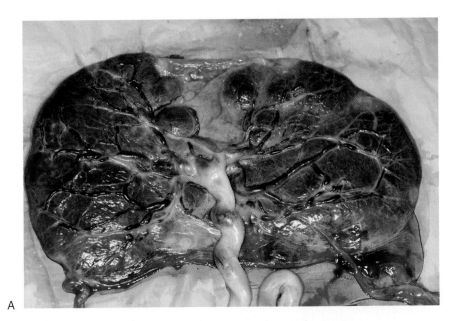

A

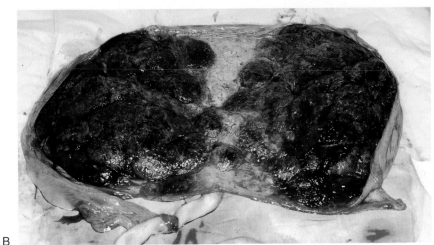

B

Figure 24. Normal variation in placental shape. **A:** The mid-portion of this placenta where the cord inserted underwent degeneration but did not form as completely a bilobed shape as the one shown in Fig. 9. The normal surface divisions of each umbilical artery going to opposite halves of the placenta are apparent. **B:** Individual cotyledons that have separated from the main mass are succenturiate lobes. Small infarcts are seen on both the maternal and fetal surfaces at the margins. None of these findings were clinically significant.

more likelihood of fusion, determining chorionicity is equally important in all same-sex multiple gestations (Fig. 24).

Fetal Surface

Examine the fetal surface and take measurements of the placental mass. Note the shape of the placenta and the presence of succenturiate lobes or accessory masses. Note the presence of cloudiness, staining, subchorionic cysts or hematomas, or nodules. If the surface is cloudy or there is a clinical suspicion of infection and cultures are desired, after blotting the blood from the surface, peel the membrane over the cloudiest area to expose the tissue under the amnion. Take cultures and then press a clean microscope slide to the exposed surface for Gram stain if desired. Note if there is any unusual odor.

Size and Shape

Placenta morphometrics are listed in Table 1. The size directly correlates with fetal weight. The shape of the placenta reflects the intrauterine shape and is normally discoid or ellipsoid. Variations occur when there is anatomic influence such as a bicornuate uterus or fibromyomas, poor blood supply such as after uterine scarring, or a low lying placenta (Fig. 25, Table 5).

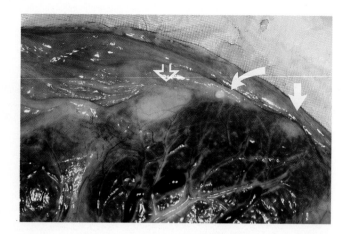

Figure 25. Normal findings. Yolk sac located between the chorion and amnion at term (*curved arrow*) and subchorionic fibrin (*straight arrow*). Found in approximately 20% of mature placentas, subchorionic fibrin (synonym *pseudo-infarct, subchorial thrombosis*) appears as a firm, white plaque under the chorion with the larger surface on cross section toward the fetal side. Most lesions are located closer to the center of the placenta but may develop anywhere. There is no compromise to fetal circulation, so this is not a true infarction and it carries no clinical significance. The larger area (*open arrow*) is an infarct that has its base on the maternal surface. When found at the margins, small infarcts have little clinical significance.

Table 5. *Placentation abnormalities*

Abnormality	Incidence (%)	Significance
Abnormal placental shape		
Extrachorial (complete, partial, combined)		
Circum-marginate	5–20	None
Circumvallate	0.5–2	Ab, IUGR, CA, premature labor, fetal malformation
Membranous (diffuse)	Rare	AP and PP hemorrhage, Ab, premature labor, IUGR, adherence
Annular (ring-shaped; girdle; collar)	Rare	AP and PP hemorrhage, IUGR
Fenestrate (zonaria)	Rare	None
Accessory (succenturiate) lobe	5–8	Fetal hemorrhage, retention
Bilobate (bipartite; duplex)	0.04–4.2	First trimester hemorrhage, adherence
Multilobate	Rare	Fetal hemorrhage
Abnormal placental invasiveness/ adherence		
Accreta, percreta, increta (total, partial, focal)	0.04	AP and PP hemorrhage, uterine rupture, 10% fetal and maternal mortality
Retroplacental hematoma (abruptio placentae)	4.5	AP hemorrhage, IUGR; includes one-third of cases of clinical abruption; one-third will have clinical abruption
Abnormal placental location		
Previa	5–28 (second trimester) 0.3–0.7 (live births)	AP hemorrhage, abruption, IUGR, 10% perinatal mortality

Ab, abortion, AP, antepartum; CA, chorioamnionitis; IUGR, intrauterine growth retardation; PP, postpartum.
From Heifetz, ref. 91, with permission.

Odor

The placenta normally has little odor other than that of fresh blood. Infection may impart an odor typical of whichever organism is involved. The presence of a foul odor suggests infection but is not pathognomonic.

The yolk sac may be seen as a yellow, flat oval on the fetal surface between the amnion and the chorion. Rarely, tiny remnants of vitelline vessels leading toward the umbilical cords may still be visible (Fig. 25).

The fetal vessels run to and from the umbilical cord across the fetal surface. There should be at least five to eight large fetal vessels apparent on the surface. Marginal or velamentous insertions have fewer branches. Relatively near the umbilical insertion the arteries have walls thick enough to be distinguishable from the veins, which ordinarily have less apparent wall thickness as long as they are not emptied of blood. If the veins are collapsed, the walls seem thicker. The earliest changes of chorioamnionitis may sometimes be best detected by the veins appearing to have walls thicker than normal. In general, arteries cross on top of veins except randomly in isolated areas in the periphery. Placentas that have a reversal of this pattern have been associated with polyhydramnios and abnormal fetal development (71).

Chorioamnionitis as defined clinically implies maternal infection with fever and dysfunctional labor but pathologically means an inflammatory reaction of the placental membranes that may be due to infection or to other irritants. It is found in the absence of infection with meconium staining of more than a few hours' duration (Fig. 13), in severe oligohydramnios (Fig. 12), or with marked membrane edema. The entire surface may be involved, or the reaction may be localized to a small segment. Early amnionitis does not have any evidence of membrane changes but progressive discoloration and cloudiness of the membranes eventually leads to opacity and obliteration of the surface anatomy on gross examination.

When placentas with changes of chorioamnionitis are cultured, the most common organisms recovered are the expected neonatal bacterial pathogens (group B streptococcus, *Escherichia coli*, staphylococci, *Pseudomonas, Proteus,* and *Klebsiella* organisms, as well as anaerobes, or *Candida albicans* and, more rarely, viruses). Chorioamnionitis is a major cause of premature labor and premature rupture of membranes (1).

Other common gross findings on the fetal surface include subchorionic fibrin deposition (Fig. 26), subamnionic hemorrhage, and subchorionic cysts, none of which are clinically significant.

Subchorionic hematoma (synonym *Breus's mole, tuberose subchorial hematoma*) is easily seen as a bulging protuberance on the fetal surface produced by nodular and red thrombus formation in the subchorionic zone. The lesions are most often limited and small but rarely may be massive, involving a large portion of the subchorionic area (Fig. 28). In contrast, subamnionic hemorrhage is flat, not well defined, and almost exclusively a delivery event (Fig. 27). The cause of subchorionic hematoma is unclear, but the source of the blood is maternal. When there is fetal compromise, it is likely because of significant interference with fetal blood flow rather than because of fetal blood loss into the blood collection.

The incidence of subchorionic hematoma varies greatly among studies from 4% to 48%, depending on the mode and timing of diagnosis (72). There are many more subchorionic fluid collections seen on early sonograms than are present on examination at delivery, but subchorionic cysts without blood are commonly seen at term. Small subchorionic hematomas tend to be more common in the first trimester and appear to add no risk to the ongoing pregnancy. Some investigators suggest that there is a causative factor in abortion or prematurity and undergrown fetuses, but there are many cases of advanced gestation as well (73,74). Conversely, subchorionic hematomas in the second trimester, particularly when associated with maternal bleeding, are often larger and may be associated with an increased risk of preterm delivery and poor fetal growth. (72–82).

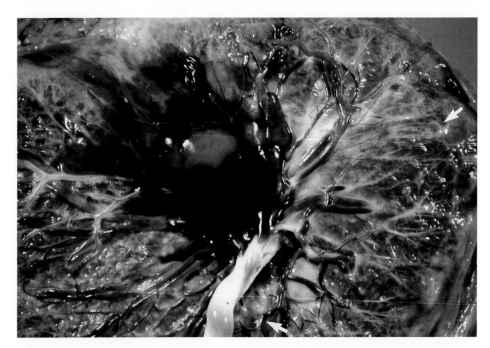

Figure 26. Subamnionic hemorrhage. The blood accumulation with ill-defined borders occurs as a result of traction on the umbilical cord most commonly after the infant is born unless there is an abnormally short umbilical cord. It has no clinical significance. Subchorionic fibrin deposition is apparent near the base of the umbilical cord as firm, white masses of variable size but limited to the subchorionic area. Several benign, small subchorionic cysts are evident (*arrow*). Bosselation is the knobby granulation apparent below the area of hemorrhage at 7 o'clock and represents surface granulation that increases with maturity but carries no clinical significance.

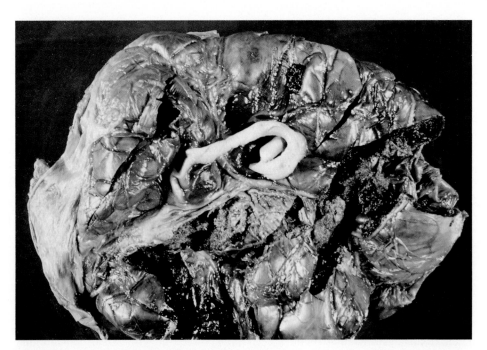

Figure 27. Massive subchorionic hematoma (Breus's mole). The fetal surface of this placenta has been cut to reveal extensive subchorionic collections of blood. In the uncut areas the tuberous swelling is evident. The presence of poor fetal growth and abnormal ultrasound findings on the placenta was diagnosed 12 weeks before the emergency delivery at 29 weeks because of poor fetal condition. This infant was undergrown at 710 g with an expected weight for gestational age of a least 900 g for 29 weeks (10th percentile). His placenta was heavy for gestational age. Although the blood accumulated in the subchorionic space is maternal, there is enough fetal compromise that this condition is often associated with fetal demise or spontaneous abortion.

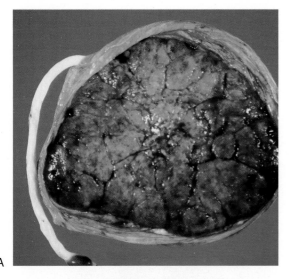

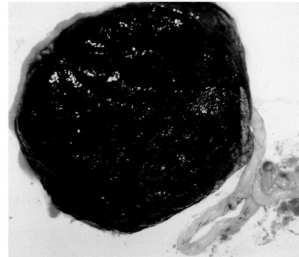

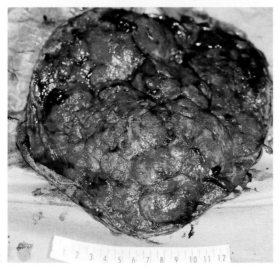

Figure 28. Maternal surface at term. **A:** Normal. The cotyledons are well defined. The color is yellowed because of the layer of normal fibrin deposition. An umbilical hematoma is evident at the cut end of the cord. **B:** Engorged. The definition of the cotyledons is somewhat obscured because of the marked swellings and engorgement of this plethoric placenta. Palpation of the maternal surface reveals a boggy firmness. Several false knots are seen in the umbilical cord. **C:** Pale. The color of the maternal surface is pale, suggesting fetal anemia or blood loss.

Maternal Surface

Turn the placenta over and examine the maternal surface for color, the presence of adherent blood clots, depressions in the surface, or areas of discoloration. Feel the surface to assess for uniformity of texture. If the placenta is not being sent to pathology, make cuts perpendicular to the maternal surface about 1 inch apart and examine the villous parenchyma for the presence of fibrin deposition, apparent thromboses or infarction, masses, and color.

It is often easier to feel for differences in texture than to see many of the gross lesions such as recent infarcts unless there has been enough change in color. Placentas that indicate an increase in blood volume look darker in color and feel boggier (Fig. 29). In converse, placental appearance after fetal exsanguination or severe fetal anemia is pale in nature. In chronic TTTS the donor twin's maternal surface appears paler. Calcium deposits in the placenta feel gritty and crunch when the placenta is cut. Depressions with adherent blood clots indicate retroplacental hemorrhage and abruption of the placenta. The absence of such a depression or adherent blood does not rule out an event just before delivery.

Infarct

These are the most common lesions seen on placental examination of the maternal surface. It is easiest to detect early infarctions by palpation. They feel firm and initially are dark red and granular, turning yellow and then yellow–gray as the infarct matures. They oc-

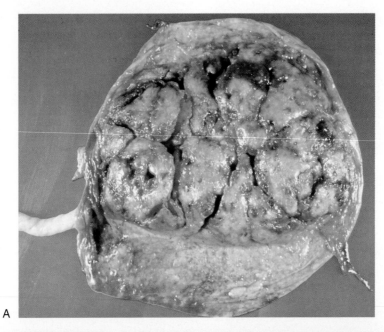

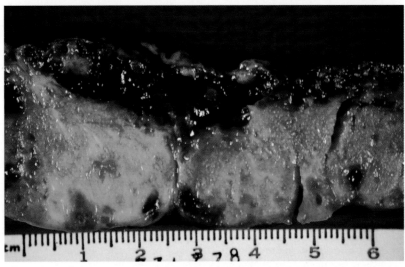

Figure 29. Maternal floor infarction in live born but growth retarded infant at term. **A:** Most of the maternal surface is covered by thick fibrin deposition. **B:** The fibrin extends far toward the fetal surface and significantly interferes with placental circulation.

cur most commonly near the edge of the placental plate but, when they are centrally located, are more highly accompanied by maternal vascular disease, particularly when found early in gestation (6). Infarcts are closely associated with abruption placenta.

Gross infarcts are found in approximately 25% of term pregnancies but generally involve less than 5% of the parenchyma (2). The frequency and extent of infarction increases with maternal vascular disease. Infarction means loss of viable tissue for fetal maternal exchange. Normally there is sufficient reserve to allow some loss without fetal compromise, but it is not possible to determine the actual flow patterns based only on gross placental examination. Clearly, multiple infarctions in the presence of a circulation compromised by hypertension or other vascular disease would be less well tolerated than as isolated events.

Maternal floor infarction is far less common but clinically more significant (Fig. 30). The thickened maternal surface is gray–yellow from massive fibrin deposition that involves the decidua basalis and the contiguous villi. The reported incidence of this condition is 0.09% to 0.5% of placentas (83,84). There is a strong association with fetal death, preterm birth, and intrauterine growth retardation with a high risk of recurrence (83). Pathological findings associated with maternal and fetal conditions are noted in Tables 6 and 7.

Worksheet for Gross Examination of the Placenta
Patient Identification:

Date and time of delivery _____ Weeks gestation _____
Clinical diagnosis: Uncomplicated   Pregnancy induced hypertension
Diabetes   Isoimmunization   Preterm labor   Prolonged rupture of membranes
Maternal infection_____   Intrauterine Growth retardation   Other _____
Infant's birth weight: _____ gm   Weight ratio of Placenta: Infant _____
Placental weight _____ gm   (Note if this is before or after fixing, with or without membranes.)

Cord   Length _____ cm   Av. Diameter _____ cm uniform
          Insertion site: central/eccentric/marginal/velamentous/furcate
          true knot   varicosities   twist: R/L/Absent   stricture
          vessels: single artery, two arteries
          Other: _____
                    (hematoma, calcification, edema, staining, extravascular markings)

Membranes: disrupted, absent, point of rupture less than 2 cm from placenta
     % Circummargination _____   % Circumvallation _____

     Multiple gestation: DiDi   MoDi   MoMo
                              If monochorionic, visible vascular communication,
                              discordant size, pallor, plethora
Fetal Surface
     Dimensions _____ × _____ × _____ cm   Bilobate _____ × _____ cm   irregular
     Subchorionic Fibrin   0/1/2/3   Subchorionic hemorrhage _____ %   old/recent
     Color: steel gray, red, green, yellow, brown
     Opacification of surface (mild, moderate, extensive)
     Amnion nodosum   Squamous metaplasia   Tessellation
     Subamniotic hemorrhage   Subchorion: cyst, fibrosis, hematoma
     Succenturiate Lobe: present, _____ number; atrophic/partial atrophy

Maternal Surface   disrupted focal/extensive
     Color: pallor, plethora, normal   Calcification: absent, mild, moderate, extensive
     Thrombus   Fresh/Recent/Old
     Infarcts: absent, less than 5% total surface; 5–15%; >25%.
     Hemorrhage Old: Retromembranous/Retroplacental/Marginal   Fresh: RM/RP/M
     Fibrin deposition: diffuse or localized
     Atrophy: diffuse or localized   pale/deep red/soft/firm

OTHER: _____

Figure 30. Worksheet for examining the placenta.

Table 6. *Salient features of the placenta in maternal disorders*

Disorders	Salient gross features	Salient microscopic features	Comment
Toxemia of pregnancy	Low weight, infarcts (>5%), retroplacental hematoma	Villi: accelerated maturation, prominent cytotrophoblastic hyperplasia, thickening of trophoblastic basement membrane; maternal arteries-acute atherosis (fibrinoid necrosis, lipid macrophages); thrombosis of vessels may be present	Placenta may be normal in mild cases; severe lesions tend to occur in severe cases; additional sections from the membranes and maternal surface of the placenta may be needed to get adequate sample of maternal arteries; HELLP syndrome shows similar but more severe lesions
Maternal hypertension	Low weight, infarcts (5%), retroplacental hematoma	Villi: same as in toxemia, except for less prominence of syncytial knots; maternal arteries—intimal hyperplasia and medial thickening	Toxemia of pregnancy may be superimposed on hypertension
Maternal diabetes	Increased weight, generalized pallor, high incidence of single umbilical artery, localized pallor due to fetal artery thrombosis	Villi: edema, variable maturity (normal, delayed, or accelerated) and vascularity obliterative endarteritis, thrombosis of fetal stem arteries	Maternal vascular lesions are not seen in diabetes without hypertension or toxemia of pregnancy; the placenta may be normal; lesions are less severe and less frequent in gestational diabetes
Abortion	Torsion, stricture and true knot of the cord, massive subchorial thrombosis, partial hydatidiform mole, maternal floor infarction	Villi: (1) normal or (2) stromal fibrosis with prominent trophoblast or (3) hydropic change with hypo- or avascularity of villi or (4) hydatidiform change when partial mole or (5) hypoplastic villi	In hydropic change, there is no circumferential trophoblastic hyperplasia: DNA analysis of the placental tissue by flow cytometry and/or image cytometry should be done if hydatidiform change is present
Premature labor and delivery	Placental findings related to associated obstetrical or maternal condition such as abruptio placentae, preeclampsia, hypertension, diabetes, chorioamnionitis	Placental findings in otherwise normal pregnancies; variable villous maturation (delayed, accelerated, or normal for the gestational age), higher incidence of fibrinoid necrosis of villi	In many cases, there is no detectable associated condition; the placenta may be normal for the gestational age
Postmaturity	Heavy placenta, infarct, and calcification (not more frequent than in term placentas)	Villi: stromal fibrosis, prominent trophoblast, thickened trophoblastic basement membrane, obliterative endarteritis of fetal stem arteries, variable vascularity (normal, hypovascular)	Some cases may be misdiagnosed due to incorrect calculation of the gestational age
Polyhydramnios	Seen in association with fetal malformations (e.g., esophageal atresia), twin transfusion syndrome, maternal diabetes, and chorangioma	No histologic changes related to polyhydramnios	Placental findings are related to the maternal or fetal condition present in the particular case (e.g., vascular anastomoses in twin transfusion syndrome)
Premature, preterm, and prolonged rupture of membranes	Retroplacental hematoma tends to occur more frequently in patients with rupture of membranes	Acute chorioamnionitis	Cultures should be taken in the delivery room in all of these cases

continued

Table 6. *Continued*

Disorders	Salient gross features	Salient microscopic features	Comment
Maternal fever		Chorioamnionitis, villitis, and funisitis related to specific viruses, bacteria, fungi, or parasites are the main lesions seen in the placenta	Malarial parasites may be present in the intervillous space in cases of maternal malaria; placenta may not show any lesion in some cases of maternal fever
Maternal substance abuse	Low weight, retroplacental hematoma, premature rupture of membranes, and meconium staining are seen with higher frequency in different types of substance abuse	Chorioamnionitis, villitis, hypovascularity of villi, and stromal fibrosis	Placenta may be normal; the lesions will vary depending on the type of substance abused
Abruptio placentae	Retroplacental hematoma with/without infarction of the overlying placental territory	Lesions associated with preeclampsia and hypertension seen when these conditions are present	Retroplacental hematoma is present in only 30% of cases of abruption placentae; the blood clot may become detached and not recognized; depression on the maternal surface, with or without an accompanying blood clot can be considered evidence of retroplacental hematoma
Systemic lupus erythematosus (SLE)	Infarct (>25%), retroplacental hematoma	Premature aging of villi, acute atherosis of maternal arteries, and obliterative changes in fetal stem arteries may occur	Acute atherosis with thrombosis also can occur in women with lupus anticoagulant in the absence of SLE; preeclampsia may be superimposed on SLE; therefore the vascular lesions probably reflect the former

From Joshi, ref. 2, with permission.

Table 7. *Salient features of the placenta in fetal disorders*

Disorder	Salient gross features	Salient microscopic features	Comment
Twin birth with MoDi placenta	Single placental disk, two amniotic sacs, of same or dissimilar size, and dividing septus attached to the fetal surface are seen; velamentous or marginal insertion and a single umbilical artery are more frequent; vascular anastomoses are present in 85% to 100% of cases; pallor of the donor and congestion of the recipient territory are seen when there is twin transfusion syndrome; amnion nodosum may be present in the donor territory.	Histologic findings reflecting the gross findings are seen; the dividing septum is composed of two amnions only, without intervening chorion.	Superficial vascular anastomoses can be visualized by naked eye examination; injection studies may be done to confirm these findings; injection studies are the only way to demonstrate deeper arteriovenous anastomoses via a shared lobule. The twin transfusion syndrome is seen in 15% to 30% of twins with MoDi placenta.
Twin birth with DiDi placenta	Two placental disks may be completely separate or fused, resembling the MoDi placenta; the fusion may be partial, with fusion of only a portion of membranes; a dividing septum is present in fused placentas. Vascular anastomoses are extremely rare.	Dividing septum shows chorion between the two amnions.	Twin transfusion is extremely rare; the pathology of separate DiDi placentas is same as that of singleton placenta.[a]
Twin birth with MoMo placenta	Only one amniotic sac and a single placental disk without a dividing septum are present; a small amniotic fold representing disrupted septum of a previously DiDi placenta may be present; vascular anastomoses are common; findings of twin transfusion syndrome described above may be seen; the cords often become entangled.	No specific features other than vascular anastomoses.	Demonstration of vascular anastomoses should be done when twin transfusion syndrome is present. This is the rarest type of twin placenta with a high incidence of fetal morbidity and mortality
Vanishing twins	Plaques of previllous fibrin, embyonic remnants on the membranes, and a second amniotic sac, with or without an embryo may be found; the embryonic remnant appears as a flattened yellow plaque, with or without ocular pigment.	The embryonic remnant shows autolyzed embryonic tissues.	There are few reports describing the pathologic features of the placenta; the placenta should be carefully examined for detection of the embryonic remnant; the twin may be lost via vaginal bleeding.
Fetus papyraceous/ fetus compressus (FP/FC)	FP/FC representing a dead twin is identifiable as a plaque of dehydrated remnant, with or without identifiable fetal parts; umbilical cord torsion or massive infarction may cause fetal death.	Histologic findings reflect the gross abnormalities; autolyzed fetal tissues are seen in the sections from FP/FC.	Careful gross examination is essential to detect FP/FC, roentgenograms may be taken to show the skeleton of FP/FC; the causes of fetal death may not be evident.
Acardiac twin	MoMo placenta with artery-to-artery and vein-to-vein anastomoses between the viable twin and acardiac twin placental territories.	No specific microscopic features other than vascular anastomoses	Vascular anastomoses should be sought; the acardiac twin has no heart or a severely malformed heart; other malformations may also be present.
Intrauterine growth retardation (IUGR)	IUGR is associated with maternal factors (preeclampsia, chronic renal disease, substance abuse, etc.), fetal factors (severe congenital anomalies chromosomal disorders, intrauterine infarctions, etc.), and placental factors (extrachorial placenta, velamentous insertion of cord, maternal floor infarctions, VUE, extensive infarction or perivillous fibrin deposition, etc.); placenta findings related to the maternal, fetal, and placental factors are seen.	Histologic findings related to fetal, maternal, and placental factors are seen.	The placenta is small, which may be a reflection rather than a cause of IUGR; the causes of IUGR may not be evident, and the placenta may be normal except for its size.

continued

Table 7. *Continued.*

Disorder	Salient gross features	Salient microscopic features	Comment
Erythroblastosis fetalis	Enlarged weight and size, pallor, intervillous thrombi	Villi: immature with persistent cytotrophoblast, numerous normoblasts in capillaries, villous edema, hemosiderin in chorionic macrophages	Severity of placental changes is related to severity of fetal anemia; the fetus is hydropic
Nonimmunologic hydrops fetalis (NIHF)	The causes of NIHF include genetic and metabolic disorders, chromosomal abnormalities, cardiac and pulmonary anomalies, thalassemia, fetomaternal hemorrhage, fetal infection, fetal tumors, arrhythmias, congenital nephrotic syndrome; placental findings related to the disorders are present.	Histologic findings related to the associated condition are seen.	In ~22% of NIHF cases, no associated condition can be found.
Chromosomal disorders (trisomy 13, 18, 21)	Small placenta, high incidence of single umbilical artery	Villi: delayed maturation, hypovascularity, large, atypical Hofbauer or trophoblastic cells.	Karyotyping may be done on the chorion or amnion.
Metabolic disorders	Large hydropic placenta	Vacuoles in the syncytiotrophoblasts, intermediate trophoblast, Hofbauer cells, endothelium and fetal WBCs in the villous capillaries.	The vacuoles represent the accumulated metabolite, which is dissolved during processing; electron microscopy may give clues regarding the precise diagnosis (e.g., Nieman-Pick disease, glycogenosis type IV); biochemical study of snap-frozen fresh placental tissue is essential for definitive demonstration of enzyme deficiency.
Antepartum stillbirth, intrauterine fetal death (IUFD).	Massive infarction, retroplacental hematoma, large chorangioma, true knot, torsion or stricture of the cord, nuchal cord, intrauterine infection, maternal floor infarction, and extensive perivillous fibrin deposition are placental lesions than may lead to IUFD.	Histologic findings reflecting these placental lesions are seen; assessment of the interval between IUFD and delivery can be made on the basis of histologic findings.	Maternal conditions (e.g., preeclampsia) and fetal conditions (e.g., erythroblastosis fetalis) may also cause IUFD; certain placental abnormalities such as stromal fibrosis, hypovascularity, thrombosis of vessels in stem villi, and villous edema are secondary to IUFD; confined placental mosaicism may occur in rare cases.

[a] Author's note: There may still be significant fetal-to-placental transfusion after delivery of the first-born twin, but true twin-to-twin transfusion is so unlikely as to necessitate looking for a different etiology should this be a consideration.

MoDi, monochorionic diamnionic; DiDi, dichorionic diamnionic; MoMo, monochorionic, monoamnionic. From Joshi, ref. 2, with permission.

GLOSSARY

Abruptio placentae Synonym *Placental abruption, ablatio placentae, accidental hemorrhage.* Separation of the normally implanted placenta from its uterine site before delivery of the fetus. It may be associated with retroplacental hematomas and vaginal bleeding. Abruption occurs in about 1% of all pregnancies with a higher incidence in conditions of poor maternal nutrition, five or more prior pregnancies, previous abruptions, maternal vascular disease, trauma, cigarette smoking, or cocaine use.

ADAM sequence *Amnionic Deformities, Adhesions, Mutilation* complex that features amputations, strangulations, or absence of body portions in association with amnionic bands (65).

Adams-Oliver syndrome Congenital absence of the lower extremities and fingers and aplasia cutis congenita. This is not the ADAM complex or sequence (85,86).

Amnion The thinnest layer of membrane, lying closest to the fetus, that is continuous over the umbilical cord (umbilical amnion), the placental surface (placental amnion), and chorion laeve (reflected amnion). It is a layer of epithelial cells and connective tissue derived from fetal ectoderm and contains no lymphatics, blood vessels, or nerves. The amnion is involved in the turnover of the amnionic fluid and is at least partly responsible for maintaining the pH of the amnionic fluid. It derives its nutrition from surrounding chorionic fluid, amnionic fluid, fetal surface vessels, or magma reticulare. Because of its avascularity, it is more translucent than the chorion. The amnion is passively attached to the chorion and held in place by intra-amnionic fluid pressure so it may be relatively easily separated from the chorion. Amnion has been used in treatment of burns. It may be considered as an appropriate temporary covering for a gastroschisis or open meningomyelocele in the delivery room.

Apt test Alkaline denaturation of hemoglobin in a pink supernatant of bloody fluid. In the presence of predominantly fetal hemoglobin, the pink color remains but in the presence of predominantly adult hemoglobin, the color changes to yellow.

Bosselation Surface granulation of the placenta that appear as little, gray–white bumps most notable at the periphery and proportionate to the length of gestation (see Fig. 26).

Chorangioma Hemangioma of the placenta that occurs in up to 1% of pregnancies. These are hamartomas that develop most commonly under the chorionic surface. Their appearance may be relatively ill defined and easily confused with other lesions such as thrombus, cysts, and large subchorionic hematomas. Infarction within will also be confusing, and only histologic examination can distinguish them. When the hemangioma acts physiologically like an arteriovenous fistula and puts enough stress on the fetal circulation leading to high output failure, chorangioma may be associated with fetal hydrops.

Chorion The tough, fibrous layer of membrane that lies adjacent to the amnion. The villi arise from its outer surface. It carries fetal blood vessels that persist up to 6 months of gestation. Between the chorion and amnion is an intermediate or spongy layer that is collagen and fibroblasts of fetal origin. There may be persistence of early trophoblastic cells as ghost villi in the chorion. The presence of vessels and opaque villi give the chorion a less transparent appearance than the amnion and helps in distinguishing the two layers.

Chorion frondosum The placenta proper; the placental disk.

Chorion laeve The membranous portion of the chorionic sac.

Circummarginate The membranes insert at some point inward from the edge of the placenta but without the typical folding described in circumvallate placentation and generally not as extensively. Clinically the term is applied when only a portion of the circumference is involved and does not likely carry any clinical significance.

Circumvallate The membranes of the chorion laeve insert with a typical folding at some inward distance from the margin of the placenta, toward the umbilical cord. Clinically the term is applied when the entire circumference is involved and there is more extramembranous placenta but pathologically partial circumvallation occurs (6). Circumvallation is associated with prenatal bleeding and premature delivery but its occurrence in at least 5% of pregnancies suggests it is not always so associated (6).

Cotyledon The lobules on the basal (maternal) surface of the human placenta that are separated by grooves (septa). There are 10 to 40 lobules, each containing several villous trees (6). At the periphery the lobules tend to have fewer villous trees and are more prone to undergo atrophy and infarction.

Dizygotic Pertaining to or derived from two separate zygotes or eggs and, therefore, "fraternal."

False knot of the umbilical cord Synonym *Nodus spurious vasculosus* or *nodus spurious gelatinosus*. Nodular swellings of the cord produced by segmental redundancy, dilatation or branching of the blood vessels, or focal excessive accumulation of Wharton's jelly. The dilated vessels are not prone to rupture or thrombosis. These should be distinguished from umbilical varices and aneurysms, which they may grossly resemble more than true knots.

Fetus papyraceous Synonym *Fetus compressus*. A stillborn fetus of long enough duration to have undergone changes of autolysis and compression with loss of amnionic fluid. When associated with a surviving twin, including situations of unrecognized twinning with loss early in the first half of pregnancy, the fetus may be retained until term when the surviving twin is delivered and be barely recognizable on placental examination as a mass or small nodule.

Funis/funiculus Umbilical cord.

Hemiacardius One of a monozygotic, monochorionic twin gestation in which only part of that twin's circulation is accomplished by its own heart. Remnants of cardiac tissue remain but the majority of its support comes from its twin.

Holoacardius One of a monozygotic, monochorionic twin gestation in which all of its circulation is supported by the remaining twin. The holoacardiac fetus will have a variable anatomy but may be completely amorphous with minimal remnants of human morphology (Fig. 21).

Kleihauer-Betke test Acid denaturation of a dried blood smear. Red blood cells containing adult hemoglobin will loose their density and appear as ghost cells but cells with fetal hemoglobin will remain intact. Results are recorded as a percentage of intact (fetal) cells compared with ghost cells (adult).

Lithopedion A dead fetus of long-standing duration that has become petrified or calcified.

Magma reticulare The gelatinous material that occupies the chorionic cavity between the amnion and the chorion until 10 to 12 weeks' gestation after which time the space is obliterated. The yolk sac is suspended in this space (Fig. 2).

Monozygotic Pertaining to or derived from a single zygote or egg and therefore "identical."

Placenta accreta An unusually adherent placenta that fails to detach after delivery of the infant. It is highly associated with placenta previa and previous uterine surgeries, including curettage, cesarean section, uterine infections, and uterine myomas (87).

Placenta increta Placental villi invade the myometrium superficially but more deeply than with placenta accreta. The associations are similar to accreta.

Placenta membranacea A very unusual type of placenta that envelops the entire or most of the gestational sac with the membranes covered on their outer aspect by villi because of failure to undergo the normal villous atrophy that should lead to formation of the chorion laeve and frondosum. There is high fetal mortality and morbidity rate with recurrent antepartum bleeding.

Placenta percreta Placental villi invade through the myometrium. The associations are similar to accreta but are clinically far more serious.

Placenta previa Implantation of the placenta in the lower uterine segment encroaching on the cervical os so impeding delivery of the fetus through the cervix and prone to bleeding. In all pregnancies the incidence is less than 3% if there has been no previous uterine surgery but the incidence increases almost linearly with the number of uterine incisions to as high as 10% with four or more surgeries (87). It is associated with uterine malformations and leiomyomas as well that inhibit normal implantation. Placenta previa is particularly prone to maternal and fetal bleeding before and with the onset of labor. Placentas that have been documented by ultrasound to be low lying early in gestation clearly seem to move away from that area.

Superfecundation Fertilization of two or more ova at different times during the same menstrual period or having two or more eggs fertilized by sperm from different males.

Superfetation Pregnancy that occurs in the presence of an already existing pregnancy, therefore with the potential for different lengths of gestation to term.

Tessellation The irregular latticelike pattern that occurs as the smallest subchorionic vessels undergo the sclerosis of maturation. It first develops at the margins of the placenta, is rarely apparent before 28 weeks, and progresses toward the center of the placenta.

Vasa previa Fetal blood vessels within the membranes that present before the fetal parts and are therefore subject to compression and rupture with fetal exsanguination.

Vernix caseosa The oily, white material found on the fetal skin that is composed of sebum, hair, desquamated cells, and other secretions from the fetal skin. It covers the fetal skin and provides some element of protection from fluid loss and bacterial invasion.

Vitelline Pertaining or belonging to the yolk sac.

Wharton's jelly The connective tissue of the umbilical cord derived from extraembryonic mesoblast. The substance is a gelatinous material composed of open-chain polysaccharides distributed in a network of microfibrils and a little collagen. It contains fibroblasts and numerous mast cells but few macrophages. Wharton's jelly contributes to the tensile strength of the cord and provides protection against compression to the other structures of the umbilical cord.

References

1. Altshuler G. Some placental considerations related to neurodevelopmental and other disorders. *J Child Neurol* 1993;8:78–94.
2. Joshi VV. *Handbook of placental pathology.* New York: Igaku-Shoin; 1994.
3. Kaplan C. Placental pathology for the nineties. *Pathol Annu* 1993;28(Pt 1):15–72.
4. Benirschke K. The placenta in the litigation process. *Am J Obstet Gynecol* 1990;162:1445–1450.
5. Salafia CM, Vintzileos AM. Why all placentas should be examined by a pathologist in 1990. *Am J Obstet Gynecol* 1990;163:1282–1293.
6. Benirschke K, Kaufmann P. Pathology of the human placenta. 2nd ed. New York: Springer-Verlag; 1990.
7. Naeye RL. Do placental weights have clinical significance? *Hum Pathol* 1987;18:387–391.
8. Naeye RL. Umbilical cord length: clinical significance. *J Pediatr* 1985;107:278–281.
9. Mills JL, Harley EE, Moessinger AC. Standards for measuring umbilical cord length. *Placenta* 1983;4:423–426.
10. Gardiner JP. The umbilical cord. *Surg Gynecol Obstet* 1922;34:252–256.
11. Miller ME, Higginbottom M, Smith DW. Short umbilical cord: its origin and relevance. *Pediatrics* 1981;67:618–621.
12. Miller ME, Jones MC, Smith DW. Tension: the basis of umbilical cord growth. *J Pediatr* 1982;101:844.
13. Moessinger AC, Blanc WA, Marone PA, Polsen DC. Umbilical cord length as an index of fetal activity: experimental study and clinical implications. *Pediatr Res* 1982;16:109–112.
14. Moessinger AC, Mills JL, Harley EE, Ramakrishnan R, Berendes HW, Blanc WA. Umbilical cord length in Down's syndrome. *Am J Dis Child* 1986;140:1276–1277.
15. Katz V, Blanchard G, Dingman C, Bowes WA Jr, Cefalo RC. Atenolol and short umbilical cords. *Am J Obstet Gynecol* 1987;156:1271–1272.
16. Soernes T, Bakke T. The length of the human umbilical cord in twin pregnancies. *Am J Obstet Gynecol* 1987;157:1229–1230.
17. Soernes T, Bakke T. The length of the human umbilical cord in vertex and breech presentations. *Am J Obstet Gynecol* 1986;154:1086–1087.
18. Giacoia GP. Body stalk anomaly: congenital absence of the umbilical cord. *Obstet Gynecol* 1992;80(3 Pt 2):527–529.
19. Gunther WM, Anderson VM, Drut RM. Torque deformation sequence associated with short umbilical cord and abdominal wall defect. *Birth Defects* 1993;29:317–333.
20. Gilbert-Barness E, Drut RM, Drut R, Grange DK, Opitz JM. Developmental abnormalities resulting in short umbilical cord. *Birth Defects* 1993;29:113–140.
21. Scheffel T, Langanke D. [Umbilical cord complications at the Leipzig University Gynecologic Clinic during 1955–1967]. *Zentralbl Gynakol* 1970;92:429–434.
22. Chasnoff IJ, Fletcher MA. True knot of the umbilical cord. *Am J Obstet Gynecol* 1977;127:425–427.
23. Lacro RV, Jones KL, Benirschke K. The umbilical cord twist: origin, direction, and relevance. *Am J Obstet Gynecol* 1987;157(4 Pt 1):833–838.

24. Strong TH Jr, Elliott JP, Radin TG. Non-coiled umbilical blood vessels: a new marker for the fetus at risk. *Obstet Gynecol* 1993;81:409–411.
25. Rana J, Ebert GA, Kappy KA. Adverse perinatal outcome in patients with an abnormal umbilical coiling index. *Obstet Gynecol* 1995;85:573–577.
26. Collins JH. Prenatal observation of umbilical cord torsion with subsequent premature labor and delivery of a 31-week infant with mild nonimmune hydrops. *Am J Obstet Gynecol* 1995;172:1048–1049.
27. Robertson RD, Rubinstein LM, Wolfson WL, Lebherz TB, Blanchard JB, Crandall BF. Constriction of the umbilical cord as a cause of fetal demise following midtrimester amniocentesis. *J Reprod Med* 1981;26: 325–327.
28. Jones TB, Sorokin Y, Bhatia R, Zador IE, Bottoms SF. Single umbilical artery: accurate diagnosis? *Am J Obstet Gynecol* 1993;169:538–540.
29. Bourke WG, Clarke TA, Mathews TG, O'Halpin D, Donoghue VB. Isolated single umbilical artery—the case for routine renal screening. *Arch Dis Child* 1993;68(5 Spec No):600–601.
30. Lilja M. Infants with single umbilical artery studied in a national registry. General epidemiological characteristics. *Paediatr Perinat Epidemiol* 1991;5:27–36.
31. Lilja M. Infants with single umbilical artery studied in a national registry. 2: Survival and malformations in infants with single umbilical artery. *Paediatr Perinat Epidemiol* 1992;6:416–422.
32. Khong TY, George K. Chromosomal abnormalities associated with a single umbilical artery. *Prenat Diagn* 1992;12:965–968.
33. Nyberg DA, Mahony BS, Luthy D, Kapur R. Single umbilical artery. Prenatal detection of concurrent anomalies. *J Ultrasound Med* 1991;10:247–253.
34. Leung AK, Robson WL. Single umbilical artery. A report of 159 cases. *Am J Dis Child* 1989;143:108–111.
35. Froehlich LA, Fujikura T. Follow-up of infants with single umbilical artry. *Pediatrics* 1973;52:6–13.
36. Saller DN Jr, Neiger R. Cytogenetic abnormalities among perinatal deaths demonstrating a single umbilical artery. *Prenat Diagn* 1994;14:13–16.
37. Saller DN Jr, Keene CL, Sun CC, Schwartz S. The association of single umbilical artery with cytogenetically abnormal pregnancies. *Am J Obstet Gynecol* 1990;163:922–925.
38. Craver RD, Baldwin VJ. Necrotizing funisitis. *Obstet Gynecol* 1992;79:64–70.
39. Fojaco RM, Hensley GT, Moskowitz L. Congenital syphilis and necrotizing funisitis. *JAMA* 1989;261: 1788–1790.
40. Benirschke K. Congenital syphilis and necrotizing funisitis. *JAMA* 1989;262:904.
41. Schwartz DA, Reef S. Candida albicans placentitis and funisitis: early diagnosis of congenital candidemia by histopathologic examination of umbilical cord vessels. *Pediatr Infect Dis J* 1990;9:661.
42. Hood IC, Desa DJ, Whyte RK. The inflammatory response in candidal chorioamnionitis. *Hum Pathol* 1983; 14:984–990.
43. Silver RK, Dooley SL, Tamura RK, Depp R. Umbilical cord size and amnionic fluid volume in prolonged pregnancy. *Am J Obstet Gynecol* 1985;157:716–720.
44. Shipp TD, Bromley B, Benacerraf BR. Sonographically detected abnormalities of the umbilical cord. *Int J Gynaecol Obstet* 1995;48:179–185.
45. Kaplan CG. *Color atlas of gross placental pathology*. 1st ed. New York: Igaku-Shoin; 1994.
46. Robinson LK, Jones KL, Benirschke K. The nature of structural defects associated with velamentous and marginal insertion of the umbilical cord. *Am J Obstet Gynecol* 1983;146:191–193.
47. Quek SP, Tan KL. Vasa Praevia. *Aust N Z J Obstet Gynaecol* 1972;12:206–209.
48. Fries MH, Goldstein RB, Kilpatrick SJ, Golbus MS, Callen PW, Filly RA. The role of velamentous cord insertion in the etiology of twin-twin transfusion syndrome. *Obstet Gynecol* 1993;81:569–574.
49. Heckel S, Weber P, Dellenbach P. [Benckiser's hemorrhage. 2 case reports and a review of the literature]. *J Gynecol Obstet Biol Reprod (Paris)* 1993;22:184–190.
50. Chenard E, Bastide A, Fraser WD. Umbilical cord hematoma following diagnostic funipuncture. *Obstet Gynecol* 1990;76(5 Pt 2):994–996.
51. Jauniaux E, Nicolaides KH, Campbell S, Hustin J. Hematoma of the umbilical cord secondary to cordocentesis for intrauterine fetal transfusion [Letter; comment]. *Prenat Diagn* 1990;10:477–478.
52. Fletcher MA, Meyer M, Kirkpatrick SE, Papelbaum S, Gluck L, Benirschke K. Myocardial infarction associated with umbilical cord hematoma. *J Pediatr* 1976;89:806–807.
53. Usher RH, Boyd ME, McLean FH, Kramer MS. Assessment of fetal risk in postdate pregnancies. *Am J Obstet Gynecol* 1988;158:259–264.
54. Miller PW, Coen RW, Benirschke K. Dating the time interval from meconium passage to birth. *Obstet Gynecol* 1985;66:459–462.
55. Fujikura T, Klionsky B. The significance of meconium staining. *Am J Obstet Gynecol* 1975;121:45–50.
56. Landing BH. Amnion nodosum: a lesion of the placenta apparently associated with deficient secretion of fetal urine. *Am J Obstet Gynecol* 1950;60:1339–1342.
57. Elchalal U, Ashkenazy M, Weissman A, Rosenman D, Blickstein I. Strangulation of the umbilical cord due to combined amnionic band and true knot. *Int J Gynaecol Obstet* 1992;38:45–47.
58. Baler J, Topper SF, Hashimoto K, Sturman S. Linear erosions in a newborn. Amnionic band syndrome. *Arch Dermatol* 1994;130:1057–1060.
59. Lage JM, VanMarter LJ, Bieber FR. Questionable role of amniocentesis in the etiology of amnionic band formation. A case report. *J Reprod Med* 1988;33:71–73.
60. Kohn G. The amnionic band syndrome: a possible complication of amniocentesis. *Prenat Diagn* 1987; 7:303–305.
61. Hughes RM, Benzie RJ, Thompson CL. Amnionic band syndrome causing fetal head deformity. *Prenat Diagn* 1984;4:447–450.
62. Bamforth JS. Amnionic band sequence: Streeter's hypothesis reexamined. *Am J Med Genet* 1992;44: 280–287.
63. Murata T, Hashimoto S, Ishibashi T, Inomata H, Sueishi K. A case of amnionic band syndrome with bilateral epibulbar choristoma. *Br J Ophthalmol* 1992;76:685–687.

64. Nishi T, Nakano R. Amnionic band syndrome: serial ultrasonographic observations in the first trimester. *J Clin Ultrasound* 1994;22:275–278.
65. Yang SS. ADAM sequence and innocent amnionic band: manifestations of early amnion rupture. *Am J Med Genet* 1990;37:562–568.
66. Wehbeh H, Fleisher J, Karimi A, Mathony A, Minkoff H. The relationship between the ultrasonographic diagnosis of innocent amnionic band development and pregnancy outcomes. *Obstet Gynecol* 1993;81:565–568.
67. Seidman JD, Abbondanzo SL, Watkin WG, Ragsdale B, Manz HJ. Amnionic band syndrome. Report of two cases and review of the literature. *Arch Pathol Lab Med* 1989;113:891–897.
68. Hunter AG, Carpenter BF. Implications of malformations not due to amnionic bands in the amnionic band sequence. *Am J Med Genet* 1986;24:691–700.
69. Irving WL, Doublestein GL. Congenital amnionic band syndrome: report of a familial recurrence. *J Am Osteopath Assoc* 1988;88:891–893.
70. Froster UG, Baird PA. Amnionic band sequence and limb defects: data from a population-based study. *Am J Med Genet* 1993;46:497–500.
71. Bhargava I, Raja PT. Arteriovenous crossings on the chorial surface of the human placenta in abnormal pregnancy and development. *Experientia* 1969;25:831–832.
72. Pearlstone M, Baxi L. Subchorionic hematoma: a review. *Obstet Gynecol Surv* 1993;48:65–68.
73. Shanklin DR, Scott JS. Massive subchorial thrombohaematoma (Breus' mole). *Br J Obstet Gynaecol* 1975;82:476–487.
74. Olah KS, Gee H, Rushton I, Fowlie A. Massive subchorionic thrombohaematoma presenting as a placental tumour. Case report. *Br J Obstet Gynaecol* 1987;94:995–997.
75. Gemer O, Zohav E, Calman D, Sassoon E, Segal S. Synchronous intrauterine and tubal pregnancies with subchorionic hematoma [see comments]. *Acta Obstet Gynecol Scand* 1993;72:495–496.
76. Fruchter O. Subchorionic hematoma and autoantibodies: is there a relation? [Letter; comment]. *Am J Obstet Gynecol* 1992;167(4 Pt 1):1150.
77. Dickey RP, Olar TT, Curole DN, Taylor SN, Matulich EM. Relationship of first-trimester subchorionic bleeding detected by color Doppler ultrasound to subchorionic fluid, clinical bleeding, and pregnancy outcome. *Obstet Gynecol* 1992;80(3 Pt 1):415–420.
78. Thomas D, Makhoul J, Muller C. Fetal growth retardation due to massive subchorionic thrombohematoma: report of two cases. *J Ultrasound Med* 1992;11:245–247.
79. Mimmo B, Boggio G, Mossetti M, Caula E, Botta G, Pagliano M. [Massive subchorionic fibrin deposit: echographic diagnosis]. *Minerva Ginecol* 1992;44:147–150.
80. Baxi LV, Pearlstone MM. Subchorionic hematomas and the presence of autoantibodies [see comments]. *Am J Obstet Gynecol* 1991;165(5 Pt 1):1423–1424.
81. Katz VL, Blanchard GF Jr, Watson WJ, Miller RC, Chescheir NC, Thorp JM Jr. The clinical implications of subchorionic placental lucencies. *Am J Obstet Gynecol* 1991;164(1 Pt 1):99–100.
82. Pedersen JF, Mantoni M. Prevalence and significance of subchorionic hemorrhage in threatened abortion: a sonographic study. *AJR* 1990;154:535–537.
83. Andres RL, Kuyper W, Resnik R, Piacquadio KM, Benirschke K. The association of maternal floor infarction of the placenta with adverse perinatal outcome. *Am J Obstet Gynecol* 1990;163:935–938.
84. Naeye RL. Maternal floor infarction. *Hum Pathol* 1985;16:823–828.
85. Adams FH, Oliver CP. Hereditary deformities in man due to arrested development. *J Hered* 1949;36:3–7.
86. Bonafede RP, Beighton P. Autosomal dominant inheritance of scalp defects with ectrodactyly. *Am J Med Genet* 1979;3:35–41.
87. Clark SL, Koonings PP, Phelan JP. Placenta previa/accreta and prior cesarean section. *Obstet Gynecol* 1985;66:89–92.
88. Hall JG, Froster-Iskenius UG, Allanson JE. *Handbook of normal physical measurements.* Oxford: Oxford University Press; 1989.
89. Molteni RA, Stys SJ, Battaglia FC. Relationship of fetal and placental weight in human beings: fetal/placental weight ratios at various gestational ages and birth weight distributions. *J Reprod Med* 1978;21:327–334.
90. Kaufmann P. Entwicklung der plazenta. In: Becker V, et al., eds. *Die Plazenta des Menschen.* Stuttgart: Thieme; 1981:13–50.
91. Heifetz SA. The placenta. In: Stocker JT, Dehner LP, eds. *Pediatric pathology.* 1st ed. Vol. 1. Philadelphia: JB Lippincott; 1992:387–423.

5

Skin

The most important tool in physical diagnosis is inspection and no organ presents itself more readily for direct inspection than the skin. This is the first area encountered for physical examination whether the approach is by region or by systems. If the general examination is approached by regions, the skin is part of each regional assessment. If by systems, its findings suggest processes in the skin itself as well as in all other body systems because it is a window to other body systems and to how well they are functioning. In some respects that window is quite transparent and allows semiquantitative assessment of blood contents by estimation of bilirubin, hematocrit, or oxygen content as examples. In other respects, the skin is only translucent and allows just enough information to filter through to suggest an internal process or malformation, for example, the neurocutaneous syndromes.

ANATOMY OF NEONATAL SKIN

The anatomy of the fetal and neonatal skin is depicted in Fig. 1.

The epidermis is the outermost layer of the skin and is composed of keratinized cells that are constantly shed and replenished from below. Keratinization occurs first and most rapidly on the palms, soles, face, and scalp.

The dermis is the inner layer that contains the vessels, sensory nerve endings, and glands, as well as the autonomic nerve fibers for the associated vessels and glands.

The hypodermis or subcutis lies under the dermis and is a layer of connective tissues and fat attaching the dermis to the underlying structures.

Within the dermis are the specialized glands and the source for the skin appendages, the hair and nails. The eccrine or sweat glands develop first in the areas where keratinization occurs the earliest. The density of glands is highest at birth but the activity is relatively low until the second or third year of life (1). In term infants, sweating is first apparent on the forehead and palms (2). The pilosebaceous glands develop in a cephalocaudad direction and become active earlier than do other glands. Keratinization of the skin at the hair follicle occurs several weeks before keratinization of skin between the follicles (3). The sebaceous glands are under the influence of maternal androgens and endogenously produced steroids. Very active at birth, they become less active over the first year of life.

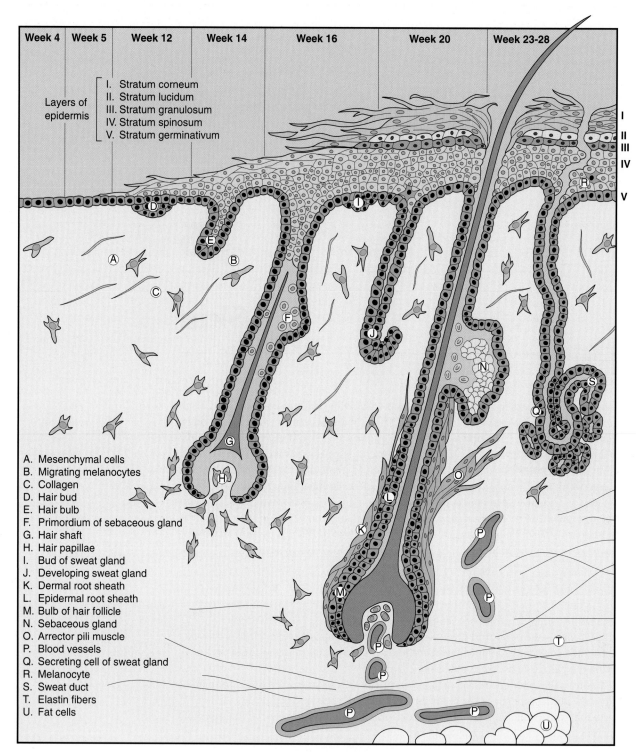

Figure 1. Anatomy of the skin.

Week 4 | Week 5 | Week 12 | Week 14 | Week 16 | Week 20 | Week 23-28

Layers of epidermis
- I. Stratum corneum
- II. Stratum lucidum
- III. Stratum granulosum
- IV. Stratum spinosum
- V. Stratum germinativum

I
II
III
IV
V

A. Mesenchymal cells
B. Migrating melanocytes
C. Collagen
D. Hair bud
E. Hair bulb
F. Primordium of sebaceous gland
G. Hair shaft
H. Hair papillae
I. Bud of sweat gland
J. Developing sweat gland
K. Dermal root sheath
L. Epidermal root sheath
M. Bulb of hair follicle
N. Sebaceous gland
O. Arrector pili muscle
P. Blood vessels
Q. Secreting cell of sweat gland
R. Melanocyte
S. Sweat duct
T. Elastin fibers
U. Fat cells

Table 1. *Comparison of the structural properties of the skin of the second trimester fetus, premature infant (third trimester), newborn infant, and older child/adult*

	Fetal (second trimester)	Premature (third trimester)	Newborn infant	Child/Adult	Ref
Full-thickness	0.5–0.9 mm	0.9 mm	1.2 mm	2.1 mm	207–209
Epidermal surface	Periderm	Cornified; some vernix caseosa	Cornified; may have some vernix caseosa	Dry; sebaceous lipids may be present	
Epidermal thickness	50–60 μ	50–60 μ	~50–60 μ	>70 μ	210
Stratum corneum thickness	NA	4–5 μ	9–10 μ	9–15 μ	209
Stratum corneum barrier	Permeable	Permeable in the fetus and preterm infant; becomes similar to the adult and full-term infant after 2–3 wks postnatal maturation	Effective permeability barrier	Effective permeability barrier	211–214
Melanocytes	Dendritic; melanogenic; ~800 cells/mm^2	Dendritic; melanogenic; ?density	Dendritic; melanogenic; 800–900 cells/mm^2	Dendritic; melanogenic; 600–700 cells/mm^2	215, 216
Pilosebaceous structures	Bulbous hair peg stage; keratinization of the hair and follicle occurs	Lanugo follicle; sebaceous gland well developed; hairs exposed	Lanugo follicle; may have second hair pelage; large, active sebaceous gland	Follicles produce vellus or terminal hairs; sebaceous glands become quiescent until later childhood	217, 218
Eccrine sweat glands	Formed only on palms and soles; primordia appear on other regions of the body later in this period	Sweat glands present; high in the dermis; sweating is unlikely to occur	Sweat glands present; still high in the dermis; not fully functional	Sweat glands become positioned deeper in the dermis; most are active within the first few years	2, 219
Hypodermis	Fine connective tissue framework of lobules; few adipocytes	Subcutaneous fat lobules	Subcutaneous fat layer; depends on nutritional status	Subcutaneous fat layer	220

Modified from Holbrook, ref. 3, with permission.

Comparison of Adult and Neonatal Skin

The skin of the neonate differs from adult skin in several ways, with variances especially pronounced in extreme prematurity. These differences are sufficient to make attention to them important both in determining general care and in interpreting physical findings (Table 1). Because it is relatively thin and less pigmented, the appearance of neonatal skin responds rapidly to environmental and internal processes, potentially providing more information about the infant's well-being than in older patients. In the first few hours and days of life, skin appearance can change dramatically as the circulation shifts from fetal pathways, jaundice develops, light bathes the surface for the first time, ambient temperatures fluctuate, and colonization of skin flora begins. No longer is the skin provided a stable and protective environment where it is constantly bathed and protected by vernix and amnionic fluid, but the skin has to assume its full responsibility for protecting the infant. The more immature the infant at birth, the less prepared the skin is to perform that function and the more subject it is to injury. Because the skin continues to develop and change in appearance after birth, lesions that are truly congenital may not be apparent at birth, may decrease in activity and size after the effect of maternal hormones subsides, or may disappear completely.

TECHNIQUE OF EXAMINATION

Steps in Examination of the Skin

Inspect and palpate skin
    Color
    Moisture
    Temperature
    Texture and creasing
    Mobility and turgor
    Lesions
        Measurements in all dimensions
        Configuration
        Elevation or depression
        Palpable characteristics (or absence)
        Color(s)
        Location(s) on body
        Pattern of distribution
Inspect and palpate fingernails and toenails
    Color
    Size
    Shape
    Lesions
Inspect and palpate the hair
    Color
    Distribution
    Pattern of growth
    Texture
    Unusual concentration
Take scraping or aspirant for stain or culture when indicated
Photograph findings as indicated

General Examination

Examination of the skin requires skill primarily in being able to describe accurately what is seen or felt. On the basis of these descriptions and the effect of time or environment, a reasonable differential diagnosis is immediately available. As it is in all phases of the examination, using clear descriptors accurately is especially important both in making the diagnosis and in communicating the findings to record for follow-up examination of the skin. The basic types of descriptors for the skin include color, quantity, size, shape and pattern of distribution, and texture. Tables 2 through 5 provide some definitions for the more commonly needed subjective appearances; others are listed in the glossary. The International League of Dermatological Societies Committee on Nomenclature has published a glossary of basic dermatology lesions to promote more standardized communication of skin findings (4).

Inspect the skin, the nails, and the hair. Examine the skin with the infant completely exposed to allow comparison between body regions. Use as much natural light as possible rather than fluorescent lighting. If the infant is under phototherapy, turn the lights off, remove any eye patches, and look at all sides, including areas hidden in skin folds or by external equipment.

A described skin color results from a combination of the light in which it is viewed, the quantity and type of pigments developed or deposited, the thickness and character of the various structures, and the perception of the observer. There are wide swings in overall color from relative pallor to erythema as an infant goes from deep sleep to vigorous crying. *Erythema neonatorum* is the generalized hyperemia that develops a few hours after birth, typically during a bath when the infant cries vigorously. It resolves within a few minutes to

Table 2. *Color variations in skin findings: localized to lesions or general hue*

Black	Melanin in highest concentration, some nevi
Blue–gray	Deep blood collection (venous malformation, deep hemangioma); dermal melanosis: blue nevus of Ota, nevus of Ito, Mongolian spot
Dark brown	Melanin near surface (melanocytic nevus)
	Exogenous chemical: silver nitrate
Pale brown	Melanin near surface; immature development of eumelanin
Muddy brown	Melanin in superficial dermis; base of lesions of transient pustular melanosis
Purple	Vascular lesions: hemangioma
Dusky blue	Reduced hemoglobin, methemoglobinemia
Bright blue	Exogenous pigment: triple dye for cord care; methylene blue, acrocyanosis
Violaceous and lilac	Early superficial hemangioma
Pink–red	Many exanthemata
	Normal neonatal skin color in light pigmented infants
Red–brown	Inflammatory reaction (lesions of congenital syphilis)
Scarlet red	Lesions with increased arterial supply: pyogenic granuloma, carbon monoxide poisoning; early superficial hemangioma
Orange	Sebaceous nevus, particularly when infant is jaundiced
Yellow–white	Xanthoma; xanthogranuloma, sebaceous nevus
Yellow	Jaundice due to elevated indirect (unconjugated) bilirubin
Green	Meconium staining; high direct bilirubin level; combination of jaundice, cyanosis, and pallor
White (or pale pink, depending on vascularity)	Loss of pigment: piebaldism, albinism, vitiligo, burns, scars, early arterial insufficiency, anemia

From Lawrence and Cox, ref. 221, with permission.

Table 3. *Distribution and quantification of skin lesions*

Single	Occurring by itself
Grouped	Multiple discrete lesions in a localized area (e.g., herpetiform); a particularly close grouping of nodules is known as agminated
Scattered	Describes widespread lesions without a uniform pattern that is further qualified as localized, regional, or generalized
Disseminated	Multiple small, uniformly distributed pattern that is further qualified as localized, regional, or generalized
Exanthematous	Multiple red and/or scaly lesions that are generally predominant on the trunk (e.g., infection and drug eruptions are frequent causes). Further descriptions include morbilliform; measles-like with blotchy pinkish–brown lesions or scarlatiniform; scarlet fever-like lesions that are tiny red papules or petechiae).
Confluent	Refers to lesions of any type and severity when they merge to cover a wider area. Erythroderma implies total redness of the skin due to confluence of lesions over a large area.
Symmetric, asymmetric	Symmetric lesions suggest an endogenous or systemic cause while asymmetric lesions suggest exogenous cause such as a skin infection or irritation. There are many exceptions to this concept.
Photosensitive	Pattern confined to light-exposed areas.
Gravitational	Developing in the most dependent regions. In neonates this pattern depends on what position the infant was in at the time of lesion formation. It may mean sacral and scapular although it can include eyelids or lower extremities. If related to vertex positioning in utero, it may mean above the neck.
Regional involvement or sparing: creases, islands, peristomal	Lesions may develop in only certain areas or with striking patterns of sparing. Typically, contact, irritant rashes spare creases, whereas candidial infections classically involve creases most heavily. There is overlap in either case. The regions typically are palms/soles, intertriginous (skin folds), diaper area, trunk only, face and neck only, scalp, dermatomal distribution, pressure areas.

These terms are relatively imprecise and more subject to individual interpretation.

Table 4. *Shapes and patterns of skin lesions found in newborn infants*

Discoid, nummular, or coin-shaped	A filled circle with fairly sharp demarcation and uniformity; coin-shaped
Annular	A ring or empty circle shape
Target	An arrangement of concentric rings (e.g., iris, bull's eye); in practice, target is used to describe rashes (lupus)
Cocade	Rosettelike; *en cocarde*; in practice, cocade is used to describe a static variant or a benign pigmented nevus that has a bull's eye appearance
Arcuate	Curved lesions with the appearance of a part, or arc, or a circle (urticaria)
Circinate	Circular although in practice applied when the circle is not quite complete (when complete, use annular; when less than $\frac{1}{2}$ complete, use arcuate) (urticaria)
Polycyclic	Interlocking or coalesced, unfilled circles; these eruptions are usually formed by enlargement of annular lesions that coalesce and enlarge further (tinea corpora or lupus)
Petaloid	Similar to polycyclic but refers to interlocking, filled circles to form a flower shape (seborrheic dermatitis)
Whorled	Roughly concentric parts of circles or spirals with a stirred appearance; lesions may follow developmental lines of Blaschko with cutting off in the midline (hypomelanosis of Ito, incontinentia pigmenti)
Stellate	Star-shaped; lesions with a radial spread but not rounded
Oval	A common shape in skin lesions often with discoid lesions in erythematous rashes; they tend to form mostly on the trunk with the long axis following dermatomal lines
Digitate	More extreme elongated ovals or finger shaped
Serpiginous	Wavy, angulated, or snakelike line; gyrate
Linear	Occurring in lines; these lines may represent blood vessels, lymphatics, developmental lines of Blaschko, tracking lines of infestations (scabies), or externally caused lesions
Dermatomal	Lesions that follow nerve dermatomes are linear on the trunk and limbs but have a more typical distribution on the face, neck, or sacrum (synonym: zosteriform)
Reticulate	Lacelike appearance describing either the overall appearance or close-up features of individual lesions (synonym: retiform)
Livedo	A lacelike pattern of erythema that follows the vascular supply to the skin
Cribriform	A pattern of strand-like scarring resembling a colander
Unusual or perfect geometric shapes	Particularly if accompanied by erosive or ulcerated components, lesions with shapes that are perfect circles, squares, or lines in neonates suggest external or iatrogenic causes
Multiform	A combination of shapes

From Lawrence and Cox, ref. 221, with permission.

an hour and only rarely recurs with the same intensity, even with further crying episodes. This event of total blushing is noteworthy in that it likely signals the successful completion of fetal to neonatal transition in the cardiopulmonary system and provides some reassurance of the health in that infant. This term is often used in literature as synonymous with erythema toxicum neonatorum, but its use should be reserved for simply the red newborn infant (5).

Comparison of colors is the best way to detect variations, and identical twins provide one of the best opportunities (Fig. 2). Natural light with neutral background allows the most accurate comparison of hue and intensity. Two of the most important colors to distinguish are the blues of true hypoxemia and the yellows of jaundice.

Cyanosis means "blue," but its clinical use is generally reserved for the appearance of the skin when the blood oxyhemoglobin content is low rather than for other conditions where the skin and mucous membranes might be blue from pigment or extravascular hemoglobin deposits (Fig. 3). It takes desaturation of approximately 5 g of hemoglobin for

Table 5. *Types of skin lesions likely to occur in newborn infants*

Papule	A papule is a small solid elevation of the skin, less than 0.5 cm in diameter. Its description may be further subdivided according to its location or character: epidermal, dermal, inflammatory, papulosquamous, or wheal.
Pustule	A visible accumulation of pus. This may develop within a pilosebaceous follicle or a sweat duct or on glabrous skin.
Vesicle	A vesicle is a circumscribed elevation of the skin less than 0.5 cm in diameter and containing a liquid.
Bulla	A bulla is circumscribed elevation of skin over 0.5 cm in diameter containing a liquid; also a bleb or a blister. The distinction between vesicle and bulla is arbitrary and depends only on size.
Dermal bulla	A bulla caused by separation of tissue components of the dermis with collection of serous fluid.
Epidermal vesicle or bulla	A blister formed within the epidermis by pathologic change in epidermal cells or cellular cohesion.
Spongiotic vesicle or bulla	An intraepidermal multilocular vesicle or blister formed by separation of epidermal cells by edema. Lymphocytes predominate in allergic contact dermatitis and neutrophilic leukocytes predominate in irritant dermatitis.
Subcorneal bulla	A bulla formed by exudate beneath the stratum spinosum, as in bullous impetigo.
Subepidermal vesicle or bulla	A vesicle or bulla formed by cleavage of the dermal-epidermal interface and with the roof of the bulla composed of the epidermis.
Excoriation	A loss of skin substance produced by scratching. Excoriations may be linear and superfiical or sharply demarcated and deep.
Erosion	A loss of epidermis that heals without scarring, commonly after a blister.
Ulcer	A defect or loss of dermis and epidermis produced by sloughing of necrotic tissue.
Fissure	Any linear gap or slit in the skin surface.
Atrophy	A loss of tissue characterized by the loss of normal skin markings. It may affect epidermis, dermis, or subcutaneous tissues.
Scale	A scale is a flat plate or flake of stratum corneum.
Colarette scale	Describes the fine, peripherally attached and centrally detached scale at the edge of an inflammatory lesion (e.g., transient pustulosis)
Furfuraceous	Describes fine and loose scales (e.g., normal postpartum scaling)
Ichthyosiform	Describes large, polygonal scales, as in fish scales (e.g., lamellar ichthyosis or post-maturity scaling)
Psoriasiform (resembling psoriasis)	Describes a silvery, white parakeratotic, lamellated scale, similar to a scale of psoriasis (neonatal lupus)
Crust	A covering consisting or dried serum and other exudates (synonym: scab)
Macule	A circumscribed alteration in the color or texture of the skin consisting of erythema (vasodilation and inflammation), blood pigments (purpura), or an excess or deficiency of melanin. A maculopapular rash consists of macules and papules.
Patch	A large macule, more than 2 cm or more in diameter.
Plaque	An elevated area of skin 2 cm or more in diameter. Plaques may have the same subdivisions as mentioned above under papules. It may be formed by the extension or coalescence of either papules or nodules.
Nodule	A solid mass in the skin that can be observed as an elevation or can be palpated. Usually 0.5 cm or more in diameter. It may involve epidermis and dermis, dermis and subcutis, or subcutis alone. It may consist of edema, inflammatory cells, or infiltrate.
Wheal	An elevated, white compressible, evanescent area produced by dermal edema. It is often surrounded by a red, axon-mediated flare.
Erythema	Redness of the skin produced by vascular congestion or increased perfusion (synonym: blush)
Ecchymosis	A macular red or purple colored hemorrhage in skin or mucous membrane more than 2 mm in diameter (synonym: bruise)
Hematoma	A localized collection of blood
Petechia	A punctate hemorrhage spot approximately 1–2 mm in diameter that is nonblanching. It resolves with degradation of the hemoglobin.
Purpura	Discoloration of the skin or mucosa due to extravasation of blood.
Telangiectasia	A visible vascular lesion formed by dilation of small cutaneous blood vessels.

From Winkelmann, ref. 4, with permission.

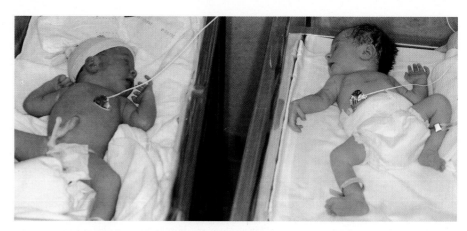

Figure 2. Twins of twin-to-twin transfusion syndrome. Hematocrit of the pale twin on the right was 32%, and that of the erythematous twin on the left was 60%.

most people to perceive a blue color. If the hemoglobin level is very high as it is in healthy term infants, cyanosis is readily seen even when the total blood oxygen content may be sufficient. In contrast, if there is severe anemia, pallor supersedes cyanosis. **Acrocyanosis** occurs when the blood flow to an area is slow enough that all available oxygen is extracted during its course through the region (Fig. 3D). Commonly found in the early hours after birth especially before erythema neonatorum develops, acrocyanosis disappears as the area is warmed and recurs with cooling.

Jaundice is best detected by compressing the skin to subtract the color contributed by hemoglobin in the blood vessels (Fig. 4). The color changes develop from the head caudally at a rate comparable with the increasing level of serum bilirubin (6). The heavier the layer of subcutaneous fat, the slower the progression, so thin, premature infants demonstrate jaundice in their lower extremities at lower serum levels and more quickly than do fat, term babies. In conditions of rapidly increasing serum bilirubin, the skin changes will lag somewhat. Deposition in the sclera is relatively late and usually indicates a bilirubin level greater than 10 mg/dl (171 μmol/L).

When hyperbilirubinemia is primarily the result of indirect or unconjugated bilirubin, jaundice gives a yellow cast to the skin and mucous membranes. If the hyperbilirubinemia has a significant portion as conjugated or direct reacting bilirubin, the jaundice appears greener. In darkly pigmented or cyanotic infants this appears muddy green.

Infants affected by intrauterine hemolytic processes with elevated amnionic levels of bilirubin have vernix and umbilical cords with a yellow stain, but the cause cannot be easily differentiated from other sources of bilirubin, such as old blood associated with abruptio placentae or prior meconium passage.

Transcutaneous estimation of bilirubin using photoelectric meters allows comparison of yellowness within an individual for paralleling serum levels but is highly affected by the basal level of skin pigmentation and amount of subcutaneous fat, so it is not as helpful for comparison among infants (7).

Phototherapy makes dermal estimation of serum bilirubin invalid. Areas unexposed during phototherapy retain their jaundice until the serum levels decrease, whereas the areas exposed to the light bleach in response to photometabolism. Besides its positive effect on the dermal metabolism of bilirubin, phototherapy has several other direct effects on the skin. Infants can develop a macular rash similar to the earliest phases of erythema toxicum neonatorum (8). There can be a marked darkening of skin due either to induction of normal pigmentation or to increased melanogenesis (9). If the darkening is due to increased melanogenesis, it can persist for months and be rather troublesome to parents, particularly if there are patches of lighter areas that were unexposed. Exposure to the drying heat of the lights aggravates the expected scaling and dehydration, particularly in premature infants (10). An increase in stooling sometimes causes perianal excoriations (11). An important skin change from phototherapy is the bronze baby syndrome that results in dark

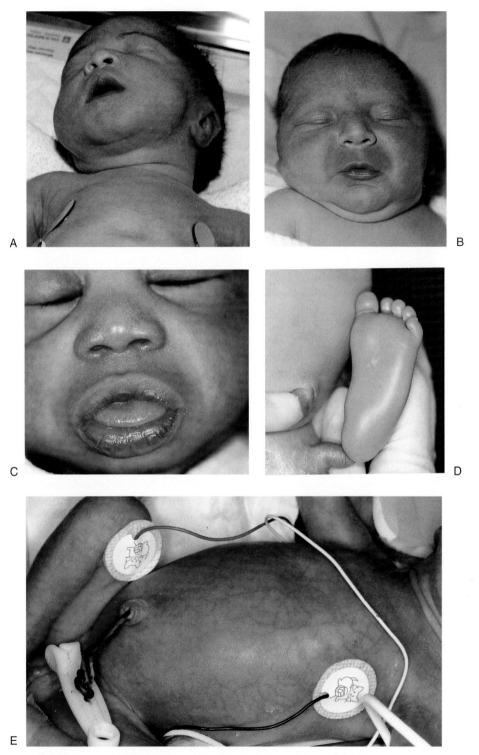

Figure 3. Cyanosis. **A:** Generalized cyanosis due to total anomalous pulmonary venous return with an oxygen saturation level of 80%. **B:** Perioral cyanosis. The mucous membranes and area over the chest remain pink in the presence of mild cyanosis above the lips. Petechiae make the forehead area appear blue. **C:** Lips appear blue from normal pigment deposition in vermilion border but the mucous membranes are pink. **D:** Acrocyanosis in the first half hour of life in a 32-week infant. **E:** Cyanosis localized to the abdominal wall. The blue color is caused by meconium peritonitis after an intrauterine bowel perforation. If peritoneal meconium is of long enough standing, a flat plat of the abdomen would show calcifications.

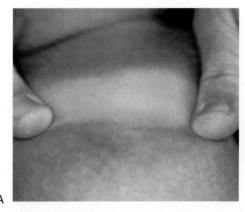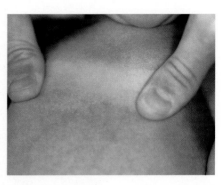

A   B

Figure 4. Jaundice pressing the red color from the skin allows better recognition of the yellow of jaundice. **A:** Infant with no appreciable jaundice at chest level. **B:** Infant with bilirubin level of 13 mg/d (222 μmol/L).

gray–brown discoloration throughout when infants with elevated conjugated bilirubin levels are under phototherapy (12–17).

   Carotenemia is a condition mimicking jaundice that is common in infancy when the diet is high in yellow vegetables so it is not seen in neonates. The skin appears slightly more orange–yellow, but the mucous membranes or sclera are not discolored.

   To distinguish vascular from extravascular blood or pigment, determine if there is blanching by diascopy. Apply pressure with a clear glass slide or plastic ruler held flat against the lesion to view the lesion and compare with the surrounding area. The pressure will cause emptying of vascular blood but will not change the appearance of ecchymoses, petechiae, or pigment deposits. When magnification is needed, a standard ophthalmoscope or magnifying otoscope is most often available, but a hand-held reading lens is easier to use. Applying oil to the skin surface may improve visibility of vessels but is usually unnecessary in neonates unless there is a lot of overlying scaling.

   Palpate the skin in several representative areas for moisture, turgor and elasticity, and temperature. Take a small fold of skin on the anterior abdomen, anterior thigh, and posterior arm and pull each fold gently away from the surface and then allow it to return. How easily it pulls away implies mobility and how quickly it returns tests turgor and elasticity. Feel for temperature using the back of the hand, especially over lesions that appear reddened, indurated, or ischemic, and compare with adjacent but normal-appearing areas. Use point pressure to detect excessive fluid (edema or lymphedema) in the eyelids, anterior shins, feet, and lumbosacral regions. Assess for redundancy of skin, particularly in the face and neck and over the abdomen (Table 6). Look at the pattern of

Table 6. *Genesis of redundant skin*

Mechanism of production	Examples
Distention of skin from within by an unusual force that has regressed	Web neck due to prior distention of jugular lymph sac
	Loose skin due to prior edema
	"Prune belly" due to prior distention of the abdomen
Compression of the skin by external forces	Loose skin, especially in the face, with oligohydramnios
	Loose skin over areas of unusual constraint in utero
Malformation of skin, with unusual overgrowth to normal forces	Cutis laxa
Idiopathic	Achondroplasia

From Smith, ref. 222, with permission.

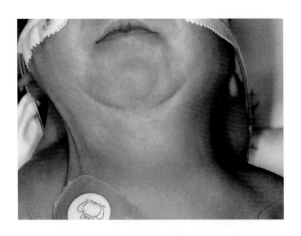

Figure 5. Redundant skin. The quantity of skin on both the anterior and posterior aspects of the neck is clearly excessive because there had been a large, fetal cystic hygroma now resolved in this infant with Noonan's syndrome.

creasing on the face, hands, feet, and buttocks. Note the presence of dimples on any unusual site. Estimate the depth and location of any lesions as epidermal (superficial), dermal (within skin), or hypodermal (deep to skin but above muscles).

The skin becomes quite dry after birth, with scaling occurring in all gestational ages. The dryness may be so marked that deep cracking develops in skin folds, leaving hemorrhagic creases. Persistent extreme dryness beyond the first 2 weeks suggests a hypohidrotic or ichthyosis syndrome, or hypothyroidism. If the skin remains in a tented pattern when pulled, it indicates decreased turgor or elasticity due to dehydration, weight loss, or hyperelastic conditions such as Ehlers-Danlos syndrome. **Redundant skin** indicates more skin than is necessary or normally found in a specific area with a primary example being the redundant skin found in the neck after resolution of nuchal cystic hygroma or in the scalp in microencephaly vera or over the abdomen in prune belly syndrome (Fig. 5).

The pattern of skin creasing at birth reflects in part alterations in shape and function of the hand and foot. Palmar creasing develops by 13 weeks' gestation and digital creasing by 10 weeks' gestation (18). Patterns in crease formation may reflect early influences such as familial tendencies, race, sex, and chromosomal markers, but even when commonly found in chromosomal syndromes, there is still a lack of specificity unless there is also a malformation or malfunction of the limbs (19).

Single palmar crease occurs unilaterally in approximately 4% and bilaterally in 1% of newborn infants and in boys twice as frequently as in girls (20). Although there is an increased frequency of single palmar creases in infants with Down's syndrome, only 45% of these infants have a simian crease (21) (Fig. 6). The locations of creases correlates for the most part with the location of interphalangeal and metacarpophalangeal joints (22). How well developed the creases are correlates with gestational age and with the function of the limb (19). With exceptions, the presence of deep creasing indicates maturity and fetal constraint (Fig. 7). Fetal constraint is a normal feature of term pregnancies as the growing fetus vies for his proportion of space. When there are multiple fetuses, uterine anomalies, or an absence of amnionic fluid, constraint can be so great that it inhibits development. Creasing greater than that expected for a given gestational age or in unusual locations suggests an extremity or region that has been abnormally folded or constrained. Absence of palmar or sole creasing indicates a lack of normal movement from the first trimester on and always requires further evaluation (see Chapter 10 Fig. 9).

Dimpling may develop at any location where the skin has been fixed to the deeper tissues or bone and the underlying tissue has not fully developed. They may represent merely a familial trait or signal an underlying defect or bony prominence. Common sites include the elbows, knees, the acromion prominence (trisomy 9p), and the sacrum. Other locations are seen after amniocentesis (23–25) or with arthrogryposis (21). When especially deep or in an unusual location, further investigation of the underlying tissues or cause may be warranted. Supernumerary nipples that are especially rudimentary and have no external resemblance to breast tissue may appear as shallow dimples in the mammary line.

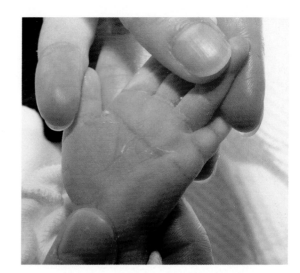

Figure 6. Single palmar crease. Down's syndrome (Trisomy 21). Because of shortening of metacarpals 3, 4, and 5, the hand has a relatively squared appearance in addition to a single palmar crease. There is also hypoplasia of the fifth mid-phalanx and clinodactyly partially obscured by the holder.

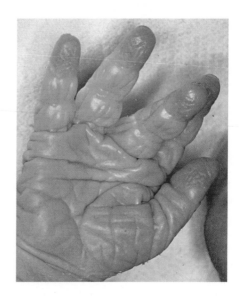

Figure 7. Creases indicating maturity. The deep creasing and dry skin belie the postmature status but the pattern of crease formation is normal.

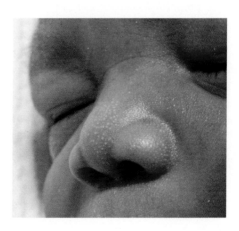

Figure 8. Sebaceous hyperplasia on the nose. The yellowish papules will gradually disappear.

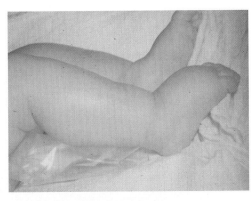 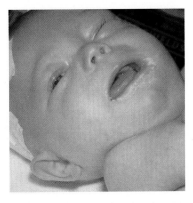

A   B

Figure 9. Generalized edema of congenital nephrotic syndrome. There is diffuse pitting edema, causing loss of bony landmarks in the lower extremities (**A**) and over the eyelids (**B**). Note the loss of anatomic creases due to the edema.

The production of **sebum** is increased during the first month of life still under the influence of maternal androgens (26), but oiliness is unlikely except over a sebaceous nevus and areas of sebaceous hyperplasia, notably the nose (Fig. 8).

Sweating is possible in response to environmental hyperthermia in all but the most premature infants and is most notable on the forehead. The amount of sweating in response to hot air is limited in infants delivered at less than 36 weeks immediately after birth but increases with postnatal age so that by 2 weeks of age, even premature infants should be capable of sweating, although with variable ability to use sweating to control their body temperature. Unless the infant is overheated by the external environment or has been crying vigorously, sweating upon mild exertion such as nursing is unusual. Sweating during sleep has been suggested to correlate with obstructive sleep apnea (27).

Edema causes stretching and loss of normal skin creases and folds, easily pits on gentle pressure, and shifts with position change. Characteristically, the overlying skin becomes shiny (Fig. 9). The pattern of swelling with lymphedema differs from peripheral edema in its tethering appearance of clefts between regions. Rather than loss of skin creases, there is accentuation in lymphedema (Fig. 10). Both edema and lymphedema have some degree of pitting. If truly localized, the location of either edema or lymphedema suggest the etiology (Figs. 11 and 12).

In neonates the most frequent association of lymphedema is with Turner's syndrome, but it is not invariably present in this condition. It is also seen in familial lymphedema, erysipelas or severe cellulitis, and in cases of amniotic band syndrome, particularly where there is constriction of an extremity (28). The pretibial myxedema of adult hypothyroidism is not detectable in the newborn period.

Palpate any lesion unless the overlying surface is open. When indicated, apply linear pressure to elicit a wheal (dermatographism) or an intraepidermal blister (Nicolsky's sign). Apply point pressure to determine capillary refill, for blanching of lesions, and for general assessment of perfusion, or to detect an underlying defect through which a nod-

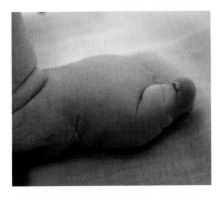

Figure 10. Lymphedema and hypoplastic great toenail in Turner's syndrome.

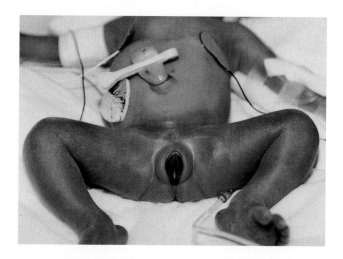

Figure 11. Marked edema and ecchymoses in premature (26 weeks) twin breech presentation. Note the loss of definition in skin folding particularly around the knees. Although edema makes up the majority of the swelling, there can be enough extravasation of blood to elevate the bilirubin significantly.

ule has herniated. Gently squeeze lesions and the surrounding tissue to determine the depth of the lesion. If a cystic lesion is suspected, use a small transilluminator light to detect differences in optical density from the surrounding tissue. Rub a lesion with an intact surface to elicit Darier's sign, smooth muscle contraction, vasodilation, or constriction. If a lesion is likely to have a major vascular component, feel for pulsation or thrills.

The skin of most neonates has some degree of dermatographism and less tolerance to rubbing than does adult skin, so gentleness is appropriate. It is possible to estimate the depth of a lesion by its response to movement or gentle squeezing. The skin will slide over deep lesions attached to or within muscle or bone. Intradermal nodules may wrinkle or dimple at the surface upon gentle squeezing. The most superficial lesions will elevate more with squeezing.

Take scrapings of scaling lesions by gently scratching the skin surface and transferring the scale to a clean slide. To culture and stain material from pustular lesions, aspirate any fluid with a 25-gauge needle. Cultures also may be obtained from injecting and aspirating nonbactericidal saline in the periphery of the lesions.

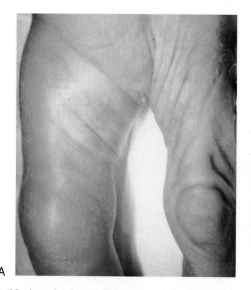
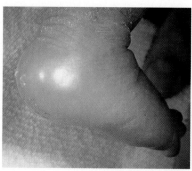

A   B

Figure 12. Local edema. Edema is easiest to detect when there is a normal area for comparison. **A:** The right thigh is shiny with loss of the skin folds defining the patella and other underlying structures after reaction to an intramuscular injection in this premature infant. **B:** Induration associated with cellulitis of the heel after multiple heel sticks for capillary blood draw. Note shininess and erythema. Increased warmth and tenderness were present. An underlying osteomyelitis is a strong possibility with these findings in neonates.

Using as much natural light as possible, photograph any lesions as indicated when the diagnosis is in question and when a baseline image will be helpful to compare in follow-up.

Many potential skin lesions occur in consequence to the birth process or care given in the newborn period. Because these patients cannot report a direct historical relationship, the examiner should consider injury as a possible cause in some instances while remembering that many congenital skin conditions may appear to be the result of trauma but are not. For example, cutis aplasia of the scalp often appears as a covered "blister" in the same spot as the site for fetal scalp monitoring; scarring after fetal scalp electrode monitoring that results in loss of tissue and hair may be confused with cutis aplasia (29). Mongolian spots appear similar to ecchymoses leading to misdiagnosis of trauma or abuse. In contrast, silver nitrate used for eye prophylaxis stains the skin tan to resemble a café-au-lait spot. If strong enough, the silver nitrate can cause blistering and crusting as well as color changes. Triple dye used for cord care stains the skin blue, and iodophors stain it orange–brown. Each of these stains will transfer to an alcohol wipe as an easy tool for distinction.

Hair and Nails

Variations in scalp hair are discussed in Chapter 6. The visibility of body hair varies under the influence of maternal androgens by gestational age, pigmentation, and genetic backgrounds. Hair shafts exit the skin at an angle and form nonspiraling sprays in streams or spiraling from central foci or whorls. Both physical and chemical factors are proposed as the determinants for the direction and location of hair streams (30). Although the total number of hair follicles is less in newborn infants, the density is increased to almost double that in adults. The number of emergent hair shafts from each follicle is lower, at only one each (31). There is also variation in density related to hair color, with lighter color tending to be less dense.

Lanugo is the very fine, unpigmented fetal hair, with two growths ending in two periods of shedding. The first shed occurs in utero at 7 to 8 months and the second occurs inconspicuously near term gestation or after birth (Fig. 13) Vellus hair, which is fine and generally poorly pigmented replaces the second shed of lanugo and continues to grow throughout life on the body and with the scalp hair. It covers all of the body except the palms and soles. Because of maternal androgens, this hair can appear coarser and more pigmented until it is initially shed (Fig. 14). Although most often not associated with significant pathology in the adrenals or ovaries, especially in breast-fed infants, hair on the genitalia in the neonatal period is abnormal and requires follow-up if an isolated finding or further investigation if other findings suggest increased androgen levels (32,33). Terminal hair refers to the thicker, pigmented hairs on the scalp, eyelashes, and eyebrows. At birth it is not as medullated or as pigmented as adult hair and, hence, is finer and likely to darken as the child ages. Until the hair erupts and the plug of keratin is lost, the pilosebaceous follicles may appear as shiny, slightly raised papules, notably over the back and extremities (Fig. 15).

The **nails** are a skin appendage that are the first areas of keratinization in the body. They are visible at the base by 17 weeks, reaching the fingertips by 32 weeks' gestation and the toetips by 36 weeks (3). Normally, the nails of neonates are thin enough to bend and tear easily, and they often appear cupped and bent on themselves. The size and shape of the nail reflects in part the size and shape of the underlying bone and resembles those of the parents

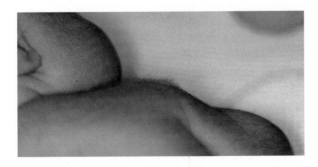

Figure 13. Lanugo. The area over the shoulder in this 36-week infant shows remnants of the second growth of lanugo. It is very fine and unpigmented. Other areas of his body had much less lanugo apparent except for isolated patches.

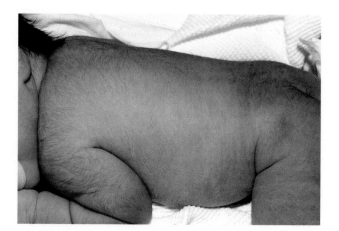

Figure 14. Neonatal hirsutism. This Latino infant shows a typical pattern of directional hair growth away from the axillae and swirling over the lumbar spine. The apparent coarseness and pigmentation will decrease after this hair is shed and the infant is no longer under the effect of maternal androgens.

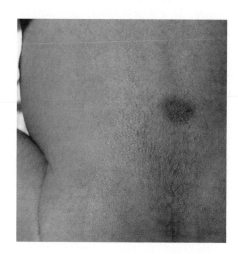

Figure 15. Preeruptive hair follicles. The lumbosacral area is covered with shiny, very slightly raised papules that may or may not have a hair protruding. The finding disappears when the keratin plug is lost. Mongolian spot is present.

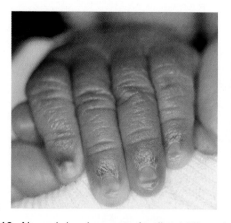
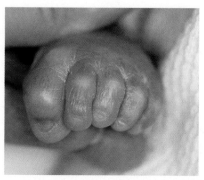

A   B

Figure 16. Normal development of nails at 37 weeks. **A:** The area at the base of the fingernails suggests the anticipated level of general skin pigmentation. The distal tip is very thin but closely adherent to the underlying skin. **B:** Hypoplasia of toenails on the same infant. Isolated hypoplasia of the toenails is a normal variation, commonly agreeing with similar patterns in a parent. If part of a constellation of signs, there may be more serious implications.

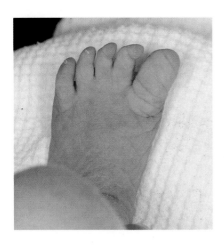

Figure 17. Anonychia. Absence of toenail on digit 1-3 bilaterally with hypoplastic nails on 4-5. The deviation and pattern of creases suggests hypoplasia or absence of the distal phalanx of these toes. There is mild dermal syndactyly between the second and third toes.

enough that they often recognize the similarity during their initial inspection. Hypoplastic toenails are most often transient variations in newborns, whereas hypoplastic fingernails may carry more significance (Figs. 16 and 17).

FINDINGS

General Newborn Findings
Lesions consequent to perinatal care
Papulosquamous eruptions
Vesicular pustular eruptions
Plaques and nodules
Flat lesions with color change

Development of Pigmentation

The degree and distribution of skin pigmentation depends on the child's race, influence of maternal androgens, maturity of the infant, compressed areas, and exposure to light (Fig. 18). Although generally concordant with parental pigmentation, there are wide variations in how much eumelanin is present, so assumption about race and parentage can be erroneous if based only on initial physical appearance of a newborn infant, especially one born prematurely. Areas of hyperpigmentation after phototherapy may take several months to

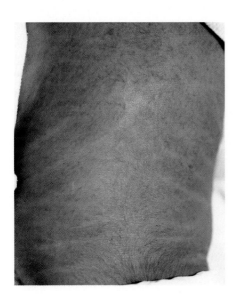

Figure 18. Irregular development of pigment within skin folds. This pattern of pigmentation will become more uniform within a few weeks. The round areas of increased pigmentation are residua of transient pustulosis.

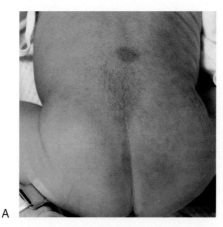
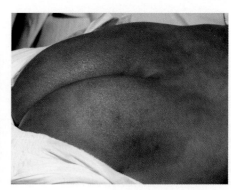

A   B

Figure 19. Mongolian spots. **A:** Two spots are present. The upper spot with more discrete borders with a nonblanching, intense blue color is likely to remain visible for life, but the more diffuse, lower one will become less apparent as the surrounding skin increases in pigmentation. **B:** Typical location for these lesions must not lead to confusion with bruising attributed to child abuse.

blend (9). A helpful algorithm for evaluation disorders of pigmentation is included toward the end of this chapter (see Fig. 71)

Mongolian spots, the most frequent "birth marks," represent dermal melanosis (Fig. 19) Because the color is developed deeply within the skin, it appears more gray–blue than more superficial melanosis would. Many of the lighter spots become less noticeable as the rest of the skin darkens, and in lighter pigmented skin tones, the color may be less intense but remains detectable. The darkest lesions are the least likely to disappear. Mongolian spots are found in approximately 95% of black, 81% of Asian-Oriental, 70% of Latino, 62% of Asian-Indian, and 10% of white infants (34–36).

Dermal melanosis over the supraclavicular, deltoid, and scapular regions may be merely widespread Mongolian spotting or considered a variant of Mongolian spotting, a nevus of Ito (37). Usually an isolated finding in blacks or Asians, the nevus of Ito may appear with a nevus of Ota, which covers the trigeminal distribution, often involving the eye. Both lesions are darker than typical Mongolian spots and have more definite borders. Neither lesion fades with time but only rarely, particularly in whites, do they undergo malignant degeneration. Ota's nevus is associated with orbital pathology, including glaucoma when there is scleral pigmentation, so those infants should undergo an ophthalmologic evaluation (38).

Milia represents miniature epidermal inclusion cysts present at birth in approximately one third of infants, less commonly in black infants (36,39) (Fig. 20A). There is no associated erythema, and the lesions generally resolve within a few weeks. Milia can develop in older infants and children after cutaneous injury (37), and premature infants not showing milia at birth may develop it at several months of age (Fig. 20B). Extensive or persistent milia is a feature of the oro-facial-digital syndrome (21). Pearls are large, generally single

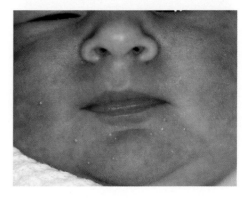

Figure 20. Milia. Usual appearance at birth.

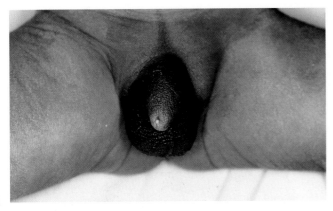
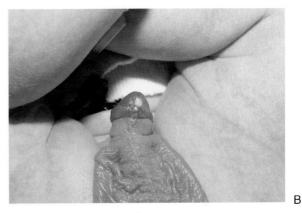

A   B

Figure 21. Pearls. Large, single lesions of milia may persist for several months although they normally disappear during the first month. There is no inflammatory reaction. **A:** Pearl at tip of penis visible before circumcision. Note the normal, dark pigmentation of the genitalia at term and a linea nigra. **B:** Pearl on dorsal surface visible only after circumcision. Note the lack of eumelanin despite mature formation of the scrotum.

lesions of milia that occur primarily on the genitalia or around the areola (Fig. 21). Like all milia, no erythema is associated with the lesions, and they are not easily removed. Pearls also occur in the mouth (Epstein's pearls).

Vernix Caseosa

This creamy white substance coats the fetal skin until the 37th to 38th week of gestation when, for the most part, it is shed into the amniotic fluid (Fig. 22). It tends to accumulate in nuchal, axillary, and inguinal folds. Its smooth, greasy consistency indicates its lipid origin from fetal sebaceous cells with secondary deposition of desquamated cells and hair. It appears to provide a moisture barrier for the fetal skin and, by analogy to sebum, it likely has antibacterial and antifungal properties (40,41). Vernix is normally white but will take on the color of intrauterine processes. Yellow vernix may indicate bile pigment from hemoglobin breakdown after chronic abruption, from immune hemolytic disease or form earlier meconium passage or nonbile pigments with chorioamnionitis.

Lesions Consequent to Perinatal Care

Healing after extreme immaturity   Intravenous infiltration
Blistering   Arterial insufficiency
Pressure   Petachiae
Tape excoriation   Ecchymoses
Self-inflicted

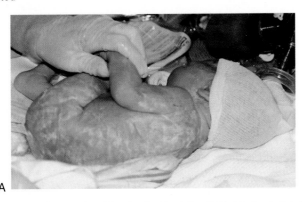
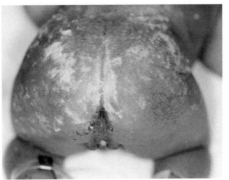

A   B

Figure 22. Vernix. **A:** Unstained. **B:** Marked staining from intrauterine meconium passage.

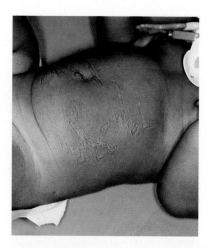

Figure 23. Irregular scarring. In her first week after birth at 23 weeks gestation, much of the skin surface appeared like second degree burns with some areas developing widespread, deep excoriations.

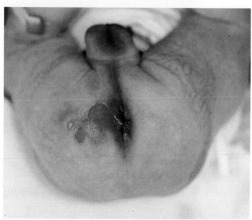

Figure 24. Blistering in normal skin with denudation and ecchymoses from prolonged pressure on the perineum after breech presentation. The scrotum is swollen and ecchymotic as well. This blistering is very superficial and dries quickly.

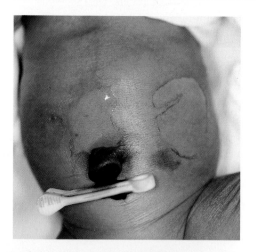

Figure 25. Excoriation upon removal of micropore tape in an otherwise healthy infant.

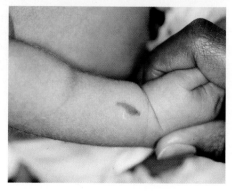

Figure 26. Sucking blisters. There are two blisters at right angles across each other: one is deeply crusted, the other is more superficial. The location is always on a surface of the lips, hand, arm, or foot that can easily be taken into the mouth in the fetal position (202). This depth of crusting is unusual. A more frequent presentation is a small flaccid bulla or excoriation.

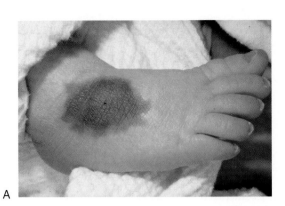
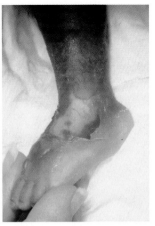
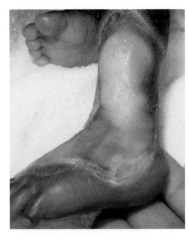

A

B, C

Figure 27. Injuries associated with intravenous therapy. **A:** This lesion is not edematous or tense and is typical of a mild chemical burn. The full extent of injury is unpredictable early in the course, but the lack of swelling suggests good perfusion and a better prognosis. **B:** Early lesion shows blistering, edema, and superficial loss of skin in a relatively limited area. The presence of blanching suggests poor perfusion. **C:** The same lesion with eschar formation that shows a far greater involvement than originally evident. [with permission (203)]

Neonatal skin is especially susceptible to trauma, increasingly so with decreased maturity. The most frequent association is the birth process itself, during which the skin is subjected to significant pressures, stretching, and rubbing. Infants themselves may inflict several types of skin injuries, most commonly scratching by their fingernails, excoriation from rubbing a bony prominence against bedding, or sucking blisters. Several examples of the types of skin trauma are included herein, but others are demonstrated in the regional discussions throughout this book (Figs. 23–28).

Collections of blood as petechiae, ecchymoses, or hematomas that appear within hours after birth suggest direct trauma (Figs. 29 and 30). They may be benign and self-limited or signs of more serious conditions (see also Chapter 6). Petechiae are pinpoint areas of hemorrhage that can develop after an abrupt increase in venous pressure or local rubbing. Small, localized areas of petechiae that appear at the same time and do not progress are rarely of concern, but progressive or widespread formations are abnormal and require full evaluation for cause and associated coagulopathy.

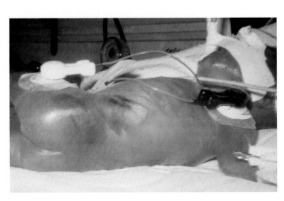
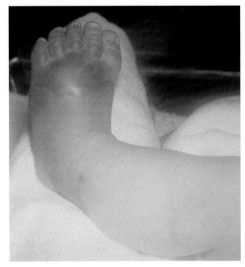

A

B

Figure 28. Skin necrosis associated with an umbilical artery catheter. Such lesions develop after vasospasm or embolization. **A:** Spinal injury may be present when ischemia involves this region. **B:** The distal part of an extremity is a common site for embolic arterial loss. The full extent of loss is unpredictable at this stage.

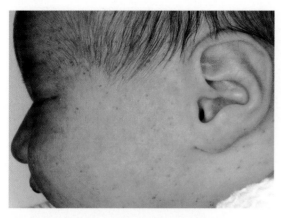

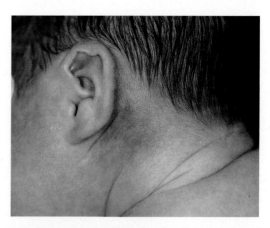

Figure 29. Petechiae limited to the head because of a tight nuchal cord. Appearing within the first 2 hours after a birth associated with a nuchal cord, the petechiae are all the same color, indicating a single showering event. Petechiae do not blanch on diascopy and go through the same color evolution as other dermal blood collections. Petechiae that appear in crops or not concurrently suggest a coagulopathy and require further evaluation.

Figure 30. Ecchymosis after subgaleal hemorrhage. The bilateral location of this blood collection away from the site of application of forceps and crossing suture lines suggests a wide area of involvement typical of a moderately large subgaleal hematoma. When accompanied by hemotympanum or frank bleeding in the canal, a unilateral collection behind the ear, particularly if there had been application of delivery forceps too far posteriorly, would suggest a basilar skull fracture.

Papulosquamous Eruptions

Normal desquamation   Contact dermatitis
Postmaturity desquamation   Seborrheic dermatitis
Collodion baby   Fungal skin infection
Harlequin baby   Syphilis

An algorithm for evaluation of papulosquamous rashes is provided in Fig. 31.

Desquamation Patterns

In healthy term infants, at birth the skin does not appear dry because it is well lubricated by vernix. After a period of 12 to 24 hours, the skin starts to dry and flake, with more marked desquamation over the feet and ankles, slightly less over the hands (Fig. 32A). Reddened fissures may develop over the ankles. If the skin is peeling at the time of birth or

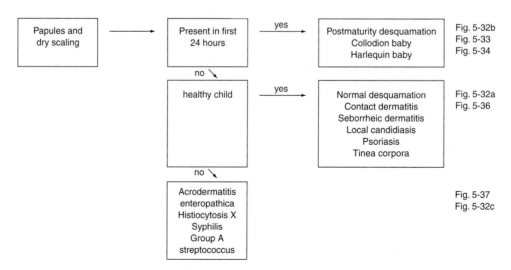

Figure 31. Algorithm for evaluation of papulosquamous rashes. Modified from Cohen (37) with permission.

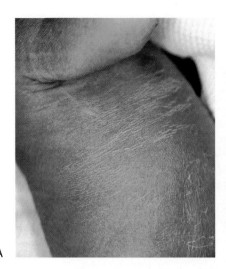
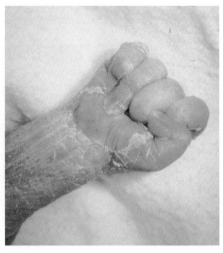
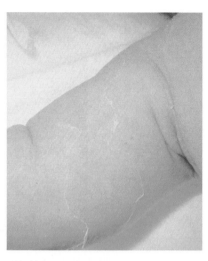

A   B, C

Figure 32. Dry skin. **A:** Normal skin dry skin at term. Peeling is normally most marked on the feet and hands and is rarely present at birth. The amount and depth of desquamation increases over the next several days, leading to deep cracking over joints. **B:** Excessive peeling in a postdates infant may be present and notable at birth. Note the long fingernails. **C:** Superficial peeling with little underlying erythema of group A streptococcus infection. In contrast to the desquamation seen because of age, the peeling associated with infection may be of skin that is not particularly dry and that leaves abnormal skin underneath.

within the first few hours, the infant is most likely to be postdates or postmature (Fig. 32B). If the gestational dates and rest of the examination eliminate postmaturity as a diagnosis, the infant may have an abnormal dry skin condition, the causes of which include infections or one of the lamellar exfoliation syndromes. The two congenital infections notable for desquamation at the time of birth are syphilis and systemic candidiasis (42–45). Other infections causing desquamation within the neonatal period but not as likely on the first day of life are similar to those causing similar symptoms in other age groups: Group A *Streptococcus* (Fig. 32C), local candidiasis, *Staphylococcus* impetigo, and ringworm (46–48).

Collodion Baby

Also known as lamellar exfoliation of the newborn (Fig. 33), this condition is apparent at birth because of the marked restriction in growth of the cartilaginous tissue, notably the nose and ears. As soon as the skin dries, it takes on the appearance of dried collodion or parchment wrapping the baby. As the shedding progresses, the infants are susceptible to dehydration through excessive transcutaneous losses and poor feeding. They may experience significant aspiration symptoms due to perinatal aspiration of the amnionic debris containing the dry exfoliation (49), and the loss of skin integrity puts them at risk for infection. Collodion baby skin is not a disease in itself but is a presenting manifestation for several conditions, and in at least 10% of cases the skin is remarkably normal after initial shedding; making a prognosis at birth is not possible (50–52). Early biopsy is not as helpful in determining severity as biopsy performed after 2 weeks. The majority of cases and the more serious forms precede the chronic lamellar ichthyosis syndromes (50–56).

Harlequin Fetus

This condition represents the most severe form of an ichthyosis syndrome, with thick, dry, hyperkeratotic skin that starts to crack immediately after birth in a pattern resembling plates of armor (Fig. 34). The majority of patients of this rare illness have died within a few hours to days from dehydration, infection, and respiratory insufficiency, but there are iso-

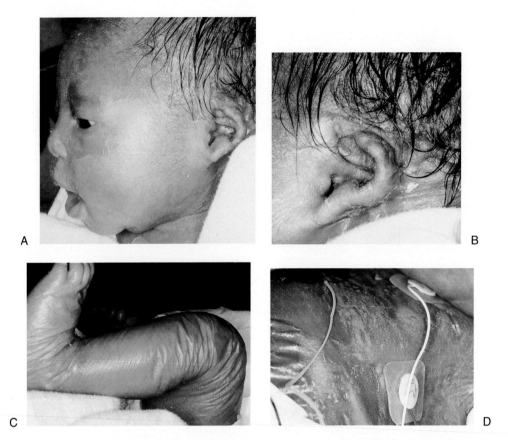

Figure 33. Collodion baby. Lamellar desquamation of the newborn. **A and C:** The infant appears encased in a covering resembling dried collodion. The face is relatively immobile, and growth of the cartilaginous nose has been restricted. Mild ectropion is present. **B:** The ears are distorted with fixation to the head. **D:** Within days after birth, the skin cracks and peels in thick sheets or scales, leaving hemorrhagic fissures and an erythematous base.

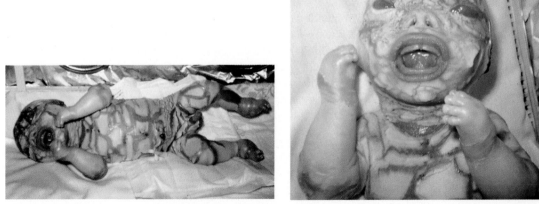

Figure 34. Harlequin fetus. **A:** There is total involvement with tight restriction in movement, including respiratory excursions. **B:** The internal mucous membranes are normal. Note the ectropion of the eyes and eclabium of the mouth, the restricted nasal and ear growth, and hypoplasia of the digits and nails.

lated reports of survivors who develop chronic ichthyosis (57). Prenatal diagnosis is possible because of its recurrent nature and typical fetal skin biopsies (58,59).

Papular Rashes with Desquamation as a Major Feature

Contact irritations are depicted in Fig. 35.

Candida

The dermal manifestations of systemic infection with *Candida* organisms depend in part on the route of spread of the fungus and the gestational age of the infant. Congenital disease localized to the skin manifests as an erythematous maculopapular rash of the trunk and extremities that desquamates extensively. Less commonly, there may be pustules, vesicles, and skin abscesses. Intrauterine infection manifests with a characteristic funisitis and yellow plaques on the cord (see Chapter 4 Fig. 7). Very low birth weight infants with congenital infection may present with a widespread dermatitis that resembles first-degree burns

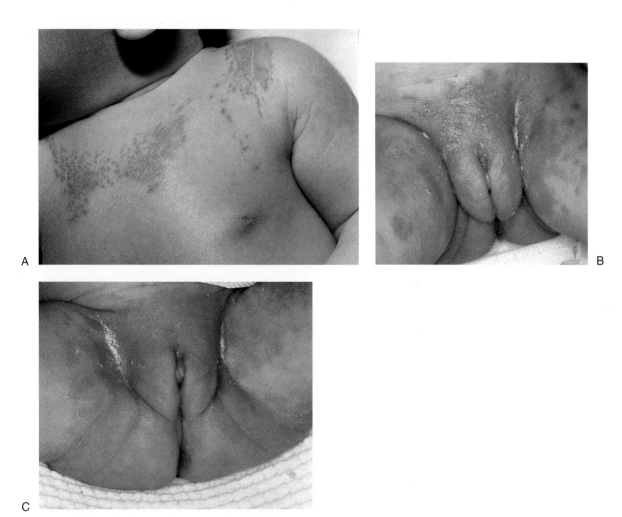

Figure 35. Contact irritation. **A:** Papulosquamous rash with appearance of contact irritation present at birth. The areas involved were in contact with a nuchal cord and the chin when the infant was put into his fetal position. Lesions became progressively less erythematous, peeled, and cleared without recurrence. **B:** Primary irritant diaper dermatitis with coincident lupus. Typically, the deepest parts of the inguinal folds are somewhat spared because of less contact with the irritant. When the intertriginous areas are involved, as in this case, causes other than contact irritation, including infection and seborrheic dermatitis, should be considered. The satellite lesions, although suggesting infection due to *Candida,* are skin manifestations of maternally transmitted lupus erythematosus. **C:** Response after 48 hours of treatment with steroids and exposure of the area.

(42). These areas desquamate in either a fine, bran-like pattern or in sheets, and commonly there are superficial moist erosions, especially in skin folds. A characteristic unpleasant odor accompanies the moist rash.

Mucocutaneous Candidiasis

Pseudomembranous candidiasis (synonym *thrush*) develops in the neonatal period as white, curdlike plaques on the mucosa of the oropharynx, extending to the posterior pharynx in severe cases. The appearance is similar to adherent milk except that candidial plaques are more tightly adherent and leave an erythematous base upon removal. Infants with thrush who suck their thumbs may autoinoculate the skin and develop papules or pustules on their fingers or hands (60).

Monilial diaper dermatitis, with or without thrush, is an intense erythematous, scaling papular rash with some formation of pustules. Characteristically, there are satellite lesions at the margins. The areas of greatest involvement are in skin folds and regions of constant moisture. In infants kept in high-humidity incubators, this rash can develop diffusely (61–63). Rarely, infantile psoriasis can develop in the neonatal period with similar desquamating erythematous plaques in regions of monilial dermatitis but, unlike for candidiasis, moisture of the diaper regions is therapeutic (43–45,64–67).

Infection with *Candida* species is the most common neonatal skin infection in residents of intensive care nurseries, but other unusual and common organisms can occur sporadically or in nosocomial outbreaks (Fig. 36). Tinea corpora or ring worm of the smooth skin is most frequently caused by *Microsporum* species, but infections with *Trichophyton* or *Epidermophyton* species are reported in the early neonatal period as well (46–48,68–70). Lesions are single or multiple, round or oval. As the scaling erythema spreads peripherally, the centers clear and the margins overlap, becoming polycyclic. Examination of smears under sodium or potassium hydroxide would reveal hyphae to confirm a fungal infection. Culture is necessary for identification of the species.

Skin Manifestations of Congenital Syphilis

The skin is affected in as few as 15% of infants with congenital syphilis so it most often appears normal at birth (Fig. 37) (71). Skin lesions may initially appear anywhere because neonatal infection is secondary or disseminated syphilis. The sites of predilection include the face, palms, and soles, with progression proximally on the extremities. Typical lesions begin as pale pink macules or papules that become more reddish brown or coppery and scaling (72). About 3% develop bullous lesions (pemphigus syphiliticus) with marked shedding of the skin. If there is thrombocytopenia, petechiae may be present. The fluid in all moist skin lesions is teaming with spirochetes and is therefore highly infectious.

Neonates with skin lesions also have hepatosplenomegaly, generalized lymphadenopathy, anemia, leukopenia, leukocytosis, thrombocytopenia, and jaundice with elevated conjugated bilirubin levels. They may have pneumonia at birth (pneumonia alba). The copious

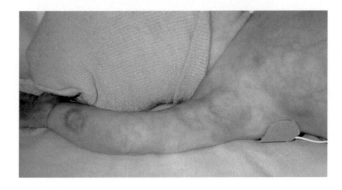

Figure 36. Tinea corpora (Synonym *Ring worm of smooth skin*) in premature infant at 1 month of age. He had been in the neonatal intensive care unit since birth at 27 weeks' gestation. His mother had a history of recurrent ring worm.

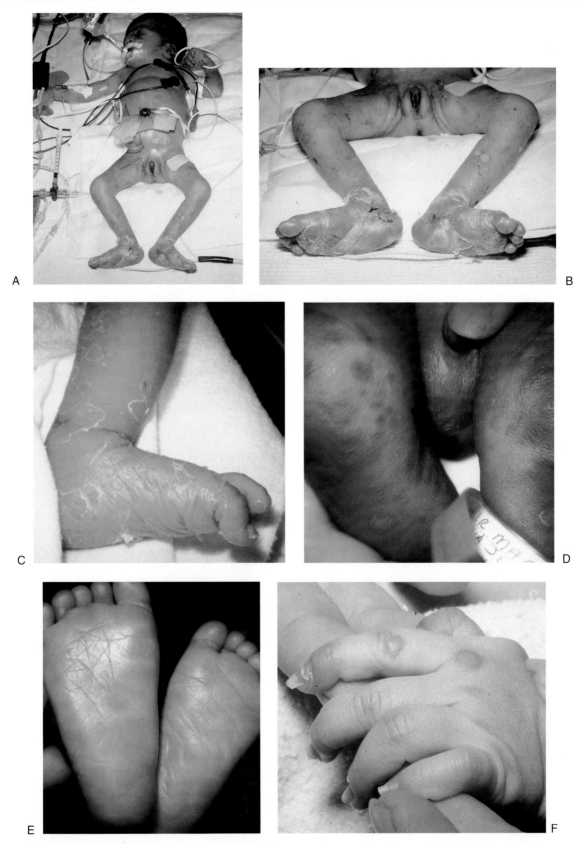

Figure 37. Congenital syphilis. **A:** Hepatosplenomegaly causing abnormal distension in growth-re-tarded infant with bullous lesions including the soles of feet. **B:** Pemphigus syphiliticus, bullae teaming with spirochetes. **C:** Peeling is quite marked in another infant with congenital syphilis, but the circular pattern does not resemble desquamation due to postmaturity. **D:** Macular lesions with coppery base on extremities. **E:** Presence of discolored macules on the soles in typical distribution. **F:** Slightly raised mac-ule at 3 weeks of age.

rhinitis known as snuffles appears after the early newborn period in untreated syphilis (71). Deep fissures and the subsequent fine scarring around infected orifices (rhagades) develop after the first 2 to 3 months.

Congenital syphilis is one of the most important causes of necrotizing funisitis, which may be the only manifestation apparent at birth but a lost sign unless the placenta and cord are examined (73).

Contact Irritation

Because of the skin fragility, many forms of contact irritation can develop with amazing rapidity in newborn infants. The expected sites for contact irritation in neonates are those over bony prominences (the elbows and knees) or on the nose and chin, where the irritation is caused by rubbing, especially in an irritable infant. Its presence in these areas is useful as a sign of irritability in assessing status during drug withdrawal. In the diaper area the irritant is more likely chemical due to change in stool pH and can develop remarkably rapidly. Beginning with erythema, the contact rash has well-demarcated erythema and mild edema progressing to dry scaling or blister formation that remains moist or crusts. The area is painful and, in causing further irritability for the neonate, may be self-propagating.

An important cause of contact irritation in intensive care patients is that associated with the chemicals used to clean the skin: alcohol and iodophors (74). Burns develop with increasing ease as the gestational age of the patient decreases. The chemicals may pool in dependent positions or creases to remain wet and prolong exposure to the irritant.

The term **seborrheic dermatitis** is applied to many rashes about the face and extremities in young infants, probably far more often than the condition actually occurs. True seborrheic dermatitis is unusual within the early neonatal period but appears within the first two months with lesions that are reddish yellow plaques with surface scaling in greasy plaques. Fissuring, maceration, and weeping develop in the most affected areas. The sites of initial presentation are the scalp and diaper areas and later in skin folds, particularly the axillae, and on the trunk and limbs (75). When located in the scalp, the adherent scaling is called cradle cap. Infection with the yeast *Pityrosporum* has been implicated (37). A less common presentation is **psoriasiform infantile seborrheic dermatitis** with drier and larger superficial scales, most often presenting in the diaper area. Erythrodermic seborrheic dermatitis, the least common clinical form in infancy, involves the entire skin surface with erythema and fine scaling. About 70% to 80% of infants with any type of infantile seborrheic dermatitis progress to other skin conditions, most commonly atopic dermatitis, ichthyosis, psoriasis, or keratosis pilaris (76). Histiocytosis X and benign variants initially appear as a severe scaling rash similar to seborrheic dermatitis but worsen to hemorrhagic erosions, particularly in the diaper area (37).

Vesicular Pustular Eruptions

Erythema toxicum neonatorum	Candidiasis
Transient neonatal pustular melanosis	Scabies
Miliaria	Staphylococcal scalded skin syndrome
Neonatal acne	Epidermolysis bullosa
Herpes simplex	Mastocytosis
Varicella	Incontinentia pigmenti
Staphylococcal pustulosis	Aplasia cutis congenita
Bullous impetigo	

An algorithm for evaluating vesicular pustular eruptions is provided in Fig. 38. A computer detailed tabulation of neonatal pustular lesions is found in Table 12 at the end of this chapter.

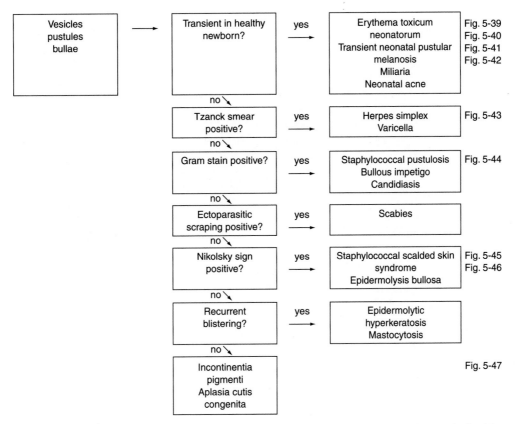

Figure 38. Algorithm for evaluation of pustular vesicular rashes. Modified from Cohen (37) with permission.

Erythema Toxicum Neonatorum

Erythema toxicum neonatorum (ETN; synonym *toxic erythema, erythema neonatorum allergicum*) is the most common neonatal papulopustular rash and occurs in up to 70% of term neonates (Fig. 39) (5,36,77–85). The major outbreak of the rash is on the 2nd and 3rd days of life but can begin or recur for several weeks after birth. Although ETN does occur in premature infants, its occurrence increases with gestational age and is uncommon enough to warrant initial consideration of the possible infectious mimickers in infants delivered after less than 34 weeks' gestation (77).

The lesions of ETN typically appear as erythematous macules that rapidly progress into central papules. They may resolve within a few hours or progress further into a yellow–white pustule that crusts before resolving. As the more transient lesions progress, the area of erythema decreases so that by the time a papule is formed, there is only a small or no erythematous base. If there is coalescence of multiple lesions or marked pustular formation, there is more erythema at the base but it invariably resolves before the pustule is fully developed. Confluent lesions persist more than the few hours that is typical of isolated lesions. Vesicles rarely form, but considerations of other etiologies is necessary. Lesions may be isolated or clustered on the face, trunk, or proximal extremities but not on the hands and feet. The lesions are composed primarily of eosinophils and are sterile (80). When the pustules are pronounced or coalescent, they mimic infectious pustular rashes, but the major distinction of ETN is in the pattern of progressively less erythema as the pustule forms.

Erythema toxicum neonatorum is not synonymous with erythema neonatorum, although many textbooks overlap the two findings. Even though ETN is benign and does not merit the implied toxicity, its use allows differentiation from the generalized erythema neonatorum (86).

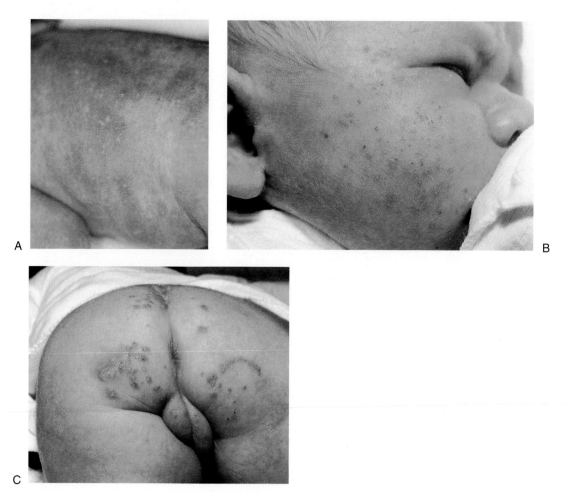

Figure 39. Erethema toxicum neonatorum (ETN). **A:** Usual pattern with most of the lesions on the trunk and face, fewer on the extremities. **B:** Crusting papules. The extremes of crusting occur in lighter skinned infants. **C:** Extreme pustule formation that resembled herpes in an otherwise healthy infant.

Transient Neonatal Pustular Melanosis

Generally observed only in term infants, transient neonatal pustular melanosis (TNP; synonym *transient neonatal pustular melanosis, transient pustulosis of the neonate*) is a short-lived eruption that may be present at birth as a fragile pustule, the top of which easily wipes off, leaving a typical halo (collarette) around the base (Fig. 40) (36,84,86–91). In infants of color, the base of the pustule will be darker than the adjacent skin. In none will there be any erythema at the base of the pustule. These are not freckles. The pigmented areas will either fade slightly or the surrounding skin will catch up in the extent of pigmentation.

The clinical presence at birth with an absence of dermal erythema makes infection unlikely in the differential diagnosis and culture of pustular content will be negative. Smears of the pustular contents show no bacteria with predominantly neutrophils in intra- or subcorneal collections and a few eosinophils. The underlying skin may be normal or have a mild perivascular and perifollicular inflammatory infiltrate. Pigmented macules demonstrate basal and suprabasal increase in pigmentation only, apparently without pigmentary incontinence.

There is some suggestion that TNP is a precursor to erythema toxicum. The two rashes are seldom present simultaneously, and infants who present with TNP can develop ETN. Ferrándiz et al. have proposed unifying transient pustular melanosis and erythema toxicum as a continuum under the name "sterile transient neonatal pustulosis" (86).

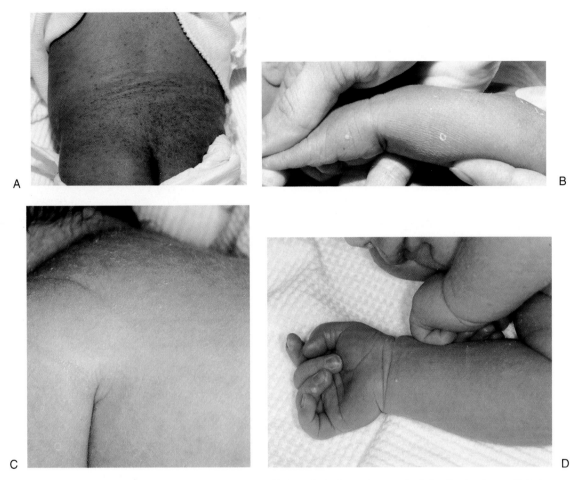

Figure 40. Transient pustulosis neonatorum. **A:** Melanotic lesions show typical distribution for multiple lesions as well as Mongolian spots. **B:** Pustules and collarettes. **C:** In infants with light skin color the collarettes will be without pigmented base. The resemblance to the appearance of miliaria after rupture of the blisters is striking but the location is inconsistent. **D:** Pustules have no erythematous base and are fragile.

Miliaria Crystallina (Sudamina) and Miliaria Rubra (Prickly Heat)

Miliaria develops when the flow from individual eccrine sweat glands is blocked. If the obstruction is in the more superficial stratum corneum, miliaria crystallina develops (Fig. 41). If the obstruction is deeper within the epidermis, miliaria rubra develops. Each vesicle

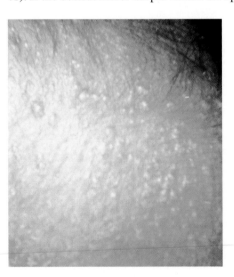

Figure 41. Miliaria crystallina alba. Immediately after birth this infant was noted to have fragile vesicles over her forehead into the scalp that disappeared with a first washing. There are a few lesions of milia on her nose that demonstrate the difference in these lesions.

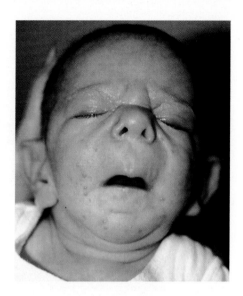

Figure 42. Neonatal acne. This infant has facies of de Lange syndrome with evidence of pustular acne over the face. Note the erythematous base to each pustule.

of miliaria crystallina measures 1 to 2 mm and has a delicate, thin roof that comes off with the gentlest of pressure. The lesions occur primarily on the forehead, neck, or upper trunk in the first 2 weeks of life. Although there are few case reports in the literature of lesions present at birth, it is likely more frequent than documented because of its transient nature, even in the absence of fever (92). The base of the lesion is nonerythematous and nonpigmented. The lesions rarely appear pustular, but there are never abnormal cellular elements in the fluid.

Miliaria rubra occurs in folds of the neck and groin, on the face, or under occlusive dressings or diapers. The lesions last 2 to 3 days and tend to recur unless the environmental conditions of heat and humidity are changed.

Neonatal Acne

Under the influence of maternal androgens, acne develops as red papules, pustules, and white heads (comedones) in up to 20% of newborn infants (Fig. 42). Open comedones or blackheads occur occasionally. The lesions develop most often after the first 2 weeks, last longer than the other more fleeting neonatal rashes, ETN or TPN, but generally resolve within a few months. Acne is more marked in breast-feeding infants, in infants with endogenous sources of androgen, and in Apert syndrome, XYY syndrome, and pseudo-Hurler polydystrophy (21).

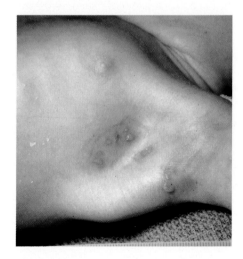

Figure 43. Herpes simplex. Appearance on day of life 12. The earliest lesions are circled; extension is apparent outside the marking.

Herpes Simplex

The lesions of neonatal herpes simplex are moist on an erythematous base, and the fluid contains multinucleated giant cells after Giemsa or Wright staining (Fig. 43). The Tzanck smear is prepared by removing the roof of a blister and scraping the base of the lesion to obtain moist debris that is spread on a slide and air dried. The giant cell typical of viral infections appears larger than other inflammatory cells and has overlapping nuclei. It should not be confused with overlapping epidermal cells. Direct fluorescent antibody testing is a rapid identification technique.

Most cases of herpes simplex type I are vertically transmitted by inoculation from lesions on the cervix or vagina and most often with a primary maternal infection, but there may be spread after birth from infected caregivers, and the infection can occur prenatally (93–95). The incubation period is 2 to 21 days, with a peak onset of symptoms at 1 week. Approximately 70% of neonatally infected infants develop the skin rash that begins as clusters of 1- to 2-mm red papulovesicles, appearing first at the site of inoculation, on the occiput in vertex presentations or on the buttocks in breech presentations. A common site for inoculation is the location of a fetal scalp monitor (96–98).

Varicella zoster transmitted from the mother just before birth also presents with vesicopustules that are clinically indistinguishable from herpes simplex, although they are generally more disseminated. The maternal history indicates a recent infection (95,99–101).

Staphylococcal Pustulosis

Skin pustules due to infection with *Staphylococcus aureus* develop in areas prone to skin trauma, such as the base of the umbilical cord, circumcision site, and the diaper area (Fig. 44). The lesions are 1- to 3-mm creamy white pustules on an erythematous base. If infection is due to phage group II strains of *Staphylococcus aureus,* bullous impetigo may develop (72). These bullae enlarge rapidly with initially clear, and later purulent, fluid. Stained preparations of contents in either conditions show typical Gram-positive cocci.

Staphylococcal Scalded Skin Syndrome

The dermal manifestations of staphylococcal scalded skin syndrome develop in response to an epidermolytic toxin made by the *Staphylococcal aureus* organism, most commonly phage group II, at a distant infection site (circumcision, umbilicus) and then transported in the blood to affect other skin areas (Fig. 45) (102–104). The rash begins as a faint, macular, orange–red scarlatiniform eruption often with accompanying conjunctivitis or rhinorrhea. Over the next 24 hours the rash spreads and becomes more confluent, edematous, and erythematous in an infant who appears quite ill. The surface wrinkles and leaves raw erosions to give the scalded skin appearance.

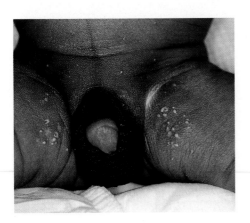

Figure 44. Superficial *Staphylococcus aureus* infection at 2 weeks of age. The pustules, concentrated in the diaper area, were on a generally erythematous area and remained moist after rupture. More distal, isolated lesions are seen spreading onto the abdomen.

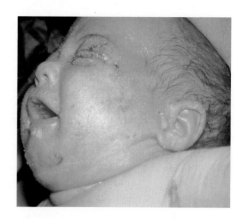

Figure 45. Staphylococcal scalded skin syndrome (SSSS) (synonym *Ritter's disease*).

Epidermolysis Bullosa

The conditions that cause recurrent blistering are a varied group that are differentiated on the basis of the inheritance pattern, clinical presentation, histopathology, and biochemical markers (Fig. 46) (105–109). The most severe forms present early, but the prognosis for each type depends on the level of cleavage of the blister. Those that are the deepest carry the worst prognosis because total blistering externally and internally can develop rapidly. The inheritance is either autosomal dominant or recessive depending on type. The most superficial blistering conditions might not result in scarring. With deeper lesions, the healing is more dystrophic, leading to atrophy, loss of skin appendages, and digital fusion. Because of internal damage, there is an association of epidermolysis bullosa with internal stenoses of the pylorus, larynx, and esophagus and with ulcerative colitis (110–113).

Incontinentia Pigmenti

Incontinentia pigmenti (IP) (Fig. 47) occurs almost exclusively in girls and presents at birth or within the first 6 weeks, with skin manifestations of patches of erythema and blisters on the scalp, trunk, and extremities arranged in swirls and lines. The blisters can recur but eventually are replaced by verrucous lesions that then become hyperpigmented. Some present at birth or shortly thereafter with swirls of hyperpigmentation. In later childhood the hyperpigmented lesions fade into hypopigmented, atrophic patches. IP is a neurocutaneous syndrome associated with a high incidence (80%) of other systemic defects: hair

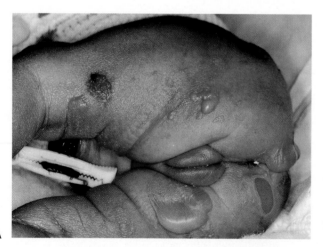

A

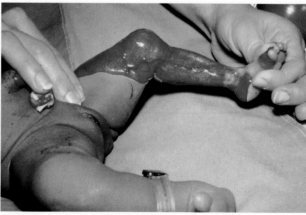

B

Figure 46. Epidermolysis bullosa. **A:** Areas of denudation are adjacent to areas of flaccid bullae. The denudation includes the base of the umbilicus. **B:** Rather than flaccid bullae, there is total denudation of the undergrown extremity showing subcutaneous anatomy.

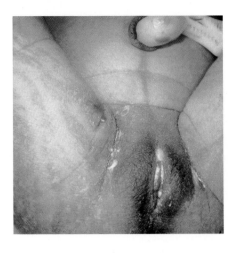

Figure 47. Incontinentia pigmenti (IP). Blistering with denudation is apparent with early hyperpigmented lines and swirls on the thighs.

(38%), nail (7%), dental (65%), ocular (35%), skeletal (14%), and neurologic (31%) (114–116).

Cultis Aplasia

Aplasia cutis congenita is a heterogeneous group of skin disorders in which there are localized or widespread foci of absent skin. In the majority of instances the absence is limited to the scalp, typically over the occiput, without other anomalies, although it may be seen in association with limb reduction defects as part of amnionic band syndrome or with epidermal and organoid nevi (107). Other areas of the body also may be involved, and it may overlie occult embryologic malformations, including spina bifida or cutaneous attachment of a fibrous tract to the dura or filum terminale (117). The complication of sagittal sinus hemorrhage is reported in a patient with large mid-line scalp defects associated with absence of the underlying cranium (118). A form of aplasia cutis congenita occurs in association with placental infarcts (119) or the in utero death of a twin fetus (120). Aplasia cutis congenita may be the presenting manifestation of epidermolysis bullosa, fetal teratogens, or intrauterine infections (107). Large scalp defects are characteristic of Trisomy 13 (21). Most cases are sporadic, but there are familial occurrences, particularly of the isolated scalp defects, and the pedigrees show an inheritance pattern consistent with autosomal dominance with reduced penetrance or autosomal recessiveness (121).

Plaques and Nodules

Lymphangioma
Hemangioma
Venous malformation
Subcutaneous fat necrosis
Juvenile xanthogranuloma

Epidermal nevus
Sebaceous nevus
Melanogenic nevus
Cutaneous smooth muscle nevus

An algorithm for evaluating plaques and nodules is depicted in Fig. 48.

Cutaneous Lymphangioma

These lesions may involve every area of skin, including fingers, scalp, umbilicus, foreskin, vulva, and ear lobe. Most commonly on the anterior and lateral chest, the thigh and buttock, neck and axilla, there is no predilection for side. Histologically the lymphangioma is identified by the presence of thin-walled, irregularly shaped vascular channels that are empty or do not contain many erythrocytes unless they are associated with complex vascular malformations (122).

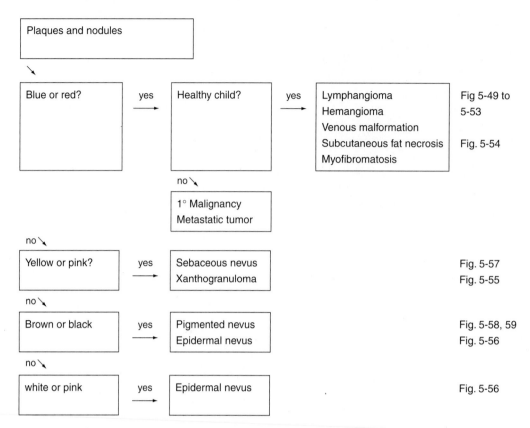

Figure 48. Algorithm for evaluation of plaques and nodules. Modified from Cohen (37) with permission.

Vascular Lesions: Hemangiomas and Venous Malformations

Identification and classification of the various types of vascular skin lesions that present within the neonatal period have been confusing, with a variety of naming systems based on appearance or histopathology but not helpful in determining clinical course. Mulliken has suggested a classification system based on the clinical characteristics and course as well as the histologic findings (123). The three broad, clinically useful categories of cutaneous vascular abnormalities are angiomatous nevi or hemangiomas, vascular malformations, and angiokeratomas, with subdivision into types of vascular malformations (Table 7). The only angiokeratoma potentially present at birth is the rare angiokeratoma circumscripta. It has a clinical appearance of a plaque of aggregated papules that are deep red to blue–black in a streaky, zosteriform configuration on one lower leg or foot that resembles lymphangioma circumscripta except in color. Characterization and comparison of hemangioma and vascular malformations as suggested by Mulliken are shown in Table 8.

The term **hemangioma** (angiomatous nevus) is reserved for lesions that are proliferative, unlike vascular malformations, meaning there is a period of increase in size and number of cells wherein the lesion grows faster than the infant, followed by an involution (Figs. 49–53). In contrast, **vascular malformations** grow at the same rate as the infant and do not decrease in size by involution (Fig. 54). Vascular malformations can decrease in size by spontaneous vascular occlusions. At birth, because the capacity to proliferate may not be clinically evident, it is more difficult to separate some of these lesions than it is by the end of the neonatal period.

In term infants the greater the number of cutaneous hemangiomas the more likely there is internal involvement. In contrast, premature infants of all races seem to have both a higher incidence and greater numbers of hemangiomas and do not have the same female

Table 7. *Translation from old terminology for vascular birthmarks into hemangioma or malformation*

Hemangioma	Old terminology	Malformation
←	Capillary	
←	Strawberry	
	Port-wine ──────→	CAPILLARY
←	Capillary-cavernous	
	Cavernous ──────↘	
	Venous ──────→	VENOUS
	Hemangio-lymphangioma ↘	
	Lymphangioma ──────↗	LYMPHATIC
	Arteriovenous ──────→	ARTERIOVENOUS

From Mulliken and Young, ref. 223, with permission.

sexual predominance, with a male-to-female ratio of only 1:1.4 (124). There does not appear to be any concordance in identical twins. Hemangiomas occur with increasing frequency with decreasing gestational age: 22.9% in infants with birth weights below 1,000 g, 15.6% in infants with birth weights below 1,500 g (124). It is unusual for hemangiomas in premature infants to require therapy, and spontaneous involution generally starts within the first year. In all infants the vascular lesions likely to require therapy are those that occlude the airway or the field of vision, that have arteriovenous fistulae leading to high-output heart failure, or that trap platelets with a microangiopathic hemolytic anemia and consumption coagulopathy (the Kasabach-Merritt syndrome) (125,126).

Table 8. *Characteristics of vascular birthmarks*

Hemangioma	Malformation
Clinical	
Usually nothing seen at birth, 30% present as red macule	All present at birth; may not be evident
Rapid postnatal proliferation and slow involution	Commensurate growth; may expand as a result of trauma, sepsis, hormonal modulation
Female:male 3:1	Female:male 1:1
Cellular	
Plump endothelium, increased turnover	Flat endothelium, slow turnover
Increased mast cells	Normal mast cell count
Multilaminated basement membrane	Normal thin basement membrane
Capillary tubule formation in vitro	Poor endothelial growth in vitro
Hematologic	
Primary platelet trapping: thrombocytopenia (Kasabach-Merritt syndrome)	Primary stasis (venous); localized consumptive coagulopathy
Radiologic	
Angiographic findings: well-circumscribed, intense lobular-parenchymal staining with equatorial vessels	Angiographic findings: diffuse, no parenchyma
	Low-flow: phleboliths, ectatic channels
	High-flow: enlarged, tortuous arteries with arteriovenous shunting
Skeletal	
Infrequent "mass effect" on adjacent bone; hypertrophy rare	Low-flow: distortion, hypertrophy, or hypoplasia
	High-flow: destruction, distortion, or hypertrophy

From Mulliken and Young, ref. 223, with permission.

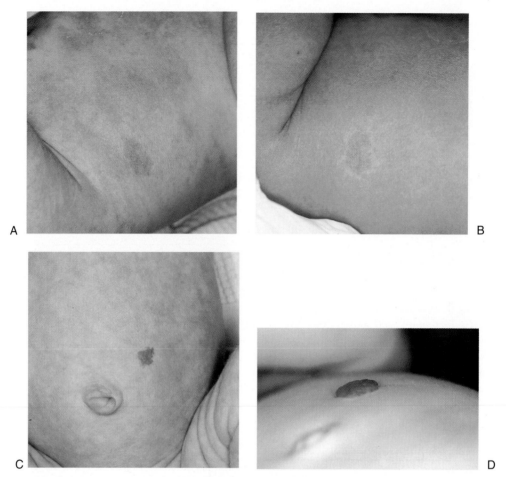

Figure 49. **A:** Early hemangioma on the abdomen appears at first glance to be an ecchymosis, but it blanches upon compression. **B:** Stroking the area causes a blanching in the periphery but dilation of the vessels in the center. The infant has marked erythema toxicum that is apparent until he starts to cry and skin becomes flushed. **C:** In a prematurely born infant at 3 weeks of age, the hemangioma appears bright red. Note the physiologic mottling. **D:** At 4 months' corrected gestational age, the hemangioma has reached its full size but has not started to involute.

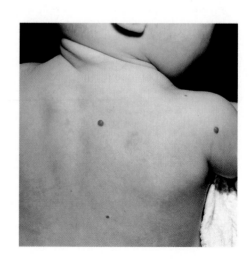

Figure 50. Premature infant with multiple hemangiomas that appeared at 40 weeks' corrected gestational age but were not apparent at birth at 27 weeks' gestation. She developed a total of 13 hemangiomas, of which these were the largest. Her nonidential twin had a single large hemangioma on an extremity. Involution was partial by 2 years of age.

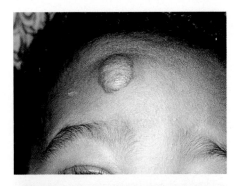

Figure 51. Hemangioma beginning to involute with softening, some loss of volume in the center, and change in color from red to gray. With further involution the mass will retract. Although there may be some residual change of stretching in the overlying skin in especially large areas, most become barely visible by school age.

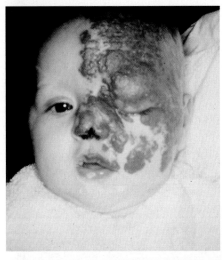

Figure 52. Aggressive hemangioma of the face likely to cause amblyopia and glaucoma of the left eye if not controlled. Although the distribution is in the trigeminal region, this is a proliferative lesion rather than a vascular stain so is not consistent with simple port-wine staining. Any vascular lesions of this magnitude would require studies of the central nervous system (204).

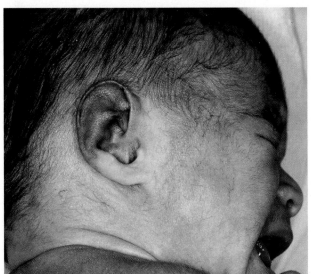

Figure 53. Complex vascular lesion of face associated with Dandy-Walker syndrome (204). At birth fine telangiectasias were present around the ear and onto the neck and anterior cheek. When the infant cried vigorously, the area did not flush compared with the adjacent normal area. The right ear had simplified folding of a thinner pinna but the left ear was well formed and of normal thickness. The lesion is developed into a typical raised hemangioma. The presence of this type of lesion would warrant neuroimaging for complete evaluation. The transillumination of this infant is shown in Chapter 6, Fig. 22.

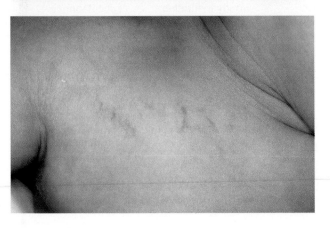

Figure 54. Venous malformation over right upper hemithorax. This lesion demonstrates prominence of superficial vessels, but often the depth of vascular malformations is so great that their vascular component is not apparent. This lesion has not changed in size or appearance over the first year.

Other Conditions Causing Plaques or Nodules in the Neonatal Period

Subcutaneous Fat Disorders

The development of subcutaneous fat is an important measure of nutritional health and maturity in the fetus. The layer of fat serves as an important insulator against trauma and cold stress, and the chemical production of heat by subcutaneous fat is critical for thermostasis in neonates. There are a limited number of disorders of subcutaneous tissues in neonates, many of which have been virtually eliminated by good perinatal care. There still are occasions when infants are born in or exposed to extreme cold or experience direct physical trauma or asphyxia severe enough to injure the subcutaneous tissue. Characteristics of the types of disorders are given in Table 9.

Juvenile Xanthogranuloma

Juvenile xanthogranuloma (JXG) is a self-limited tumor that grows into yellow papules, plaques, or nodules 0.5 cm to 4.0 cm in diameter (Fig. 55). About half of JXGs are isolated

Table 9. *Disorders of the subcutaneous fat in neonates[a]*

Feature	Cold panniculitis	Neonatal cold injury	Sclerema	Subcutaneous fat necrosis
Frequency	Uncommon	Previously common, now rare	Rare, usually seen in neonatal intensive care units	Uncommon generalized, most common in very small areas (buccal fat pad)
Patient	Any aged patient can develop cold panniculitis, but the younger the patient, the shorter the necessary time exposure	Full-term neonates, often small-for-dates, born out of the hospital and exposed to low environmental temperature	Usually severely ill neonates often preterm or small-for-dates, commonly with sepsis and poor perfusion syndromes	Healthy infants, usually full-term or post-term or after hypothermia for cardiac surgery. When over wide area, associated with hypercalcemia in late phase (224, 225)
Onset	Within hours or days of exposure. Occurs almost always after exposure of cheeks to cold air. Application of ice for 50 seconds can cause panniculitis.	During the first week	Almost always during the first week	1–6 weeks
Sites	Cheeks or any area in direct contact with extreme cold	Extremities, spreading centrally	Lower limbs initially, become generalized	Trunk, buttocks, thighs, arms, face
Appearance	Indurated, warm, red subcutaneous plaques and nodules that quickly resolve with warming although there may be residual hyperpigmentation	Pitting edema initially with erythema or cyanosis of face and extremities	Diffuse yellow-white woody induration with immobility of limbs	Firm reddish–violet subcutaneous nodules that undergoes liquefaction
Histology	Lymphohistiocytic infiltrate around the blood vessels at the junction of dermis and subcutaneous fat	Thin panniculus	Subtle; thickened connective tissue trabeculae; radial needle-like clefts	Granulomatous inflammation and fat necrosis
Prognosis	Self-resolving	Mortality rate around 25%	Poor, mortality greater than 50%	Generally excellent

[a] These conditions are separate entities often although with clinical overlap.
  Data from Kruse (224), Thomsen (225), Molteni (226), Vonk (227), Chen (228), Fretzin (229), Megilner (230), Silverman (231), Norwood-Galloway (232), Shackelford (233), Hughes (234), Warwick (235), and Hicks (236).

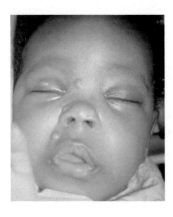

Figure 55. Juvenile xanthogranuloma. Three lesions appear near the midline. A fourth is on the right eyelid.

or they may be scattered, but the sites tend to be on the head and neck, with the trunk and extremities affected less often. Giant xanthogranuloma with complicated course is extremely rare (127). After a period of proliferation, the lesions spontaneously regress. Recurrence is most likely in adult onset (128). Biopsies show lipid-laden histiocytes, but serum lipid levels are normal. JXGs are associated with extracutaneous symptoms, including spontaneous hemorrhage of the anterior chamber of the eye (128).

Nevi

Epidermal Nevus

Epidermal nevi (synonym *nevus unius lateralis*) derive from pleuripotential ectodermal cells that can evolve into a variety of cell types (Fig. 56). Classifications of the epidermal nevi are based on what type of cell predominates. In the immediate newborn period it is not always possible nor particularly important to distinguish clearly what final form an epidermal nevus will take. What is more important is predicting a clinical course to determine the course of follow-up or to recognize patterns of nevi that are associated with multisystem syndromes or defects, particularly in the skeletal and central nervous systems.

Epidermal Nevus Syndrome

Several epidermal nevus syndromes are described in the literature that reflect skeletal and neurologic associations (129–132). The epidermal nevus syndrome (ENS) was originally described with sebaceous nevi, but the association is often made with any combination of epidermal nevus with any single significant skeletal, neurologic, or ocular abnor-

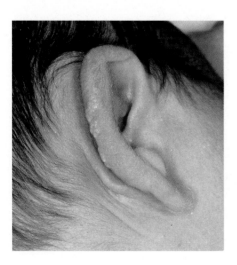

Figure 56. Epidermal nevus on ear. There is normally little color associated with epidermal nevus unless an infant is sufficiently jaundiced to cause it to yellow.

Table 10. *Defects associated with epidermal nevus syndrome*

Cutaneous	Skeletal	Neurologic (50% of cases)	Ocular (~33%)	Other
Angiomatous	Kyphosis	40% mental retardation	Eyelid nevus	Bilateral sensorineural deafness
Nevus flammei	Scoliosis	30% seizures	Coloboma of lid, iris, retina	Endocrine disease
Hypochromic nevi	Cystic and lytic changes	Spastic hemiparesis	Conjunctival lipodermoids and choristomas	Cardiac disease
Café au laitmacules	Hypertrophy	Spastic tetraparesis	Cortical blindness	Genitourinary disease
Congenital melanocytic nevi	Atrophy	Cerebral vascular malformation and secondary changes after hemorrhage	Microphthalmia	Higher incidence of systemic malignancies
Dermatomegaly	Short limbs		Macrophthalmia	
Dental enamel hypoplasia	Syndactaly		Anophthalmia	
Hypodontia	Vitamin D resistant rickets	Encephalocele	Corneal opacities and cataracts	
Malformation of teeth				

mality. As many as 10% of children with epidermal nevi may have ENS with the likelihood higher, the larger and more widespread the nevus. Any nevus associated with ENS has the same potential for malignancy as it does outside the syndrome. There appears to be a higher incidence of systemic malignancies at an early age in the ENS (131). The defects associated with ENS are shown in Table 10.

Sebaceous Nevus

The most common type of epidermal nevus present at birth, sebaceous nevus (synonym *sebaceous nevus of Jadassohn*), is found in about 0.3% of all neonates (Fig. 57) (133). Most occur sporadically, with occasional familial cases (134,135). The nevus may first come to attention as a bald spot in the scalp, devoid of hair or with occasional hair follicles. The lesions vary from 1 to 10 cm, are round, oval, or linear, and rarely are found at more than one site. The slightly raised, pebbly surface is distinctly oily or velvety in texture in the early neonatal period, betraying the sebaceous gland origin. The color is pink, yellow, or orange, increasing in yellowness if the infant is jaundiced.

After the newborn period the lesions feel less oily and appear more verrucous. Tumors that are either local, invasive, or malignant may develop within the sebaceous nevus but generally not until after puberty. The proportion of sebaceous nevi diagnosed in newborn

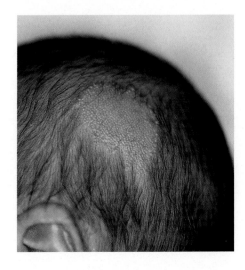

Figure 57. Sebaceous nevus on scalp. Initially pale pink or yellow, the surface feels waxy and has little or no hair. After the neonatal period, the color will fade and there will be no increase in area. With the pubertal growth spurt there may be a more rapid growth and nodularity with syringo-cystadenomatous changes.

Table 11. *Lesions in differential diagnosis of sebaceous nevus at birth*

Nevus	Pinker surface
syringocystadenomatosis	More individual nodules
papilliferous	Not waxy
	Hair follicles interspersed
Cutis aplasia	Surface covering, if present, is more paperlike
	Lesion is an erosion, not raised
	Family history more likely
Solitary mastocytoma	Lesion demonstrates wheal and may blister
	More commonly located on extremities or trunk
Early juvenile	Pinker
xanthogranuloma	Evolves into domed, papular, or nodular lesion
	Not commonly present at birth (127, 128, 237)
Encephalocele or heterotopic brain tissue with overlying bald spot (238)	Circular, hemispherically elevated, dull reddish surface

infants that develop into tumors is unknown (136). The lesions that may appear similar to sebaceous nevus in the newborn period are compared in Table 11.

Congenital Melanocytic Nevi

Congenital melanocytic nevi (CMNs) are grouped by their adult size as giant, larger than 20 cm; intermediate, 2 to 20 cm; and small, under 2 cm (Figs. 58 and 59). Giant CMNs are uncommon, occurring in fewer than one in 20,000 infants and in more girls than boys (137). These nevi develop typically over the posterior trunk with irregular topography, including coarse hair, irregular pigmentation, and tumor nodules, with satellite nevi often present. When located on the limbs, the extremity may be undergrown. If covering the head or posterior midline of the back, there may be neural melanosis leading to increased intracranial pressure, seizures, and developmental delay, and carrying a poor prognosis (138). When associated early with rapid growth, intracranial extension may be present (139). The reported estimation of malignant conversion of giant CMNs ranges from 3% to 45%, but the true risk is probably between 5% and 15%, with a higher risk in early childhood (140–143). Close follow-up is clearly indicated.

Small CMNs occur in about 1% of the general population, with a higher incidence in darkly pigmented populations (35,133,144–146). At birth small CMNs are difficult to distinguish from other pigmented lesions, so it is best to document the appearance and size for accurate comparison in follow-up. There is a relationship that is less clear between small CMNs and melanoma but, for the most part, treatment, if necessary, is generally delayed a

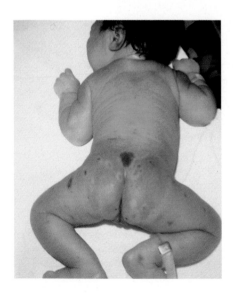

Figure 58. Congenital melanocytic nevus. The location and size of this nevus necessitates consideration of spinal bifida occulta and an associated tethering of the spinal cord. Other lesions that correlate with underlying spinal defects are hemangiomas, lipomas, skin tags, or a faun-tail nevus that has long tufts of hair (205,206). There is an absence of Mongolian spotting around these pigmented nevi. The darker lesions are likely to darken and develop more prominent hair during the first 2 years. One cannot determine at birth if light lesions will darken. When multiple areas are involved, the differential diagnosis includes dermal extramedullary hematopoiesis, congenital primary melanoma, and metastatic melanoma, but biopsy may be necessary to distinguish the cause.

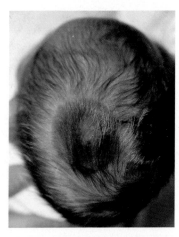

Figure 59. Congenital melanocytic nevus. The round appearance in this location might suggest the corona of ecchymosis seen after vacuum extraction or prolonged engagement of the fetal head, but it is a giant nevus with variable pigmentation as seen by the smaller dark point near the center. The size and location of this nevus in a lightly pigmented infant is of concern for the potential association with neurologic involvement.

few years. Candidates for surgical removal are patients with deeply or irregularly pigmented nevi, those with light skin who have a family history of melanoma, and those with nevi in an abnormal pattern (147). Use of the following mnemonic may help determine which lesions should be removed (148,149):

*A*symmetry
*B*order irregularity
*C*olor variation
*D*iameter greater than 6 mm or changing size of atypical area
*E*levation with firm nodules

Congenital Pilar and Smooth Muscle Nevus

This rare lesion is an organoid nevus that has smooth muscle bundles in the dermis and a prominence of vellus hairs (Fig. 60) (150,151). An estimated prevalence is about one in 2,600 live births, with a slight male predominance (152). The lesions typically appear off the midline in the lumbosacral area in an oval plaque of 2 to 4 cm that is either nonpigmented or only slightly discolored but remarkable for the presence of more prominent hair. The lesion feels indurated but superficial. Upon stroking, the skin wrinkles and hair stands erect momentarily (pseudo Darier's phenomenon). Because the skin may redden with rubbing and appear edematous as the muscles contract, it can resemble a mastocytoma, but

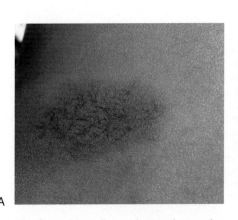
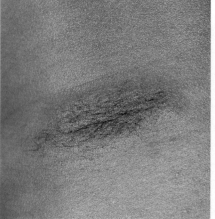

A   B

Figure 60. Congenital pilar and smooth muscle nevus (150). **A:** Undisturbed, the well-defined area on the left flank of this 4-month-old infant appears only slightly darker than the surrounding skin with coarser, more pigmented hair. **B:** After stroking, the nevus becomes more wrinkled and slightly raised as the hair follicles erect.

there is no blistering or wheal formation with stimulation (153). The lesions enlarge slightly as the infant grows but become less prominent. There does not appear to be any increased risk of malignant transformation (152).

Lesions with Pigment Change as Primary Finding

Vascular stains
   salmon patch
   port wine stain
Cutis marmorata
Vascular collapse
Purpura fulminans

Cutis marmorata telangiectatica congenita
Lupis
Harlequin sign
Café-au-lait spot
Ash leaf spots

An algorithm for evaluating flat lesions with color change is provided in Fig. 61.

Vascular Stains: Telangiectatic Nevi

Salmon Patch

The lesions of salmon patch (synonym *erythema nuchae, Unna's nevus, stork bite, angel's kiss, nevus flammeus nuchae, medial telangiectatic nevus, nevus simplex*) are dull, pinkish red, irregularly shaped, blanching macules often with fine telangiectasia visible on close inspection (Fig. 62). They occur most often on the nape of the neck (hence, the name stork bite) but also on the eyelids, glabella, forehead, and upper lip (angel's kiss). They can be found in 22% to 40% of children of all races, with the higher incidence reported in white neonates (34–36,154–156). Some appear to have an autosomal-dominant pattern of inheri-

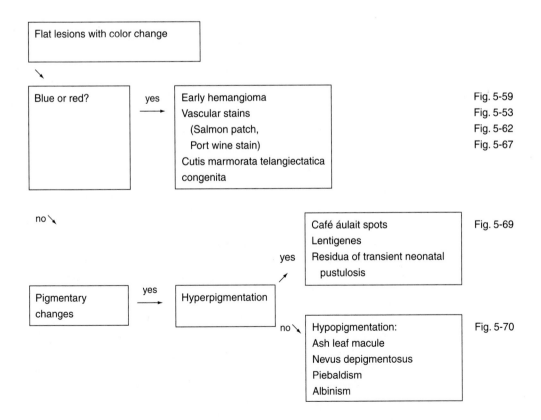

Figure 61. Algorithm for evaluation of flat lesions with color change only. Modified from Cohen (37) with permission.

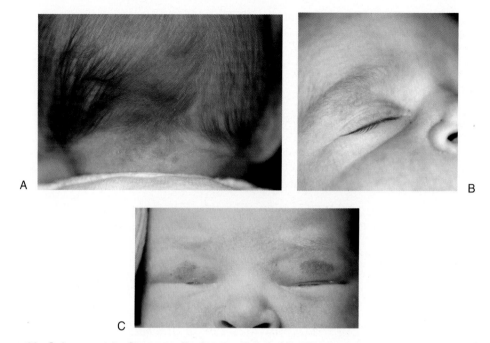

Figure 62. Salmon patch. Synonym *Erythema nuchae, Unna's nevus, nevus flammeus simplex.* **A:** Nuchal salmon patch at hairline. **B:** Stain on eyelid with telangiectasia. **C:** Ecchymoses on eyelids resembling salmon patch but without the characteristic blanching. It is important to recognize the difference because ecchymoses on the lids may indicate injury to the underlying eye.

tance (157,158). Most lesions except those on the neck disappear by 1 year of age (159). Lesions on the glabella may lighten with age but become more visable with anxiety or activity.

Port-Wine Staining

Port-wine staining (PWS; synonym *nevus flammeus, lateral telangiectatic nevus*) is a vascular malformation of developmental origin characterized by persistent macular erythema (Fig. 63). Although present at birth, it may initially be relatively pale and hard to discern. These lesions range in size from a few millimeters to many centimeters. They are most frequently unilaterally located on the face, but also appear on the upper trunk, back, and extremities in decreasing frequency.

The lesions rarely increase in area but grow with the infant. With time, the pink macular lesions progress to dark red to purple, particularly when they are located on the face; when on the limbs, they have a greater tendency to fade with time. Some stains become more nodular and cobblestoned in appearance, with small angiomatous nodules present within the affected area.

The reported incidence in the newborn is from 0.1% to 2% with no significant sexual predilection (34–36,154,160,161). There is no pattern of inheritance, except when PWS is part of an associated syndrome such as hereditary neurocutaneous angioma, in which case it is autosomal dominant (162), or part of a familial disorder involving hydrocephalus, posterior cerebellar agenesis, or mega cisterna magna, in which case it is autosomal dominant with variable expression (163).

Port-wine stains are not hemangiomas. At birth the histologic abnormalities are minimal. There is a progressive dilatation of mature dermal blood vessels, starting most superficially and increasing more deeply although always remaining predominantly in the upper dermis. Only the diameter of the vessels, not the total number, is likely increased. Therefore this is not a true nevus or hemangioma. There is a diminished density of perivascular nerves in the cutaneous superficial vascular plexus (164).

Port-wine stains can occur either in isolation or with structural abnormalities, particularly in those underlying the birthmark itself.

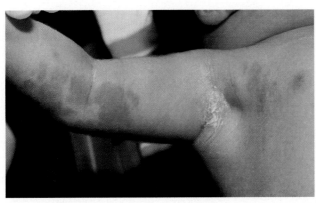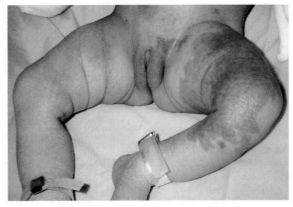

A   B

Figure 63. Vascular staining of thigh and leg. **A:** Subtle mark of a vascular stain likely to fade. **B:** More dramatic port-wine stain that will not fade. At the time of birth, it is difficult to say with certainty which lesions are vascular stains that will not increase in size and which are hemangiomas that will undergo proliferation. By the end of the neonatal period, the distinction will be easier.

Port-Wine Stain Associations

Eye: glaucoma

Face: angiomatosis of the leptomeningeal vessels in the brain, causing seizures (Sturge-Weber syndrome) when bilateral, or involving the ophthalmic and maxillary division of the trigeminal nerve (161,165)

Segmental distribution of the spinal nerves: hemangioma of the cord at the corresponding level, causing weakness and loss of sensation below the lesion (Cobb syndrome) (166)

Lumbosacral region: spina bifida occulta; lumbosacral hemangiomas are more often associated with spina bifida occulta than with PWS (167–170)

Trunk or extremities: underlying venous and lymphatic abnormalities (Klipple-Trenaunay syndrome) with or without bony overgrowth

Oral mucosa, gingivae, lip, or eyelid: soft-tissue swelling of underlying tissue

Other Vascular Skin Changes

Cutis Marmorata

Immature skin shows a normal tendency to mottle, especially when exposed to cold (Fig. 64A). Cutis marmorata (synonym *cutaneous marbeling*) is greatest on the extremities but is present on the trunk as well. It is most noticeable on lightly pigmented infants. If mot-

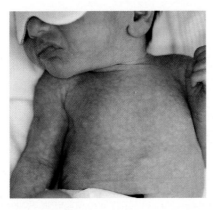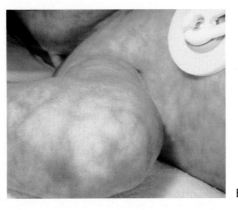

A   B

Figure 64. A: Normal mottling in premature infant. The prominent xiphoid is a normal finding in thin infants. **B:** Exaggerated mottling due to severe hypertension. Cutaneous marbling is seen in a variety of conditions, including congenital hypothyroidism, de Lange syndrome, trisomies 18 and 21, Coffin-Lowry syndrome, and Adams-Oliver syndrome (21).

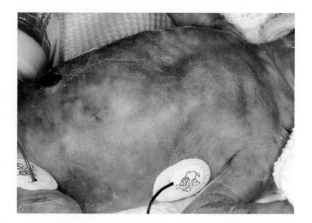

Figure 65. Evidence of extreme vascular constriction in an infant with Gram-negative sepsis. Areas of pooling are adjacent to areas of blanching. The arterial blood oxygen saturation was much higher than the level of skin cyanosis would suggest because the slow circulation through the skin allowed almost complete extraction of oxygen from the capillary blood.

tling is excessive, does not improve with warming, or persists past the first few months, other conditions may be involved, including cardiovascular hypertension (Fig. 64B) and hypothyroidism. Some infants with Down's syndrome have a tendency to have exaggerated mottling throughout infancy.

Vasomotor collapse

Extreme vascular markings on the skin occur in conditions of vascular collapse when the circulation to the skin is irregularly restricted (Fig. 65). Some areas are blanched, with other areas showing marked cyanosis in the low flow to dermal capillaries. When circulation is completely restricted by capillary thrombosis, purpura fulminans may develop rapidly, leading to localized areas of purpuric lesions that result in skin necrosis and ulceration (Fig.

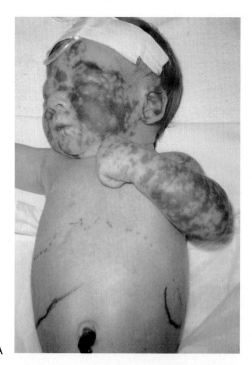

A

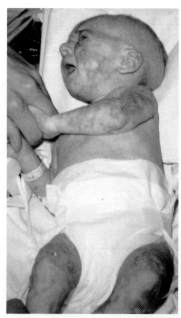

B

Figure 66. Purpura fulminans. **A:** The acute phase of hepatosplenomegaly and disseminated intravascular coagulopathy with marked purpuric lesions distally and sparing of the trunk. **B:** Recovery phase at 1 month of age shows areas of necrosis apparent over the arm, cheeks, and pinna corresponding with the acute lesions most deeply purpuric. Infants who develop this degree of purpura should be tested for protein C deficiency, either as a result of overwhelming sepsis or congenital deficiency (171).

66). Bacterial infections, particularly with *Pseudomonas* and other Gram-negative rods and protein C deficiency, have been implicated (171).

Cutis Marmorata Telangiectatica Congenita

Cutis marmorata telangiectatica congenita (synonym *congenital generalized phlebectasia, nevus vascularis reticularis, congenital livedo, reticulate vascular nevus*) is a rare condition that is a combination of a capillary and venous vascular malformation characterized by a persistence of reticulate erythema in an area ranging from a few centimeters to large portions of the extremities or a generalized condition (Fig. 67). Involvement of the limbs is more common than of the trunk or face, and the distribution is segmental and asymmetric although not strictly unilateral. The skin in the area may be atrophic or ulcerated in linear erosions. Telangiectasia is visible within the hyperemic areas (172).

When the face is involved, the lesions are similar to PWS, and there is a high risk for glaucoma (173). In addition to underlying atrophy of the skin, there is risk for facial hemiatrophy or reduced growth of affected limbs. Occasionally hypertrophy of the affected limb may develop (174). Gradually, most lesions fade except those particularly prominent or associated with marked ulceration (172,175–178). If the lesions are uniform bilaterally or prominent on the head, they more likely represent congenital lupus with atrophy and telangiectasia.

Congenital Lupus Erythematosus

Neonatal lupus is a reaction to a transplacentally transmitted material, most likely the ssA(Ro) or ssB(La) antibodies, in a manner similar to Sjögren's syndrome in adults with those antibodies (179–183) (Fig. 68). The major symptoms include congenital heart block and variable effect on the reticuloendothelial system with hepatosplenomegaly, thrombocytopenia, leukopenia, anemia, and lymphadenopathy. The symptoms last for weeks to months until the level of circulating antibodies decreases. The third-degree congenital heart block normally is permanent (184,185), but reversal of fetal heart block after maternal therapy with steroids has been reported (186). Results of testing for ssA(Ro) or ssB(La) antibodies by immunodiffusion in the neonate are not always positive, but other antibodies will be detected (187). The skin manifestations of maternally transmitted lupus erythematosus are a vascular reaction that may be present at birth but more commonly appears at any time up to several months after birth. The rash may be composed of small areas of atrophy with overlying telangiectasis, much like cutis marmorata telangiectatica congenita, or as scaling discoid erythematous plaques with telangiectasia, atrophy, and pigmentary changes. Telangiectasia and atrophy may persist, although most show some improvement or disappear completely (188). Newborn infants may have signs of lupus without their mothers showing any symptoms of the disease as long as the necessary antibodies have been transmitted (189).

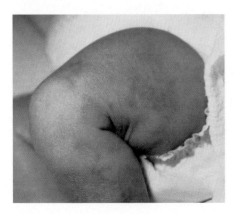

Figure 67. Cutis marmorata telangiectatica congenita. Present on the left leg and arm, the mottled appearance was accompanied by underlying atrophy at birth.

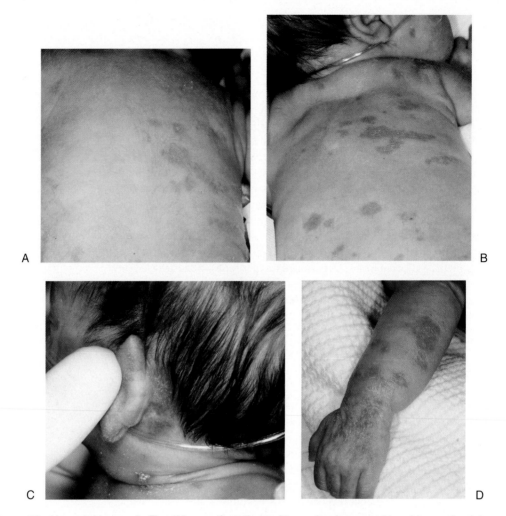

Figure 68. Neonatal lupus. **A:** The skin manifestations of lupus begin as nonblanching, pale pink macules randomly distributed over all skin surfaces but maximum in intertriginous areas. In this infant born at 28 weeks, the first lesions developed at 1 month of age. **B:** In 48 hours the lesions increased in intensity of erythema and distribution. **C:** The intertriginous areas showed the maximum scaling with skin breakdown. **D:** Arrest of the process was rapid after systemic steroids were initiated for severe thrombocytopenia and deteriorating liver function. Forty-eight hours into a short course of treatment the erythema began to subside, the platelets became normal, and the liver function improved. A recurrence of the skin lesions after the systemic steroids were stopped quickly responded to local steroid therapy.

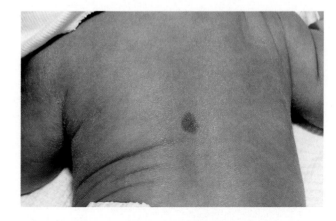

Figure 69. Café-au-lait spot. This flat spot is expected to grow proportionately with the infant. The hyperpigmentation in the café-au-lait spot is epidermal melanosis and thus light brown, whereas the melanosis in the lesion over the shoulder is deeper and, therefore, appears slate gray or blue.

Harlequin Sign

Another vascular phenomenon unique to neonates is the dramatic but fleeting harlequin sign. The harlequin color change presents with a distinct line of demarcation along the midline, including the face in side-lying infants. The dependent half is a deep red, and the upper half pale. The color differentiation lasts a few seconds or up to a half hour and in some infants reverses when the infant's position is changed. Single episodes are the rule, although some recurrences may be present in the neonatal period, particularly in more premature infants (190,191). The one hypothesis advanced regarding immature hypothalamic control of vascular tone remains untested (192). When the color changes recur or persist, associated cardiac disease should be considered (193).

Disorders of Pigmentation

Café-au-Lait Spot

One percent to 20% of normal infants have café-au-lait spots varying in size from pinpoints to 20 cm or more (Fig. 69) (160). These lesions are regions of increased epidermal melanosis, so they are a lighter tan or brown than pigmented nevi. The appearance of the café-au-lait spot is no different from the surrounding skin except in color. Spots are far more common in normal infants of color, with an incidence of less than 2% in Japanese infants (35). White infants rarely have more than one spot greater than 5 mm. The presence of six or more spots, regardless of size or race, particularly if located in the axillae, is abnormal and suggests an associated neurocutaneous syndrome: neurofibromatosis, Bannayan-Riley-Rubalcaba syndrome, multiple lentigines syndrome, or fibrous dysplasia (194).

Hypopigmented Lesions

About 0.1% of normal newborns have hypopigmented macules (ash-leaf macules) that measure 2 mm to 3 cm, but they should be followed for possible tuberous sclerosis because 70% to 90% of such individuals have similar lesions (Fig. 70). The majority of infants with one or two hypopigmented macules will have simple nevus depigmentosus with no other signs of neurocutaneous disease (160). Rarely there may be poor intellectual development and hemihypertrophy but without tuberous sclerosis.

Apparently depigmented lesions should be rubbed to cause hyperemia. If the lesion remains blanched while the surrounding skin reddens with vasodilation, the lesion is likely a nevus anemicus. On diascopy the lesion blends with the blanched surrounding skin. At birth these lesions can appear pinker than surrounding skin and then become paler. There is no histologic abnormality in the skin but rather a localized increase in reactivity to catecholamines (195,196). Nevus anemicus is frequently associated with PWS (197,198).

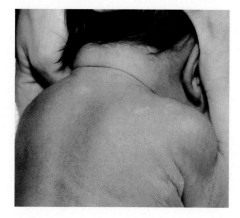

Figure 70. Hypopigmented lesions on shoulder and crossing the mid-line. Because the development of pigment may be somewhat irregular at the time of birth, continued absence of pigmentation should be documented over the next several weeks before diagnosing true ash leaf spots or other unpigmented lesions.

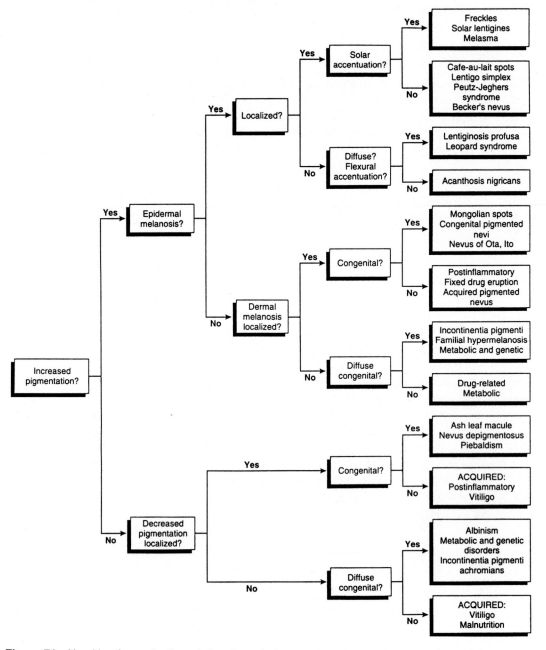

Figure 71. Algorithm for evaluation of disorders of pigmentation. Reprinted from Cohen (37) with permission.

Table 12. *Neonatal pustular lesions*

Disease	Usual age	Skin: morphology	Skin: usual distribution	Clinical: other	Diagnosis/findings
Infectious causes					
Staphylococcal impetigo	Few days to weeks	Pustules, bullae, occasional vesicles	Mainly diaper area, periumbilical	More prevalent in boys than in girls; may be in epidemic setting	Gram stain: PMNs; gram + cocci in clusters; bacterial culture
Staphylococcal scalded skin syndrome	3 to 7 days; occasionally older	Erythema, cutaneous tenderness; superficial blisters, erosions	Generalized, begins on the face; blistering and erosions in areas of mechanical stress	Irritability, fever	Skin biopsy: separation of upper epidermis. Bacterial cultures: blood, urine, etc.
Group A streptococcus	Few days to weeks	Isolated pustules, honey-crusted areas	No specific area predisposed	Moist umbilical stump: cellulitis, meningitis, pneumonia occasionally	Gram stain: Gram + cocci in chains; bacterial culture
Group B streptococcus	At birth or first few days	Vesicles, bullae, erosions, honey-crusted lesions	No specific area predisposed	Pneumonia, bacteremia	Gram stain: gram + cocci chains; bacterial culture
Listeria monocytogenes	Usually at birth	Hemorrhagic pustules and petechiae	Generalized, especially trunk and extremities	Septic; respiratory distress; maternal fever	Gram stain: gram + rods, bacterial cultures
Hemophilus influenzae	Birth or first few days	Vesicles and crusted areas	No specific are predisposed	Bacteremia; meningitis may be present	Gram stain: small gram without bacilli; bacterial culture
Congenital syphilis	Usually at birth	Blisters or erosions on dusky or hemorrhagic base	Palms, soles, knees, abdomen, groin, buttocks	Low birth weight, hepatosplenomegaly, metaphyseal dystrophy	Dark field or FA of involved skin; serial serology
Congenital candidiasis	At birth or first week	Erythema and fine papules evolves into vesicles and pustules	Any part of body; palms and soles often involved	Prematurity, foreign body cervix, uterus risk factors	KOH: Hyphae, budding yeast
Neonatal candidiasis	Weeks to months	Scaly red patches with satellite papules and pustules	Diaper area or intertriginous areas	Usually none; previous antibiotic therapy	KOH: Hyphae, budding yeast
Neonatal herpes simplex	Usual: 5 to 14 days	Vesicles, crusts, erosions; may be grouped or not. May follow dermatome	Anywhere: scalp monitor site, torso, oral lesions are frequent sites	Signs of sepsis; irritability and lethargy; eye, CNS frequent disease	Tzanck; FA slide test; viral culture
Intrauterine herpes simplex	At birth	Vesicles, widespread bullae, erosions, scars, missing skin	Anywhere on body; skin involved in 90%	Low birth weight; microcephaly, chorioretinitis	Tzanck; FA; viral culture
Fetal varicella infection	At birth	Usually scarring, limb hypoplasia, erosions	Anywhere; usually extremities	Maternal varicella first trimester	Tzanck; FA; viral culture
Neonatal varicella	0 to 14 days	Vesicles on an erythematous base; may be very numerous	Generalized distribution	Maternal varicella 4 days before to 2 days after delivery	Tzanck, FA, viral culture
Cytomegalovirus infection	Birth (one case)	Vesicles	Forehead; ? other	Prematurity, jaundice, hepatosplenomegaly	Urine culture; IgM to cytomegalovirus
Scabies	3 to 4 weeks or later	Papules, nodules, crusted areas, vesicles	Generalized with increase in insteps of feet, axillae	Others in family with itching or rash	Scabies prep: mites eggs, feces
Sporadic conditions: common causes					
Erythema toxicum neonatorum	Most 24 to 48 hours	Erythematous macules, papules, pustules	Buttocks, torso, proximal extremities, no palms, soles	Usually term infants over 2,500 g	Wright's stain: eosinophils
Neonatal pustular melanosis	At birth	Pustules without erythema; hyperpigmented macules: some have collarette of scale	Anywhere: most common on forehead, behind ears, neck, back, fingers, toes	Term infants; more common in black infants	Wright's stain: PMNs occasional eosinophil
Miliaria crystallina	Usually 1st week of life	Dew drop-like vesicles, very superficial; no erythema	Forehead, upper trunk, volar forearms most common sites	May be history of warm incubator, occlusive clothing, dressings	Usually clinical; Wright, Gram stain negative

continued

Table 12. *Continued.*

Disease	Usual age	Skin: morphology	Skin: usual distribution	Clinical: other	Diagnosis/findings
Miliaria rubra	Days to weeks	Erythematous papules with superimposed pustules	Same as miliaria crystallina	Same as miliaria crystallina	Usually clinical; skin biopsy if doubt
Acropustulosis of infancy	Birth of first days or weeks	Vesicles and pustules	Hands and feet, especially medial palms and soles	Severe pruritus; lesions come in crops	Clinical; skin biopsy: intraepidermal pustule
Neonatal acne	3 to 4 weeks	Comedones, papules, pustules	Mainly cheeks, forehead	Comedones clue to diagnosis	Clinical diagnosis
Sporadic conditions: rare causes					
Histiocytosis X	Usually at birth	Erythematous papules, pustules	Generalized distribution	Check lymph nodes, liver, spleen, blood	Skin biopsy: large histiocytes
Diffuse cutaneous mastocytosis	Birth, first weeks of life	Bullae, infiltrated skin, hives, dermographism	Generalized distribution	Wheezing, diarrhea, bleeding diatheses	Skin biopsy: infiltrate of mast cells
Maternal bullous disease	At birth	Tense or flaccid bullae or erosions	Generalized distribution	Graft-versus-host disease; *Klebsiella* sepsis, etc.	Skin biopsy: full-thickness necrosis
Erosive and vesicular dermatosis	Birth	Vesicles and erosions	Generalized, over 75% of body	? Infection or placental infarctions	? Skin biopsy
Eosinophilic pustular folliculitis	Birth or later	Multiples pustules, crusted areas	Scalp, hands, feet	Frequent eosinophilia	Skin biopsy: Folliculitis with eosinophilia
Genetic causes					
Epidermolysis bullosa (EB)	Birth, rarely later	Bullae or erosions; milia nail dystrophy in dystrophic EB; occasional aplasia cutis	Anywhere; especially extremities, mucosa	Other epithelial tissues; i.e., GI, GU, cornea, trachea, may be affected	Skin biopsy for electron microscopy or IF mapping
Epidermolytic hyperkeratosis	Birth	Bullae, erosions, ichthyotic areas of skin	Generalized; blisters more on hands and feet	Family history may be positive	Skin biopsy; large keratohyaline granules
Incontinentia pigmenti	Birth or first weeks	Linear streaks of erythematous papules and vesicles	Generalized following Blaschko's lines	Family history may be positive; eye, CNS, and other abnormalities	Skin biopsy; eosinophilic spongiosis and dyskeratosis
Acrodermatitis enteropathica	Weeks to months	Sharply demarcated psoriasiform plaques, sometimes vesicles and bullae	Periorificial and acral	Diarrhea, irritability, alopecia, history of hyperalimentation	Serum zinc level less than 50 mcg/dl
Hyperimmuno-globulin E syndrome	Days to weeks	Multiple vesicles, grouped and individual	Generalized distribution	Recurrent *S. aureus* infection, eosinophilia	? Clinical (IgE not usually high in newborn period)
Blister like aplasia cutis congenita	At birth	One or multiple membrane-covered, depressed areas of skin	Usually scalp	May be associated with epidermal nevus	Clinical or skin biopsy
Ectodermal dysplasias (ED)	Congenital or early infancy	Vesicles or bullae	Depends on specific kind; acral in some; Blaschko's lines in Goltz syndrome	Sweating, limb, oral abnormalities, vary with specific kind of ED	Usually clinical
Erythropoietic porphyria	Early infancy	Vesicles or bullae	Photodistribution	Hemolytic anemia, pink urine	High porphyrins in blood, urine
Protein C deficiency	Birth or first days of life	Hemorrhagic bullae and cutaneous infarctions	May be focal or generalized	Blood picture consistent with DIC	Absent protein C in blood

From Frieden, ref. 239, with permission.

GLOSSARY

Abscess   A localized collection of pus in a cavity formed by disintegration or necrosis of tissues.

Alopecia   Synonym *Baldness.* Absence of hair from a normally hairy area.

Aphtha   Synonym *Canker sore.* Small ulcer of the mucous membranes.

Atrophy   A loss of tissue characterized by the loss of normal skin markings. It may affect epidermis, dermis, or subcutaneous tissues.

Bulla   A circumscribed elevation of skin over 0.5 cm in diameter containing a liquid. Also a bleb or a blister. The distinction between vesicle and bulla is arbitrary and depends only on size. *Dermal bulla*: A bulla caused by separation of tissue components of the dermis with collection of serous fluid. *Epidermal vesicle or bulla*: A blister formed within the epidermis by pathologic change in epidermal cells or cellular cohesion. *Spongiotic vesicle or bulla*: An intraepidermal multilocular vesicle or blister formed by separation of epidermal cells by edema. *Subcorneal bulla*: A bulla formed by exudate beneath the stratum spinosum, as in bullous impetigo. *Subepidermal vesicle or bulla:* A vesicle or bulla formed by cleavage of the dermal–epidermal interface and with the roof of the bulla composed of the epidermis.

Burrow   A small tunnel in the skin that houses a metazoal parasite, such as the scabies acarus.

Callus   A localized hyperplasia of the stratum corneum

Carbuncle   A necrotizing infection of the skin and subcutaneous tissue composed of a group of furuncles (boils).

Cellulitis   An inflammation of cellular tissue, particularly purulent inflammation of dermis, subcutaneous tissue, and soft tissue.

Cobb syndrome   Synonym *Cutaneomeningospinal angiomatosis.* Port-wine stains in a segmental distribution with hemangiomas of the spinal cord at the corresponding level (166).

Comedo   Synonym *Blackhead.* A plug of keratin and sebum in a dilated pilosebaceous orifice.

Crust   Synonym *Scab.* A covering consisting of dried serum and other exudates.

Cyst   Any closed cavity or sac (normal or abnormal) with an epithelial, endothelial, or membranous lining and containing fluid or semisolid material.

Darier's sign   Formation of a wheal and flare upon stroking; indicates a histamine release from mast cells within the lesion and lasts 30 to 60 minutes. Seen in solitary mastocytomas in neonates.

Diascopy   A technique of pressing a transparent slide against the skin to force blood out of the surface. Vascular lesions will blanch and allow better visualization of pigment otherwise obscured by the red color; purpura or blood outside vessels will not blanch. Any pressure decreases the blood flow so that lesions associated with vasodilatation and erythema will also blanch.

Ecchymosis   Synonym *Bruise.* A macular red or purple or colored hemorrhage in skin or mucous membrane more than 2 mm in diameter.

Erosion   Loss of the epidermis which heals without scarring.

Erythema   Redness of the skin produced by vascular congestion or increased perfusion.

Erythroderma   A generalized redness of the skin. It is often associated with desquamation, as in exfoliate dermatitis.

Excoriation   A loss of skin substance produced by scratching. Excoriations may be linear and superficial or sharply demarcated and deep.

Exfoliation   Synonym *Desquamation.* The splitting off of the epidermal keratin in scales or sheets.

Fibrosis   The formation of excessive fibrous tissue.

Fissure   Any linear gap or slit in the skin surface.

Fistula   An abnormal passage from a deep structure to the skin surface or between two structures. It is often lined with squamous epithelium.

Furuncle   Synonym *Boil.* A localized pyogenic infection originating in a hair follicle.

Gangrene   Death of tissue, usually due to loss of blood supply.

Granuloma   Chronic inflammatory tissue composed of macrophage, fibroblasts, and granulation tissue.

Gumma   A necrotic granuloma of tertiary syphilis.

Hamartoma, cutaneous   Indicates a tumorlike but primarily non-neoplastic malformation showing an abnormal mixture of a tissue's usual components. A particular tissue component may be absent from its normal site or it may be anatomically normal but abnormal in function.

Harlequin fetus   Ichthyosis congenita.

Harlequin phenomenon   The transient appearance of an infant where there is a distinct line in the sagittal plane when the infant is side lying with the upper side blanched pale and the lower side flushed. The finding are reversed when the infant is turned to the opposite side (190,191).

Hematoma   A localized, tumorlike collection of blood.

Hereditary neurocutaneous angioma   The presence of one or more port wine stains at various sites, associated with localized vascular malformations within the CNS that have a marked tendency to hemorrhage (162). Transmission is autosomal dominant.

Horn   A keratosis which is taller than it is broad.

Infarct   An area of coagulation necrosis due to local ischemia.

Keloid   An elevated progressive scar formation without regression.

Keratoderma   Hyperplasia of the stratum corneum.

Keratosis   Horny thickening of the skin.

Kerion   A nodular, inflammatory, pustular lesion, due to a fungus infection.

Lichenification   A chronic thickening of the epidermis with exaggeration of its normal markings, often as a result of scratching or rubbing.

Livido reticularis   An exaggeration of vascular mottling that never completely disappears on warming. It follows the normal vascular supply of the skin.

Macule   A circumscribed alteration in the color or texture of the skin consisting of erythema (vasodilation and inflammation), blood pigments (purpura), or an excess or deficiency of melanin.

Maculopapular rash   Changes consisting of both macules and papules.

Milium   A tiny white cyst containing lamellated keratin.

Necrosis   Death of tissue or cells.

Nevus, segmental   Describes a nevus that appears to follow a dermatomal distribution.

Nikolsky's sign   Blistering or separation of the superficial epidermis occurring after mild pressure or stroking. In infants this is seen in association with infections, notably *Staphylococcus aureus.*

Nodule   A solid mass in the skin which can be observed as an elevation or can be palpated. Usually 0.5 cm or more in diameter. It may involve epidermis and dermis, dermis and subcutis, or subcutis alone. It may consist of edema, inflammatory cells, or infiltrate.

Nummular   Synonym *Discoid or coin-shaped.* A filled circle that is fairly sharply demarcated and uniform across its surface.

Papilloma   A nipplelike mass projecting from the surface of the skin.

Papule   A small solid elevation of the skin, less than 0.5 cm in diameter. *Epidermal papule:* A papule composed of localized thickening of the epidermis or of the stratum corneum. *Dermal papule:* A papule composed of a localized, solid thickening of the dermis produced by augmentation of normal structures, deposition of metabolic products, concentrations of cells, or other pathologic changes. *Inflammatory papule:* A papule produced by inflammation of the dermis, epidermis, or both. *Papulosquamous lesion:* A papule that develops a reactive or degenerative epithelial component resulting in desquamation, which is the loss of epithelial cells or of stratum corneum (scaling). *Wheal:* An elevated compressible, transitory, white or pink papule or plaque of dermal edema.

Patch   A large macule, more than 2 cm or more in diameter.

Petechia   A punctate, nonblanching, hemorrhagic spot 1 to 2 mm in diameter.

Phakomatosis   A developmental malformation syndrome involving the eye, skin, and central nervous system.

Plaque An elevated area of skin 2 cm or more in diameter. Plaques may have the same subdivisions as mentioned above under papules. It may be formed by the extension or coalescence of either papules or nodules.

Poikiloderma A dermatosis characterized by variegated cutaneous pigmentation, atrophy, and telangiectasia.

Pruritus Synonym *Itching*. An irritating skin sensation that elicits the scratch response. In neonates, irritability and restlessness are possible symptoms of pruritus.

Pseudo Darier's sign Contraction of muscle within lesion that causes a drawing up similar to a wheal but without any change in color. Lasts only a few minutes.

Purpura Discoloration of the skin or mucosa due to extravasation of blood.

Pustule A visible accumulation of pus in the skin.

Pyoderma Pyoderma is any purulent skin disease, either bacterial or nonbacterial in origin.

Scale A flat plate or flake of stratum corneum. *Collarette scale:* Describes the fine, peripherally attached, and centrally detached scale at the edge of an inflammatory lesion (example: transient pustulosis). *Furfuraceous:* Describes fine and loose scales (example: normal postpartum scaling). *Ichthyosiform:* Describes large, polygonal scales, as in fish scales (example: lamellar ichthyosis or postmaturity scaling). *Psoriasiform (resembling psoriasis):* Describes a silvery, white, parakeratotic, lamellated scale, similar to a scale of psoriasis (example: neonatal lupus).

Scar Synonym *Cicatrix*. A scar is the fibrous tissue replacing normal tissues destroyed by injury or disease. *Atrophic scar:* Papyraceous, or cigarette paper scar, describes the wrinkled scars. *Cribriform scar:* Describes a scar perforated with multiple small apertures or pits. *Hypertrophic scar:* An elevated scar with excessive growth of fibrous tissue.

Sclerosis Diffuse or circumscribed induration of the subcutaneous tissues. It also may involve the dermis when the overlying epidermis is atrophic.

Sinus A cavity or channel; a channel that permits the escape of pus or fluid.

Skin ulcer A loss of dermis and epidermis, often with loss of underlying tissues, produced by sloughing of necrotic tissue.

Stria A streak or band of linear, atrophic, pink, purple, or white lesions of the skin due to changes in connective tissue.

Sturge-Weber syndrome The association of port-wine stains on the face and ipsilateral leptomeningeal angiomatosis leading to underlying cerebral atrophy, calcifications, and seizures (199). CNS lesions may be bilateral. The eyes may be involved with glaucoma. The facial lesions are often large and bilateral or virtually always involve the eyelids and forehead (first division of the trigeminal nerve) (161,165).

Sydney line The proximal transverse crease extends across the entire palm, as in a simian line, but the distal transverse crease is also present. This appears to be at least twice as common as simian lines and should not be confused as it is a variant without any established clinical correlation (200,201).

Telangiectasia A visible vascular lesion formed by dilation of small cutaneous blood vessels.

Tourniquet test Synonym *Hess test*. To assess capillary fragility or platelet defects, select a 5 cm diameter circle without petechiae on the forearm. Apply a sphygmomanometer cuff to the upper arm at between systolic and diastolic pressure for 5 minutes and then release the pressure. Count the number of petechiae. More than five is considered abnormal.

Tumor A swelling. Generally used to imply enlargement of tissue by a normal or pathological material or cells that form a mass. It may be inflammatory or noninflammatory, benign or malignant.

Ulcer A skin ulcer is a defect or loss of dermis and epidermis produced by sloughing of necrotic tissue.

Vegetation A growth of pathological tissue consisting of multiple closely set papillary masses.

Verruca   A verruca is an epidermal tumor caused by a papilloma virus. Verrucous describes a lesion with a warty surface.

Vesicle   A vesicle is a circumscribed elevation of the skin less than 0.5 cm in diameter and containing a liquid.

Vibex   A narrow linear mark, usually hemorrhagic, from scratching.

Wallace's lines   A line of demarcation between the skin of the sole and of the upper part of the foot that limits most rashes, the notable exception of which is syphilis which extends onto the soles.

Wheal   An elevated white compressible, evanescent area produced by dermal edema. It is often surrounded by a red, axon-mediated flare.

References

1. Sinclair JD. Thermal control in premature infants. *Ann Rev Med* 1972;23:129–148.
2. Green M. Comparison of adult and neonatal eccrine sweating. In: Maibach HI, Boisits EK, eds. *Neonatal skin structure and function.* New York: Marcel Dekker; 1982:35–66.
3. Holbrook KA. Structural and biochemical organogenesis of skin and cutaneous appendages in the fetus and neonate. In: Polin RA, Fox WW, eds. *Fetal and neonatal physiology.* 1st ed. Vol. 1. Philadelphia: WB Saunders; 1991:527–551.
4. Winkelmann RKe. *Glossary of basic dermatology lesions.* Supplement 130. Uppsala: International League of Dermatological Societies, Committee on Nomenclature and Acta Derm Venereol; 1988.
5. Harris R, Schick B. Erythema neonatorum. *Am J Dis Child* 1956;92:27–33.
6. Kramer LI. Advancement of dermal icterus in the jaundiced newborn. *Am J Dis Child* 1969;118:454–458.
7. Amit Y, Jabbour S, Arad ID. Effect of skinfold thickness on transcutaneous bilirubin measurements. *Biol Neonate* 1993;63:209–214.
8. Giunta F. Bilirubin rash in the newborn. *JAMA* 1969;208:1703.
9. Woody NC, Brodkey MJ. Tanning from phototherapy for neonatal jaundice. *J Pediatr* 1973;82:1042–1043.
10. McDonagh AF, Lightner DA. "Like a shrivelled blood orange"—bilirubin, jaundice, and phototherapy. *Pediatrics* 1985;75:443–455.
11. Sivan Y, Dinari G, Goodman C, Merlob P, Nitzan M. Small intestine transit time and lactose absorption during phototherapy. *Biol Neonate* 1985;48:10–14.
12. Ashley JR, Littler CM, Burgdorf WHC, Brann BS. Bronze baby syndrome. Report of a case. *J Am Acad Dermatol* 1985;12:325–328.
13. Clark CF, Torii S, Hamamoto Y, Kaito H. The "bronze baby" syndrome: postmortem data. *J Pediatr* 1976;88:461–464.
14. Kopelman AE, Brown RS, Odell GB. The "bronze baby syndrome": a complication of phototherapy. *J Pediatr* 1972;81:466–472.
15. Onishi S, Itoh S, Isobe K, Togari H, Kitoh H, Nishimura Y. Mechanism of development of bronze baby syndrome in neonates treated with phototherapy. *Pediatrics* 1982;69:273–276.
16. Purcell SM, Wians FH, Ackerman NB, Davis BM. Hyperbiliverdinemia in the bronze baby syndrome. *J Am Acad Dermatol* 1987;16:172–177.
17. Rubaltelli FF, Jori G, Reddi E. Bronze baby syndrome: a new porphyrin related disorder. *Pediatr Res* 1983;17:327–330.
18. Stevens CA, Carey JC, Shah M, Bagley GP. Development of human palmar and digital flexion creases. *J Pediatr* 1988;113(1 Pt 1):128–132.
19. Schaumann BA, Kimura S. Palmar, plantar, and digital flexion creases: morphologic and clinical considerations. *Birth Defects* 1991;27:229–252.
20. Davies PA. Sex and the single transverse palmar crease in newborn singletons. *Dev Med Child Neurol* 1966;8:729–734.
21. Jones K, ed. *Smith's recognizable patterns of human malformation.* 4th ed. Philadelphia: WB Saunders; 1988.
22. Bugbee WD, Botte MJ. Surface anatomy of the hand. The relationships between palmar skin creases and osseous anatomy. *Clin Orthop* 1993;296:122-126.
23. Raimer SS, Raimer BG. Needle puncture scars from mid-trimester amniocentesis. *Arch Dermatol* 1984;120:1360–1362.
24. Bruce S, Duffy JO, Wolf JE. Skin dimpling associated with midtrimester amniocentesis. *Pediatr Dermatol* 1984;2:140–142.
25. Broome DL, Wilson MG, Weiss B, Kellogg B. Needle puncture of fetus: a complication of second-trimester amniocentesis. *Am J Obstet Gynecol* 1976;126:247–252.
26. Agache P, Blanc D, Barrand C, et al. Sebum levels during the first year of life. *Br J Dermatol* 1980;103:643–649.
27. Kahn A, Groswasser J, Sottiaux M, et al. Clinical symptoms associated with brief obstructive sleep apnea in normal infants. *Sleep* 1993;16:409–413.
28. Chen H, Gonzalez E. Amniotic band sequence and its neurocutaneous manifestations. *Am J Med Genet* 1987;28:661–673.
29. Ashkenazi S, Metzker A, Merlob P, Ovadia J, Reisner SH. Scalp changes after fetal monitoring. *Arch Dis Child* 1985;60:267–269.
30. Smith DW, Gong BT. Scalp hair patterning as a clue to early fetal brain development. *J Pediatr* 1973;83:374–380.
31. Barth JH. The hair in infancy and childhood. In: Rook A, Dawber RP, eds. *Diseases of the hair and scalp.* Oxford: Blackwell Scientific; 1991:51–70.

32. Slyper AH, Esterly NB. Nonprogressive scrotal hair growth in two infants [see comments]. *Pediatr Dermatol* 1993;10:34–35.

33. Diamond FB, Shulman DI, Root AW. Scrotal hair in infancy. *J Pediatr* 1989;114:999–1001.

34. Jacobs AH, Walton RG. The incidence of birthmarks in the neonate. *Pediatrics* 1976;58:218.

35. Hidano A, Purwoko R, Jitsukawa K. Statistical survey of skin changes in Japanese neonates. *Pediatr Dermatol* 1986;3:140–144.

36. Nanda A, Kaur S, Bhakoo ON, Dhall K. Survey of cutaneous lesions in Indian newborns. *Pediatr Dermatol* 1989;6:39–42.

37. Cohen BA. *Atlas of pediatric dermatology.* 1st ed. London: Wolfe; 1993.

38. Gellis S, Feingold M, Fikar CR, Lee MA. Picture of the month: Ota's nevus. *Am J Dis Child* 1980;134:1083–1084.

39. Gordon I. Miliary sebaceous cysts and blisters in the healthy newborn. *Arch Dis Child* 1949;24:286–288.

40. Joglekar VM. Barrier properties of vernix caseosa. *Arch Dis Child* 1980;55:817–819.

41. Aly R, Maibach HI, Rahman R. Correlation of human in vivo and in vitro cutaneous antimicrobial factors. *J Infect Dis* 1975;131:579–583.

42. Baley JE, Silverman R. Systemic candidiasis: cutaneous manifestations in low birth weight infants. *Pediatrics* 1988;82:211–215.

43. Rudolph N, Tariq AA, Reale MR, Goldberg PK, Kozinn PJ. Congenital cutaneous candidiasis. *Arch Dermatol* 1977;113:1101–1103.

44. Gellis SS, Feingold M. Picture of the month: congenital cutaneous candidiasis. *Am J Dis Child* 1976;130:291–292.

45. Kam LA, Giacoia GP. Congenital cutaneous candidiasis. *Am J Dis Child* 1975;129:1215–1218.

46. Snider R, Landers S, Levy ML. The ringworm riddle: an outbreak of *Microsporum canis* in the nursery. *Pediatr Infect Dis J* 1993;12:145–148.

47. Bereston EW, Robinson HM. Tinea capitis and corporis in an infant 4 weeks old. *Arch Dermatol Syphilol* 1953;68:582.

48. Jacobs AH, Jacobs PH, Moore N. Tinea facei due to *Microsporum canis* in an eight-day-old infant. *JAMA* 1972;219:1476.

49. Perlman M, Bar-Ziv J. Congenital ichthyosis and neonatal pulmonary disease. *Pediatrics* 1974;53:573–575.

50. De Dobbeleer G, Heenen M, Song M, Achten G. Collodion baby skin: ultrastructural and autoradiographic study. *J Cutan Pathol* 1982;9:196–202.

51. Frenk E, de Techtermann F. Self-healing collodion baby: evidence for autosomal recessive inheritance. *Pediatr Dermatol* 1992;9:95–97.

52. Frenk E. A spontaneously healing collodion baby: a light and electron microscopical study. *Acta Derm Venereol (Stockh)* 1981;61:168–171.

53. Bloom D, Goodfried MS. Lamellar ichthyosis of the newborn. The "collodion baby": a clinical and genetic entity; report of a case and review of the literature with special consideration of the pathogenesis and classification. *Arch Dermatol* 1962;86:336–342.

54. Finlay HVL, Bound JP. Collodion skin in the neonate due to lamellar ichthyosis. *Arch Dis Child* 1952;27:438–441.

55. Lentz CL, Altman J. Lamellar ichthyosis: the natural clinical course of collodion baby. *Arch Dermatol* 1968;97:3–13.

56. Sandberg NO. Lamellar ichthyosis. *Pediatr Rev* 1981;2:213–216.

57. Lawlor F. Progress of a harlequin fetus to nonbullous ichthyosiform erythroderma. *Pediatrics* 1988;82:870–873.

58. Esterly NB, Elias S. Antenatal diagnosis of genodermatoses. *J Am Acad Dermatol* 1983;8:655–662.

59. Elias S, Mazur M, Sabbagha R, Esterly NB, Simpson JL. Prenatal diagnosis of harlequin ichthyosis. *Clin Genet* 1980;17:275–280.

60. Resnick SD, Greenberg RA. Autoinoculated palmar pustules in neonatal candidiasis. *Pediatr Dermatol* 1989;6:206–209.

61. Jordan WE, Lawson KD, Berg RW, Franxman JJ, Marrer AM. Diaper dermatitis: frequency and severity among a general infant population. *Pediatr Dermatol* 1986;3:198–207.

62. Dixon PN, Warin RP, English MP. Alimentary *Candida albicans* and napkin rashes. *Br J Dermatol* 1972;86:458–462.

63. Weston WL, Lane AT, Weston JA. Diaper dermatitis: current concepts. *Pediatrics* 1980;66:532–536.

64. Farber EM, Jacobs AH. Infantile psoriasis. *Am J Dis Child* 1977;131:1266–1269.

65. Hebert AA, Esterly NB. Bacterial and candidal cutaneous infections in the neonate. *Dermatol Clin* 1986;4:3–21.

66. Baley JE. Neonatal candidiasis: the current challenge. *Clin Perinatol* 1991;18:263–280.

67. Chapel TA, Gagliardi C, Nichols W. Congenital cutaneous candidiasis. *J Am Acad Dermatol* 1982;6:926–928.

68. Yesudian P, Kamalam A. Epidermophyton floccosum infection in a three week old infant. *Trans St Johns Hosp Dermatol Soc* 1973;59:66–67.

69. Stepanova Z, V., Livanova NK. [Microsporia of the scalp in a 10-day-old girl]. *Vestn Dermatol Venerol* 1971;45:84–85.

70. Alden ER, Chernila SA. Ringworm in an infant. *Pediatrics* 1969;44:261–262.

71. Saxoni F, Lapaanis P, Pantelakis SN. Congenital syphilis: a description of 18 cases and re-examination of an old but ever-present disease. *Clin Pediatr (Phila)* 1967;6:687–691.

72. Atherton DJ. The neonate. In: Champion RH, Burton JL, Ebling FJG, eds. *Rook, Wilkinson, Ebling Textbook of Dermatology.* Vol. 1. 5th ed. Oxford: Blackwell Scientific; 1992:381–444.

73. Fojaco RM, Hensley GT, Moskowitz L. Congenital syphilis and necrotizing funisitis. *JAMA* 1989;261:1788–1790.

74. Schick JB, Milstein JM. Burn hazard of isopropyl alcohol in the neonate. *Pediatrics* 1981;68:587–588.

75. Yates VM, Kerr RE, Frier K, Cobb SJ, MacKie RM. Early diagnosis of infantile seborrhoeic dermatitis and atopic dermatitis—total and specific IgE levels. *Br J Dermatol* 1983;108:639–645.

76. Menni S, Piccinno R, Baietta S, Ciuffreda A, Scotti L. Infantile seborrheic dermatitis: seven-year follow-up and some prognostic criteria. *Pediatr Dermatol* 1989;6:13–15.
77. Carr JA, Hodgman JE, Freedman RI, Levan NE. Relationship between toxic erythema and infant maturity. *Am J Dis Child* 1966;112:129–133.
78. Duperrat B, Bret AJ. Erythema neonatorum allergicum. *Br J Dermatol* 1961;73:300–302.
79. Eitzman DV, Smith RT. The non-specific inflammatory cycle in the neonatal infant. *Am J Dis Child* 1959;97:326–334.
80. Freeman RG, Spiller R, Knox JM. Histopathology of erythema toxicum neonatorum. *Arch Dermatol* 1960;82:586–589.
81. Keitel HG, Yadav V. Etiology of toxic erythema. *Am J Dis Child* 1963;106:306–309.
82. Levy HL, Cothran F. Erythema toxicum neonatorum present at birth. *Am J Dis Child* 1962;103:617–619.
83. Lüders D. Histologic observations in erythema toxicum neonatorum. *Pediatrics* 1960;26:219–224.
84. Marino LJ. Toxic erythema present at birth. *Arch Dermatol* 1965;92:402–403.
85. Taylor WB, Bondurant CP. Erythema neonatorum allergicum. *Arch Dermatol* 1957;76:591–594.
86. Ferrándiz C, Coroleu W, Lorenzo JD, Natal A. Sterile transient neonatal pustulosis is a precocious form of erythema toxicum neonatorum. *Dermatology* 1992;185:18–22.
87. Ramamurthy RS, Reveri M, Esterly NB, Fretzin DF, Pildes RS. Transient neonatal pustular melanosis. *J Pediatr* 1976;88:831–835.
88. Merlob P, Metzker A, Reisner SH. Transient neonatal pustular melanosis. *Am J Dis Child* 1982;136:521–522.
89. Auster B. Transient neonatal pustular melanosis. *Cutis* 1978;22:327–328.
90. Barr RJ, Globerman LM, Werber FA. Transient neonatal pustular melanosis. *Int J Dermatol* 1979;18:636–638.
91. Wyre HW, Murphy MO. Transient neonatal pustular melanosis. *Arch Dermatol* 1979;115:458.
92. Arpey CJ, Nagashima-Whalen LS, Chren MM, Zaim MT. Congenital miliaria crystallina: case report and literature review. *Pediatr Dermatol* 1992;9:283–287.
93. Light IJ. Postnatal acquisition of herpes simplex virus by the newborn infant: a review of the literature. *Pediatrics* 1979;63:480–482.
94. Hutto C, Arvin A, Jacobs R, et al. Intrauterine herpes simplex virus infections. *J Pediatr* 1987;110:97–101.
95. Whitley RJ, Corey L, Arvin A, et al. Changing presentation of herpes simplex virus infections in neonates. *J Infect Dis* 1988;158:109–116.
96. Kaye EM, Dooling EC. Neonatal herpes simplex meningoencephalitis associated with fetal monitor scalp electrodes. *Neurology* 1981;31:1045–1046.
97. Parvey LS, Ch'ien LT. Neonatal herpes simplex virus infection introduced by fetal monitor scalp electrodes. *Pediatrics* 1980;65:1150–1153.
98. Golden SM, Merenstein GB, Todd WA, Hill JM. Disseminated herpes simplex neonatorum: a complication of fetal monitoring. *Am J Obstet Gynecol* 1977;129:917–918.
99. Borzyskowski M, Harris RF, Jones RW. The congenital varicella syndrome. *Eur J Pediatr* 1981;137:335–338.
100. Paryani SG, Arvin AM. Intrauterine infection with varicella-zoster virus after maternal varicella. *N Engl J Med* 1986;314:1542–1546.
101. Glover MT, Atherton DJ. Congenital infection with herpes simplex virus type 1. *Pediatr Dermatol* 1987;4:336–340.
102. Melish ME, Glasgow LA, Turner MD. The staphylococcal scalded skin syndrome; isolation and partial characterisation of the exfoliative toxin. *Br J Dermatol* 1982;125:129–140.
103. Annunziata D, Goldblum LM. Staphylococcal scalded skin syndrome: a complication of circumcision. *Am J Dis Child* 1978;132:1187–1188.
104. Artman M, Shanks GD. Staphylococcal scalded skin syndrome after herniorrhaphy. *Am J Dis Child* 1981;135:471–472.
105. Cohen BA, Patel HP. Blistering eruption in healthy newborns. Case 2. Junctional epidermolysis bullosa. *Arch Dermatol* 1986;122:212,214–216.
106. Fine JD, Bauer EA, Briggaman RA, et al. Revised clinical and laboratory criteria for subtypes of inherited epidermolysis bullosa. A consensus report by the Subcommittee on Diagnosis and Classification of the National Epidermolysis Bullosa Registry [see comments]. *J Am Acad Dermatol* 1991;24:119–135.
107. Frieden IJ. Aplasia cutis congenita: a clinical review and proposal for classification. *J Am Acad Dermatol* 1986;14:646–660.
108. Lin AN, Carter DM. Epidermolysis bullosa: when the skin falls apart. *J Pediatr* 1989;114:349–355.
109. Rabinowitz LG, Esterly NB. Inflammatory bullous diseases in children. *Dermatol Clin* 1993;11:565–581.
110. Ramadass T, Thangavelu TA. Epidermolysis bullosa and its E.N.T. manifestations. Two case reports. *J Laryngol Otol* 1978;92:441–446.
111. Smith PK, Davidson GP, Moore L, et al. Epidermolysis bullosa and severe ulcerative colitis in an infant. *J Pediatr* 1993;122:600–603.
112. ElShafie M, Stidham GL, Klippel CH, Katzman GH, Weinfeld IJ. Pyloric atresia and epidermolysis bullosa letalis: a lethal combination in two premature newborn siblings. *J Pediatr Surg* 1979;14:446–449.
113. Adashi EY, Louis FJ, Vasquez M. An unusual case of epidermolysis bullosa hereditaria letalis with cutaneous scarring and pyloric atresia. *J Pediatr* 1980;96:443–446.
114. el-Benhawi MO, George WM. Incontinentia pigmenti: a review. *Cutis* 1988;41:259–262.
115. Watzke RC, Stevens TS, Carney RG Jr. Retinal vascular changes of incontinentia pigmenti. *Arch Ophthalmol* 1976;94:743–746.
116. Carney RG. Incontinentia pigmenti. A world statistical analysis. *Arch Dermatol* 1976;112:535–542.
117. Higgenbottom MC, Jones KL, James HE, Bruce DA, Schut L. Aplasia cutis congenita: a cutaneous marker of occult spinal dysraphism. *J Pediatr* 1980;96:687–689.
118. Schneider BM, Berg RA, Kaplan AM. Aplasia cutis congenita complicated by sagittal sinus hemorrhage. *Pediatrics* 1980;66:948–950.

119. Levin DL, Nolan KS, Esterly NB. Congenital absence of skin. *J Am Acad Dermatol* 1980;2:203–206.
120. Dror Y, Gelman-Kohan Z, Hagai Z, Juster-Reicher A, Cohen RN, Mogilner B. Aplasia cutis congenita, elevated alpha-fetoprotein, and a distinct amniotic fluid acetylcholinesterase electrophoretic band. *Am J Perinatol* 1994;11:149–152.
121. Sybert VP. Aplasia cutis congenita: a report of 12 new cases and review of the literature. *Pediatr Dermatol* 1985;3:1–14.
122. Flanagan BP, Helwig EB. Cutaneous lymphangioma. *Arch Dermatol* 1977;113:24–30.
123. Mulliken JB. Classification of vascular birthmarks. In: Milliken JB, Young AE, eds. *Vascular birthmarks: hemangiomas and malformations.* Philadelphia: WB Saunders; 1988:24–37.
124. Amir J, Metzker A, Krikler R, Reisner SH. Strawberry hemangioma in preterm infants. *Pediatr Dermatol* 1986;3:331–332.
125. Esterly NB. Kasabach-Merritt syndrome in infants. *J Am Acad Dermatol* 1983;8:504–513.
126. Larsen EC, Zinkham WH, Eggleston JC, Zitelli BJ. Kasabach-Merritt syndrome: therapeutic considerations. *Pediatrics* 1987;79:971–980.
127. Caputo R, Ermacora E, Gelmetti C, Gianni E. Fatal nodular xanthomatosis in an infant. *Pediatr Dermatol* 1987;4:242–246.
128. Cohen BA, Hood A. Xanthogranuloma: report on clinical and histologic findings in 64 patients. *Pediatr Dermatol* 1989;6:262–266.
129. Rogers M, McCrossin I, Commens C. Epidermal nevi and the epidermal nevus syndrome. *J Am Acad Dermatol* 1989;20:476–488.
130. Solomon LM, Fretzin DF, Dewald RL. The epidermal nevus syndrome. *Arch Dermatol* 1968;97:273–285.
131. Solomon LM, Esterly NB. Epidermal and other congenital organoid nevi. *Curr Probl Pediatr* 1975;6:1–56.
132. Solomon LM. Epidermal nevus syndrome. *Mod Probl Paediatr* 1975;17:27–30.
133. Alper J, Holmes LB, Mihm MCJ. Birthmarks with serious medical significance: nevocellular nevi, sebaceous nevi, and multiple café au lait spots. *J Pediatr* 1979;95:696–700.
134. Monk BE, Vollum DI. Familial naevus sebaceus. *J R Soc Med* 1982;75:660–661.
135. Benedetto L, Sood U, Blumenthal N, Madjar D, Sturman S, Hashimoto K. Familial nevus sebaceus. *J Am Acad Dermatol* 1990;23:130–132.
136. Jones EW, Heyl T. Naevus sebaceus. A report of 140 cases with special regard to the development of secondary malignant tumours. *Br J Dermatol* 1970;82:99–117.
137. Kopf AW, Bart RS, Hennessey P. Congenital nevocytic nevi and malignant melanomas. *J Am Acad Dermatol* 1979;1:123–130.
138. Kadonaga JN, Frieden IJ. Neurocutaneous melanosis: definition and review of the literature. *J Am Acad Dermatol* 1991;24(5 Pt 1):747–755.
139. Gooneratne S, Hughson MD, Othersen HB, Kurtz SM. Multicentric giant pigmented nevi of the scalp with local invasion of the cranium and dura mater. *J Pediatr Surg* 1982;17:55–58.
140. Symposium. The management of congenital nevocytic nevi. *Pediatr Dermatol* 1984;2:143–156.
141. Gari LM, Rivers JK, Kopf AW. Melanomas arising in large congenital nevocytic nevi: a prospective study. *Pediatr Dermatol* 1988;5:151–158.
142. Rhodes AR, Wood WC, Sober AJ, Mihm MC Jr. Nonepidermal origin of malignant melanoma associated with a giant congenital nevocellular nevus. *Plast Reconstr Surg* 1981;67:782–790.
143. Rhodes AR, Melski JW. Small congenital nevocellular nevi and the risk of cutaneous melanoma. *J Pediatr* 1982;100:219–224.
144. Osburn K, Schosser RH, Everett MA. Congenital pigmented and vascular lesions in newborn infants. *J Am Acad Dermatol* 1987;16:788–792.
145. Kroon S, Clemmensen OJ, Hastrup N. Incidence of congenital melanocytic nevi in newborn babies in Denmark. *J Am Acad Dermatol* 1987;17:422–426.
146. Walton RG, Jacobs AH, Cox AJ. Pigmented lesions in newborn infants. *Br J Dermatol* 1976;95:389–396.
147. Williams ML, Pennella R. Melanoma, melanocytic nevi, and other melanoma risk factors in children. *J Pediatr* 1994;124:833–845.
148. Krowchuk DP, Tunnessen WWJ, Hurwitz S. Pediatric dermatology update. *Pediatrics* 1992;90:259–264.
149. Eichenfield LF, Honig PJ. Difficult diagnostic and management issues in pediatric dermatology. *Pediatr Clin North Am* 1991;38:687–710.
150. Gvozden AB, Barnett NK, Schron DS. Congenital pilar and smooth muscle nevus. *Pediatrics* 1987;70:1021–1022.
151. Goldman MP, Kaplan RP, Heng MD. Congenital smooth muscle hamartoma. *Int J Dermatol* 1987;26:448–452.
152. Zvulunov A, Rotem A, Merlob P, Metzker A. Congenital smooth muscle hamartoma. Prevalence, clinical findings, and follow-up in 15 patients. *Am J Dis Child* 1990;144:782–784.
153. Gagne EJ, Su WP. Congenital smooth muscle hamartoma of the skin. *Pediatr Dermatol* 1993;10:142–145.
154. Rivers JK, Frederiksen PC, Dibdin C. A prevalence survey of dermatoses in the Australian neonate. *J Am Acad Dermatol* 1990;23:77–81.
155. Metzker A, Shamir R. Butterfly-shaped mark: a variant form of nevus flammeus simplex. *Pediatrics* 1990;85:1069–1071.
156. Fries MH, Goldstein RB, Kilpatrick SJ, Golbus MS, Callen PW, Filly RA. The role of velamentous cord insertion in the etiology of twin-twin transfusion syndrome. *Obstet Gynecol* 1993;81:569–574.
157. Merlob P, Reisner SH. Familial nevus flammeus of the forehead and Unna's nevus. *Clin Genet* 1985;27:165–166.
158. Pasyk KA, Wlodarczyk SR, Jakobczak MM, Kurek M, Aughton DJ. Familial medial telangiectatic nevus: variant of nevus flammeus—port-wine stain. *Plast Reconstr Surg* 1993;91:1032–1041.
159. Fox H. Pathology of the placenta. In: Bennington JL, ed. *Major problems in pathology.* Vol. VII. London: WB Saunders; 1978.
160. Alper JC, Holmes LB. The incidence and significance of birthmarks in a cohort of 4641 newborns. *Pediatr Dermatol* 1983;1:58–66.
161. Tallman B, Tan OT, Morelli JG, et al. Location of port-wine stains and the likelihood of ophthalmic and/or central nervous system complications. *Pediatrics* 1991;87:323–327.

162. Zeremba J, Stepien M, Jelowicka M, et al. Hereditary neurocutaneous angioma: a new genetic entity? *J Med Genet* 1979;16:443–447.

163. Nova HR. Familial communicating hydrocephalus, posterior cerebellar agenesis, mega cisterna magna and port wine nevi. *J Neurosurg* 1979;51:862–865.

164. Smoller BR, Rosen S. Port-wine stains: a disease of altered neural modulation of blood vessels? *Arch Dermatol* 1986;122:177–179.

165. Enjolras O, Riche MC, Merland JJ. Facial port-wine stains and Sturge-Weber syndrome. *Pediatrics* 1986;76:48–51.

166. Cobb S. Haemangioma of the spinal cord associated with skin naevi of the same metamere. *Ann Surg* 1915;62:641–649.

167. Eid K, Hochberg J, Saunders DE. Skin abnormalities of the back in diastematomyelia. *Plast Reconstr Surg* 1979;63:534–539.

168. Tavafoghi V, Ghandchi A, Hambrick GW, Udverhelyi GB. Cutaneous signs of spinal dysraphism: report of a patient with a tail-like lipoma and review of 200 cases in the literature. *Arch Dermatol* 1978;114:573–577.

169. Harris H, Miller O. Midline cutaneous and spinal defects: midline cutaneous abnormalities associated with occult spinal disorders. *Arch Dermatol* 1976;112:1724–1728.

170. Goldberg NS, Hebert A, Esterly NB. Sacral hemangiomas and multiple congenital abnormalities. *Arch Dermatol* 1986;122:684–687.

171. Gladson CL, Groncy P, Griffin JH. Coumarin necrosis, neonatal purpura fulminans, and protein C deficiency. *Arch Dermatol* 1987;123:1701–1706.

172. Shipp TD, Bromley B, Benacerraf BR. Sonographically detected abnormalities of the umbilical cord. *Int J Gynaecol Obstet* 1995;48:179–185.

173. Cook V, Weeks J, Brown J, Bendon R. Umbilical artery occlusion and fetoplacental thromboembolism. *Obstet Gynecol* 1995;85(5 Pt 2):870–872.

174. South DA, Jacobs AH. Cutis marmorata telangiectatica congenita (congenital generalized phlebectasia). *J Pediatr* 1978;93:944–949.

175. Picascia DD, Esterly NB. Cutis marmorata telangiectatica congenita: report of 22 cases [see comments]. *J Am Acad Dermatol* 1989;20:1098–1104.

176. Fitzsimmons JS, Starks M. Cutis marmorata telangiectatica congenita or congenital generalized phlebectasia. *Arch Dis Child* 1970;45:724–726.

177. Kurczynski TW. Hereditary cutis marmorata telangiectatica congenita. *Pediatrics* 1982;70:52–53.

178. Spraker MK, Stack C, Esterly NB. Congenital generalized fibromatosis: a review of the literature and report of a case associated with porencephaly, hemiatrophy, and cutis marmorata telangiectatica congenita. *J Am Acad Dermatol* 1984;10(2 Pt 2):365–371.

179. Alexander EL, McNicholl J, Watson RM, Bias W, Reichlin M, Provost TT. The immunogenetic relationship between anti-Ro(SS-A)/La(SS-B) antibody positive Sjogren's/lupus erythematosus overlap syndrome and the neonatal lupus syndrome. *J Invest Dermatol* 1989;93:751–756.

180. Buyon JP. Neonatal lupus and congenital complete heart block: manifestations of passively acquired autoimmunity. *Clin Exp Rheumatol* 1989;7(suppl 3):199–203.

181. Buyon JP, Slade SG, Reveille JD, Hamel JC, Chan EK. Autoantibody responses to the native 52-kDa SS-A/Ro protein in neonatal lupus syndromes, systemic lupus erythematosus, and Sjogren's syndrome. *J Immunol* 1994;152:3675–3684.

182. Dugan EM, Tunnessen WW, Honig PJ, Watson RM. U1RNP antibody-positive neonatal lupus. A report of two cases with immunogenetic studies. *Arch Dermatol* 1992;128:1490–1494.

183. Franceschini F, Bertoli MT, Martinelli M, et al. The neonatal lupus erythematosus associated with isolated LA(SSB) antibodies [Letter]. *J Rheumatol* 1990;17:415–416.

184. Korkij W, Soltani K. Neonatal lupus erythematosus: a review. *Pediatr Dermatol* 1984;1:189–195.

185. Buyon JP. Neonatal lupus syndromes. *Curr Opin Rheumatol* 1994;6:523–529.

186. Ishimaru S, Izaki S, Kitamura K, Morita Y. Neonatal lupus erythematosus: dissolution of atrioventricular block after administration of corticosteroid to the pregnant mother. *Dermatology* 1994;189(suppl 1):92–94.

187. Horng YC, Chou YH, Tsou Yau KI. Neonatal lupus erythematosus with negative anti-Ro and anti-La antibodies: report of one case. *Acta Paediatr Sin* 1992;33:372–375.

188. Bourke JF, Burns DA. Neonatal lupus erythematosus with persistent telangiectasia and spastic paraparesis. *Clin Exp Dermatol* 1993;18:271–273.

189. Buyon JP. Neonatal lupus syndromes. *Am J Reprod Immunol* 1992;28:259–263.

190. Mortenson O, Stougard-Andresen P. Harlequin colour change in the newborn. *Acta Obstet Gynecol Scand* 1959;38:352–358.

191. Neligan GA, Strang LB. A "harlequin" colour change in the newborn. *Lancet* 1952;2:1005–1007.

192. Herlitz G. Unilateral skin vessel crises in the newborn. *Acta Paediatr Scand* 1953;42:506–513.

193. Pearson HA, Cone TE. Harlequin color change in a young infant with tricuspid atresia. *Pediatrics* 1957;50:609–612.

194. Korf B. Diagnostic outcome in children with multiple café au lait spots. *Pediatrics* 1992;90:924–927.

195. Fleisher TL, Zeligman I. Nevus anemicus. Arch Dermatol 1969;100:750–755.

196. Greaves MW, Birkett D, Johnson C. Nevus anemicus: a unique catecholamine-dependent nevus. *Arch Dermatol* 1970;102:172–176.

197. Weber FP, Harris KE. A case of widely distributed superficial telangiectatic naevus (capillary haemangiectatic naevus) associated with areas of naevus anaemicus. *Br J Dermatol* 1932;44:77–83.

198. Hamm H, Happle R. Naevus vascularis mixtus. *Hautarzt* 1986;37:388–392.

199. Alexander GL, Norman RM. *The Sturge-Weber syndrome.* Bristol, England: John Wright; 1960.

200. Alter M. Variation in palmar creases. *Am J Dis Child* 1970;120:424–431.

201. Dar H, Schmidt R, Nitowsky HM. Palmar crease variants and their clinical significance: a study of newborns at risk. *Pediatr Res* 1977;11:103–108.

202. Murphy WF, Langley AL. Common bullous lesions, presumably self-inflicted, occurring in utero in the newborn infant. *Pediatrics* 1963;32:1099–1101.

203. Fletcher MA, MacDonald MG, eds. *Atlas of procedures in neonatology.* 2nd ed. Philadelphia: JB Lippincott; 1993.

204. Reese V, Frieden IJ, Paller AS, et al. Association of facial hemangiomas with Dandy-Walker and other posterior fossa malformations. *J Pediatrics* 1993;122:379–384.

205. Hall DE, Udvarhelyi GB, Altman J. Lumbosacral skin lesions as markers of occult spinal dysraphism. *JAMA* 1981;246:2606–2608.

206. Prendiville J, Esterly NB. When congenital nevi signal underlying disease. *Contemp Pediatr* 1987;4:24–52.

207. Kazancera ND. Growth characteristics of skin thickness in children and its significance in free skin grafts. *Acta Chir Plast* 1969;11:71.

208. Holbrook KA, Smith LT. Ultrastructural aspects of human skin during the embryonic, fetal, premature, neonatal and adult periods of life. In: Blandau RJ, ed. *Morphogenesis and malformations of the skin.* New York: Liss; 1981:9–38.

209. Holbrook KA. A histologic comparison of infant and adult skin. In: Maibach HI, Boisits EK, eds. *Neonatal skin structure and function.* New York: Marcel Dekker; 1982:3–31.

210. Foster CA, Bertram JF, Holbrook KA. Morphometric and statistic analyses describing the in utero growth of human epidermis. *Anat Rec* 1988;222:201–206.

211. Nachman RL, Esterly NB. Increased skin permeability in preterm infants. *J Pediatr* 1971;79:628–632.

212. Evans NJ, Rutter N. Development of the epidermis in the newborn. *Biol Neonate* 1986;49:74.

213. Evans NJ, Rutter N. Percutaneous respiration in the newborn infant. *J Pediatr* 1986;108:282.

214. Lane AT. Development and care of the preterm infant's skin. *Pediatr Dermatol* 1987;4:1.

215. Hamada H. Age changes in melanocyte distribution of the normal, human epidermis. *Jpn J Dermatol* 1972; 82:223.

216. Holbrook KA, Underwood RA, Vogel AM, Gown AM, Kimball H. The appearance, density and distribution of melanocytes in human embryonic and fetal skin revealed by the anti-melanoma monoclonal antibody, HMB-45. *Anat Embryol (Berl)* 1989;180:443–455.

217. Pinkus H. Embryology of Hair. In: Montagna W, Ellis RA, eds. *The hair growth.* New York: Academic; 1958:1–32.

218. Holbrook KA, Dale BA, Williams ML, et al. The expression of congenital ichthyosiform erythroderma in second trimester fetuses of the same family: morphologic and biochemical studies. *J Invest Dermatol* 1988; 91:521.

219. Hashimoto K. The ultrastructure of human embryo skin. 2. The formation of intradermal portion of the eccrine sweat duct and secretory segment during the first half of embryonic life. *J Invest Dermatol* 1966;46: 513.

220. Fujita H, Asagami C, Oda Y, Mori T, Suetomi Y. Electron microscopic studies of the differentiation of fat cells in human fetal skin. *J Invest Dermatol* 1969;53:122.

221. Lawrence CM, Cox NH. *Physical signs in dermatology. Color atlas and text.* 1st ed. London: Mosby-Year Book Europe; 1993.

222. Smith DW. Commentary: redundant skin folds in the infant—their origin and relevance. *J Pediatr* 1979;94: 1021–1022.

223. Mulliken JB, Young AE. *Vasular birthmarks. Hemangioma and malformations.* 1st ed. Philadelphia: WB Saunders; 1988.

224. Kruse K, Irle U, Uhlig R. Elevated 1,25-dihydroxyvitamin D serum concentrations in infants with subcutaneous fat necrosis. *J Pediatr* 1993;122:460–463.

225. Thomsen RJ. Subcutaneous fat necrosis of the newborn and idiopathic hypercalcemia. *Arch Dermatol* 1980; 116:1155–1158.

226. Molteni RA, del Rosario Ames M. Sclerema neonatorum and joint contractures at birth as a potential complication of chronic in utero hypoxia. *Am J Obstet Gynecol* 1986;155:380–381.

227. Vonk J, Janssens PMW, Demacker PNM, Folkers E. Subcutaneous fat necrosis in a neonate, in association with aberrant plasma lipid and lipoprotein values. *J Pediatr* 1993;123:462–464.

228. Chen TH, Shewmake SW, Hansen DD, Lacey HL. Subcutaneous fat necrosis of the newborn. *Arch Dermatol* 1981;117:36–37.

229. Fretzin DF, Arias AM. Sclerema neonatorum and subcutaneous fat necrosis of the newborn. *Pediatr Dermatol* 1987;4:112–122.

230. Mogilner BM, Alkalay A, Nissim F, et al. Subcutaneous fat necrosis of the newborn. *Clin Pediatr* 1981;20: 748–750.

231. Silverman AK. Panniculitis in infants. *Arch Dermatol* 1985;121:834.

232. Norwood-Galloway A, Lebwohl M, Phelps RG, et al. Subcutaneous fat necrosis of the newborn with hypercalcemia. *J Am Acad Dermatol* 1987;16:435–439.

233. Shackelford GD, Barton LL, McAlister WH. Calcified subcutaneous fat necrosis in infancy. *J Can Assoc Radiol* 1975;26:203–207.

234. Hughes WE, Hammond ML. Sclerema neonatorum. *J Pediatr* 1948;32:676–692.

235. Warwick W, Ruttenberg HD, Quie PG. Sclerema neonatorum—a sign, not a disease. *JAMA* 1963;184: 680–683.

236. Hicks MJ, Levy ML, Alexander J, Flaitz CM. Subcutaneous fat necrosis of the newborn and hypercalcemia: case report and review of the literature. *Pediatr Dermatol* 1993;10:271–276.

237. Ossoff RH, Levin DL, Esterly NB, Tucker GF. Intraoral and cutaneous juvenile xanthogranuloma. *Ann Otol Rhinol Laryngol* 1980;89(3 Pt 1):268–270.

238. Tanii T, Hamada T. A variant of encephalomeningocele: heterotopic brain tissue on the scalp. *Dermatologica* 1984;169:354–358.

239. Frieden IJ. Blisters and pustules in the newborn. *Curr Probl Pediatr* 1989;19:551–614.

Head and Neck Region

6

Head and Neck Region

The head and neck region is the area to which our eyes are initially drawn by the constellation of facial features that renders each baby a unique blending of the parents. This region naturally comes first in the examination and merits careful attention because it is also the region where the majority of malformations, deformations, and variations of normal occur. Up to 90% of congenital anomalies that are visible at birth occur in the head and neck region (1). However, many facial features considered diagnostic of syndromes are not as obvious at birth as they are in later infancy or childhood. Some of these characteristic features reflect abnormal growth of specific regions and, in newborn infants, may not have had enough time to deviate outside the ranges of normal variation. Further complicating interpretation of features of the head region are the many variations that reflect transient deformation, molding, or soft-tissue swelling, or racial, sexual, and familial traits.

This chapter discusses the head and neck region except for the detailed examinations of the eyes and ears, which are covered in separate chapters. The order of examination is not necessarily as listed below but should include each subregion with emphasis as directed by individual findings.

SUMMARY OF EXAMINATION OF THE HEAD AND NECK REGION

Inspect the head for the following:

Shape, size, and position of the bony landmarks
Soft-tissue swelling, discoloration, openings or lack of continuity of skin over the scalp, face, and neck
Hair distribution and patterning, color, and density

Palpate the head for the following:

Firmness and continuity of the bones over the cranial vault
Movement and spacing of the sutures
Location, size, and tension of the fontanels
Texture and consistency of the hair
Soft-tissue masses

Measure the head circumference.

Auscult for the following:

Bruits over both temporal regions, the anterior fontanel, and the neck if there is a heart murmur, tachycardia, or visible vascular malformation.
Extrathoracic sounds in the presence of respiratory distress
Character of cry or other vocalization

Transilluminate the skull over the anterior and posterior fontanels as indicated by other findings
Inspect the facial structures and relate their position, size, and shape to each other:

Observe facial expression and relate it to the general infant activity.
Measure any individual parts of the region that appear out of proportion.

Assess nose and nasal cavities for the following:

Size and shape
Masses or clefts
Secretions
Patency, air flow, and flaring

Inspect the mouth for the following:

Size, shape, and continuity of lips, gums, tongue, palate, and all mucosal surfaces
Presence of anomalous structures
Response of rooting reflex, strength of suck, gag reflex

Inspect the ears:

For size, shape, position and rotation, presence of a canal, and any anomalous structures
For recoil and firmness of the pinna
For response to sound
With an otoscope to observe the tympanic membrane and middle ear landmarks

Inspect the eyes for the following:

Shape and regularity of the lid margins
Discharge or matting
Configuration of lashes and eyebrows
Ability to open and close both eyelids
Position and size of the orbits, irides, and pupils
Color and continuity of the conjunctiva, sclera, and irides
Movement in response to an appropriate stimulus
Clarity of the structures in the anterior chamber and the fundus
Presence of bilateral red reflex

Inspect or palpate the neck for the following:

Position of the head and neck
Appearance of skin
Symmetry of cervical musculature
Range of movement of cervical spine
Flexion, anterior and lateral, extension, and rotation
Presence of masses
Presence of lymphadenopathy
Presence and size of thyroid gland
Position of trachea
Continuity of the clavicles

ANATOMY

The head is composed of the neurocranium and the face (Figs. 1 and 2). In the fetus, the development of the head prevails over that of the face and that of the cranial vault over the

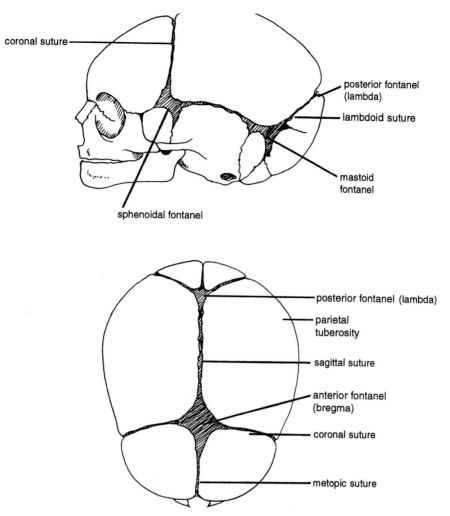

Figure 1. Major sutures and fontanels in newborn skull.

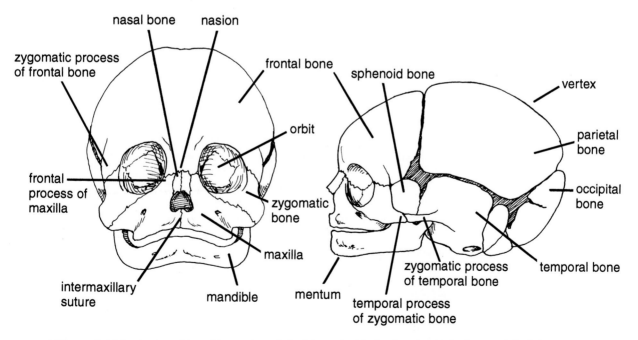

Figure 2 Major bones of head in newborn infant for palpable landmarks. Note the craniofacial proportions with relative underdevelopment of the lower face, particularly the region that will comprise the lower one third by adulthood.

base. Compared with other body regions, the head is proportionately bigger during the fetal and neonatal periods than in any other developmental epoch. Similarly, the neurocranium is comparatively larger than the face. The proportions of the face differ markedly from the adult. In the adult, the eyes are at a level roughly correlating with a line transecting the upper and middle thirds. In the neonate that line transects roughly the mid-point of the vertical axis. It is primarily the lower half of the face that grows to form the eventual adult proportions.

DETAILS OF EXAMINATION OF THE HEAD

Head Shape and Size

Inspect the head for shape and its size relative to the rest of the body and face. Look at it from all aspects, including the front, back, both sides, and top in order to appreciate the entire contour. Note the key landmarks (Fig. 2). Look for any abnormal prominence, depressions, or flattening. If there is any flattening or apparent decrease in volume of one area (plagiocephaly), compare the shape in diagonally opposite corners of the head. Evaluate for range of motion or any masses in the neck to detect a torticollis associated with plagiocephaly. Measure the head circumference in its largest plane above the ears and plot on appropriate growth charts. If either the shape or circumference is abnormal, measure the width and length as well (see Chapter 2 for these techniques).

In assessing the appearance of the head in a neonate, we can make some reasonable conclusions about brain development, fetal position and engagement, and route of delivery. After the immediate neonatal period we can see the effects of brain growth and infant activity or lack thereof because the size and shape of the cranial vault reflect an interaction of internal and external forces and growing bone. The bony structure of the developing calvarium is pliable and responds to applied forces relatively quickly as long as the sutures remain open. These forces accrue from the anatomy, shape, and volume of the brain combined with intracranial pressure interacting against intra- or extrauterine pressures applied to the skull.

Head Shape

Normal intrauterine molding in a vertex presentation leads to a narrowed biparietal diameter with a maximum occipitomental dimension; in a breech presentation, the molding leads to accentuation of the occipitofrontal dimension with parietal flattening, an occipital shelf, and apparent frontal prominence (Fig. 3). After either vertex or breech presentation, the overall contour, particularly when viewed only in profile, may be remarkable enough to suggest intracranial pathology. Normal molding resolves within a few weeks, but pathologic aberrations progress. In infants who failed to engage in a vertex presentation or to descend in labor, the examination should rule out pathologic conditions that inhibit normal molding of the fetal head such as premature synostosis or macrocephaly.

Evaluation of shape also includes noting the position in which the infant holds his head at rest because, in the early neonatal period, the position of comfort suggests the likely fetal position (Fig. 4). Normal fetal position is with anterior neck flexion regardless of the intrauterine position. If the infant prefers a position of neck extension or consistent neck rotation, other fetal positions are suggested (Table 1).

Head Size

The biparietal diameter of the fetus may be measured as early as 8 to 9 weeks' gestational age, although more reliably from 12 to 13 weeks. This diameter is measured on the transverse section of the fetal cranium at the level of the thalamic nuclei. The fetal head circumference is assessed in the same plane as the biparietal diameter. Normal values for biparietal diameter and head circumference of the developing fetus are well established so that many instances of abnormal head size are predicted before birth (2,3).

Aberrations in head size require explanation. A first step in an evaluation is to use growth curves that reflect a similar population, gestation, and chronologic age. In up to 50% of cases, deviations from the normal ranges of the commonly used curves generated by Nellhaus are benign, familial variations (4,5). However, because a number of pathologic con-

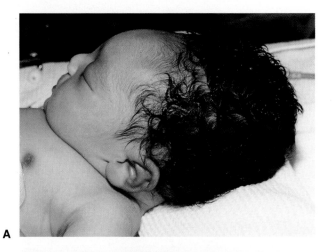

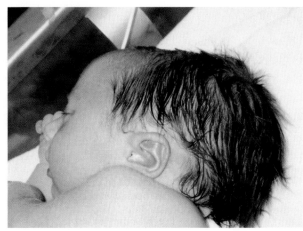

A   **B**

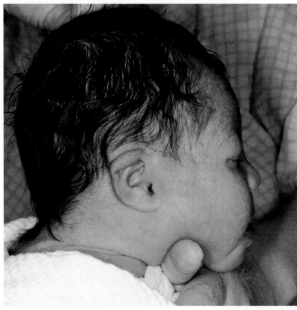

C

Figure 3. Examples of cranial molding. **A:** Occipitomental molding associated with vertex fetal presentation. The maximal dimension is from the back of the head to the chin, minimizing head width to facilitate descent through the pelvic outlet. This degree of deformation is marked but normal and will resolve within a few weeks. With this much molding, one might expect also to find a caput succedaneum or craniotabes. **B:** Occipitofrontal molding due to breech fetal presentation. The maximal dimension is from the back of the head to the forehead. Note the relative prominence of the forehead and occiput with flattening across the top of the head. This dolichocephaly will resolve within a few weeks if it is secondary only to fetal breech position and not premature synostosis. Some fetuses remain in breech because the shape, size, or noncompliance of the skull will not allow the vertex to fit into the smaller, more inferior portion of the uterus. Examination of infants with this type of molding should include evaluation of suture patency and volume of the cranial vault as well as a careful check for congenital hip dislocation also associated with extended breech positioning. **C:** Flat occiput in newborn infant with Down's syndrome. The brachycephaly is only partly due to molding with most of it due to the occipital plagiocephaly characteristic of infants with trisomy 21. The posterior hair line extends low onto the neck. The unruliness and sparse nature of the hair that is characteristic of older infants with Down's syndrome is not a unique identifier in the neonate, nor is the characteristic short neck. This small ear is relatively square with folding of the angulated upper helix.

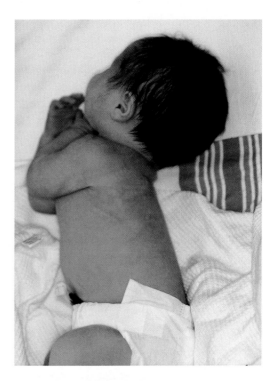

Figure 4. Head and neck position after face presentation. Infant's resting position of comfort is with neck markedly extended. Although the position is called opisthotonus fetalis during parturition, this is not accompanied by high tone elsewhere, as shown with the straight back and flexed hips and shoulders, and it resolves as the neck gradually stretches. Initially, this infant will feed best with the neck extended but should be encouraged into flexion by back lying for sleep. Expected associations after face presentation are facial edema and ecchymoses, with a range of severity sufficient to cause nasal obstruction, facial cyanosis, massive palpebral edema, and scleral hemorrhage.

ditions of aberrant head size are recurrent in families, there is indication for further investigation and follow-up if there are other physical findings or historical factors present.

The terms used to describe abnormalities in size of the head and brain should be applied thoughtfully because there is considerable overlap in the literature. Strictly defined, microcephaly or macrocephaly imply various measurements of the head falling outside 2 standard deviations (2 SD) determined from a comparable population regardless of cause, whereas micrencephaly and macrencephaly imply aberrant brain size. In more neurology-specific literature, the terms "micrencephaly" and "macrencephaly" refer to disorders of neuronal proliferation, and the term "microcephaly" implies a destruction and loss of neuronal tissue (6–9). In the most extreme cases of aberrant brain size, mental retardation is presumed, but this is not always a correlation in some of the reported familial cases (6–9).

Sutures and Fontanel

Palpate the head, feeling for firmness of the bones, the size and configuration of the fontanels and sutures, and the presence of any swelling, masses, or defects in the bones. Run a fingertip from the glabella to the occiput along the metopic and sagittal sutures, from one temporal region to the other along the coronal sutures, and over the occipitoparietal junction to define the lambdoid sutures. Determine that the sutures are open by gently applying alternating pressure on either side of the suture line. Be gentle to avoid rupturing underlying vessels.

Table 1. *Position of comfort in neonate relating to fetal presentation*

Resting position of head and neck	Suggested cause
Flexed in midline	Normal vertex presentation or floating
Extended	Face presentation or some breech presentations
Tilted	Asynclitic
Turned	Away from side of sternocleidomastoid shortening or toward side with plagiocephaly or because of poor muscle strength

The cranial bones provide protection to the underlying cranial vessels and brain during the process of labor and delivery. If these bones are firm and their configuration molded into a narrow taper for descent through the vaginal canal, under normal circumstances there is sufficient protection against vessel rupture or brain contusion. When a vertex presentation is oblique as suggested by marked asymmetry in molding or if the bones are relatively soft, there is more likelihood of brain contusion or of rupture of underlying subdural vessels. The likelihood increases when the descent in the second stage of labor is either precipitous or difficult.

Depending on the extent and direction of molding, there is variable overlap in the sutures, occasionally making it difficult to determine if the sutures are fused or open but overlapping. Overlapped bones can be compared with a cliff with a rise on one side and sharp drop on the other; premature synostosis would be more like a glacial mountain range with a rise on both sides. In craniosynostosis, fused sutures will not move freely when alternate sides are gently pressed. Reevaluation in a few days should allow time for molding and overlap to improve enough to differentiate between the two conditions.

Any suture, but most often the metopic and sagittal sutures, may be wide in the absence of increased intracranial pressure, particularly in premature infants; the exception is a widened lambdoid suture, which ordinarily indicates increased pressure in term infants. The sagittal and metopic sutures are normally wider in black infants. Palpably increased tension in the anterior fontanel is a late indicator of cranial hypertension in the neonate because there are so many compliant areas in the neonatal skull that allow rapid diffusion of pressure. The exception is with rapid increases in pressure developing before they can be diffused or exceeding the diffusion capacity. A visibly bulging fontanel, especially in the upright position, is abnormal (Fig. 5).

Palpation of the parietal bones near the sagittal suture may reveal a collapse and recoil similar to that felt when pressing on an aluminum can or a ping-pong ball. This finding in-

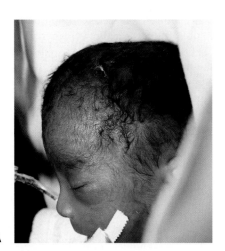

A

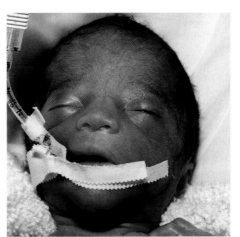

B

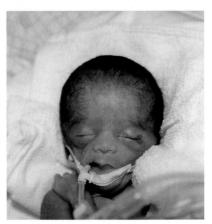

C

Figure 5. Rapid alteration in head shape due to acquired hydrocephalus. The acute increase in intracranial pressure is associated with massive intraventricular hemorrhage in a 24 weeks' gestation infant. On day 1 there is notable bulging of the anterior fontanel seen when comparing lateral (**A**) and frontal (**B**) views. **C:** Within 18 hours there is more diffusion of the pressure, with widening of the sutures and a broadening of the forehead. The infant's pallor suggests a marked anemia.

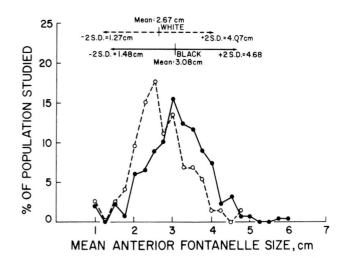

Figure 6. Distribution of mean anterior fontanel size in white (*hatched line*) and black (*solid line*) term, appropriately grown, healthy newborn infants (n = 73 white and n = 293 black infants studied after 48 hours of age). Reprinted with permission (130).

dicates craniotabes (synonym *craniomalacia*), which is found most often in infants who have been engaged in a vertex presentation for a prolonged period of at least 5 weeks (10,11). The likely cause in most cases is pressure of the fetal skull against the maternal pelvis, causing either a delayed ossification or a resorption of the bone (12,13). In more unusual cases where prolonged pressure is not an apparent factor, there may be a variation in maternal calcium metabolism but this suggested cause has not been confirmed (12,13). Craniotabes may recur in siblings, but it is not genetically transmitted, nor does it indicate neonatal rickets. The process normally resolves spontaneously within a few weeks (12,13). Because of its proximity, craniotabes might be confused with an enlarged posterior fontanel and sagittal suture and therefore suggest a pathologic condition such as hypothyroidism, hypophosphatasia, osteogenesis imperfecta, or rickets. Compared with other areas in the skull, areas with craniotabes provide less protection to the underlying structures, making them more susceptible to contusion injury. In the absence of other signs and symptoms suggesting intracranial pathology, there need be no further evaluation.

Macewen's sign has been described as an indication of open sutures in infants and older patients. To elicit the sign that is described as a "cracked pot" sound, the parietal bones are percussed (14). Another variation in technique is to use the fingers on one hand to percuss or drum gently on one side of the skull while the other hand rests on the opposite side of the head to feel an increased resonance, indicating open sutures (1). Percussion is unlikely to suggest a diagnosis of widely opened sutures or increased intracranial pressure in neonates in the absence of other more obvious or specific signs. Similarly, the absence of Macewen's sign is not helpful to detect premature closure of sutures.

Assess the tension of the fontanel with the infant in the recumbent position and, when possible, in an upright position as well. To monitor serial changes in size, measure the fontanel in the transverse diameter (15). If heart murmurs are present, auscult over the anterior fontanel and the temporal bones for bruits (16).

Measurement of the fontanel is not useful as part of a single, routine assessment because of wide variation in size and poor reproducibility, but it is helpful in following infants at risk for developing intracranial hypertension and subsequent widening of the fontanel (Fig. 6). There is little clinical application for measurements in otherwise normal infants because head growth can occur during infancy despite apparently closed fontanels; the rate of closure is independent of other growth parameters and bone age (15) (Fig. 7). At birth, apparently closed fontanels associated with immobile, ridged sutures suggest premature synostosis. Although aberrantly large fontanels are seen in genetic syndromes and metabolic and endocrine diseases, they are not pathognomonic of any condition. Racial variations are considerable.

Transillumination of the Head

Transilluminate the skull by holding a strong but cool light against the anterior fontanel and bony areas. The light source must seal against the scalp and allow no light to escape. Take time to allow for eye accommodation in a darkened room. Make sure that the light source is bright enough to provide accurate transillumination but not hot enough to burn the skin (17).

Extracranial determinants of transillumination size or the width of the corona around the light source include thickness of the scalp and subcutaneous fat layer, color and density of skin and hair, and collections of subcutaneous fluid such as intravenous infiltrate or caput succedaneum. There is spurious increase in the glow of illumination across suture lines, fontanels, and areas of craniotabes (12). The thickness of the skull also affects the transillumination with no light transmitted across a skull with a thickness of more than 2.5 mm. The skull is normally less than 2.5 mm in thickness at term birth. Transillumination does not necessarily increase in proportion to prematurity, as some investigators suggest (18). Swick found the opposite to be true, with an increase in transillumination size as premature infants approached term corrected age (12,17,19,20).

Intracranial factors enhancing transillumination (18):

Subdural
　Effusion
Subarachnoid
　Communicating hydrocephalus
　Cerebral destruction
　Cerebral anomaly (underdevelopment)
　Arachnoidal cyst
Cerebral-intraventricular
　Noncommunicating hydrocephalus
　Hydranencephaly
　Schizencephaly
　Porencephaly
Posterior fossa
　Dandy-Walker malformation and variants
　Cerebellar hypoplasia
　Trapped fourth ventricle
　Enlarged cisterna magna
　Arachnoidal cyst
　Alobar holoprosencephaly

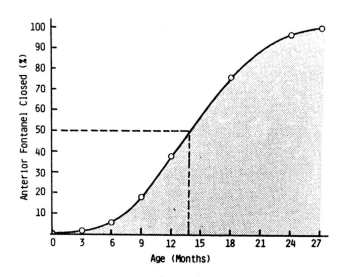

Figure 7. Age at closure of anterior fontanel (cumulative percentage). Reprinted with permission (15).

Scalp

While examining the head, carefully inspect and palpate the head, particularly when there is abundant dark hair to obscure the underlying skin. Assess for any scalp lesions or for swelling that suggests a caput succedaneum, cephalohematoma, or subgaleal hemorrhage.

The scalp, like the rest of normal neonatal skin, will be quite dry and flaking in the neonatal period. This early scaling is not related to the seborrheic dermatitis or cradle cap that might appear at several weeks of age, and it requires no treatment. Superficial ecchymoses and abrasions of the scalp are common after vaginal deliveries, especially after artificial rupture of membranes by an amnihook or extraction by forceps or vacuum. Incision sites for fetal scalp electrodes or blood sampling should be small and inconsequential, although some require closure (Fig. 8). These sites should be distinguished from congenital cutis aplasia (Fig. 9).

Lesions associated with fetal scalp electrodes:

Laceration
Blistering
Ulceration (1%) (21)
Abscess formation (0.2–4%) (21–23)
   Organisms are aerobic or anaerobic from the cervical flora
   Incidence relates to duration of scalp monitoring
   Osteomyelitis (24)
Necrotizing fasciitis (25)
Herpes meningoencephalitis (26,27)

CLINICAL EXAMPLES

Aberrations in Shape of the Head

Extracerebral Fluid Collections (Fig. 10)

Caput Succedaneum
Cephalohematoma
Subgaleal hematoma

Caput Succedaneum

See Fig. 11.

Location: In scalp at point of contact with cervix. Can extend across suture lines.
Characteristic findings:
   Vaguely demarcated, pitting edema that shifts within hours in response to gravity.
   Contents of edema, serum, or blood.
   Overlying petechiae, erythema, or ecchymosis should not be confused with a cephalohematoma.
Time of presentation: Maximum size and firmness at birth.
Clinical time course: Softens progressively from birth and resolves within 48 to 72 hours.
Volume of blood: Minimal in the absence of coagulopathy.
Treatment: None.
Incidence: Very common, particularly after prolonged engagement or labor.
Associations: Infection after use of internal scalp electrodes may be increased in the presence of significant caput.

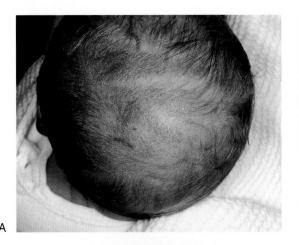

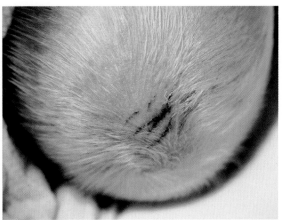

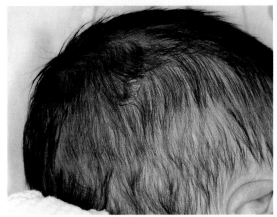

Figure 8. Scalp changes after vaginal delivery. **A:** Purpuric erythema in a linear pattern, indicating pleating of the scalp from compression. Superficial scalp laceration is due to insertion of fetal scalp electrode. **B:** Multiple superficial lacerations from amnihook used to rupture membranes. **C:** Blistering and ecchymoses may be marked after vacuum or forceps extraction. Superficial lesions dry within 12 to 24 hours and require no therapy. Differential diagnosis includes pressure-induced blistering, cutis aplasia, and epidermolysis bullosa. Infectious causes are unlikely, but herpetic lesions presenting at birth may be confusing (131).

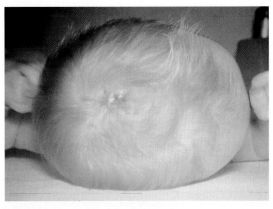

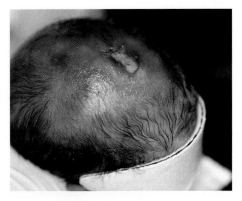

Figure 9. Cutis aplasia of the scalp. **A:** Healing lesion. Some lesions of cutis aplasia may be covered by a superficial layer of skin without hair and appear to be a simple blister. The absence of hair and depth of the defect is typical (compare with Fig. 8C). When a superficial covering is absent, as in this infant, the absence of several layers of skin is evident. The margins may appear rolled with granulation from the periphery. With time, the area and depth of the lesions may lessen, but the alopecia persists. There is a familial association, but cutis aplasia of the scalp is associated with a number of chromosomal syndromes, most notably trisomy 13. **B:** Acute lesion. The appearance of the area of cutis aplasia and the adjacent scalp suggest the etiology of vascular insufficiency, in this case likely associated with the fetal death of the twin. When the scalp defect is deep and located over the anterior fontanel, detachment of an eschar can be associated with catastrophic hemorrhage from a ruptured sagittal sinus.

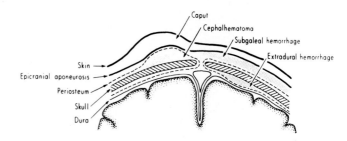

Figure 10. Types of extradural fluid collections seen in newborn infants. Reprinted with permission (18). Data from Pape and Wigglesworth (132).

Cephalhematoma or Cephalohematoma

See Fig. 12.

Location: Bleeding between the skull and the periosteum (28). Over one or both parietal bones; rarely over occipital or frontal bones.

Characteristic findings:
Does not cross suture lines.
Rarely any overlying discoloration.
Has distinct margins.
Initially firm, becoming more fluctuant after 48 hours.

Time of presentation: Increasing size after birth for the first 12 to 24 hours and then stable. Becomes more apparent at the time a caput would lessen.

Time of resolution: 2 to 3 weeks.

Volume of blood: Rarely is volume loss severe.

Treatment: None unless complicated by infection. Surgical correction of large, calcified cephalhematomas for cosmetic reasons are reported, but most resolve spontaneously given enough time (29,30).

Incidence:
0.4% to 2.5% of births.
Most frequent after prolonged or difficult labor or use of forceps or vacuum extraction with most likely spontaneous cause being a buffeting of fetal skull against maternal pelvis.
Higher in primiparous mothers.
Increasing frequency with higher application of forceps: 4.3% with outlet forceps; 7.4% with low forceps; 9.5% with mid-forceps (31,32).
Occurs prenatally (33).
Occurs after cesarean section or unassisted vaginal deliveries (34).

Associated problems: Linear skull fracture in 5.4% to 25% that are rarely of clinical significance. There is a low potential for formation of leptomeningeal cysts (35,36).
Hyperbilirubinemia (37).
Infection (sepsis and osteomyelitis) (38–40).
Epidural hematoma (rare) (41,42).

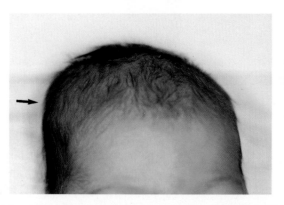
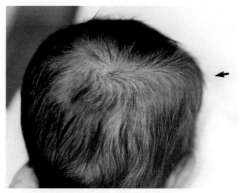

A   B

Figure 11. Caput succedaneum. **A:** The apparent tilt to the calvarium is due to mild edema over the right parietal region, a caput succedaneum (*arrow*). **B:** When viewed 24 hours after birth, the edema can be seen to shift to a dependent position. Because this infant was kept in a right side-lying position for sleeping, the caput edema layered as a ridge on the right side of the head (*arrow*). The area would be expected to pit easily upon compression.

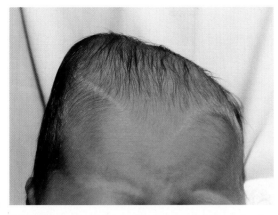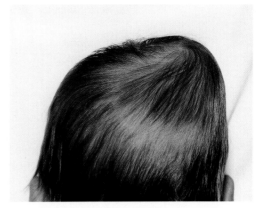

A   B

Figure 12. Cephalohematoma over right parietal area. **A:** Anterior view. **B:** Posterior view. There is a discrete margin in the reflected periosteum that on palpation sometimes leads to a false impression of a depression in the skull bone. Cephalohematomas are only rarely present at the time of delivery and increase in size during the hours after birth. They do not cause pitting edema unless coincidentally proximate to a caput.

Subgaleal Hematoma

See Fig. 13.

Location: Bleeding beneath the epicranial aponeurosis that connects the frontal and occipital components of the occipito-frontalis muscle. Unconfined expansion allows wide spreading.

Characteristic findings: Firm to fluctuant mass that may extend onto the neck or forehead but with ill-defined borders. A crepitant sensation may be present, particularly at the periphery. Softer lesions have fluid waves.

Time of presentation: Progressive increase from birth.

Time of resolution: 2 to 3 weeks.

Volume of blood: May be massive, particularly when there is an accompanying coagulation defect.

Treatment:

Correction of coagulopathy.

Replacement of blood volume as required.

Incidence:

Occur primarily after prolonged application of vacuum extraction (43).

Large collections are unusual. Smaller collections may be undetected and far more frequent.

Associated problems:

Hypovolemia with massive collections.

Hyperbilirubinemia.

Linear skull fracture.

Suture diastasis (43).

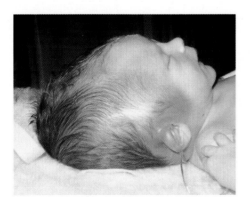

Figure 13. Large subgaleal hematoma. There is a discoloration and swelling that extends across suture lines onto the neck, even onto the ear, causing protuberance of the pinna. There may be some degree of crepitation to palpation, particularly at the margins. The area containing blood can advance well down the forehead and neck because there is little inhibition and there can be major blood extravasation.

Abnormal Shape of Skull

Plagiocephaly
Craniosynostosis

Plagiocephaly

See Figs. 14 and 15.

Description: As originally derived, the term means an oblique head. The appearance is asymmetrical, most often flattened, and accompanied by compensatory changes in the rest of the skull, particularly with fullness over a diagonally opposite corner. Parietal flattening with diagonal fullness leads to facial asymmetry that may include one ear lying more anterior to the other when the head is viewed from above, as well as unilateral epicanthal folding (44). Unfortunately, the unilateral epicanthal folding does not always predict which side is flattened. When flattening is due to positioning either before or after birth, the shape normalizes when the external forces resolve. If it is due to underlying brain maldevelopment or to craniosynostosis, the distortion increases with time.

Associations:

1. Torticollis. Because of limited rotation in the neck, constant positioning of the head on one side leads to flattening.
2. Customary resting position. Young infants, who spend the majority of their sleep and wake times on their backs, have some degree of occipital plagiocephaly but it generally crosses suture lines. A common form of plagiocephaly develops in premature infants, who do not turn their heads as readily as term infants and tend to keep them turned on the side or toward whatever environmental stimuli are most interesting to them.

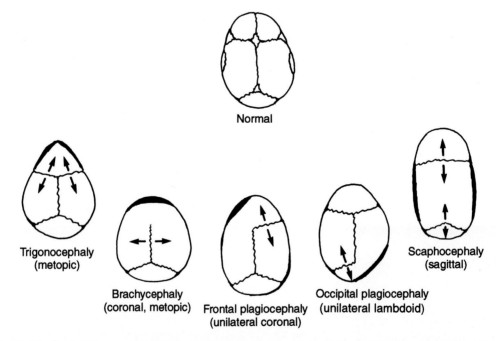

Figure 14. Skull shapes associated with premature closure of single sutures (in parentheses). The heavy lines denote the area of maximal flattening. The arrows indicate the direction of continued growth across the sutures that remain open. More complex shapes occur when combinations of sutures are closed (see Table 2).

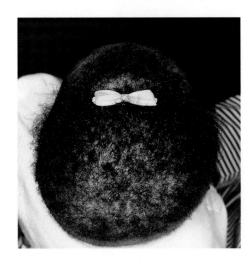

Figure 15. Mild occipital plagiocephaly due to craniosynostosis of the right lambdoid suture. The barrette is placed over the anterior fontanel in line with the coronal suture to illustrate the asymmetry. There is no significant contralateral frontal bulging as would be seen with more significant restriction of occipital growth.

3. Premature closure of sutures. Flattening due craniosynostosis will be in a plane parallel to the closed suture because growth is restricted perpendicular to the suture and unrestricted in the other planes (Fig. 14).
4. Localized brain hypoplasia. Plagiocephaly due to flattening from external pressure will generally have associated fullness on the diagonally opposite corner while flattening due to decreased volume of the underlying brain should have no compensation.

Craniosynostosis

See Figs. 14 and 16.

Description: Premature closure of one or several of the cranial sutures. The resultant restriction in growth perpendicular to the affected suture(s) is accompanied by compensated overgrowth in unrestricted regions, giving characteristic shapes (Table 2).

Etiology: The sutures are growth zones rather than primary growth centers. Sutural bone is laid down as a secondary response to capsular tensions from the expanding brain and the independent growth of the skull base. Premature fusion may be secondary to an arrest of brain growth as in micrencephaly; as an effect of metabolic disease such as rickets or hyperthyroidism (45) or overtreatment with thyroid hormone; or to chronic fetal head constraint (46); or as a primary congenital disorder of skull growth.

Predilection for sex: Some patterns of craniosynostosis are more common in male than in female infants, especially scaphocephaly (4:1 male:female) and trigonocephaly (47). Frontal plagiocephaly is more common in females (47).

Inheritance pattern: Most cases of craniosynostosis represent isolated congenital anomalies without family history, although 10% to 20% have an inherited pattern (47).

Associations: Isolated craniosynostosis occurs in 0.6 of 1,000 live births, with affected sutures in decreasing frequency being sagittal/metopic, 50%; sagittal, 28%; coronal, 16.5%; and lambdoid, 5.5% (48).

Further evaluation and course: Some patterns of synostosis are accompanied by restricted brain growth (craniostenosis) or hydrocephalus and require prompt intervention to minimize brain damage. Others require timely intervention for cosmetic correction. Most of the syndromes in which craniosynostosis is a major sign have other manifestations, particularly of the facial structures and extremities. These are genetically transmitted.

The aberrations in skull shape due to untreated premature cranial synostosis increase after birth while changes that are due to intrauterine deformation resolve.

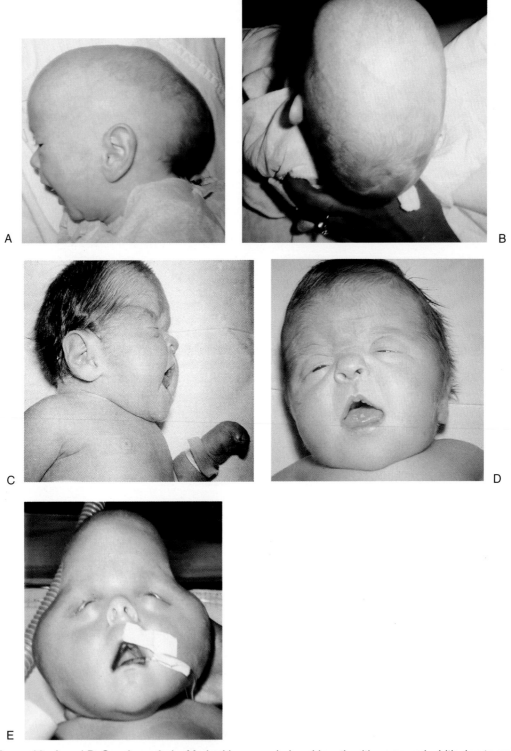

Figure 16. A and B: Scaphocephaly. Marked increase in head length with narrowed width due to premature fusion of sagittal suture. Premature infants allowed to remain with the head in a side-lying position develop scaphocephalic changes but with more flattening of the side or sides of the skull. **C:** Premature closure of bilateral coronal and basial sphenofrontal and frontoethmoidal sutures in an infant with Apert's syndrome (acrosyndactyly) leads to turricephaly if left uncorrected. **D:** The length of the head is markedly shortened (brachycephaly) due to craniosynostosis of the coronal sutures. The characteristic facies of Apert's syndrome derive in part from craniosynostosis of the basial sutures and mid-face hypoplasia: shallow orbits, small nose, maxillary hypoplasia, supraorbital horizontal groove. The palate is narrow with a median cleft. The ears appear relatively large compared with the undergrown mid-face. Syndactyly and shortening of the fingers and a short thumb are visible. **E:** Kleeblattschädel. Cloverleaf skull caused by craniosynostosis of all sutures forcing brain growth through the anterior and temporal fontanels. This most severe form of restricted skull growth has the poorest prognosis due to a combination of craniostenosis and hydrocephalus.

Table 2. *Skull shapes associated with premature synostosis*

Description of shape	Skull configuration	Chief sutures involved	Occurrence (nonsyndromic)	Comments
Scaphocephaly (dolichocephaly)	Elongated configuration in the AP axis	Sagittal	45–50%	80% males; sagittal suture feels like a bony keel
Frontal plagiocephaly	Flattening over frontal area on one side with marked facial asymmetry, elevation and recession of the eyebrow and orbital margin, prominence of the ipsilateral ear with bony bulge on contralateral parietal vault.	Unilateral coronal and sphenofrontal	20–25%	More females; Saethre-Chotzen syndrome
Occipital plagiocephaly	Flattening over one occiput with prominence of ipsilateral frontal region but with little facial deformation; sometimes with prominence of ipsilateral ear. The resulting shape is a parallelogram.	Unilateral lambdoid	2–10%	Findings are similar to positional deformations after prematurity, torticollis, spinal tumors, cervico-occipital abnormalities, or without discernible cause. It becomes less noticeable with age and rarely involves brain so does not require surgical treatment.
Trigonocephaly	Triangular shape with prowlike forehead	Metopic	5%	There is a median ridge representing the fused metopic suture. Males affected more than females. Similar facial appearance develops with bilateral frontal lobe dysplasia but without bony keel. Optiz syndrome
Turricephaly (acrocephaly)	Broad, tower-shaped skull with absence of anterior fontanel	Bilateral coronal, sphenofrontal, and frontoethmoidal	5–10%	Crouzon (most common pattern); Apert (variable with additional anomalies at the skull base)
Oxycephaly	Conical shape with forehead sloping to a bony boss at the bregma	Multiple	Rare	
Triphyllocephaly (Kleeblattschädel)	Cloverleaf with bilateral temporal bulges and a medial bregmatic bulge	Multiple sutures	Rare	
Pachycephaly	Flattened back of head with brachycephalic skull	Bilateral lambdoid	Rare	
Brachycephaly	Broad skull with reduction of AP diameter	Bilateral coronal	12%	Seen in Apert, Antley-Bixler, Pfeiffer syndromes

Data from Simpson P (47).

Conditions with Aberrations in Head Size

Micrencephaly (Fig. 17)
Microcephaly
Macrencephaly (Fig. 18)
Hydrocephalus (Fig. 19)
Hydranencephaly (Fig. 20)
Holoprosencephaly (Fig. 21)
Dandy-Walker cyst (Fig. 22)

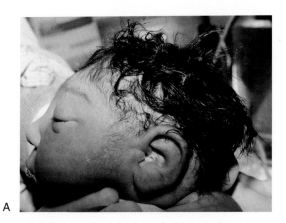
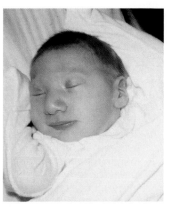

Figure 17. Micrencephaly vera. The designation of micrencephaly vera generally reflects diminished neuronal proliferation rather than a result of intrauterine or early postnatal destruction of neuronal tissue or abnormal development in induction, cleavage, or migration of neurons. The brain is formed but small. At birth most infants with micrencephaly vera do not show the abnormal neurologic function typical of destructive microcephaly, such as seizures or motor defects, nor is there hydrocephalus ex vacuo. The brain is fully covered with a firm skull with little suture mobility and small or absent fontanels. **A:** This infant demonstrates an extremely small cranial vault. She was able to feed well and had no notable findings on neurologic examination. Note the fleshy ear that on first appearance seems long but is proportionate with her mid-face. The apparent unruliness of her hair at this hour shortly after birth is insignificant. **B:** Less severe micrencephaly. The craniofacial disproportion makes the normally sized nose and mouth seem too large, but it is the cranium that is too small. Typically, the head circumference falls more than 2 SD below normal, whereas the weight and length are closer to the mean. The possible etiologies of micrencephaly and microcephaly include familial (autosomal-dominant, autosomal-recessive, X-linked recessive, and other undefined familial types); teratogenic (irradiation, alcohol, cocaine, maternal hyperphenylalaninemia, anticonvulsant drugs, organic mercurials, and excessive intake of vitamin A or its analogues); infection (rubella and less commonly early onset cytomegalovirus and HIV); or sporadic. Depending on the etiology, not all cases of micrencephaly vera are associated with retardation, particularly those transmitted by autosomal dominance.

Disorders of neuronal proliferation associated with micrencephaly (18,49) (Fig. 17):

Presumed diminished number of proliferative units: radial microbrain
Presumed diminished size of proliferative units: micrencephaly vera
Familial
    Autosomal recessive
    Autosomal dominant
    X-linked recessive
    Genetics unclear with ocular abnormalities
    Chromosomal translocation
Teratogenic
    Irradiation
    Metabolic-toxic
        Fetal alcohol syndrome
        Cocaine
        Hyperphenylalaninemia
    Infection (early onset)
        Rubella
        Cytomegalovirus
Sporadic
    Nonfamilial with unknown cause

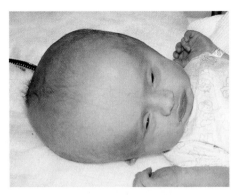
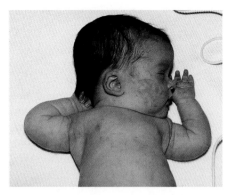

A

B

Figure 18. Macrencephaly. **A:** This infant had a dysmorphic, enlarged brain without hydrocephalus. Macrencephaly represents an increase in the size of the brain, generally due to aberration in neuronal proliferation, not secondary to hydrocephalus. It may be familial, sporadic, associated with other growth abnormalities, a component of a neurocutaneous syndrome, or chromosomal. **B:** Macrocephaly associated with macrencephaly of achondroplasia. The head is relatively large for the chest circumference with a prominent forehead despite occipito-mental molding. Note the depressed nasal bridge, short humerus, and trident shape of her left hand. Her head did not measure more than 2 SD above a circumference expected for her gestational age, but it was greater than two quartiles above her weight and length with mild craniofacial disproportion. Although not present at birth, she is at risk for craniostenosis and hydrocephalus related to basial skull changes of achondroplasia.

Disorders of neuronal proliferation associated with macrencephaly (18,49) (Fig. 18):

Isolated macrencephaly
    Familial
        Autosomal dominant: related to benign enlargement of extracerebral spaces or external hydrocephalus
        Autosomal recessive
    Sporadic
Associated disturbance of growth
    Cerebral gigantism
    Beckwith syndrome
    Achondroplasia
Neurocutaneous syndrome
    Multiple hemangiomatosis
        Pseudopapilledema (Riley-Smith)
        Lipomas, lymphangiomas (Bannayan-Zonana)
        Asymmetrical hypertrophy ± scoliosis (Klippel-Trenaunay-Weber)
        Asymmetrical hypertrophy ± scoliosis, telangiectatic lesions, flame nevus of the face (cutis marmorata telangiectatica congenita)
    Neurofibromatosis (tuberous sclerosis, Sturge-Weber)
    Linear nevus sebaceous (unilateral macrencephaly)
Chromosomal disorders
    Fragile-X syndrome (relative macrencephaly)
    Klinefelter syndrome
Unilateral macrencephaly (hemimegalencephaly)

Note that some of these conditions involve enlargement of the head or brain without affecting the size or number of the neurons. Internal hydrocephalus is excluded. In many of these processes macrencephaly is not present at birth or within the neonatal period.

Hydrocephalus, Congenital or Acquired

See Figs. 5 and 19.

Description: By convention, the term "hydrocephalus" is used to mean increase in both fluid and intracranial pressure. When there is increased fluid but without elevated pressure as found in cerebral atrophy, the term "hydrocephalus ex vacuo" is used.

The clinical presentation of hydrocephalus is evidence of increased intracranial pressure in the presence of progressive macrocephaly: a full anterior fontanel with separated sutures, prominent scalp veins, abnormal tone (generally low), lethargy, vomiting, poor feeding, unilateral or bilateral sixth nerve palsies, a setting-sun sign, and, especially in premature infants, apnea. There may be an excessive increase of the head circumference, but the widely used criterion of growth of greater than 2 cm per week is a late indicator of acquired hydrocephalus (50). On ultrasonography, ventricular width greater than 1.5 cm in premature infants is suggested as an early indicator of developing posthemorrhagic hydrocephalus (50).

Etiology: Among the causes of hydrocephalus (18,51) are increased production of cerebral spinal fluid (CSF) (choroid plexus papilloma), obstruction to CSF pathways (tumor, aqueductal stenosis, Arnold-Chiari malformation, Dandy-Walker malformation, intraventricular hemorrhage, or ventriculitis), and impaired absorption of CSF (post-subarachnoid hemorrhage or meningitis, abnormal arachnoid villi or decreased venous drainage).

Acquired hydrocephalus can develop very soon after birth, making it difficult to separate all cases from congenital hydrocephalus. The onset can be rapid or quite gradual. The most common causes of acquired neonatal hydrocephalus are intraventricular hemorrhage in

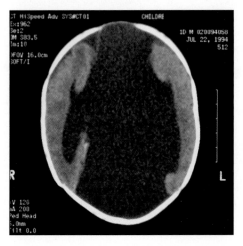

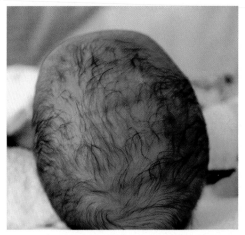

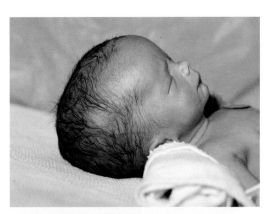

A

B

C

Figure 19. Congenital hydrocephalus. **A:** Marked craniofacial disproportion, but with normal facial structures. Not visible was his hand that showed shortening of the first metacarpal and holding of the thumb across the palm (cortical thumb), suggesting a most likely cause of X-linked aqueductal stenosis. **B:** Transillumination is strongly positive except to the sides of the head. **C:** CT scan correlates with transillumination showing remaining mantle of cortical tissue.

premature infants and meningitis. Acquired hydrocephalus is not associated with other brain anomalies, although delayed manifestation of congenital hydrocephalus may suggest otherwise.

Incidence: In a retrospective case study in Australia the incidence of obstructive congenital hydrocephalus was 0.6 ± 0.2 per 1,000 live and stillbirths (52).

Predilection for sex: Three-fifths of cases are male with X-linked aqueductal stenosis the most frequent cause (52).

Associations: When hydrocephalus is associated with the fetal onset of ventriculomegaly, there is a high incidence of associated anomalies, with 80% having either extraneural or central nervous anomalies or both (18): 40% to 50% have major extraneural anomalies, and 60% to 65% have major central nervous system anomalies. More than half the cases of hydrocephalus diagnosed at birth are associated with aqueductal stenosis or myelomeningocele with Arnold-Chiari malformations (53,54).

In X-linked aqueductal stenosis, approximately 50% of the male infants have a deformity of the thumbs in which there is a short metacarpal and adduction of the thumb over the palm (cortical thumb) (52).

Most cases of hydrocephalus caused by chronic intrauterine infection result in hydrocephalus ex vacuo and have other systemic findings of infection: hepatosplenomegaly, chorioretinitis, skin rash, and small weight for dates.

Comments: In neonates and young infants with early hydrocephalus, the white matter of the brain is more damaged by the increased intracranial pressure than is the gray matter; in older patients, the gray matter is more affected (51). If there is permanent damage from congenital or neonatal hydrocephalus, there is a likelihood of motor impairment (cerebral palsy) as a consequence.

In the absence of other neurologic anomalies, the prognosis for hydrocephalus is worse in premature infants of less than 28 weeks gestational age than in term infants (55,56). Most of the cases in premature infants are associated with intracranial hemorrhage, which is more destructive than simple obstructive hydrocephalus. The prognosis for all infants depends on what anomalies are associated, with intracranial anomalies such as the Dandy-Walker malformation having the worst prognosis (54). The width of the cortical mantle visible before shunting gives some indication of potential outcome (54).

The outcome for antenatally diagnosed ventriculomegaly seems to be worse than that reported in the neurosurgical literature for children treated with simple, congenitally diagnosed hydrocephalus. A favorable outcome of normal mental development is present in cases with borderline, nonprogressive, isolated ventriculomegaly or cases in which ventriculomegaly resolved in utero (57).

Hydranencephaly

See Fig. 20.

Description: Hydranencephaly is an extreme form of loss of neuronal tissue where most or all of both hemispheres is reduced to nothing but transparent membranous sacs containing fluid. If the cavitation is limited to one hemisphere with a mantle of cerebral cortex persisting at the margins, the term "porencephaly" applies. In porencephaly, the defect is in contact with either the ventricle or the cerebral surface. If loss is diffuse in multiple cavities, the term "multicystic encephalomalacia" is appropriate (18).

Embryology: Congenital hydranencephaly is most commonly the result of bilateral cerebral infarction of both cortex and cerebral white matter in the distribution of both carotid arteries. The area most consistently damaged is in the distribution of the middle cerebral arteries and to a lesser extent, the anterior cerebral arteries. Because true thromboses have not been found in the carotid arteries, vascular insufficiency probably results from severe maternal hypotension, general placental or cord catastrophes, death of a twin, or severe viral infections, hyperthermia, or endotoxemia (51,58,59). By comparison to animal models, an insult sufficient to cause hydranencephaly most likely occurs early in the second half of the second trimester (60). Insults resulting in multicystic changes occur later in the second and

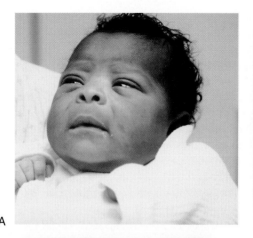

A

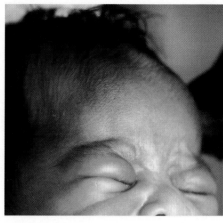

B

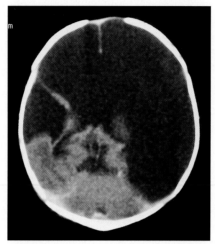

C

Figure 20. Hydranencephaly. **A:** Normal facies without craniofacial disproportion. Macrocephaly is often not present at birth. This infant was able to eat well and had the expected primitive reflexes but did not extinguish her Moro reflex. She was mildly jittery and did not self-console well. She developed macrocephaly after the neonatal period. **B:** Positive transillumination in the frontal and parietal regions even in the presence of copious dark hair and bright ambient light. **C:** CT scan correlates with transillumination and indicates typical findings of hydranencephaly with loss of most of the distribution of the anterior and middle cerebral arteries and preservation of posterior brain structures.

third trimesters (51). Porencephaly and multicystic changes also can develop after insults up to several months of age, notably from hemorrhage, infection, or ischemia.

Predilection for sex: None.

Inheritance pattern: In the vast majority of cases, these are isolated events. There are reports of affected siblings, suggesting either a maternal proliferative vasculopathy or a genetic disorder (61,62). Rarely, isoimmune thrombocytopenia is a possible cause of fetal intracranial hemorrhage resulting in hydranencephaly (63,64).

Associations: The event causing hydranencephaly is often undetermined unless there was a known catastrophic event such as death of a monochorionic twin or intrauterine infection.

Expected course or treatment: Many infants with hydranencephaly appear remarkably normal at birth because the brain stem functions are intact. When closely tested on neurologic examination, there is poor self-consolation, irritability, and jitteriness. They are able to feed sufficiently for some time until spasticity develops.

Holoprosencephaly

See Fig. 21 (65–77).

Description: The major feature is a single-sphered cerebral structure with a common ventricle, a membranous roof over the third ventricle, absence of the olfactory bulbs and tracts, and variable hypoplasia of the optic nerve. The third ventricle may be markedly enlarged as a posterior cyst. Microcephaly is more common than macrocephaly unless there is significant hydrocephalus from accumulation in the posterior cyst.

Mid-line facial anomalies range in severity as listed in Table 3.

Embryology: Holoprosencephaly is a monotopic developmental field defect caused by failure of the migration and differentiation of mesoderm into the forebrain and mid-line facial structures. The onset is by at least the 5th to 6th weeks of gestation. In the brain's development, the telencephalon fails to cleave into hemispheres. If cleavage is absent, there is alobar holoprosencephaly; if partial, lobar or semilobar holoprosencephaly results.

Predilection for sex: None.

Inheritance pattern: The frequency is approximately 1 in 15,000 live births but is much higher in spontaneously aborted embryos (65,66). There is a strong association with chromosomal anomalies or familial occurrence. The most severe defects tend to be associated with chromosomal disorders, with chromosome 13 the most frequently affected. Recurrence risk of sporadic, nonchromosomal, and nonsyndromic holoprosencephaly is approximately 6%. (65).

Associations: The most severe facial anomalies are associated with the most severe forms of holoprosencephaly, but up to 30% of severe cases do not have facial anomalies.

Facial anomalies in holoprosencephaly:

Nasal malformations
    Absence of nasal structure
    Single proboscis, sometimes above the eye
    Absence of nasal septum or bridge, partial or complete
    Flat nose
Ocular
    Orbital hypotelorism
    Single median eye
    Ocular hypotelorism
    Ocular hypertelorism (rare)
Oral
    Mid-line cleft lip and palate, absent philtrum
    Bilateral cleft lip and palate
    Single mid-line maxillary incisor

Anomalies found in other organ systems (in 75% of cases, especially when associated with chromosomal disorders) include those of the cardiac, skeletal, genitourinary, and gastrointestinal systems.

Neurologic findings in holoprosencephaly:

Apnea
Seizures
Stimulus-sensitive tonic spasms
Abnormalities of hypothalamic function (lack of temperature regulation, diabetes insipidus, inappropriate antidiuretic hormone secretion)
Failure of neurodevelopment
Positive transillumination due either to hydrocephalus or a large posterior cyst

Further evaluation: Family history and examination of parents is critical to look for the presence of familial mental retardation or associated physical findings, such as single central incisor, hypotelorism, mid-face hypoplasias or deficiencies including cleft lip, anosmia, microcephaly.

Expected course: The most severely affected infants die in the early neonatal period, but some milder cases without facial anomalies remain undetected until later in infancy when there is failure to develop normally.

Genetic associations in holoprosencephaly:

Chromosomal
    Chromosome 2, 3, 7, 13–15, 18, 21
        Ring
        Deletions
        Trisomies
    Triploidy: 69, XX

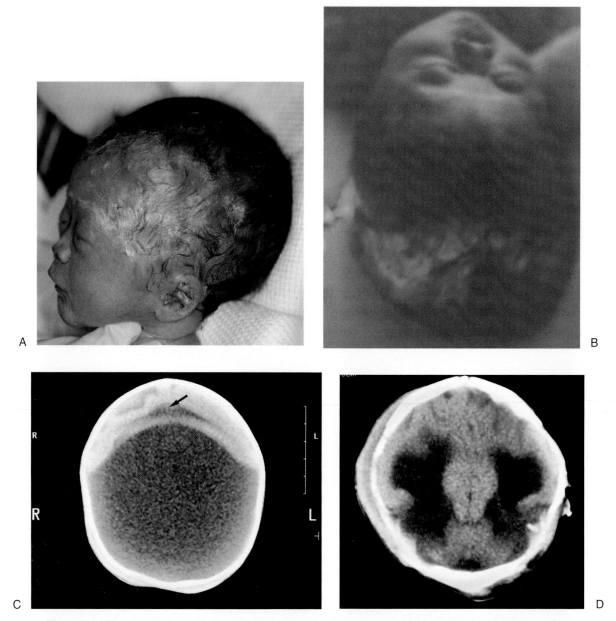

Figure 21. Macrocephaly and facies in infant with alobar holoprosencephaly. **A:** Marked flattening of the nose due to absence of nasal bridge and hypoplastic columella nasi and an increase in craniofacial disproportion. A transillumination light in normal room light shows a positive result seen as a red glow in the scalp behind the coronal suture. **B:** Positive transillumination in a lower ambient light shows a strong glow in the area of the large posterior cyst seen on CT scan (**C**). The lack of transillumination anteriorly correlates with the presence of the severely malformed underlying brain in the typical boomerang brain shape. The single ventricle is noted by the arrow. **D:** The mid-line fusion of the basal ganglion and thalami confirms the diagnosis suggested by the facies and transillumination.

Table 3. *Severe degrees of holoprosencephaly (arrhinencephaly)*

Type of facies	Facial features	Cranium and brain
Cyclopia	Single eye or partially divided eye in single orbit; arrhinia with proboscis	Microcephaly Alobar holoprosencephaly
Ethmocephaly	Extreme orbital hypotelorism but separate orbits; arrhinia with proboscis	Microcephaly alobar holoprosencephaly
Cebocephaly	Orbital hypotelorism, proboscis like nose with single nostril, but no media cleft of lip	Microcephaly; usually has alobar holoprosencephaly
With median cleft lip	Orbital hypotelorism, flat, hypoplastic nose; absence of median portion of upper lip	Microcephaly and sometimes trigonocephaly; usually has alobar holoprosencephaly
With medial philtrum–premaxilla anlage	Orbital hypotelorism, bilateral lateral cleft of lip with median process representing philtrum–premaxilla anlage	Microcephaly and sometimes trigonocephaly; semilobar or lobar holoprosencephaly

Modified from Hengerer, ref 69 with permission.

Familial
    Autosomal dominant (with variable penetrance)
    Autosomal recessive
    X-linked recessive
    With chromosomal disorder
Normal karyotype and family history
    Infant of diabetic mother

Dandy-Walker Malformation

See Fig. 22.

Description: Cystic dilation of the fourth ventricle, complete or partial agenesis of the cerebellar vermis, and hydrocephalus. There is enlargement of the posterior fossa with lifting of the tentorium that leads to a typical cranial appearance of occipital prominence. Hydrocephalus is only rarely pronounced at birth and may not develop for years.

Embryology: The foramen of Magendie either fails or delays to open, contributing to an impairment of CSF flow that persists even in the presence of normal foramina of Luschka. The most likely embryologic timing for this malformation is the second and third months of gestation, during which time neuronal migration overlaps.

Inheritance or recurrence patterns: Not established.

Associations: Approximately 70% have associated brain abnormalities (18):

Agenesis of the corpus collosum (20–30%)
Cerebral neuronal heterotopias (15%)
Cerebral gyral abnormalities (10%)
Aqueductal stenosis (5–10%)
Abnormalities of inferior olivary and/or dentate nuclei (20%)
Occipital encephalocele (10–15%)
Syringomyelia (5–10%)

The earlier in the fetal or the neonatal period the malformation manifests and is diagnosed, the more likely it is to be associated with other extraneural malformations (60–80%). These malformations include primarily cardiac and urinary tract defects. Approximately 20% to 30% of cases diagnosed postnatally have associated extraneural anomalies (18). There is an association of aggressive facial hemangiomas and Dandy-Walker malformation (78).

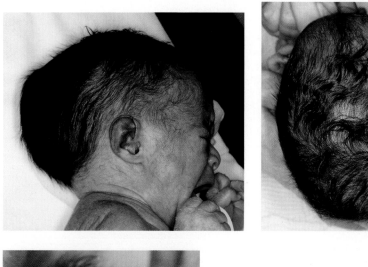

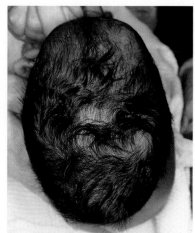

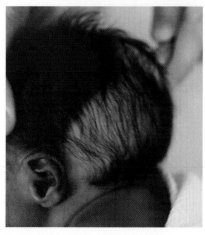

Figure 22. **A:** Occipital prominence due to a cyst in the posterior fossa. (Dandy-Walker cyst). Note the telangiectatic vessels around the ear that are harbingers of a large facial hemangioma, the development of which is reported as associated with Dandy-Walker brain malformations (78). **B:** The increase in the posterior cranial vault contents causes an occipital prominence with a widening of the lambdoid sutures. The elongated appearance of this view suggests scaphocephaly, but rather than the head width being narrowed as in true scaphocephaly, the head length is increased. **C:** Transillumination is positive in the posterior region corresponding to the cyst.

Differential diagnosis of posterior fossa collections of fluid and positive transillumination:

Dandy-Walker syndrome
Familial vermian agenesis
Trapped fourth ventricle
Enlarged cisterna magna
Arachnoidal cyst

Disorders of Primary Neurulation

See Tables 4 and 5.

Craniorrhachischisis totalis (Fig. 23)
Anencephaly (Fig. 24)
Myeloschisis
Encephalocele (Fig. 25)
Myelomeningocele, Arnold-Chiari malformation (Fig. 26)

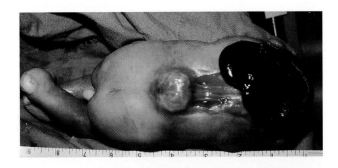

Figure 23. Craniorrhachischisis totalis. There is complete failure of primary neurulation, leaving an open skull with little brain formation and a spine with an unfolded spinal cord.

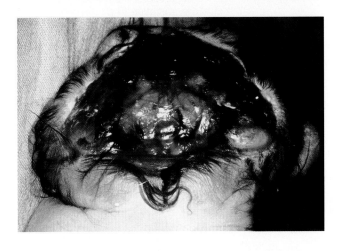

Figure 24. Anencephaly. There is complete failure of closure of the anterior neural tube without skull formation and a fully exposed, hemorrhagic mass of neural tissue with no definable structure. The orbital ridges are seen at their normal level but protruding above the top of the remnant anteriorly to give the characteristic froglike appearance. Infants with anencephaly possess brain stem function to varying degrees, including spontaneous respirations, but most die within 48 hours unless there is active intervention. The lack of a protective covering to the brain makes it susceptible to the environment and infection.

Table 4. *Disorders of primary neurulation in order of decreasing severity*

Disorder	Description	Associations
Craniorrhachischisis totalis (see Fig. 23)	Essentially complete failure results in no overlying bone or skin from the brain down the spine.	Onset is by 20–22 days after conception. Most cases abort early
Anencephaly (cranioschisis) (see Fig. 24)	The severely malformed brain tissue is a mass of fibrotic, degenerated neurons and glia with little definable structure. There is absence of the frontal bones above the supraciliary ridge, the parietal bones, and the squamous part of the occipital bone. There is usually a rudimentary brain stem present.	Anterior neuropore closure normally occurs by the 25th day of gestation (173) Up to 75% are stillborn More common in whites than in blacks, in females, and in mothers either older or younger than average. The incidence of live births with anencephaly is decreasing with better prenatal diagnosis with maternal alpha-fetoprotein and sonography screening and with prevention of folate deficiency.
Myeloschisis (rachischisis)	After failed closure of the posterior neural tube, the result is a flat, open spinal structure with no overlying vertebrae or skin.	Posterior neuropore closure normally occurs by the 26th day of gestation (173). There are often associated cranial defects.
Encephalocele (see Fig. 25)	Variable portions of the brain that herniate outside the cranial cavity most often in the occipital midline but also frontal or rarely the transsphenoidal temporal and parietal regions. This may represent abnormal anterior neural tube closure or it may reflect a primary mesodermal defect that developes after neurulation.	Most commonly posteriorly located, the occipital lobe is most frequently involved. The scalp is often intact with hair on the scalp. 50% associated with hydrocephalus 10–20% of the occipital lesions contain no neural elements (meningoceles).
Myelomeningocele, (spina bifida cystica, spina bifida occulta) (see Fig. 26)	The posterior neural tube fails to close completely. In the majority, the result is a protruding dorsal sac of neural tissue. The vertebral arches are absent with a widened spinal canal. The covering is most often a thin membrane but can be intact skin.	The time of formation is controversial but most likely develops at no later than 26 days of gestation (173). There is almost uniform association with Arnold-Chiari and high incidence of other brain malformations (174). Most myelomeningoceles are in the thoracolumbar, lumbar, and lumbosacral areas, with 90% of these developing hydrocephalus.

Table 5. *Major milestones in brain development*

Developmental event	Age
Neural plate	18 days PCA
Neural tube	22 days PCA
Anterior neuropore closure	24 days PCA
Posterior neuropore closure	28 days PCA
Caudal neural tube	28–32 days PCA
Diverticulation	5–6 wk PCA
Neuronal proliferation	2–4 mo PCA
Neuronal migration	3–5 mon PCA
Neuronal organization and maturation	Late gestation to infancy
Myelination	Late gestation to adolescence

PCA, postconceptual age.
Reprinted from Becker, ref. 51, with permission.

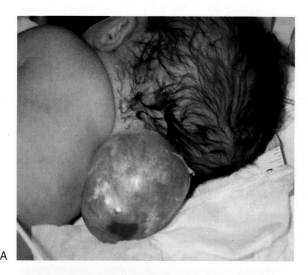

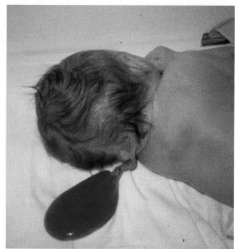

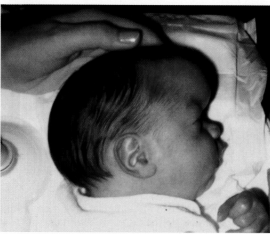

Figure 25. A: Occipital encephalocele. This sac contains extensive neural tissue in a typical central occipital nuchal location. The size generally correlates inversely with the prognosis. **B:** Occipital meningocele containing no neural elements. **C:** Anterior encephalocele. This location is uncommon in the United States, where 80% are occipital, but much more common in Southeast Asia (133).

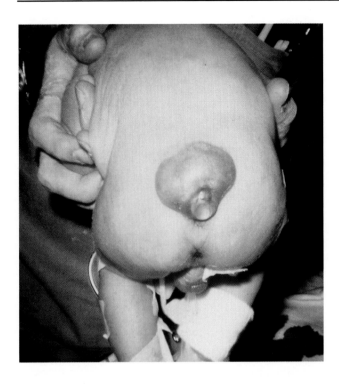

Figure 26. Spina bifida cystica (meningomyelocele). The appearance of a meningomyelocele can vary from a very small, completely covered mid-line mass to an open, large mass involving many levels of the spinal vertebral column. This mass is low and partially skin covered. Lesions at this low level may have encouragingly good neurologic function at birth but carry a high association with hydrocephalus.

HAIR

Evaluate the hair for quantity, length, continuity, texture, color, direction of growth, position and number of hair whorls, and the anterior and posterior hairlines.

Although hair color changes during childhood, at birth there should be racial concordance with the parents. For example, reddish or blond hair in an infant whose parents are dark may suggest some degree of albinism, but there can be wide variations with a familial tendency to darkening hair in adulthood. Similarly, the hair color should be fairly uniform, although many infants have a beautiful blend of light (vellus) and dark (terminal) hair that is uniformly distributed (Fig. 27A). Random patches of white hair are familial or sporadic and inconsequential (Fig. 27B), whereas white forelocks with other pigment defects in the eyes or skin are sometimes associated with deafness and retardation (79).

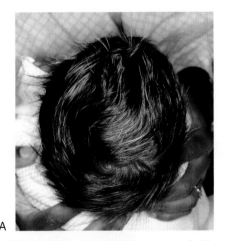
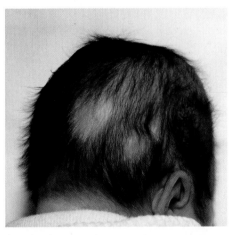

A   B

Figure 27. Variable pigmentation in hair. **A:** Natural temporary "frosting" in hair that represents a blend of vellus (light) and terminal (dark) hair. Note the typical (95%), single parietal hair whorl that is clockwise 80% of the time (80,81). **B:** Three occipital white patches. Congenital absence of hair pigment may be associated with abnormal pigmentation of the irides. Most often these areas of depigmentation are sporadic or autosomally transmitted and are isolated findings, but they may be part of other pigmentation syndromes (79,134–136).

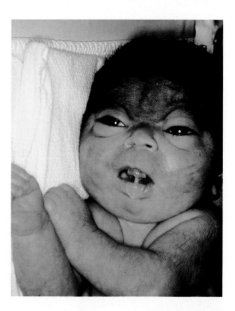

Figure 28. The position of the anterior hairline is variable, but there is normally a separation from the eyebrows. **A:** This SGA infant with Cornelia de Lange syndrome has diffuse hirsutism and cutis marmorata. Her typical facies include small nose with anteverted nostrils, proptosis and inner epicanthal folds, long eyelashes, thin lips with a mid-line beak and downward curve at the angles, micrognathia, and low-set ears. She has only mild micromelia and flexion contractures at the elbows.

The texture of hair at birth is relatively fine, with more immature infants having the finest hair. The straightness or curliness at birth does not always signal the adult tendency. Most of the conditions associated with abnormal textures or fragility are not apparent in the newborn period.

The anterior hairline varies. Normal but hirsute infants have pigmented hair well onto the forehead but without true blending with or across the eyebrows (synophrys) (Fig. 28). The posterior hair line has a more consistent limitation, so that hair roots below the neck creases, particularly at the lateral margins, suggest syndromes associated with short or webbed neck (Fig. 3C).

Neonatal hair initially appears quite disheveled, but its growth direction normally is consistent. There is usually only a single, off-center but variably positioned, parietal hair whorl, 80% of which grows in a clockwise pattern (80) (Fig. 29). Black infants with short, curly hair tend not to have any hair whorl (90%) (80). The location of the whorl does not correlate with handedness (80).

Smith et al. suggested that the pattern of hair development correlated with underlying brain development. Abnormally placed or more than two hair whorls and unruly hair could be external indicators of abnormal underlying brain (81). Hair is considered to be unruly if it stands up over the top of the head from the area of the posterior parietal whorl toward the frontal hairline despite attempts at grooming. When found in the presence of unusual facies, microcephaly, turricephaly, or small size for gestational age, there may be poor brain growth of early fetal onset, as is typical of a number of genetic syndromes, including Cornelia de Lange and Down's syndromes (81). Many normal newborn infants have hair re-

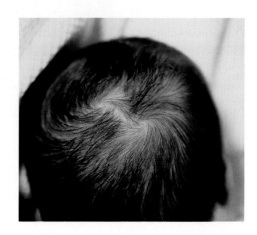

Figure 29. Double hair whorl found normally in parietal region in 5% of the population (80). More than two whorls or abnormal positioning of the whorls may indicate aberrant brain development (81).

Table 6. *Development of hair*

Week of gestation	Developmental event
8	Hair follicle begins as a cylindric down budding of the epidermis
9	Hair follicles appear on face in region of eyebrows, upper lip, and chin
10	Follicles uniformly form over scalp
11	Follicles sharply angulate to epidermis
17	Hair shafts emerge on brow
18–20	Anagen hair shafts are visible over entire scalp Development of follicles spreads in cephalocaudal direction Formation of lanugo hair
24	Beginning development of vellus hair to continue throughout life
26–28	Scalp hair roots change to catagen and then telogen in progressive wave from frontal to parietal regions over 7–10 days
28–32	Primary lanugo is shed; second, short lanugo develops
Perinatal period	Second lanugo is shed followed by growth of vellus hair
3–7 mo after birth	Intermediate scalp hair develops rapidly but is lost by 2 yr

sistant to grooming for several weeks to months after birth until more fully medullated hair develops, so describing hair as abnormally unruly should be reserved until after the newborn period.

During fetal and early neonatal life, adjacent hair follicles are essentially synchronized in the stages of the growth cycle so that waves of growth and loss occur (Table 6). This is in contrast to the postneonatal mosaic patterning in which growth and loss are more random over the scalp hair. At birth there are two consecutive waves of hair growing from the forehead to the nape of the neck. The newer wave is only anagen hair, whereas the older wave is converting to a telogen stage and, therefore, will be shed first. The frontal region is maximally telogen phase with a predominance of anagen hairs in the occipital region. The hairs in the occipital region do not enter telogen until after birth and so they fall out at about 8 to 12 weeks, commonly causing a localized alopecia, mistakenly attributed to the infant's rubbing of only that area. A similar localization of telogen hairs over the parietal regions also may cause alopecia there. The loss of primary hair proceeds caudally from the vertex so that the last hair is lost at the nape of the neck. Infants with darker complexions have a slower rate of transition to the telogen phase and, therefore, tend to have more abundant hair at birth (82) (Fig. 30). In any individual infant the length of the hair is fairly uniform over the scalp, but among infants it varies significantly. Any longer tufts may indicate an underlying nevus.

Alopecia, or absence of hair from its normal location, is not at all unusual in neonates because of the synchronized waves of hair growth as compared with more diffuse and unsynchronized patterns in older children, but there are a number of conditions that accentuate the process. Graduates of intensive care nurseries may have lost their hair to a razor blade, but other causes should be considered in infants who have been ill.

Conditions associated with neonatal alopecia:

Congenital-localized:
    Cutis aplasia congenita
    Focal dermal hypoplasia
    Nevus sebaceous
    Epidermal nevi
    Incontinentia pigmenti
Congenital-diffuse:
    Hidrotic and anhidrotic ectodermal dysplasia
    Hereditary hypotrichosis
    Cartilage hair hypoplasia
    Monilethrix (Beaded hair)
    Menkes kinky hair syndrome
    Pili torti (twisted hair)

Bamboo hair (Netherton's disease)
Ichthyosis
Acquired-localized:
    Scars after infection
    Scars after trauma
    Infection: ring worm
    Trauma
    Neonatal anagen delay
Acquired-diffuse:
    Alopecia totalis and universalis
    Nutritional deficiency
    Metabolic deficiency
    Endocrine: hypo- or hyperthyroidism

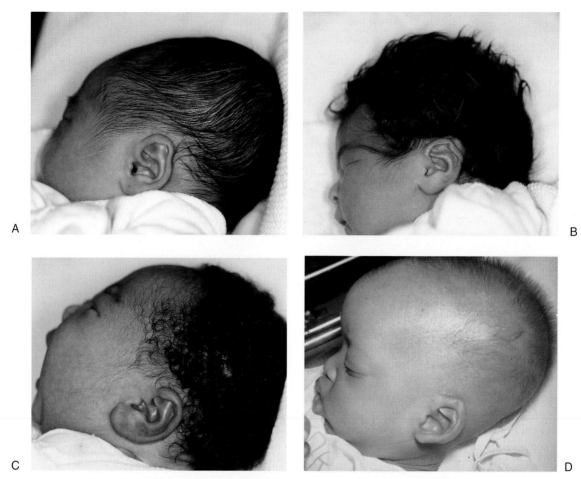

Figure 30. Variations in quantity of scalp hair. The density of hair follicles is highest at birth, but because the phase of hair growth may be primarily telogen frontally and a mixture of telogen and anagen posteriorly, the appearance is that of thinner hair anteriorly and more hair posteriorly. **A:** Moderate quantity of hair in Asian newborn infant, more pronounced occipitally, showing the frontal to occipital wave of hair density. **B:** Thick, luxuriant, softly curled hair in black newborn infant. The progression of hair growth from anagen to telogen is somewhat delayed in infants with dark complexion, so they appear to have more abundant hair at birth (137). **C:** Abundant, tightly curled hair posteriorly with thinner hair anteriorly. **D:** Sparse hair of ectodermal dysplasia (X-linked or autosomal recessive). The hair is hypochromic and uniformly sparse. Note the typical facies of low nasal bridge, small nose, full forehead, and prominent lips. There is a fine papular rash over the scalp and face. The inability to sweat normally would lead to hyperthermia.

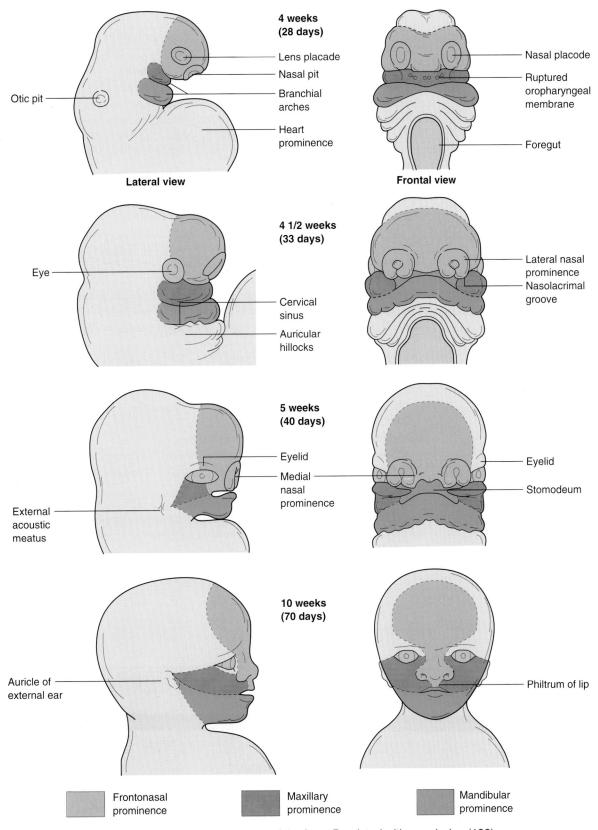

4 weeks (28 days)

Lens placade — Nasal pit — Branchial arches — Heart prominence

Otic pit —

Lateral view

Nasal placode — Ruptured oropharyngeal membrane — Foregut

Frontal view

4 1/2 weeks (33 days)

Eye —

Cervical sinus — Auricular hillocks

Lateral nasal prominence — Nasolacrimal groove

5 weeks (40 days)

Eyelid — Medial nasal prominence

External acoustic meatus —

Eyelid — Stomodeum

10 weeks (70 days)

Auricle of external ear —

Philtrum of lip

Frontonasal prominence   Maxillary prominence   Mandibular prominence

Figure 31. Embryologic development of the face. Reprinted with permission (138).

FACIES

The embryologic development of the face is diagrammed in Fig. 31.

Examine the face by looking at it from a directly frontal view, in profile, and in a tangential plane from the top of the head (Fig. 31). Assess the overall appearance by looking for symmetry, size, shape, and relationships of all the individual components of the face, how they relate to each other, and how the infant holds or uses them. Look for evidence of anxiety, pain, irritability, or fretfulness, stereotypic activity such as repetitive sucking activity, particularly at an inappropriate age or condition, and jitteriness of the jaw (Fig. 32). Be sure to observe the facial tone and strength with the infant at rest and crying or yawning (Fig. 33).

An unusual appearance dictates analyzing the individual components of the facies to decide if the constellation represents malformation, deformation, a syndrome, or merely a normal familial appearance. It is an untrained eye that perceives all babies to look alike but newborn infants do have many facial characteristics that are more similar to each other than they are to an adult. Their features are not as sculpted or as sharply defined, but, nonetheless, they demonstrate sexual, familial, and racial similarities, as well as differences. The infant's face becomes more expressive during the neonatal period, with the commonly recognized milestone of a social smile occurring toward the end of that period for term infants. Premature infants will be slower to use their facial muscles in a directed communication but will demonstrate some of the emotional extremes and conditions of illness well before 40 weeks' corrected gestational age. The degree of facial expressiveness is relatively narrow compared with that of an older infant, but the neonate can still demonstrate discomfort or pain, anger, irritability, hunger, anxiety, apathy, somnolence, or weakness and can communicate a sense of illness or health. Being able to understand the language communicated by the newborn's face helps one to interpret many of the accompanying physical signs.

The competent examiner is able to describe what it is about a face that makes it unusual or abnormal, particularly when the findings are more subtle. It is easy to say a face looks abnormal or strange, but that alone is not a meaningful description. Specific measurements of individual features may improve the description. A photograph provides the best means of documenting and communicating to others.

The first step in interpreting the facial structure is understanding the relationship of the individual parts to the whole and how that relationship changes with time. When one describes facial features as being immature, it generally means that the features are underdeveloped in size or in definition. They are not as sharply chiseled but are softer and more rounded as well as smaller. This impression is correct for some but not all of the facial features: the eyes are relatively large, whereas the nose is small. The mid-face from the max-

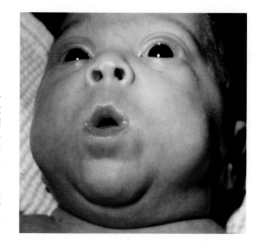

Figure 32. Whistling micturition reflex. Identical female twins made a consistent facial expression of lip pursing before urination. The movements were first observed in the intensive care nursery at 29 weeks' gestational age and thought to be possible seizure activity until the parents reported identical behavior in their three older girls for the first 4 months of life. The size of the mouth and facial expressions were normal, except as a warning of micturition. A similar reflex has not been previously reported, although infants frequently cry, fuss, and become restless as they are trying to urinate. This pattern was not a learned response but was observed to be consistent from birth until 4 to 5 months in all five siblings. This does not represent the whistling face syndrome of craniocarpotarsal dysplasia (139).

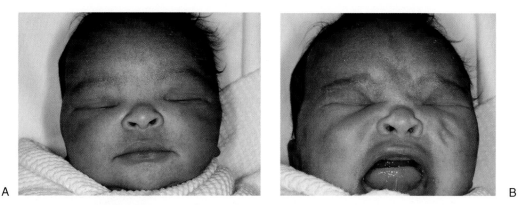

Figure 33. Accentuation of facial features with crying. **A:** Infant at rest with apparently normal facial structure. **B:** Crying brings out the presence of unusual dimples, indicating abnormal tethering of the skin.

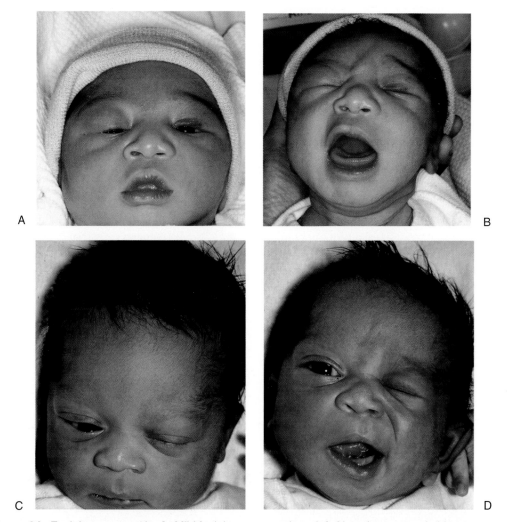

Figure 34. Facial nerve paresis. **A:** Mild facial nerve paresis on left. Note the unremarkable appearance at rest (**A**) that becomes evident with crying (**B**). The infant is unable to close the left eye tightly, but the apparent difference in size of the palpebral opening is compounded by significant edema of the right eyelids. Both sides of the mouth depress to roughly the same degree, but there is absence of a nasolabial fold on the left, and the right side of the mouth lifts further. This weakness resolved within 24 hours. **C:** More severe facial nerve paresis on right. The infant is unable to close the right eye at rest (**C**). On crying (**D**), the asymmetry becomes more evident in its effect on eye closure, flattening of the nasolabial fold, and inability to move the lips. An expected finding would be drooling of a feed from the right side with difficulty in effecting a seal around the nipple.

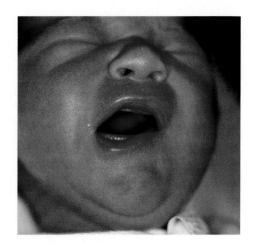

Figure 35. Absence of left depressor anguli oris (asymmetrical crying facies). Note the tight closure of both eyes and the well-defined nasolabial folds. The corner of the mouth fails to move downward and outward with crying or grimace. It is the nondepressed side that is abnormal. All other actions of lips and perioral region will be normal. As an isolated finding there is a familial recurrence and a poorly defined relationship to cardiac septal defects (140–147).

illa down has the proportionately greatest amount of growing to do before the adult facial proportions are reached (Fig. 2).

Examine the facial skin as suggested in Chapter 5. If there are forceps marks apparent, determine if the surface is intact and palpate for induration. Note the location of the forceps marks, particularly in regards to underlying structures, the eyes, or the expected course of the facial nerve. Look for equality in the buccal skin folds and the shape of the opened mouth (Figs. 34 and 35).

Immediately after a delivery in which forceps were applied, there may be few or no marks apparent. In a few hours, erythema and blistering and induration may develop. These findings should subside within 24 to 48 hours (Fig. 36). If there has been enough compression of the subcutaneous fat, the tissue may hydrolyze or harden (subcutaneous fat necrosis) and take weeks to resolve fully. No intervention is indicated, but because of the location, the areas that appear as firm masses may be mistaken for septic abscesses or lymph nodes.

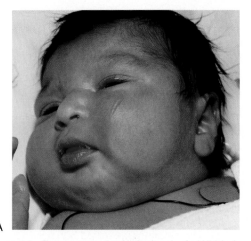

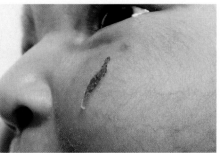

A   B

Figure 36. Forceps mark of left cheek. **A:** Within hours after birth, the early lesion shows outline of forceps edge with erythema, induration, and a superficial blister. **B:** After 24 hours, the other changes have subsided, with only a crusted blister to resolve completely.

NOSE

Development of the Nose

See Fig. 31. The major events in the development of the nose from gestation to puberty are summarized in Table 7.

External Landmarks of the Nose

See Fig. 37.
Steps in Examining the Nose:

Assess the nose and nasal cavities for:
size and shape
masses or clefts
secretions
patency, air flow, and flaring
Assess size and shape by evaluating the components individually and as the nose relates to the rest of the facial structures:
Nasofrontal angle: normal, flat, deep
Nasal root protrusion: average, high, low
Nasal bridge: high, low, broad, beaked, or bulbous
Nasal tip: normal, flat, bifid
Shape of each nasal ala: normal, slightly flat, markedly flat, angles slightly or markedly
Nasal ala configuration: cleft, hypoplastic, hypotrophic, presence of coloboma
Size of the nostrils: symmetric or asymmetric

The width of the alae nasi should be greater than the base of the nose. The distance from the bottom of the alae nasi to the arch of the orbit normally closely approximates the length of the ear. The overall development of the bridge of the nose, best viewed in profile, correlates with gestational age and serves as an indicator of mid-face development. Its undergrowth, taking into consideration racial variances, indicates a possibility of central nervous system or basal skull undergrowth. Iatrogenic causes of nasal undergrowth include extended use of nasal prongs for continuous positive airway pressure. (83) (Fig. 38). Pressure necrosis from nasal prongs can result in loss of the nasal tip or collapse of the columella of the septum. Prolonged nasotracheal intubation is associated with local necrosis of the nasal ala or septum, vestibular stenosis, and mid-face hypoplasia (84–88).

Inspect for visible deformities such as skin lesions, fistulae, swellings, and deviations. Determine the patency first by looking for apparent obstruction from an intrinsic or extrinsic factor such as swollen mucosa, a mass, or secretions. Elevate the tip of the nose to inspect the vestibule and septum. Evaluate air flow by holding a thin cotton thread in front of each nostril and watch for bending of the fiber with inhalation and exhalation. Compare the degree of deflection between both nostrils. As an alternative, hold a cool mirror beneath the nostrils and observe the formation of two areas of fogging. Auscult over both nostrils if there is poor air flow or any extrapulmonary sound. If no air flow is demonstrated, pass a small suction or feeding catheter through the posterior choanae.

Fetal compression sufficient to cause some degree of nasal deformation is a frequent physical finding on early newborn examinations and normally resolves in much the same time as does other forms of molding (Figs. 39). In some instances, intrauterine forces or pressure applied during delivery cause a true septal dislocation (Figs. 40). The occurrence of such septal deviations ranges from less than 1% to 4% (89,90). The otolaryngology literature suggests that true septal dislocations should be relocated within a few days after they occur for best outcome because they are not likely to relocate spontaneously (91). One needs to distinguish between a deviation of the nasal septum that represents a dislocation and the far more common simple deformations that require no intervention (90). Compres-

Table 7. *Development of the nasal structures in the fetus and child*

Time of event	Development
Fetal period	
3 wk	Olfactory placodes appear in frontonasal process.
4 wk	Olfactory placodes become nasal pits.
5 wk	Nasal pits deepen into clefts separated by primitive septum (frontonasal process). Vomeronasal organ appears.
6 wk	Oronasal membranes rupture, forming primitive choanae. Primitive palate forms by fusion of maxillary process with medial and lateral nasal processes. Upper lip forms by fusion of medial nasal and lateral nasal maxillary processes. Nasooptic furrow disappears in forming lacrimal apparatus. Maxillary and ethmoidal folds appear to start formation of turbinates.
7 wk	Definitive septum begins growth. Second ethmoidal fold appears.
8 wk	Olfactory nerve bundles appear. Palatine processes fuse in mid-line anteriorly. Uncinate process and ethmoidal infundibulum appear.
3 mo	Palate fusion completed. Maxillary sinus outpouching appears. Cartilaginous nasal capsule forms from mesenchymal condensation. Nasal glands appear.
4 mo	Ethmoidal sinus and sphenoidal sinus outpouchings appear. Bulla ethmoidalis becomes well defined.
5 mo	Vomeronasal organ begins degeneration.
6 mo	Cartilaginous nasal capsule divides into alar, lateral, and septal cartilages. Maxillary ossification begins.
7 mo	Maximal development of ethmoidal turbinates occurs with initiation of coalescence.
Term	Frontal sinus furrows appear. Only two to three ethmoidal turbinates remain. Craniofacial ratio is 8:1
Infancy and childhood periods	
6 mo	Nares double their birth dimensions.
1 yr	Maxillary sinus reaches infraorbital nerve.
2 yr	Frontal sinuses reach frontal bone. Ethmoidal sinuses approximate each other and lamina papyracea.
3 yr	Nasal growth spurt occurs. Ossified union occurs between perpendicular plate of ethmoid, lamina papyracea, cribriform plate, and vomer.
4 yr	Sphenoidal sinus begins invasion of sphenoid bone.
5 yr	Craniofacial ratio is 4:1.
6 yr	Frontal sinuses are visible on radiographs in frontal bone. Sphenoidal sinus is pneumatized to vidian canal. Nasal growth spurt occurs.
7 yr	Nose doubles its birth length. Maxillary sinus begins inferiorly directed growth. Ethmoidal sinuses extend beyond boundaries of ethmoids.
8 yr	Maxillary sinus approximates inferior nasal meatus. Frontal sinus reaches level of orbital roof in 50% of children.
9 yr	Maxillary sinus pneumatizes zygomatic process.
12 yr	Floor of maxillary sinus is level with floor of nose.
Puberty	Accelerated nasal and maxillary growth occurs. Nose triples its birth length. Adulthood craniofacial ratio is 2:1.

Reprinted from Fairbanks, ref. 175, with permission.

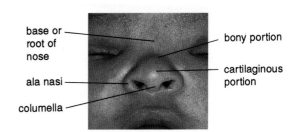

Figure 37. Landmarks of nasal anatomy.

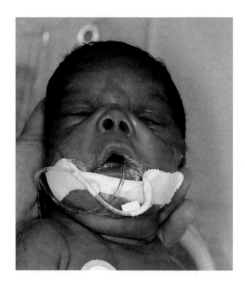

Figure 38. Nasal compression after nasal CPAP. Prolonged pressure applied against the nasal septum can cause necrosis and loss of tissue or hypoplasia of the cartilaginous structure. In this infant the extra fold of fatty tissue over the nasal bridge signals the prolonged compression, which can be expected to resolve over the next several months.

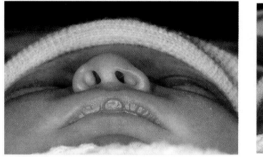
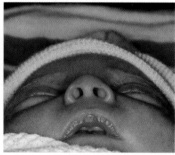

Figure 39. Nasal compression without septal deviation. **A:** Shortly after birth the nose is asymmetrical from simple compression with an angled septum at rest. **B:** The septum assumes its normal angle. Note the sucking pad on the upper lip.

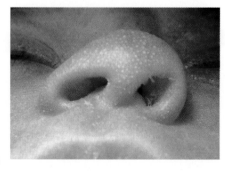
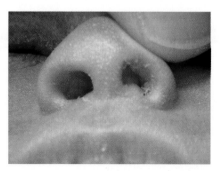

Figure 40. **A:** At rest it is difficult to distinguish a true deviation. **B:** Attempts to restore normal anatomy are unsuccessful as the septum remains deviated at the base.

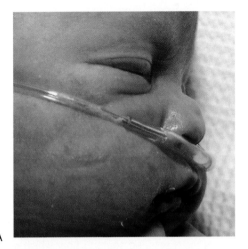
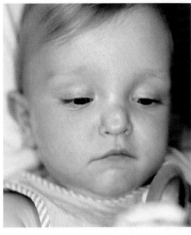

A   B

Figure 41. Congenital nasal mass. **A:** The small, firm, mid-line mass was present at birth after 26 weeks' gestation. There was no sinus tract or tuft of hair associated. The mass did not transilluminate or, upon compression, increase the pressure in the anterior fontanel. Crying or change in position did not affect the mass. The differential diagnosis includes a dermoid, nasal encephalocele, and nasal glioma (see Table 8). **B:** The mass grew at the same size as the rest of the nasal features, but there was loss of some of the columellar size. The diagnosis at this time is mild frontonasal dysplasia with a normal MRI of the internal cranium.

sion of the tip of the nose will further move a dislocated septum off the mid-line, whereas simple deformation will curve into the chamber but not move at the base.

Malformations of the nose are rare but are rarely isolated developments, often indicating more severe combinations of malformations (69,92,93) (Figs. 41 and 42, Table 8). In contrast, deformations of the nose are quite common in the newborn period.

It is rarely necessary to assess patency using a catheter, although this step is often part of the first examination in the delivery room. A finding of air flow confirms patency but not passage size and therefore does not rule out stenosis. Careful auscultation over each nostril with the bell of a stethoscope may show a variance in pitch between the two sides, with the

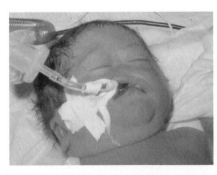
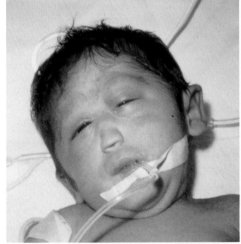

A   B

Figure 42. Holoprosencephaly with various nasal configurations. The severity of the nasal malformation correlates directly with the severity of the cerebral malformation. **A:** Arhinia with mid-line cleft. The bony nasal structures are completely absent. Hypotelorism is evident. **B:** Single nostril.

stenotic side having a higher pitch or more whistling character. A 5-French catheter should pass through both posterior choanae (94). It is important to direct such a lubricated feeding tube or catheter caudally after entering the naris in order to obtain the correct direction. Causes of nasal obstruction seen in the neonatal period are listed in Table 9.

Infants are not obligate nasal breathers but are strongly preferential for the first 4 to 6 months (95,96). If obstructed, term infants can learn to breathe through the mouth within a few days after birth, but preterm infants take longer. The nasal preference is based in large part on the anatomic factors that create a partially obstructed oral airway, principally close apposition of the relatively large tongue to the palate. Head position and mild accumulation of secretions easily affects the air flow simply because it takes less to obstruct a narrow airway that already has high resistance (97,98). In a small study using a technique of acoustic reflections, the size of the nasal cavity related weakly to birth weight and length but did not correlate with sex, race, other physical measurements, or duration of gestation (99). The area of the nasal cavity in neonates increases some 600% in area during normal facial growth to reach adult proportions (99).

Nasal flaring is a relatively frequent finding in infants seeking to decrease airway resistance and improve their airway stability, particularly in premature infants. The use of alae nasi activation in otherwise healthy premature infants varies with the activity and sleep states so by itself cannot be used as a sign of respiratory distress (100).

The nasal mucosa should be pink and slightly moist, without pallor, cyanosis, or other discoloration. Normal secretions are thin, clear, and very scanty in the newborn period unless there is unusual irritation or infection in the area. Many infants have markedly swollen mucosa in the first few days and congested nasal breathing that responds to saline drops or increased ambient humidity. Combined with the presence of sneezing as a reflex reaction to dried mucus or amniotic debris, the findings of stuffy breathing wrongly suggest a cold to their parents. Sneezing may occur as a reflex response to a bright light or during drug withdrawal (101,102). The occurrence of isolated episodes of sneezing is frequent enough in normal neonates, particularly when ambient humidity is low, that one should be cautious in associating sneezing with drug withdrawal in the absence of other signs.

Table 8. *Differential diagnosis of congenital midline nasal masses*

Variant	Encephalocele	Glioma	Dermoid
Cell origin	Neurogenic origin with glial tissue	Neurogenic origin with glial tissue	Only ectodermal and mesoderma elements
Relationship to subarachnoid space	Has CSF connection to subarachnoid space	No CSF connection to subarachnoid space	None
Age	Infants, children	Infants, children	Usually children
Gender predilection	None	M:F = 3:1	M:F = slightly higher
Associated abnormalities	30–40%		
Location of mass	Intranasal and extranasal	Intranasal (30%); extranasal (60%); combination (10%)	Intranasal and extranasal
Appearance	Soft, bluish, compressible	Reddish-blue, smooth, firm noncompressible	Solid, dimple with hair follicle. Pit may be located anywhere between the glabella and columella of the nose.
Pulsation	Yes	No	No
Transillumination	Yes	No	No
CSF leak	Yes	Rarely	Rarely
Furstenburg test	Positive	Negative	Negative
Cranial defect	Yes	Rarely	Rarely
Previous history	Meningitis	Rarely meningitis	Local infection

Furstenburg test: expansion of the mass with compression of the jugular veins indicating communication with the subarachnoid space.

Reprinted from Hengerer, ref. 69.

Table 9. *Causes of nasal obstruction in the neonatal period*

Time of presentation	Neonatal presentation
Congenital	Choanal atresia (176–179)
	Choanal stenosis (180, 181)
	Anterior nasal stenosis (pyriform aperture stenosis) (182)
	Congenital midline mass (183)
	Glioma
	Meningoencephalocele
	Dermoid
	Hemangioma
	Nasal malformation (69, 71, 92)
	Castillo (178)
	Total nasal agenesis (68)
	Proboscis lateralis
	Mandibulofacial dysostoses (93)
	Treacher-Collins syndrome
	Crouzon disease
	Coronal craniosynostosis (93)
	Cleft palate (93)
	Congenital cyst of nasal cavity
	Dermoid
	Nasoalveolar
	Dentiginous
	Mucous cysts of floor of nose
	Nasolacrimal mucocele (184–191)
	Pharyngeal bursa (Tornwald)
Inflammatory	Upper respiratory tract infection
	Allergic rhinitis
	Congenital syphilis
	Chlamydia infection
	Adenoid hypertrophy
	Nasopharyngeal or gastroesophageal reflux
Iatrogenic	Nasotracheal tube trauma (85)
	Nasal CPAP trauma (83)
	Rhinitis medicamentosa (maternal or neonatal)
	Fetal alcohol syndrome (192)
Metabolic	Hypothyroidism (193)
Trauma	Intrauterine pressure (89, 90)
	Birth injury
Neoplastic	Hemangioma
	Hemangiolymphoma
	Lymphoma
	Rhabdomyosarcoma
	Hamartomas (194)
	Craniopharyngioma (194)
	Chordomas (194)
	Teratoid tumors (163)
	Epignathus (161, 162, 195)

MOUTH

The embryology of the mouth is depicted in Fig. 31. The landmarks in anatomy of the mouth are depicted in Fig. 43.

Technique of Examination

Steps in examining the mouth:

Inspect the mouth, perioral region and oral pharynx for:
   size, shape, color, and continuity of philtrum, lips, gums, palate, buccal mucosa, tongue, and tonsils
   presence of anomalous structures or masses

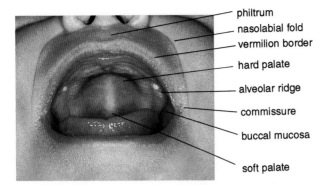

philtrum
nasolabial fold
vermilion border
hard palate
alveolar ridge
commissure
buccal mucosa
soft palate

Figure 43. Landmarks of the mouth.

Determine response and intensity of rooting reflex, the sequencing of suck, propulsion and
swallowing, and the gag reflex

*Observe the mouth and perioral region with the infant both at rest and in crying. As-
sess for size and shape of all the components, individually, and as they relate to the entire mouth and face as a whole (Fig. 44). When the infant cries or yawns, observe the position and symmetry of the structures, particularly the lower lip, the angle of the
mandible relative to the maxilla, and the tongue. Because crying or yawning is the
neonatal equivalent to an older, cooperative patient saying "ah," observe the elevation of
the soft palate (cranial nerves IX and X) when the opportunity presents itself.*

*Judge the shape, size, and thickness of the lips in their entirety, including the philtrum.
Assess for resting position, which is normally comfortably closed.*

The lateral margins of the lips at rest generally align with the nasal margin of the iris (Fig.
45). The lips should be uniform with a close approximation in size to each other. A central
swelling with a callus, more often on the upper lip, indicates a sucking pad. Shallow com-
missural lip pits occur in up to 3% of infants (Fig. 46) (103), but when found away from
the commissure they may represent a sinus tract or a subepithelial cleft (104,105). Sinus
tracts of the lower lip are rare but when associated with cleft lip or palate suggest most commonly one of four syndromes: the Van der Woude syndrome, popliteal pterygium syndrome, orofacial digital syndrome, or the ankyloblepharon filiform adnatum syndrome
(106).

The normal width or thickness of the lips is highly related to race and family but especially thick lips are unusual in the early newborn period. Swellings, in the absence of birth
injury, are abnormal and might indicate masses such as vascular malformations, cysts, or
congenital double lip (107). An upper lip that is particularly thin, especially when associated with a flat philtrum, suggests fetal alcohol syndrome but is seen in other conditions as
well, including submucous clefts or defects of the orbicularis oris muscle (105).

The intrauterine position may cause a deformation of the lower jaw by pushing toward
one side as the head is flexed against the chest. The deformation leads to an unequal angle
in the jaws as they open and occasionally makes feeding on one side more difficult than on

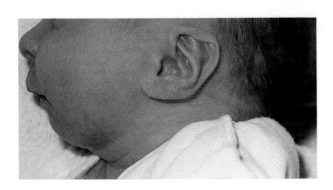

Figure 44. Retrognathia with a low-set ear. The lower lip re-
cedes well behind the upper lip. The jaw is clearly disproportionately small and behind a plane determined by the forehead
and cheeks. A line connecting the two medial canthi and extended posteriorly lies well above the ear, signaling its low set.
The ear is also posteriorly rotated with its vertical axis more than
20° off the axis of the coronal suture.

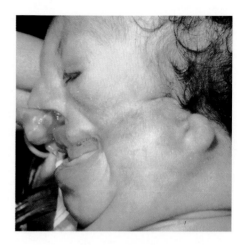

Figure 45. Oral clefting in a defect of formation of the first and second branchial arch structures (facio-auriculo-vertebral spectrum). Besides the major clefting of the upper lip, there is also a lateral cleft in the lips. The lateral margins of the lips are far too wide, and there is discontinuity in the vermilion border. The maxilla is markedly hypoplastic on the left side only, as is the ear, with only regions of the third arch having developed. When epibulbar dermoid or upper lid colobomas and vertebral anomalies are present, the eponym Goldenhar's syndrome is applied (148). Each of these conditions may just represent a continuum and degree of defect in the first and second arch structures. Compare the affected areas to the maxillary prominence of fetal development in Fig. 30.

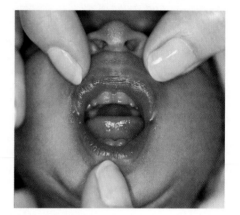

Figure 46. Lateral lip pits are not unusual in infants of color, but they are shallow and not associated with sinuses. The alveolar ridges are extraordinarily well demarcated but normal in this infant.

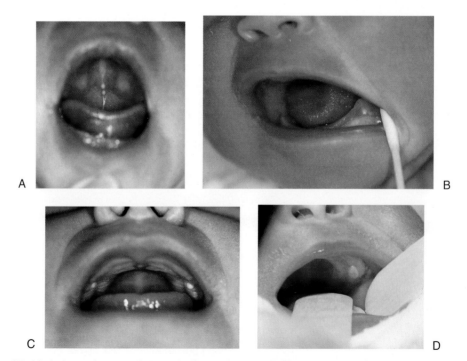

Figure 47. Variations of mucosal cysts. **A:** Epstein's pearl. **B:** Bohn's nodule. **C:** Gingival cysts. **D:** Alveolar cysts.

the other. Instead of opening in parallel, the jaws open at an angle. The infant's unimpeded position at rest will demonstrate the compression by the chest wall and shoulder. When the deformation forces in utero have been applied long enough, there is often an associated depression under the ear where the shoulder was pressed against the bony structures.

Absence of the depressor anguli oris muscle presents with unequal opening of the mouth, mimicking the appearance of muscle weakness due to facial nerve paralysis except that the nasolabial folds will be normal. The lip feels thinner when the muscle is missing. Unlike weakness due to facial nerve palsy, there is no difficulty with sucking due to absence of this muscle (Fig. 35).

Estimate the state of hydration from the quantity and quality of the secretions and dryness of the lip and tongue surfaces. Look for excessive bubbling or drooling of secretions. In premature infants at birth, if bubbles form at the lips, estimate their stability by observing how big they become and how long they last before popping. Sense and characterize any odor from the mouth.

The oral secretions should be thin and clear. In the first hours after birth, the presence in the oral secretions of only very small bubbles that do not last more than a second or two may indicate unstable or insufficient pulmonary surfactant. There has not been any clinical study to make this a truly scientific observation, but the observation of long-lasting bubbles is somewhat reassuring that the infant has the capability at that time to produce and secrete normal surfactant.

Drooling of secretions (sialorrhea) is often noted in neonates as excessive secretions or bubbling. Drooling in a supine infant suggests an overflow of secretions that are not handled by swallowing: the differential diagnosis includes an overproduction, an inability to swallow, or a pharyngeal or esophageal obstruction, notably esophageal atresia. The same differential applies in an upright infant with a further consideration of low oral tone and muscle weakness from facial nerve paresis. Infants with low oral tone or strength notably have the inability to effect a tight seal around a nipple and drool during their feedings. The causes of overproduction of saliva in neonates include most commonly a foreign body (feeding tube, nasal or endotracheal tube) or infection. Unlikely causes in neonates would be Wilson's disease, familial dysautonomia, epiglottitis (108), or pseudodiverticulum (109).

Unless the infant has just had a formula feeding, the presence of any discernible mouth odor is so unusual that it should be taken as an indicator of either a metabolic disorder, gastroesophageal reflux, or oropharyngeal infection.

Look at the alveolar ridges for the presence of alveolar cysts or lymphangiomas (laterally), dental eruptions (anteriorly), Bohn's nodules or other masses (Figs. 47–50).

Bohn's nodules are equivalent to milia on the skin and Epstein's pearls on the palate (Fig. 47). They are epithelial inclusion cysts that develop on the buccal or alveolar surface of the gums and appear as firm, white, irregularly shaped papules in isolation or small groups. Cysts that appear on the alveolar ridge are the same type of epithelial inclusions as Bohn's nodules or Epstein's pearls, in which case they are flat and white (110). Alveolar lymphangiomas are more elevated masses sometimes large enough to interfere with comfortable sucking. They appear as isolated, bluish, firm cysts of 3 to 10 mm on the alveolar ridge. The reported incidence in blacks is less than 4% and even less in white infants at birth (111). Although there may be more than one present, there is never more than one in each of the four lateral quadrants. These cysts slowly regress or become more fibrous; they contain no dental material (111).

Dental eruptions appear in the region of the central incisors, most commonly bilaterally on the mandible (Figs. 48 and 49). If the tooth has not erupted at the time of birth, a dental cyst contains a palpable tooth. The tooth is a normal primary incisor that erupts prematurely either before birth (natal tooth) or within the first weeks of life (neonatal tooth). Natal or neonatal teeth that are loose or cause trauma in feeding should be removed. Most teeth appearing in the neonatal period require extraction (112,113).

Look for the presence of any frenulum between the lips and the gums (labial frenulum) or under the tongue (lingual frenulum).

The presence of a labial frenulum in the mid-line is normal, but multiple or hypertrophied frenulae are not and suggest the presence of a multisystem syndrome, particularly in-

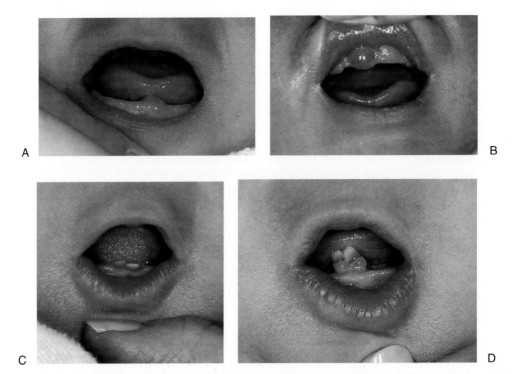

Figure 48. Dental cysts. **A and B:** Typical sites for dental cysts involving the central incisors at different stages of development. **C:** Natal teeth. **D:** Natal teeth on pedicles demonstrating poor dentin formation and loose connections, making dislodging and aspiration more likely.

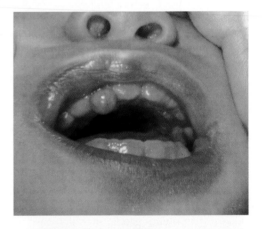

Figure 49. This cystic structure is not in the central incisor location that is typical of simple dental cysts, so the differential diagnosis widens to include alveolar lymphangioma, alveolar cyst, and epulis. Epulis is a benign granular cell tumor arising from the alveolar ridge, most often in the area of the maxillary incisors and more often in females (149–156). When large enough to interfere with feeding or to protrude from the mouth, removal is indicated (157,158). Spontaneous regression over the first year does occur (159).

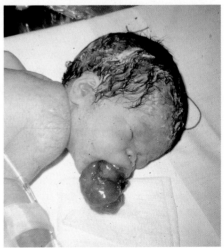

Figure 50. Epignathus. The large, smooth-surfaced tumor is a rare type of teratoma. Most epignathi attach to the base of the skull in the posterior nasopharynx near the site of Rathke's pouch (160–163). This tumor may extend into the cranial cavity and in some cases represents an oral encephalocele (164).

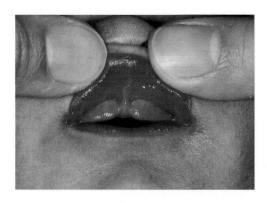

Figure 51. Normal mid-line maxillary cleft and frenum in otherwise healthy black infant whose mother had identical findings. Diastema of the central incisors will be permanent.

volving the skeletal system (114). Hypertrophied mid-line maxillary frenulum is reported to be associated with a hypoplastic left heart (115), but this association is likely stronger in white than in black infants, particularly only when there is no familial tendency. A significant mid-line labial frenulum may be associated with an alveolar cleft that predicts a widened incisor space (diastema) and with potentially impaired dental hygiene because the frenulum inhibits brushing (116) (Fig. 51).

A small lingual frenulum is normally present, but a short frenulum that limits tongue mobility is abnormal. Such limitation would be evident in crying when the tip of the tongue would form an inverted V shape (Fig. 52).

Assess cyanosis or pallor or jaundice in the mucous membranes.

The perioral vessels are easily visible in many fair-skinned, newborn infants, and they tinge the area blue, potentially creating a false impression of cyanosis. Although the perioral region may be cyanosed, the mucous membranes themselves will remain pink in the absence of desaturated hemoglobin. Similarly, more darkly pigmented lips may appear blue–gray on their external surface but will be pink inside (see Chapter 5 Fig. 3C). Any yellow or yellow–green discoloration can be attributed to an increase in tissue bilirubin.

With a gloved hand, palpate for texture, consistency, and continuity the lips, the buccal fat pad, the tongue, and the hard and soft palates. Feel for any increase due to subtle hemangiomas or other tumors and for any loss of mass or submucous clefts. Push the buccal mucosa away from the gums, lift the tongue from the floor and push the tongue away from the palate to visualize all its margins and surfaces and the adjacent structures. Touch only the anterior two thirds of the tongue surface to avoid eliciting the gag reflex.

The tongue is relatively smooth on all surfaces in neonates with less well-developed papillae. Its color is pink but may be discolored from a recent feeding. In darkly pigmented infants the presence of leukoplakia is normal (Fig. 53). Wharton's ducts from the submaxillary gland are easily seen, as are the blood vessels. A large tongue is often suggested by the way a particular infant holds his mouth with his tongue protruding because of decreased

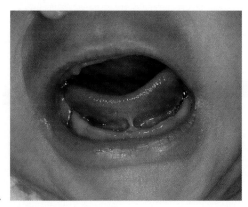

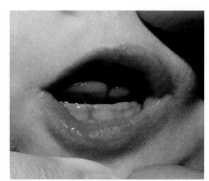

A

B

Figure 52. Lingular frenulum. **A:** Normal and nonrestrictive frenulum. **B:** Mildly restrictive, causing a V-shaped indentation to the tip of the tongue with protrusion. There is no significant restriction in tongue mobility.

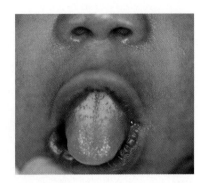

Figure 53. Leukoplakia. The white coating on this tongue is a normal finding in infants of dark pigment but should be distinguished from a recently fed formula or oral candidiasis (thrush).

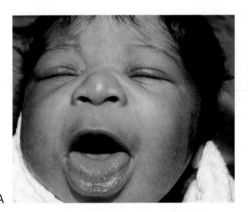

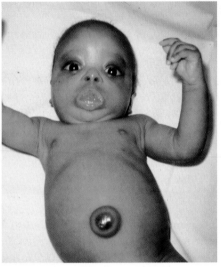

A   B

Figure 54. Large tongue. **A:** Large but normal tongue that did not interfere with mouth closure or feeding. **B:** True macroglossia. Infant of a diabetic mother at 2 months of age whose tongue interfered with effective nursing. Note also the large umbilical hernia.

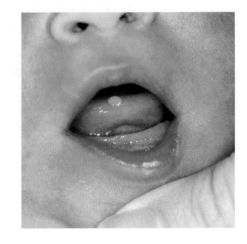

Figure 55. Tongue cyst. This small, superficial cyst persisted for several weeks before spontaneously regressing. Sucking blisters similar to those found on the lips or extremities may appear at this location on the tongue. Large and deeper cysts of the tongue are a rare cause of macroglossia.

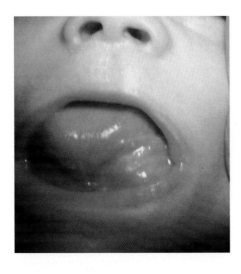

Figure 56. Ranula. The enlargement under the tongue represents a large, lateralized retention cyst of the floor of the mouth, usually caused by obstruction of the sublingual salivary gland duct. The lesion is covered by normal mucosa. Its name comes from its translucent, bluish-white appearance that resembles a frog's belly. The differential diagnosis includes stones in the salivary gland, inflammation of the gland, obstruction of Wharton's duct, thyroglossal duct cyst, cystic hygroma, branchial cleft cyst, cellulitis, benign tumors (lipoma, fibroma, hemangioma), teratoid cysts, ectopic thyroid, and excess submental fat mass.

lower facial tone. In general, if the mouth can close comfortably, macroglossia is not present (Fig. 54). The tongue appears large when there are masses or cysts within or under the tongue (Figs. 55 and 56).

Major malformations of the tongue are unusual as isolated findings and are generally part of more complex syndromes (117).

Major malformations of the tongue:

Aglossia, microglossia, or hemiatrophy
Macroglossia (Fig. 54) or hemihypertrophy
Long tongue or increased mobility
Ankyloglossia (118)
Glossoptosis
Cleft or bifid tongue (Fig. 57)

The buccal fat pad should be well developed so that the cheeks are full and rounded. Flat cheeks indicate poor nutritional fat stores. As very low birth weight infants start to grow well, deposition of buccal fat is one of the earliest visible signs that weight gain is nutritional and not fluid retention.

Look at the uvula and the elevation of the soft palate as well as the posterior faucial structures. Keep the head in the mid-line while assessing the posterior structures to avoid creating a false sense of asymmetry that might occur with tensing of the parapharyngeal muscles on the same side as the head is turned.

The soft palate forms an anterior pillar with a less well defined posterior pillar behind it. The tonsils that occupy the space between the pillars are normally very small and inconspicuous in neonates. The uvula is normally quite short in neonates.

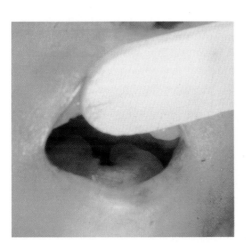

Figure 57. Mid-line posterior split in the tongue of an infant with severe micrencephaly.

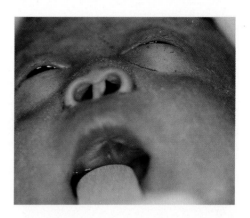

Figure 58. Abnormal palate. This term infant with holoprosencephaly has broad alveolar ridges and a moderately high but intact palate with a prominent central ridge. She had a weak suck. Note the mid-face hypoplasia with absent nasal bridge and hypoplasia of the columella typical of holoprosencephaly.

The shape of the palate should be softly rounded and smooth. When narrowed or with a high arch, there may not have been the normal action of the tongue against an intact palate during development. Causes of an abnormal but intact palate include primarily decreased neuromotor activity and prolonged orotracheal intubation (Fig. 58).

A bifid uvula usually indicates an associated submucous cleft in the palate (119). Because the uvula is very soft and compliant in the neonate, it is often seen to bend and stick to itself in such a way to suggest falsely a deviation due to nerve weakness.

Clefting of the lips and palate occur in isolation or in combination with other malformations. Approximately one half of the cases are cleft lip and palate together, one quarter are cleft lip alone, and one quarter are cleft palate alone (Figs. 59 and 60).

Assess the strength of the suck by allowing the infant to suck on a gloved finger. Feel for a coordinated propulsion in three phases from the lips to the oropharynx with each suck. Observe the overall effect of sucking on the general state of the infant: he should open his eyes and relax within a few sucks.

Because the infant cannot be asked to demonstrate the activity and strength of the muscles involved in lip, tongue, and jaw movements, it is necessary to observe how they function at rest and in the various activities likely to occur during examination, including rooting, yawning, crying, and sucking (Fig. 60). After a term birth, failure to calm down and initiate a regular, strong suck propulsion suggests increased irritability. If jitteriness persists during sucking, it may indicate abnormal neurologic irritability, most often due to drug withdrawal (120). An infant's sucking pattern will depend on his or her environment, behavior state, day of life, gestational age, and associated illness. In an infant who is in a behavior state favorable to feeding and without evidence of respiratory distress, the sucking pattern is a valid indicator of neuromotor integrity. The peristaltic tongue movements should be synchronized with the jaw movements and the force strong enough to propel the feed. The sucking pattern varies with gestational age (121). Term infants consume more formula with each suck with a stronger pressure and wider suck width. Additionally they use more sucks in succession (121).

In a newborn infant the larynx sits so much higher than it does in adults that it is relatively easy to see the epiglottis and the surrounding structures with an oral laryngoscope by little more than depressing the base of the tongue. In comparison, it is not feasible to use a

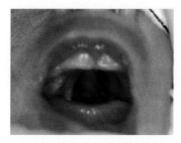
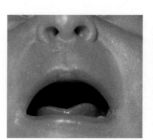
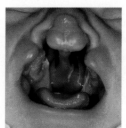

A   B, C

Figure 59. Variations of cleft palate. **A:** Isolated cleft of hard and soft palate. **B:** Cleft soft palate. **C:** Large cleft of the palate with bilateral cleft lip. This infant had an associated absence of the corpus callosum.

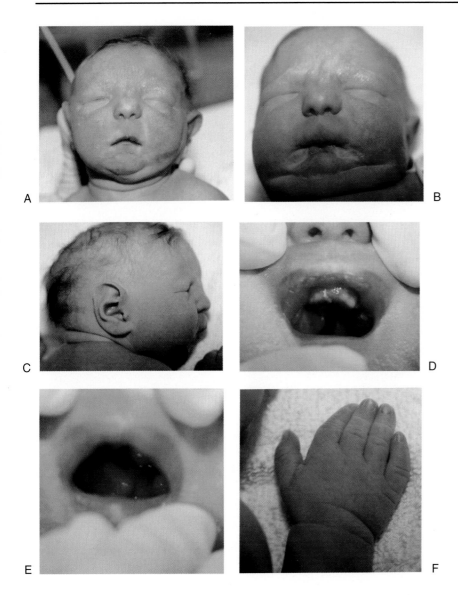

Figure 60. Oral facial digital syndrome. **A:** Facies with small alae nasi, bulbous nose, broad and flat philtrum. This infant has some milia at this stage but would be expected to develop more in the next month as a feature of this syndrome. **B:** Oral retractions with inhalation. On exhalation her perioral tissues puffed out. This finding was probably secondary to relative anterior nasal stenosis in the presence of a cleft palate and low facial tone. **C:** Profile demonstrating large ear with a simplified pinna, retrognathia, and microcephaly. **D:** Irregular and adherent vermilion bordermicrocephaly, multiple labial frenula with alveolar clefts, cleft of soft palate, and posterior hard palate. **E:** Multiple clefts of the tongue. **F:** hypoplasia of digits with deviations of the second and fifth digits and hypoplasia of the fingernail on the second digit.

mirror and light for indirect visualization. When full visualization of the larynx or pharynx is needed, using a flexible fiberoptic scope small enough to pass through the nostrils is the best technique (122).

NECK

Steps in examining the neck:

Inspect or palpate the neck for:
    position of head and neck
    appearance of skin
    symmetry of cervical musculature
    range of movement of cervical spine
        flexion, anterior and lateral
        extension
        rotation
    presence of masses
    presence of lymphadenopathy
    presence and size of thyroid gland
    position of trachea

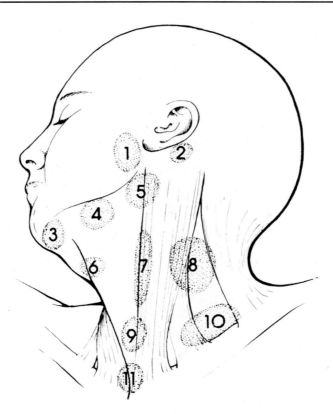

Figure 61. Identification of neck masses by location. Modified with permission (165).

Area 1: Parotid (preauricular). Congenital: Cystic hygroma, hemangioma, venous malformation. Inflammatory: Lymphadenitis secondary to upper face and anterior scalp infections.

Area 2: Postauricular. Congenital: First brachial cleft (cystic, inflamed, or both). Inflammatory: Lymphadenitis secondary to posterior scalp inflammation.

Area 3: Submental. Congenital: Thyroglossal duct cyst, cystic hygroma, dermoid cyst, venous malformation. Inflammatory: Lymphadenitis secondary to perioral, anterior oral, or nasal cavity inflammation.

Area 4: Submandibular. Congenital: Cystic hygroma, hemangioma, ranula. Inflammatory: Lymphadenitis of submandibular gland secondary to cheek and/or mid-oral cavity inflammation. Cystic fibrosis, gland enlarged without inflammation.

Area 5: Jugulodigastric (tonsil node). Normal structures: Transverse process of C2, styloid process. Congenital: First or second brachial cleft, hemangioma, cystic hygroma. Inflammation: Lymphadenitis secondary to oropharyngeal inflammation.

Area 6: Mid-line neck. Normal structures: Hyoid, thyroid isthmus, thyroid cartilage. Congenital: Thyroglossal duct cyst, dermoid cyst. Inflammatory: Lymphadenitis.

Area 7: Anterior border sternocleidomastoid muscle. Normal structures: Hyoid, thyroid cartilage, carotid bulb. Congenital: Brachial clefts I, II, III (IV rare), laryngocele hemangioma, lymphangioma, hematoma (fibroma) of sternocleidomastoid muscle.

Area 8: Spinal accessory. Inflammation: Lymphadenitis secondary to nasopharyngeal inflammation.

Area 9: Paratracheal. Thyroid, parathyroid, esophageal diverticulum, metastatic.

Area 10: Supraclavicular. Normal structure: Fat pad, pneumatocele from apical lobe due to defect in Gibson fascia (prominent mass with Valsalva maneuver). Congenital: Cystic hygroma. Neoplastic: Lipoma.

Area 11: Suprasternal. Thyroid, lipoma, dermoid, thymus, mediastinal mass

Inspect the neck first in a resting position to assess the natural head position. Next, fully extend the neck to allow visualization of all areas anteriorly. Palpate along the sternocleidomastoid muscles. Locate the thyroid isthmus in the suprasternal notch. Evaluate for suprasternal retractions. Determine range of motion in the cervical spine, particularly if there is cranial asymmetry. Inspect and palpate the posterior neck for length, masses, and skin folds (Figs. 61–64).

The possible causes for masses or defects in the neck region relate to the arches, grooves, and pouches that form the neck and facial structures. Even though many of the conditions are due to an embryologic variation, they will not present in the neonatal period. The most common tumors in newborn infants arise from abnormal lymphatic tissue, vascular malformations, teratomas, or dermoids. Probably the most frequent mass is the 1- to 2-cm

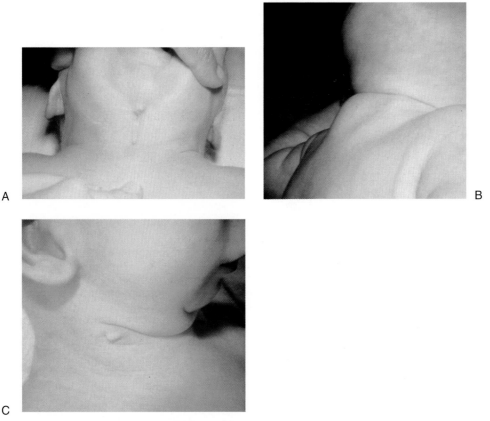

Figure 62. Small neck masses. **A:** Mid-line. Thyroglossal duct cyst is one of the most frequent congenital anomalies of the neck (125). It has a typical mid-line appearance most often inferior to the hyoid bone (approximately 70%) but may be lateral or superior to the hyoid (166). Thyroglossal duct cysts are generally sporadic, but there are rare reports of a familial occurrence (167). They represent a failed disappearance of the embryologic connection of the thyroid gland to the foramen cecum of the tongue and require surgical excision. Less frequent but often confused are mid-line cervical clefts representing failure of the branchial arch to fuse. This appears as a reddened, weeping 2-cm strip of atrophic skin 5 mm in width at a level between the chin and the sternal notch. There is always an underlying fibrous cord cephalad to the defect and variable in prominence that may cause webbing. Often there is a nipplelike projection at the upper end of the fissure and an associated sinus tract at the caudal aspect that may discharge mucoid material. Cervical clefts occur most often in white females (168). **B:** Cervical hernia seen as a soft mid-line bulge in the sternal notch that represents a benign pulmonary herniation (169). It increases in size with crying or other increase in intrathoracic pressure and is soft and fluctuant. The differential diagnosis includes enlarged thyroid, cervical thymic cyst, lipoma, dermoid, teratoma, or potentially any anterior mediastinal structure (165). **C:** Cervical tab that is a cartilaginous remnant of the branchial arch (synonym *Wattle*). The typical location is along the anterior border of the sternocleidomastoid muscle. These may be bilateral or unilateral and are not associated with fistulous tracts. Unlike accessory auricles, there are no pilosebaceous units or sweat glands. Micrognathia is present, suggesting there is hypoplasia of the mandibular prominence (see Fig. 31).

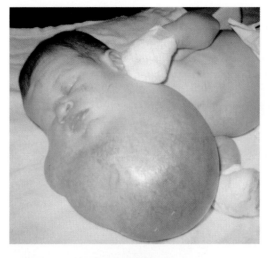

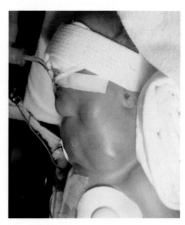

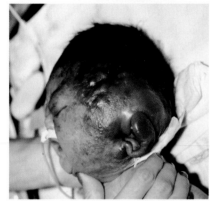

Figure 63. Large neck masses. **A:** Massive cystic hygroma with typical origin in submandibular region that will transilluminate. Origin may be submandibular, submental, preauricular, or supraclavicular, and the mass may extend onto the lower face but originates on one side. **B:** Thyroid teratoma. This tumor is more central in origin, firm, and does not transilluminate. **C:** Large deep and superficial angiomatous nevus (hemangioma) of the head and neck, originating in a typical location in the preauricular region. Although disfiguring, the major concerns at this stage would be obstruction to and consequent loss of vision in the left eye, as well as potential for platelet consumption or skin ulceration. Complete or almost complete resolution is expected in 95% of such lesions, with about 75% by the seventh birthday. Lesions on the nose, ears, and lips are least likely to show complete resolution. Although angiomatous nevus can occur on any site, about 60% occur on the head and neck (170,171). Aggressive hemangiomas on the face are associated with intracranial extension or malformations, particularly the Dandy-Walker cyst (78).

round or ovoid, firm, immobile, fibrous mass found in a sternocleidomastoid muscle associated with a torticollis (fibromatosis colli) (123–125). This may be present at birth or develop prenatally in some cases but is most often detected at 2 to 3 weeks of age. Infants with this condition hold their head turned away from and tilted toward the affected side (Table 1).

Subcutaneous emphysema in the neck resulting from severe intrathoracic air leaks, particularly tension pneumomediastinum, presents as a soft, crackling swelling in the supraclavicular region spreading in the anterior and lateral neck. Because the desperately ill infants who develop this air leak require high oxygen pressures, the nodular accumulation may look pinker than the skin color elsewhere. Nuchal emphysema develops rapidly after traumatic intubation and perforation of the trachea.

Anomalies of the skin of the neck may be localized or part of a generalized ectodermal defect (Fig. 64). Pterygium colli (wing neck) is a general term for an excessive amount of skin that presents as a flat fold extending from the region of the mastoid process to the point of the shoulders. It is found in Turner's syndrome, the multiple lentigines or leopard syndrome, Noonan's syndrome, and the multiple pterygium syndrome. Other anomalies of the nuchal skin that might present in the newborn period are seen in cutis laxa in which the skin is hanging and in cutis hyperelastica (Ehlers-Danlos syndrome).

The neck in most neonates appears relatively short. True decrease in neck length such that the head appears to sit directly on the shoulders with decreased range of rotation suggests the Klippel-Feil syndrome. In contrast, necks appear longer when there is a decrease in subcutaneous fat after poor intrauterine nutrition or when the fetal position has been in neck extension or with multiple loops of a nuchal cord.

It is convenient to examine the clavicles while palpating the neck structures. Standing at the infant's feet and using two fingers of each hand, palpate both clavicles simultaneously. Compare the definition of the borders and how much pressure is needed to feel the edges. Using alternating pressure between the two fingers, rock along the clavicles to detect movement or crepitation. Inspect for swelling, discoloration, pain or pressure, and decreased movement in the arms. Extend the infant's arm above his shoulder to detect pain or change in configuration with movement of each clavicle.

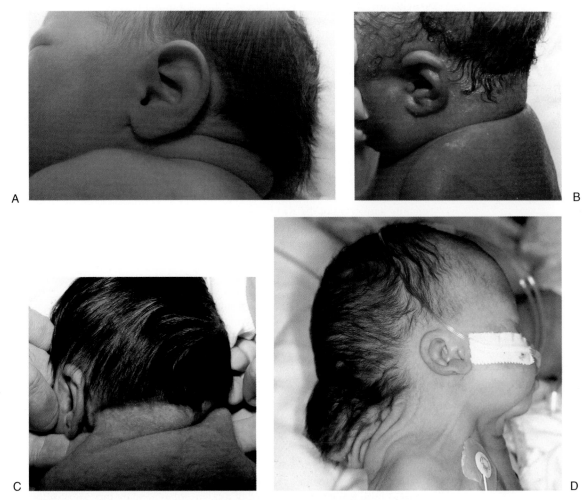

Figure 64. Patterns of nuchal skin folding. **A:** Extra folds in plump infant representing increased fat stores. **B:** Extra-deep fold in premature infant due to significant edema. **C:** Extra skin of mild webbing in infant with Turner's syndrome. This hairline is only minimally low, but the side-sweeping hair pattern originates at an abnormally placed whorl. **D:** Marked increased extra skin folds anteriorly and posteriorly with very low hairline in infant with Noonan syndrome. The ears are posteriorly rotated and low set. Although empty to palpation at the time of birth, the marked redundancy indicates the probable presence in utero of a very large cystic hygroma (172). A nuchal encephalocele could be similarly well covered by skin.

Clavicular fractures occur most often in large infants after vaginal delivery. The delivering staff often can report having heard a cracking sound at the time. Because of pain, some infants refuse to nurse on the breast opposite the fracture and are uncomfortable lying on the side of the fracture (126). Most infants with fractured clavicle have no symptoms and minimal physical findings (127).

GLOSSARY

Anagen   First stage of a hair follicle during which time growth of the hair occurs. Its duration varies according to body location. The length of the uncut hair is proportional to the duration, so may vary from several years on the adult scalp to less than 1 month on the thigh.

Ankyloglossia   As most often applied, ankyloglossia means tongue-tied with a lingular frenulum restricting extension of the tongue. When discussed as a major malformation, ankyloglossia superior refers to extensive adhesion of the tongue to the palate (glossopalatal ankylosis). The more severe malformations of oral synechiae are associated with skeletal limb anomalies (118).

Aphonia   Inability to vocalize.

Asynclitism   An oblique presentation of the fetal head in labor.

Bannayan's syndrome   An autosomal-dominant neurocutaneous syndrome characterized by macrencephaly, alterations of linear growth, and benign mesodermal hamartomas. Affected individuals are at risk for developing intracranial neoplasm (128). This may overlap the Riley-Smith syndrome, which includes pseudopapilledema.

Brachycephaly   Broadening of the skull with reduction of anteroposterior diameter; bilateral stenosis of coronal sutures usually associated with recessed lower forehead.

Calvarium   The skullcap; the superior portion of the cranium composed of the superior portions of the frontal, parietal, and occipital bones.

Catagen   A short intermediate transitional stage of the hair follicle lasting only a few days, during which time matrix cell growth ceases, the terminal portion of the hair retracts, becomes club-shaped, and rises up the follicle.

Dolichocephaly   Synonym scaphocephaly. An increase in head length, usually accompanied by narrowing of the width but not necessarily due to craniosynostosis of the sagittal suture. This head configuration occurs most frequently in premature infants who have been allowed to lie with their head in a side position.

Double lip   An apparent doubling of the lip where there is a redundancy of mucosal lining. This occurs as an isolated finding in families or as part of Ascher's syndrome of double lip, blepharochalasis, and nontoxic thyroid enlargement.

Epignathus   Any mass present at birth and attached to the jaw or jaws, the hard palate, or both. This term has been variously used to describe hamartomas, choristomas, or teratomas of the region present at birth. These may be monozygotic in origin or represent incomplete dizygotic twinning.

Epulis   Literally means "on the gum"; this term is variably applied. Congenital epulis indicates granular cell tumor. The term "epulis" has been clinically used to refer to any localized, fleshy, small- to moderate-size gingival mass regardless of its cause or histologic characteristics.

Fibromatosis colli   Congenital fibrous tumor of the sternocleidomastoid associated with torticolis.

Frenulum   Diminutive of Latin *fraenum*. Frenum and frenulum may be used synonymously, although frenulum is more often used.

Frenulum labii inferioris   The fold of mucous membrane on the inside of the middle of the lower lip, connecting the lip with the gums.

Frenulum labii superioris   The fold of mucous membrane on the inside of the middle of the upper lip, connecting the lip with the gums.

Frenulum linguae   Synonym *Frenum of the tongue*. The vertical fold of mucous membrane under the tongue, attaching it to the floor of the mouth. When marked, it limits the movements of the tongue, causing mandibular ankyloglossia (tongue-tie).

Furstenburg test Expansion of a mass on the cranium with compression of the jugular veins indicating communication of mass with intracranial pressure.

Glossoptosis Downward displacement or retraction of the tongue, as seen in Pierre-Robin syndrome of early mandibular hypoplasia.

Inion The most prominent point of the external occipital protuberance.

Intermediate scalp hair Scalp hair that develops rapidly at about 3 to 7 months and lasts to 2 years. It has a fragmented medulla and is coarser and more pigmented than lanugo.

Lanugo Fine, soft, poorly pigmented hair that lacks a central medulla. It is the first hair formed by the fetal hair follicle and is normally shed by 7 to 8 months of gestation. Primary lanugo is longer and more noticeable than secondary lanugo.

Macewen's sign As originally described, on percussion of the skull behind the junction of the frontal, temporal, and parietal bones, there is a more resonant note than normal in ventricular hydrocephalus. Other interpretations suggest increased resonance with open cranial sutures.

Macrencephaly Overgrowth of the brain.

Macrocephaly Excessive size of the head.

Macrocrania An abnormal increase in the size of the skull, the facial area being disproportionately small.

Macroglossia An abnormally large tongue. In neonates this usually means that the tongue is too large to fit inside a closed mouth. If the mouth itself is of normal size, then such a relationship implies that the tongue is too large. Failure to keep a tongue inside may indicate poor neuromotor tone or a small mouth rather than an extraordinarily large tongue. Macroglossia is seen in Down's syndrome, lymphangioma or hemangioma of the tongue, and Beckwith-Wiedemann syndrome.

Macrostomia Likely represents a form of facial clefting. This malformation is often seen in conjunction with mandibulofacial dysostosis (Treacher Collins syndrome) and oculoauriculovertebral dysplasia (Goldenhar's syndrome).

Median rhomboid glossitis The result of abnormal development of the posterior one third of the tongue with tissue free of papilla appearing in the posterior medial aspect of the tongue.

Micrencephaly Undergrowth of the brain.

Micrencephaly vera Small brain size without evidence of destruction of brain tissue either pre- or postnatally or derangement of developmental events. There is generally a decrease in the neurons of layers II and III and the amount of germinal matrix present by 26 weeks' gestation (49).

Microcephaly Abnormally small size of the head.

Neurocranium The portion of the cranium that encloses the brain.

Occipitofrontal Pertaining to a line from the back of the head to the forehead.

Occipitomental Pertaining to a line from the back of the head to the chin.

Oxycephaly Synonyms *Acrocephaly, tower head, turricephaly.* Pointed top of the head.

Ping-pong a. A benign, transient condition that describes the compliant sensation of neonatal craniotabes. b. A depressed skull fracture.

Plagiocephaly Flattening of the skull. When associated with craniosynostosis, the unilateral suture involved may be the lambdoid (occipital plagiocephaly) or cranial (frontal plagiocephaly).

Prognathism Projecting jaw.

Radial microbrain A rare disorder with an extremely small brain (5–15% expected weight) without evidence of a destructive process but with normal gyri, germinal matrix, and cortical lamination. There are approximately 30% the expected number of cortical neurons and a decrease in the number of cortical neuronal columns (49).

Retrognathism Synonym *Retrogenia* (although seen in the literature, this word is a combination of Latin and Greek). The line of the jaw is well behind the plane of the forehead. Because this relationship may be normally seen in neonatal cranial molding, the definition is applied primarily when there is a relatively small jaw (micrognathia).

Stensen's duct The duct that drains from the parotid onto the buccal mucosa opposite the second upper molar, often with a small papilla at the opening.

Subcutaneous emphysema   Characterized by a distinctive crepitant sensation on palpation of the neck associated with swelling of the tissues. In neonates it most commonly indicates a dissection of air from a severe pulmonary air leak.

Synophrys   Meeting of the eyebrows in the mid-line.

Telogen   The resting phases of the hair follicle that lasts up to several months depending on the site. The hair is shed at the end of telogen by a new anagen hair shaft ascending the follicle. The telogen stage is shorter in children than in adults.

Terminal hair   Thicker, often pigmented hair that typically grows on the scalp, eyebrows, and lashes before puberty and at the characteristic secondary sexual sites at puberty. It comprises 75% to 94% of scalp hair.

Torticollis   A wryneck; a twisting of the neck with the head in an unnatural position. In neonates and young infants this may be due to a shortening of the contralateral sternocleidomastoid muscle or to plagiocephaly of the ipsilateral occiput.

Trigonocephaly   Triangular shape with prowlike forehead; premature closure of metopic suture. Associated with a prominent vertical ridge of the mid-forehead.

Turricephaly   Synonyms *Acrocephaly, hypsicephaly, oxycephaly, tower-shaped skull.* Premature fusion of coronal, lambdoid, and metopic sutures. (Commonly misspelled turrencephaly).

Van der Woude's syndrome   A syndrome combining lip pits and cleft lip with or without cleft palate or uvula that is autosomal dominant, with 80% to 100% penetrance and variable expression (106). A higher incidence of natal teeth is associated with this syndrome (129).

Vellus hair   Fine, medullated, poorly pigmented hair that is best seen on the face and forearms but constitutes 6% to 25% of the scalp population. It continues to develop throughout life, although when noticeable at birth by its lighter pigment, does not remain as prominent in appearance because the terminal hair color predominates.

Wharton's duct   Synonym *Ductus submandibularis.* Ducts of the submaxillary glands that course under the tongue (the same Dr. Wharton described the umbilical cord jelly).

References

1. Aase JM. *Diagnostic dysmorphology.* New York: Plenum; 1990.
2. Davis RO, Cutter GR, Goldenberg RL, Hoffman HJ, Cliver SP, Brumfield CG. Fetal biparietal diameter, head circumference, abdominal circumference and femur length. A comparison by race and sex. *J Reprod Med* 1993;38:201–206.
3. Guihard-Costa AM, Larroche JC. Growth velocity of some fetal parameters. II. Body weight, body length and head circumference. *Biol Neonate* 1992;62:317–324.
4. Nellhaus G. Head circumference from birth to eighteen years. Practical composite international and interracial graphs. *Pediatrics* 1968;41:106–114.
5. Weaver DD, Christian JC. Familial variation of head size and adjustment for parental head circumference. *J Pediatr* 1980;96:990–994.
6. Haslam RH, Smith DW. Autosomal dominant microcephaly. *J Pediatr* 1979;95:701–705.
7. Hecht F, Kelly JV. Little heads: inheritance and early detection. *J Pediatr* 1979;95:731–732.
8. Merlob P, Steier D, Reisner SH. Autosomal dominant isolated ("uncomplicated") microcephaly. *J Med Genet* 1988;25:750–753.
9. Rossi LN, Candini G, Scarlatti G, Rossi G, Prina E, Alberti S. Autosomal dominant microcephaly without mental retardation. *Am J Dis Child* 1987;141:655–659.
10. Swischuk LE. The normal newborn skull. *Semin Roentgenol* 1974;9:101–113.
11. Swischuk LE. The normal pediatric skull. Variations and artefacts. *Radiol Clin North Am* 1972;10:277–290.
12. Graham JM, Smith DW. Parietal craniotabes in the neonate; its origin and significance. *J Pediatr* 1979;95:114–116.
13. Kokkonen J, Koivisto M, Lautala P, Kirkinen P. Serum calcium and 25-OH-D3 in mothers of newborns with craniotabes. *J Perinatol Med* 1983;11:127–131.
14. Bates B. A guide to physical examination and history taking. 5th ed. Philadelphia: JB Lippincott; 1991.
15. Duc G, Largo RH. Anterior fontanel: size and closure in term and preterm infants. *Pediatrics* 1986;78:904–908.
16. Cohen M, Levin SE. Significance of intracranial bruits in neonates, infants, and young children. *Arch Dis Child* 1978;53:592–594.
17. Dodge PR, Porter P. Demonstration of intracranial pathology by transillumination. *Arch Neurol* 1961;5:30–41.
18. Volpe JJ. Neurology of the newborn. 3rd ed. Philadelphia: WB Saunders; 1995.
19. Swick HM, Cunningham MD, Shield LK. Transillumination of the skull in premature infants. *Pediatrics* 1976;58:658–664.

20. Vyhmeister N, Schneider S, Cha C. Cranial transillumination norms of the premature infant. *J Pediatrics* 1977;91:980–982.
21. Ashkenazi S, Metzker A, Merlob P, Ovadia J, Reisner SH. Scalp changes after fetal monitoring. *Arch Dis Child* 1985;60:267–269.
22. Okada DM, Chow AW, Bruce VT. Neonatal scalp abscess and fetal monitoring: factors associated with infection. *Am J Obstet Gynecol* 1977;129:185–189.
23. Cordero L, Anderson CW, Zuspan FP. Scalp abscess: a benign and infrequent complication of fetal monitoring. *Am J Obstet Gynecol* 1983;146:126–130.
24. McGregor JA, McFarren T. Neonatal cranial osteomyelitis: a complication of fetal monitoring. *Obstet Gynecol* 1989;73:490–492.
25. Siddiqi SF, Taylor PM. Necrotizing fasciitis of the scalp. *Am J Dis Child* 1982;136:226–228.
26. Kaye EM, Dooling EC. Neonatal herpes simplex meningoencephalitis associated with fetal monitor scalp electrodes. *Neurology* 1981;31:1045–1046.
27. Parvey LS, Ch'ien LT. Neonatal herpes simplex virus infection introduced by fetal monitor scalp electrodes. *Pediatrics* 1980;65:1150–1153.
28. Potter EL, Craig JM. *Birth trauma. Pathology of the fetus and the infant.* 3rd ed. Chicago: Year Book Medical; 1975:105.
29. Kaufman H, Hochberg J, Anderson R, Schochet SJ, Simmons GJ. Treatment of calcified cephalohematoma. *Neurosurgery* 1993;32:1037–1039.
30. Chung KC, Buchman SR, Maher HA, Dauser RC. Surgical management of calcified cephalhematoma and associated skull defect in infancy. *Ann Plast Surg* 1995;34:99–102.
31. Churchill JA, Stevenson L, Habhab G. Cephalhematoma and natal brain injury. *Obstet Gynecol* 1966;27:580–584.
32. Hagadorn-Freathy AS, Yeomans ER, Hankins GD. Validation of the 1988 ACOG forceps classification system. *Obstet Gynecol* 1991;77:356–360.
33. Winter TD, Mack L, Cyr D. Prenatal sonographic diagnosis of scalp edema/cephalohematoma mimicking an encephalocele. *AJR* 1993;161:1247–1248.
34. Neiger R, Sacks LM. An unusual neonatal case presentation. Cephalohematoma with underlying skull fracture in a neonate delivered by cesarean section. *J Perinatol* 1988;8:160–162.
35. Zelson C, Lee SJ, Pearl M. The incidence of skull fractures underlying cephalhematomas in newborn infants. *J Pediatr* 1974;85:371.
36. Kendall N, Wolloshin H. Cephalhematoma associated with fracture of the skull. *J Pediatr* 1952;41:125.
37. Bansal A, Bothra GC, Verma CR. Hyperbilirubinemia due to massive cephalhematoma. *Indian Pediatr* 1985;22:619–621.
38. Mohon RT, Mehalic TF, Grimes CK, Philip AG. Infected cephalhematoma and neonatal osteomyelitis of the skull. *Pediatr Infect Dis* 1986;5:253–256.
39. Nightingale LM, Eaton CB, Fruehan AE, Waldman JB, Clark WB, Lepow ML. Cephalhematoma complicated by osteomyelitis presumed due to Gardnerella vaginalis. *JAMA* 1986;256:1936–1937.
40. Meignier M, Renaud P, Robert R, Roze JC, Rigal E, Mouzard A. Cephalhematoma infection in neonatal septicemia]. *Pediatrie* 1989;44:27–29.
41. Tada M, Echizenya K, Satoh M. Communication between epidural hematoma and cephalhematoma in a neonate. *Hokkaido Igaku Zasshi* 1986;61:244–248.
42. Okuno T, Miyamoto M, Itakura T, et al. [A case of epidural hematoma caused by a vacuum extraction without any skull fractures and accompanied by cephalohematoma]. *No Shinkei Geka* 1993;21:1137–1141.
43. Govaert P, Vanhaesebrouck P, De Praeter C, Moens K, Leroy J. Vacuum extraction, bone injury and neonatal subgaleal bleeding. *Eur J Pediatr* 1992;151:532–535.
44. Jones MD. Unilateral epicanthal fold: diagnostic significance. *J Pediatr* 1986;108:702.
45. Johnsonbaugh RE, Bryan RN, Hierlwimmer UR, Georges LP. Premature craniosynostosis: a common complication of juvenile thyrotoxicosis. *J Pediatr* 1978;93:188–191.
46. Graham JM Jr, deSaxe M, Smith DW. Sagittal craniostenosis: fetal head constraint as one possible cause. *J Pediatr* 1979;95:747–750.
47. Simpson P. Craniosynostosis. In: Hoffman HJ, Epstein F, eds. *Disorders of the Developing Nervous System: Diagnosis and Treatment.* Vol. 1. Oxford: Blackwell Science; 1986:327.
48. Shuper A, Merlob P, Grunebaum M, Reisner SH. The incidence of isolated craniosynostosis in the newborn infant. *Am J Dis Child* 1985;139:85–86.
49. Evrard P, de Saint-Georges P, Kadhim HJ, et al. Pathology of prenatal encephalopathies. In: French JH, Harel S, Casaer P, eds. *Child Neurology and Developmental Disabilities.* Baltimore: Paul H Brookes; 1989:153–176.
50. Muller WD, Urlesberger B. Correlation of ventricular size and head circumference after severe intra-periventricular haemorrhage in preterm infants. *Childs Nerv Syst* 1992;8:33–35.
51. Becker LE. The nervous sytem. In: Stocker JT, Dehner LP, eds. *Pediatric Pathology.* 1st ed. Vol. 1. Philadelphia: JB Lippincott; 1992:425–464.
52. Halliday J, Chow C, Wallace D, Danks D. X linked hydrocephalus: a survey of a 20 year period in Victoria, Australia. *J Med Genet* 1986;23:23–31.
53. Mealey J Jr, Gilmor RL, Bubb MP. The prognosis of hydrocephalus overt at birth. *J Neurosurg* 1973;39:348–355.
54. McCullough DC, Balzer-Martin LA. Current prognosis in overt neonatal hydrocephalus. *J Neurosurg* 1982;57:378–383.
55. Fernell E, Hagberg B, Hagberg G, Hult G, von Wendt L. Epidemiology of infantile hydrocephalus in Sweden: a clinical follow-up study in children born at term. *Neuropediatrics* 1988;19:135–142.
56. Fernell E, Hagberg B, Hagberg G, von Wendt L. Epidemiology of infantile hydrocephalus in Sweden. III. Origin in preterm infants. *Acta Paediatr Scand* 1987;76:418–423.
57. Gupta JK, Bryce FC, Lilford RJ. Management of apparently isolated fetal ventriculomegaly. *Obstet Gynecol Surv* 1994;49:716–721.

58. Norman MG. Central nervous system. In: Dimmick JE, Kalousek DK, eds. *Developmental Pathology of the Embryo and Fetus.* 1st ed. Vol. 1. Philadelphia: JB Lippincott; 1992:341–423.

59. Hutto C, Arvin A, Jacobs R, et al. Intrauterine herpes simplex virus infections. *J Pediatr* 1987;110:97–101.

60. Myers RE. Cerebral ischemia in the developing primate fetus. *Biomed Biochim Acta* 1989; 48(suppl):137–142.

61. Fowler M, Dow R, White TA, Greer CH. Congenital hydrocephalus-hydrencephaly in five siblings, with autopsy studies: a new disease. *Dev Med Child Neurol* 1972;14:173–188.

62. Harper C, Hockey A. Proliferative vasculopathy and an hydranencephalic-hydrocephalic syndrome: a neuropathological study of two siblings. *Dev Med Child Neurol* 1983;25:232–239.

63. Zalneraitis EL, Young RS, Krishnamoorthy KS. Intracranial hemorrhage in utero as a complication of isoimmune thrombocytopenia. *J Pediatr* 1979;95:611–614.

64. Naidu S, Messmore H, Caserta V, Fine M. CNS lesions in neonatal isoimmune thrombocytopenia. *Arch Neurol* 1983;40:552–554.

65. Cohen MJ. Perspectives on holoprosencephaly: Part I. Epidemiology, genetics, and syndromology. *Teratology* 1989;40:211–235.

66. Cohen MJ. Perspectives on holoprosencephaly: Part III. Spectra, distinctions, continuities, and discontinuities. *Am J Med Genet* 1989;34:271–288.

67. Collins AL, Lunt PW, Garrett C, Dennis NR. Holoprosencephaly: a family showing dominant inheritance and variable expression. *J Med Genet* 1993;30:36–40.

68. Durmus Aydogdu S, Yakut A, Oner U, Aksit MA, Tel N. Holoprosencephaly anomaly with nasal and premaxillar agenesis (possibly autosomal recessive type). *Turk J Pediatr* 1994;36:157–162.

69. Hengerer AS, Newburg JA. Congenital malformations of the nose and paranasal sinuses. In: Bluestone C, Stool, SE, Scheetz, MD, eds. *Pediatric Otolaryngology.* Vol. 1. Philadelphia: WB Saunders; 1990:718–728.

70. Hennekam RC, van Noort G, de la Fuente AA. Familial holoprosencephaly, heart defects, and polydactyly. *Am J Med Genet* 1991;41:258–262.

71. Hennekam RC, Van Noort G, de la Fuente FA, Norbruis OF. Agenesis of the nasal septal cartilage: another sign in autosomal dominant holoprosencephaly [Letter; comment]. *Am J Med Genet* 1991;39:121–122.

72. Leech RW, Shuman RM. Holoprosencephaly and related midline cerebral anomalies: a review. *J Child Neurol* 1986;1:3–18.

73. Leech RW, Bowlby LS, Brumback RA, Schaefer GB Jr. Agnathia, holoprosencephaly, and situs inversus: report of a case [Comments]. *Am J Med Genet* 1988;29:483–490.

74. Ramos-Arroyo MA, de Miguel C, Valiente A, Moreno-Laguna S. Further delineation of pseudotrisomy 13 syndrome: a case without polydactyly. *Am J Med Genet* 1994;50:177–179.

75. Shiota K. Teratothanasia: prenatal loss of abnormal conceptuses and the prevalence of various malformations during human gestation. *Birth Defects* 1993;29:189–199.

76. Tsukamoto H, Sakai N, Taniike M, et al. Case of ring chromosome 7: the first report of neuropathological findings. *Am J Med Genet* 1993;46:632–635.

77. Young ID, Zuccollo JM, Barrow M, Fowlie A. Holoprosencephaly, telecanthus and ectrodactyly: a second case. *Clin Dysmorphol* 1992;1:47–51.

78. Reese V, Frieden IJ, Paller AS, et al. Association of facial hemangiomas with Dandy-Walker and other posterior fossa malformations. *J Pediatr* 1993;122:379–384.

79. Waardenburg PJ. A new syndrome combining developmental anomalies of the eyelids, eyebrows and nose root with pigmentary defects of the iris and head hair and with congenital deafness. *Am J Hum Genet* 1951; 3:195.

80. Wunderlich RC, Heereman NA. Hair crown patterns of human newborns: studies on parietal whorl locations and their direction. *Clin Pediatr* 1974;14:1045–1049.

81. Smith DW, Gong BT. Scalp hair patterning as a clue to early fetal brain development. *J Pediatr* 1973;83: 374–380.

82. Holbrook KA. Structural and biochemical organogenesis of skin and cutaneous appendages in the fetus and neonate. In: Polin RA, Fox WW, eds. *Fetal and Neonatal Physiology.* 1st ed. Vol. 1. Philadelphia: WB Saunders; 1991:527–551.

83. Loftus BC, Ahn J, Haddad JJ. Neonatal nasal deformities secondary to nasal continuous positive airway pressure. *Laryngoscope* 1994;104:1019–1022.

84. Godar K, Bull MJ, Schreiner RL, Lemons JA, Gresham EL. Nasal deformities in neonates. *Am J Dis Child* 1980;134:954–957.

85. Baxter RJ, Johnson JD, Goetzman BW, Hackel A. Cosmetic nasal deformities complicating prolonged nasotracheal intubation in critically ill newborn infants. *Pediatrics* 1975;55:884–887.

86. Jung AL, Thomas GK. Stricture of the nasal vestibule: a complication of nasotracheal intubation in newborn infants. *J Pediatr* 1974;85:412–414.

87. Pettett G, Merenstein GB. Nasal erosion with nasotracheal intubation. *J Pediatr* 1975;87:149–150.

88. Rotschild A, Dison PJ, Chitayat D, Solimano A. Midfacial hypoplasia associated with long-term intubation for bronchopulmonary dysplasia. *Am J Dis Child* 1990;144:1302–1306.

89. Podoshin L, Gertner R, Fradis M, Berger A. Incidence and treatment of deviation of nasal septum in newborns. *Ear Nose Throat J* 1991;70:485–487.

90. Silverman SH, Leibow SG. Dislocation of the triangular cartilage of the nasal septum. *J Pediatr* 1975;87: 456–458.

91. Jeppesen F, Windfeld J. Dislocation of nasal septal cartilage in the newborn. *Acta Obstet Gynecol Scand* 1972;51:5–8.

92. Castillo M. Congenital abnormalities of the nose: CT and MR findings. *AJR* 1994;162:1211–1217.

93. Duncan NO, Miller RH, Catlin FL. Choanal atresia and associated anomalies. *Int J Pediatr Otorhinolaryngol* 1988;15:129–135.

94. Coates H. Nasal obstruction in the neonate and infant. *Clin Pediatr* 1992;January:25–29.

95. Rodenstein DO, Perlmutter N, Stanescu D. Infants are not obligatory nasal breathers. *Am Rev Respir Dis* 1985;131:343.

96. Miller MJ, Martin RJ, Carlo WA, Fanaroff AA. Oral breathing in response to nasal trauma in term infants. *J Pediatr* 1987;111:899–901.
97. Stocks J, Godfrey S. Nasal resistance in infancy. *Respir Physiol* 1978;34:233–246.
98. Martin RJ, Siner B, Carlo WA, Lough M, Miller MJ. Effect of head position on distribution of nasal airflow in preterm infants. *J Pediatr* 1988;112:99–103.
99. Pedersen OF, Berkowitz R, Yamagiwa M, Hilberg O. Nasal cavity dimensions in the newborn measured by acoustic reflections. *Laryngoscope* 1994;104:1023–1028.
100. Carlo WA, Martin RJ, Bruce EN, Strohl KP, Fanaroff AA. Alae nasi activation (nasal flaring) decreases nasal resistance in preterm infants. *Pediatrics* 1983;72:338–343.
101. Anderson RB, Rosenblith JF. Photic sneeze reflex in the human newborn. *Dev Psychobiol* 1968;1:65.
102. Reddy AM, Harper RG, Stern G. Observations on heroin and methadone withdrawal in the newborn. *Pediatrics* 1971;48:353–358.
103. Sawyer DR, Taiwo EO, Mosadomi A. Oral anomalies in Nigerian children. *Commun Dent Oral Epidemiol* 1984;12:269–273.
104. Wang M, Macomber WB. Congenital lip sinuses. *Plast Reconstr Surg* 1956;18:319–328.
105. Martin RA, Jones KL, Benirschke K. Extension of the cleft lip phenotype: the subepithelial cleft. *Am J Med Genet* 1993;47:744–747.
106. Srivastava S, Bang RL. Congenital sinuses of the lower lip: reappraisal of Van der Woude syndrome on the basis of nine patients. *Ann Plast Surg* 1989;22:316–320.
107. Reddy KA, Roa AK. Congenital double lip: a review of seven cases. *Plast Reconstr Surg* 1989;84:420–423.
108. Rosenfeld RM, Fletcher MA, Marban SL. Acute epiglottitis in a newborn infant. *Pediatr Infect Dis J* 1992; 11:594–595.
109. Myer CMI. Sialorrhea. *Pediatr Clin North Am* 1989;36:1495–1500.
110. Fromm A. Epstein's pearls, Bohn's nodules and inclusion-cysts of the oral cavity. *J Dent Child* 1967;34: 275–287.
111. Levin LS, Jorgenson RJ, Jarvey BA. Lymphangiomas of the alveolar ridges in neonates. *Pediatrics* 1976; 58:881–884.
112. Chawla HS. Management of natal/neonatal/early infancy teeth. *J Indian Soc Pedod Prev Dent* 1993;11: 33–36.
113. Jasmin JR, Jonesco-Benaiche N, Muller-Giamarchi M. [Natal and neonatal teeth. Management]. *Ann Pediatr (Paris)* 1993;40:640–641.
114. Martinot VL, Manouvrier S, Anastassov Y, Ribiere J, Pellerin PN. Orodigitofacial syndromes type I and II: clinical and surgical studies. *Cleft Palate Craniofac J* 1994;31:401–408.
115. Lovell MA, McDaniel NL. Association of hypertrophic maxillary frenulum with hypoplastic left heart syndrome. *J Pediatr* 1995;127:748–750.
116. Swenson HM. ABC's periodontics. F is for the frenum. *J Indiana Dent Assoc* 1984;63:27–28.
117. Emmanouil-Nikoloussi E, Kerameos-Foroglou C. Congenital syndromes connected with tongue malformations. *Bull Assoc Anat (Nancy)* 1992;76:67–72.
118. Gartlan MG, Davies J, Smith RJ. Congenital oral synechiae. *Ann Otol Rhinol Laryngol* 1993;102(3 Pt 1):186–197.
119. Shprintzen RJ, Schwartz RH, Daniller A, Hoch L. Morphologic significance of bifid uvula. *Pediatrics* 1985; 75:553–561.
120. Linder N, Moser AM, Asli I, Gale R, Livoff A, Tamir I. Suckling stimulation test for neonatal tremor. *Arch Dis Child* 1989;64:44–52.
121. Medoff-Cooper B, Weininger S, Zukowsky K. Neonatal sucking as a clinical assessment tool: preliminary findings. *Nurs Res* 1989;38:162–165.
122. Schmidt HJ, Fink RJ. Flexible fiberoptic bronchoscopy. In: Fletcher M, MacDondal MG, eds. *Atlas of Procedures in Neonatology*. 2nd ed. Vol. 1. Philadelphia: JB Lippincott; 1993:300–308.
123. Schullinger JN. Birth trauma. *Pediatr Clin North Am* 1993;40:1351–1358.
124. Bergman KS, Harris BH. Scalp and neck masses. *Pediatr Clin North Am* 1993;40:1151–1160.
125. Guarisco JL. Congenital head and neck masses in infants and children. Part II. *Ear Nose Throat J* 1991;70: 75–82.
126. Waninger KN, Chung MK. A new clue to clavicular fracture in newborn infants? [Letter]. *J Pediatr* 1991; 88:657.
127. Joseph PR, Rosenfeld W. Clavicular fractures in neonates. *Am J Dis Child* 1990;144:165–167.
128. Higginbottom MC, Schultz P. The Bannayan syndrome: an autosomal dominant disorder consisting of macrocephaly, lipomas, hemangiomas, and risk for intracranial tumors. *Pediatrics* 1982;69:632–635.
129. Hersh JH, Verdi GD. Natal teeth in monozygotic twins with Van der Woude syndrome. *Cleft Palate Craniofac J* 1992;29:279–281.
130. Faix RG. Fontanelle size in black and white term newborn infants. *J Pediatr* 1982;100:304–306.
131. Honig PJ, Brown D. Congenital herpes simplex virus infection initially resembling epidermolysis bullosa. *J Pediatr* 1982;101:958–960.
132. Pape KE, Wigglesworth JS. *Haemorrhage, Ischaemia and the Perinatal Brain*. Philadelphia: JB Lippincott; 1979.
133. Richards CGM. Frontoethmoidal meningoencephalocele. A common and severe congenital abnormality in Southeast Asia. *Arch Dis Child* 1992;67:717–719.
134. De Jong G, Fryns JP. Oculocerebral syndrome with hypopigmentation (Cross syndrome): the mixed pattern of hair pigmentation as an important diagnostic sign. *Genet Couns* 1991;2:151–155.
135. Findlay GH. An optical study of human hair colour in normal and abnormal conditions. *Br J Dermatol* 1982; 107:517–527.
136. Rook A. Disorders of the hair. *Practitioner* 1973;211:593–599.
137. Barth JH. Normal hair growth in children. *Pediatr Dermatol* 1987;4:1173–1184.
138. Moore KL, Persaud TVN, Shiota K. *Color Atlas of Clinical Embryology*. 1st ed. Philadelphia: WB Saunders; 1994.

139. Marasovich WA, Mazaheri M, Stool SE. Otolaryngologic findings in whistling face syndrome. *Arch Otolaryngol Head Neck Surg* 1989;115:1373–1380.
140. Millen SJ, Baruah JK. Congenital hypoplasia of the depressor anguli oris muscle in the differential diagnosis of facial paralysis. *Laryngoscope* 1983;93:1168–1170.
141. Kolandaivelu G. Depressor Anguli Oris syndrome [Letter]. *Indian Pediatr* 1982;19:553–554.
142. Levin SE, Silverman NH, Milner S. Hypoplasia or absence of the depressor anguli oris muscle and congenital abnormalities, with special reference to the cardiofacial syndrome. *S Afr Med J* 1982;61:227–231.
143. Miller M, Hall JG. Familial asymmetric crying facies. Its occurrence secondary to hypoplasia of the anguli oris depressor muscles. *Am J Dis Child* 1979;133:743–746.
144. Alexiou D, Manolidis C, Papaevangellou G, Nicolopoulos D, Papadatos C. Frequency of other malformations in congenital hypoplasia of depressor anguli oris muscle syndrome. *Arch Dis Child* 1976;51:891–893.
145. Papadatos C, Alexiou D, Nicolopoulos D, Mikropoulos H, Hadzigeorgiou E. Congenital hypoplasia of depressor anguli oris muscle. A genetically determined condition? *Arch Dis Child* 1974;49:927–931.
146. Vitti M, Correa AC, Fortinguerra CR, Berzin F, Konig B Jr. Electromyographic study of the musculus depressor anguli oris. *Electromyogr Clin Neurophysiol* 1972;12:119–125.
147. Nelson KB, Eng GD. Congenital hypoplasia of the depressor anguli oris muscle: differentiation from congenital facial palsy. *J Pediatr* 1972;81:16–20.
148. Feingold M, Baum J. Goldenhar's syndrome. *Am J Dis Child* 1978;132:136–138.
149. Hamada Y, Hamano H, Chen SH, et al. [Statistical study of epulis, especially in general pathology]. *Shikwa Gakuho* 1989;89:1507–1515.
150. Bernhoft CH, Gilhuus-Moe O, Bang G. Congenital epulis in the newborn. *Int J Pediatr Otorhinolaryngol* 1987;13:25–29.
151. Friend GW, Harris EF, Mincer HH, Fong TL, Carruth KR. Oral anomalies in the neonate, by race and gender, in an urban setting. *Pediatr Dent* 1990;12:157–161.
152. Kameyama Y, Mizohata M, Takehana S, Murata H, Manabe H, Mukai Y. Ultrastructure of the congenital epulis. *Virchows Arch [A]* 1983;401:251–260.
153. Lifshitz MS, Flotte TJ, Greco MA. Congenital granular cell epulis. Immunohistochemical and ultrastructural observations. *Cancer* 1984;53:1845–1848.
154. Subramaniam R, Shah R, Kapur V. Congenital epulis. *J Postgrad Med* 1993;39:36.
155. Chindia ML, Awange DO. Congenital epulis of the newborn: a report of two cases. *Br Dent J* 1994;176:426–428.
156. Damm DD, Cibull ML, Geissler RH, Neville BW, Bowden CM, Lehmann JE. Investigation into the histogenesis of congenital epulis of the newborn. *Oral Surg Oral Med Oral Pathol* 1993;76:205–212.
157. Eppley BL, Sadove AM, Campbell A. Obstructive congenital epulis in a newborn. *Ann Plast Surg* 1991;27:152–155.
158. Blinkhorn AS, Attwood D. Congenital epulis interfering with feeding in a day-old baby girl. *Dent Update* 1990;17:346.
159. Jenkins HR, Hill CM. Spontaneous regression of congenital epulis of the newborn. *Arch Dis Child* 1989;64:145–147.
160. Ang AT, Ho NK, Ong CL. Giant epignathus with intracranial teratoma in a newborn infant. *Australas Radiol* 1990;34:358–360.
161. Senyuz OF, Rizalar R, Celayir S, Oz F. Fetus in fetu or giant epignathus protruding from the mouth. *J Pediatr Surg* 1992;27:1493–1495.
162. Todd DW, Votava HJ, Telander RL, Shoemaker CT. Giant epignathus. A case report. *Minn Med* 1991;74:27–28.
163. Valente A, Grant C, Orr JD, Brereton RJ. Neonatal tonsillar teratoma. *J Pediatr Surg* 1988;23:364–366.
164. Carlan SJ, Angel JL, Leo J, Feeney J. Cephalocele involving the oral cavity. *Obstet Gynecol* 1990;75(3 Pt 2):494–496.
165. May M. Neck masses in children: diagnosis and treatment. *Pediatr Ann* 1976;5:518–535.
166. Ward PH, Strahan RW, Acquarelli M, Harris PF. The many faces of cysts of the thyroglossal duct. *Trans Am Acad Ophthalmol Otolaryngol* 1970;74:310–318.
167. Issa M, deVries P. Familial occurrence of thyroglossal duct cyst. *J Pediatr Surg* 1991;26:30–31.
168. Maddolozzo J, Frankel A, Holinger LD. Midline cervical cleft. *Pediatrics* 1993;92:286–287.
169. Friedberg J. Pharyngeal cleft sinuses and cysts, and other benign neck lesions. *Pediatr Clin North Am* 1989;36:1451–1469.
170. Mulliken JB. Classification of vascular birthmarks. In: Milliken JB, Young AE, eds. *Vascular birthmarks: Hemangiomas and Malformations.* Philadelphia: WB Saunders; 1988:24–37.
171. Atherton DJ. Naevi and other developmental defects. In: Champion RH, Burton JL, Ebling FJG, eds. *Rook, Wilkinson, Ebling Textbook of Dermatology.* 5th ed. Vol. 1. Oxford: Blackwell Scientific; 1992:445–526.
172. Smith DW. Commentary: redundant skin folds in the infant—their origin and relevance. *J Pediatr* 1979;94:1021–1022.
173. Lemire RJ. Variations in development of the caudal neural tube in human embryos (Horizons XIV–XXI). *Teratology* 1969;2:361–369.
174. Gilbert JN, Jones KL, Rorke LB, Chernoff GF, James HE. Central nervous system anomalies associated with meningomyelocele, hydrocephalus, and the Arnold-Chiari malformation: reappraisal of theories regarding the pathogenesis of posterior neural tube closure defects. *Neurosurgery* 1986;18:559–564.
175. Fairbanks DNF. Embryology and Anatomy. In: Bluestone C, Stool, SE, Scheetz, MD, eds. *Pediatric Otolaryngology.* Vol. 1. Philadelphia: WB Saunders; 1990:605–631.
176. Handler SD. Upper airway obstruction in craniofacial anomalies: diagnosis and management. *Birth Defects* 1985;21:15–31.
177. Kaplan LC. The CHARGE association: choanal atresia and multiple congenital anomalies. *Otolaryngol Clin North Am* 1989;22:661–672.
178. Morgan DW, Evans JN. Developmental nasal anomalies. *J Laryngol Otol* 1990;104:394–403.
179. Stahl RS, Jurkiewicz MJ. Congenital posterior choanal atresia. *Pediatrics* 1985;76:429–436.
180. Blake K. Congenital nasal stenosis in newborn infants. *J Pediatr* 1993;121:831.

181. Leiberman A, Carmi R, Bar-Ziv Y, Karplus M. Congenital nasal stenosis in newborn infants. *J Pediatr* 1992; 120:124–127.
182. Arlis H, Ward RF. Congenital nasal pyriform aperture stenosis. Isolated abnormality vs developmental field defect. *Arch Otolaryngol Head Neck Surg* 1992;118:989–991.
183. Kennard CD, Rasmussen JE. Congenital midline nasal masses: diagnosis and management. *J Dermatol Surg Oncol* 1990;16:1025–1036.
184. Demaerel P, Casteels I, Peene P, et al. Unilateral congenital nasolacrimal mucocele. *Pediatr Radiol* 1991; 21:511.
185. Denis D, Saracco JB, Triglia JM. Nasolacrimal duct cysts in congenital dacryocystocele. *Graefes Arch Clin Exp Ophthalmol* 1994;232:252–254.
186. Edmond JC, Keech RV. Congenital nasolacrimal sac mucocele associated with respiratory distress. *J Pediatr Ophthalmol Strabismus* 1991;28:287–289.
187. Grin TR, Mertz JS, Stass-Isern M. Congenital nasolacrimal duct cysts in dacryocystocele. *Ophthalmology* 1991;98:1238–1242.
188. Castillo M, Merten DF, Weissler MC. Bilateral nasolacrimal duct mucocele, a rare cause of respiratory distress: CT findings in two newborns. *Am J Neuroradiol* 1993;14:1011–1013.
189. Mazzara CA, Respler DS, Jahn AF. Neonatal respiratory distress: sequela of bilateral nasolacrimal duct obstruction. *Int J Pediatr Otorhinolaryngol* 1993;25:209–216.
190. Righi PD, Hubbell RN, Lawlor PP Jr. Respiratory distress associated with bilateral nasolacrimal duct cysts. *Int J Pediatr Otorhinolaryngol* 1993;26:199–203.
191. Yee SW, Seibert RW, Bower CM, Glasier CM. Congenital nasolacrimal duct mucocele: a cause of respiratory distress. *Int J Pediatr Otorhinolaryngol* 1994;29:151–158.
192. Usowicz AG, Edabi M, Curry C. Upper airway obstruction with fetal alcohol syndrome. *Am J Dis Child* 1986;140:1039.
193. Tachman ML, Guthrie Jr GP. Hypothyroidism: diversity of presentation. *Endocr Rev* 1984;5:456.
194. Stanjevich JF, Lore Jr JM. Tumors of the nose, paranasal sinuses, and nasopharynx. In: Bluestone CD, Stool SE, eds. *Pediatric Otolaryngology.* 2nd ed. Philadelphia: WB Saunders; 1990:78–792.
195. Lodeiro JG, Feinstein SJ, McLaren RA, Shapiro SL. Antenatal diagnosis of epignathus with neonatal survival. A case report. *J Reprod Med* 1989;34:997–999.

7

The Eyes

Selected elements of a complete eye examination serve to screen most neonates in an initial assessment. A full ophthalmologic evaluation is neither practical nor indicated unless the screening examination shows ocular pathology or the general clinical presentation suggests that a more complete examination would provide specific information. Because of many postnatal changes in the eyes, the adnexa, and their functional control, an appropriate evaluation may be staged over the first several weeks after birth as long as there are no initial indicators of serious pathology. In a premature infant, parts of the evaluations are delayed until that infant has reached at least 32 weeks corrected gestational age for the anterior structures, until 5 to 8 weeks after birth for the retina, until at least 40 to 44 weeks corrected gestational age for assessment of visual awareness, and for several months for visual acuity and interest. Aggressively examining premature eyes before there can be meaningful information is potentially harmful because of both direct damage to the eyes or systemic side effects (1,2). In otherwise healthy term infants who do not give evidence of decreased vision, assessment of visual acuity is delayed until, as young children, they can cooperate to give appropriate responses. Nevertheless, the general physical assessment of each neonate includes an examination of the eyes appropriate to that infant's condition.

The initial screening examinations determine the structural development and the relationship of the eyes to the overall facies, whereas later evaluations more fully assess both motor and sensory functions. Only rarely in neonates are major structural abnormalities of the eyes the exclusive clues to an underlying disorder, although they may suggest a diagnosis of a suspected syndrome or multi-system sequence. Similarly, the absence of pathology does not eliminate a possible diagnosis of a congenital condition in which eye findings are part of the total constellation either because many of these findings are not present or evident in the newborn period or because eye involvement is variable.

The eye examination provides a good opportunity to observe an infant's resting state and his or her ability to transition from one state to another in both stimulated and unstimulated environments. Observations that give information about the infant's general well-being and maturity include apparent awareness of surroundings with visual interest as opposed to abnormal staring or absent visual fixation, the type and extent of response to contact and stimulation, and an ability to self-console when the examination is completed.

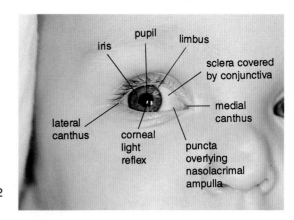

Figure 1. Normal external landmarks of the eye. The light spot at 2 o'clock on the iris is a reflection artifact.

The following steps in the examination appear to be more detailed than indicated for the majority of infants, but most of the steps are quickly combined as part of a cursory examination with observations of normalcy made during general inspection.

NORMAL ANATOMY

The normal ocular anatomy of an infant is illustrated in Fig. 1 (eyes with basic structures) and Fig. 2 (diagram of the globe).

EMBRYOLOGY

The retina arises from the neuroectoderm of the forebrain, the vascular and sclerocorneal layers of the eyeball differentiate from the mesoderm surrounding the developing retina, and the lens develops from the surface ectoderm of the head (Table 1 and Fig. 3) (3,4).

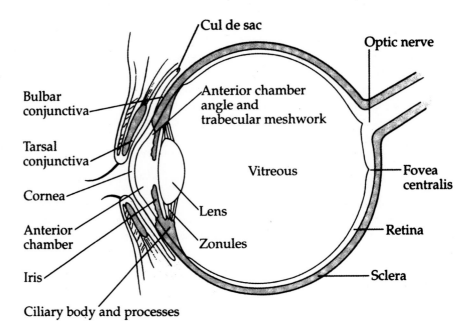

Figure 2. Cross-sectional anatomy of the globe and adnexa. Reprinted with permission (139).

Table 1. *Embryologic and fetal development of the eye*

Timing	Event
22 days	Optic primordia appears in neural fold (1.5–2 mm)
25 days	Optic vesicle evaginates; neural crest cells migrate to surround vesicle
28 days	Vesicle induces lens placode
2nd mo	Invagination of optic and lens vesicles
	Hyaloid artery fills embryonic fissure
	Closure of embryonic fissure begins
	Pigment granules appear in retinal pigment epithelium
	Primordia of lateral rectus and superior oblique grow anteriorly
	Lid folds appear
	Retinal differentiation begins with nuclear and marginal zones
	Migration of retinal cells begins
	Neural crest cells of corneal endothelium migrate centrally
	Corneal stroma follows
	Cavity of lens vesicle is obliterated
	Secondary vitreous surrounds hyaloid system
	Choroidal vasculature develops
	Axons from ganglion cells migrate to optic nerve
	Glial lamina cribrosa forms
	Bruch's membrane appears
3rd mo	Precursors of rods and cones differentiate
	Anterior rim of optic vesicle grows forward, and ciliary body starts to develop
	Sclera condenses
	Vortex veins pierce sclera
	Lid folds meet and fuse
4th mo	Retinal vessels grow into nerve fiber layer near optic disk
	Folds of ciliary processes appear
	Descemet's membrane forms
	Canal of Schlemm appears
	Hyaloid system starts to regress
	Glands and cilia develop in lids
5th mo	Photoreceptors develop inner segments
	Choroidal vessels form layers
	Iris stroma is vascularized
	Lids begin to separate
6th mo	Ganglion cells thicken in macula
	Recurrent arterial branches join the choroidal vessels
	Dilator muscle of iris forms
7th mo	Outer segments of photoreceptors differentiate
	Central fovea starts to thin
	Fibrous lamina cribrosa forms
	Choriodal melanocytes produce pigment
	Circular muscle forms in ciliary body
8th mo	Iris sphincter develops
	Chamber angle completes formation
	Hyaloid system disappears
9th mo	Retinal vessels reach the periphery
	Myelination of fibers of optic nerve is complete to lamina cribrosa
	Pupillary membrane disappears

Reprinted from Torczynski, ref. 3, with permission.

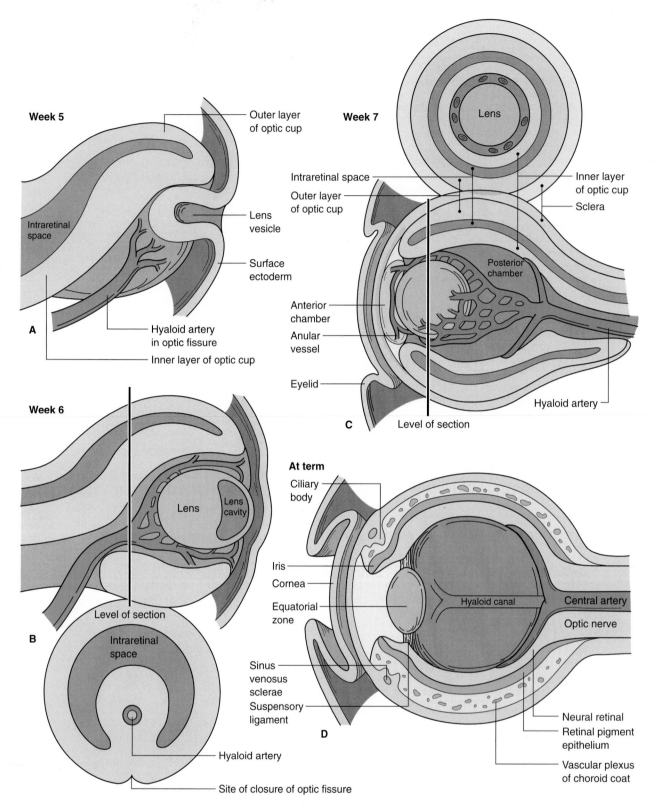

Figure 3. Development of the fetal eye from the fifth week to term (**A–D**). The intraretinal space between the inner (primordium of neural retina) and outer (primordium of the retinal pigment epithelium) layers of the optic cup disappears as the eye develops. Trauma may separate the layers of the retina in this area. The hyaloid artery supplies the developing lens, but most of it disappears. Its proximal part forms the central artery of the retina. The hyaloid canal in the vitreous body indicates the former site of the distal part of the hyaloid artery. Reprinted with permission (4).

EXAMINATION STEPS

The structural items are assessed in the following general order. The evaluation of function intermingles with the structural examination, or it may come at any point earlier in the process of the general physical examination whenever the infant's state is appropriate.

Structure
  Periorbital anatomy
  Spacing and size
  Eyelids, lashes, eyebrows
  Nasolacrimal puncta and duct pathway
  Palpebral fissures
  Conjunctiva
  Sclera
  Anterior segment
    Cornea
    Irides
    Lens
  Funduscopic examination
Function: assessed throughout examination of structure
  Visual acuity
  Pupil reactivity
  Extraocular muscle activity

General Examination Conditions and Technique

Conduct the eye exam in a room that is not brightly lit and where the immediate lights can be dimmed. Before touching the infant, inspect the eyes at rest for as many elements as possible. Next, recognize the infant's state and, if necessary, help him (or her) transition to the quiet alert state that is compatible with spontaneous eye opening. If the infant is deeply asleep, gently raising the lids should either arouse him enough to open his eyes or allow you to examine each eye as it is slowly moving while he continues sleeping. If the infant's state is light sleep or awake and quiet, he may open his eyes with a simple change in position. Gently turn him from side lying to supine, raise his head to an upright sit or held position, or, conversely, if held upright, lower his head. Be careful not to change the position abruptly to induce a Moro reflex or startle. If the infant's state is crying and very active, quiet him by swaddling, stimulating sucking on a pacifier, talking, and holding him.

Be patient in getting the infant to open his eyes spontaneously. If a spontaneous opening cannot be elicited, separate the lids using gauze pads or tissue to cover the fingers of your nondominant hand. If necessary, have an assistant grasp the lids close to their margins at the base of the lashes. Finally, if other findings or history suggest that a more detailed examination is indicated, instill one to two drops of a topical anesthetic such as 0.5% proparacaine hydrochloride (Ophthaine HCl, Squibb Mark, Princeton, NJ) and use self-retaining lid retractors to open the lids.

Forcefully opening the lids may induce Bell's phenomenon so that the anterior structures will not be visible or it may irritate him enough to squirm and cry only to close them tightly. When an infant has marked lid edema or blepharospasm from crying or bright lights, forcefully opening the lids often results in eversion of the upper lid and an even stronger reactive closure. It is prudent to wait until the edema or crying resolves to try again. Infants react so negatively to bright light that the most effective way of getting spontaneous opening is to dim the room lights and to speak comfortingly while holding the swaddled infant in one hand and the penlight or ophthalmoscope in the other.

In a true emergency, when the eyelids are swollen and an immediate examination is important but there are no lid forceps available, bending the rounded end of a paper clip or using a small laryngoscope blade provides makeshift retractors (5). This technique is not recommended because all eye instruments should be smooth and sterile.

Anatomic Position and Measurements

Inspect each eye. Estimate and compare its size to the other eye and in relation to other facial structures. Estimate the position in the vertical axis by viewing the infant en face. Estimate depth and protrusion by viewing in lateral profile and from above. Compare the symmetry of the eyes. Gently palpate the globe if you cannot visualize the eye well enough to assess the size. Measure the various distances and sizes with calipers or a transparent ruler when there appears to be a discrepancy between eyes or as part of an evaluation of unusual facies.

Abnormalities of the eyes:

Position
 Hypotelorism
 Hypertelorism
  Shallow orbits
 Size
  Nanophthalmia
  Microphthalmos
  Microcornea
  Megalocornea
  Buphthalmos
  Prominent supraorbital ridges
 Number
  Anophthalmos
  Cyclopia
  Synophthalmia
  Cryptophthalmia

The globe is approximately 70% and the cornea 80% of its adult size in a baby born at term, so the eyes appear disproportionately large (6). They maintain a relatively constant relationship in size and spacing such that the artists' rule of 1-1-1 applies and allows a simple visual inspection to be sufficient in most cases. Each eye as estimated by the palpebral fissure width and the space between the eyes occupy approximately one third the total distance between the outer canthi. In other words, the space between the inner and outer canthus of one eye approximates the width between the two inner canthi.

Part of the difficulty in determining if the globe is too small lies in the general association of microphthalmia with a small palpebral fissure, inhibiting good direct visualization, and, therefore, measurement of the globe itself. Because the easily measured length of the

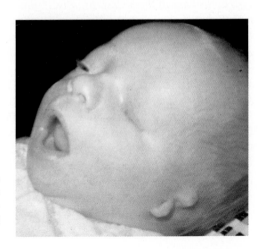

Figure 4. Microphthalmia with blepharophimosis. The right eye is normal although not widely opened in this view. The length of the palpebral fissure normally suggests the size of the globe, but sonography may be needed to determine what eye structure is present. Complete anophthalmia is more often bilateral. Microtia of the left ear is also apparent.

Table 2. *Expected size at term of ocular structures*

Structure (ref.)	Normal size at 40 wk
Palpebral fissure length (7)	
White (8)	18.5 ± 1.3 mm
Oriental (9)	19.4 ± 1.7 cm
Hispanic (10)	19.5 ± 2.0 mm
Black (10)	20.0 ± 2.2 mm
Pupil diameter without mydriasis (11)	3 mm (range 2–4 mm)
Pupil diameter after mydriasis (11)	6.7 mm
Corneal diameter (external diameter of horizontal base)	9.5–10.5 mm
Axial diameter of globe	17 mm
Palpebral area (12)	18 × 12 mm

palpebral fissure approximates the diameter of the globe except in isolated blepharophimosis, a truly short palpebral fissure indicates a need for full evaluation for microphthalmia (Fig. 4). Gentle palpation of the two globes may confirm a significant discrepancy in size, but excessive pressure causes direct trauma or cardiac bradyarrhythmia. Normally, there is a direct correlation between the diameters of the corneas and globe, but each may vary independently. Ultrasonographic measurements of the globe are both accurate and noninvasive and yield interior information as well when there are anterior opacities interfering with visualization. Any suspected deviation from the expected size dictates further evaluation Table 2 lists the expected size at term of ocular structures (7–12). The sizes of various ocular structures at different gestational ages are provided in Appendix (Figs. 15–19).

The presence of telecanthus or epicanthal folds contributes to false impressions of hypertelorism. The interpupillary distance reflects the ocular position along the horizontal plane more so than do the inner and outer canthal distances. In an infant who is not alert or who will not maintain a gaze on a stable object as most newborn infants will not, it is difficult to measure the interpupillary distance. It is easier to measure the distance from a midpoint on the nose to the mid-pupil of one eye at a time with each eye directed forward and then sum the results.

Adnexa

Eyelids
Palpebral fissures
Eyelashes, eyebrows
Nasolacrimal puncta and duct pathway

Inspect the lids for continuity, color and overlying markings, edema or ecchymoses, masses, folds, and position at rest and on movement. Determine the plane of an imaginary line drawn between the inner and outer canthus. Assess the configuration and quantity of the lashes and eyebrows. Locate the puncta on the medial margin of the lower lid. Inspect and palpate the nasolacrimal tract for swelling. Note the presence of epiphoria.

Eyelids and Palpebral Fissures

The anatomy of the eyelids is illustrated in Fig. 5.
Abnormalities of the eyelids:

Position
    Telecanthus
Direction
    Upslanting palpebral fissures
    Downslanting palpebral fissures
Size
    Blepharoptosis, ptosis

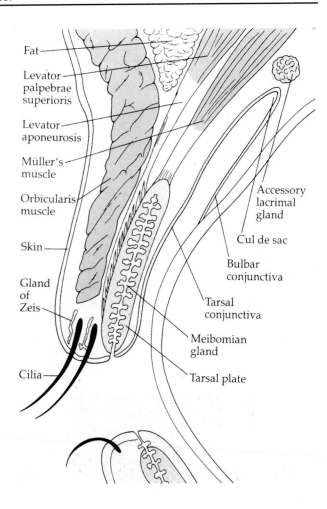

Figure 5. Anatomy of the eyelid. Reprinted with permission (139).

Blepharophimosis
Shape and continuity
   Ectropion
   Ankyloblepharon
   Coloboma
Consistency
   Edema

The upper lid is more curved than the lower lid when opened and should touch the lower lid throughout its margin when closed. There should be no coloboma or irregularities along the margin. Gross ectropion, especially when associated with other lid anomalies such as coloboma, may be detected (see Chapter 5 Fig. 34B for close-up view of harlequin fetus with severe ectropion).

When open, the upper lid of the neonate still covers much of the cornea, so rarely is the superior sclera visible if the eye is in a neutral position. Ptosis is more difficult to define in neonates unless there is unilateral involvement and asymmetry between the eyelids. The lid should open to at least above the mid-point of the pupil with the eye neutrally positioned.

Ecchymoses of the lids commonly indicate either local trauma, particularly when coupled with abrasions or clear forceps marks, or increased venous pressure associated with tight nuchal cords (13). Telangiectasia and simple flame nevus on the lids are common at birth. One of the most frequent causes of discoloration to the eyelids is the tannish brown stain from silver nitrate that develops several hours after application. The color will transfer to a moist pad when rubbed and fades by 2 weeks of age.

The lid has a relatively large potential space created by redundancy of eyelid skin and loose subcutaneous tissues, making it prone to fluid accumulation and distention. If edema is inflammatory, associated signs such as redness, warmth, or exudate will likely be pre-

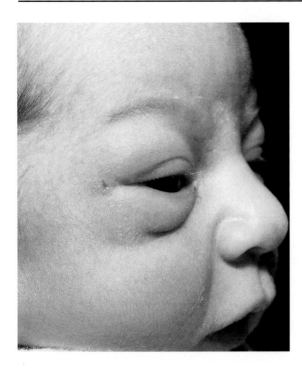

Figure 6. Edema of eyelids secondary to silver nitrate. The edema should resolve within 24 to 48 hours. The small abrasion at the lateral canthus from a forceps application denotes a close enough proximity to the globe to indicate a careful examination for ocular trauma.

sent. Noninflammatory edema indicates trauma, venous obstruction, generalized fluid retention, inadequate lymphatic drainage, or, more likely in older patients, infiltrative tumor (14).

Epicanthal folding, which is a vertical fold of skin on either side of the nose, sometimes covering the inner canthus, is an expected finding in many newborn infants, even when not an expected racial characteristic. It is the result of flattening of the nasal bridge, so it tends to resolve if the nose develops a more prominent shape as an adult. Unilateral epicanthal folding occurs more often ipsilateral to the flattened side in plagiocephaly, but this is not a consistent finding (15).

The slant of the palpebral fissures indicates mid-face architecture that is primarily racially determined. Discordant or accentuated variations are typical of a number of syndromes. If a line connecting the lateral and medial angles is oblique, with the lateral margin more than 2 mm higher than the medial margin, the slant is upward. If the medial margin is higher, it is a downward slanted palpebral fissure (Figs. 7 and 8).

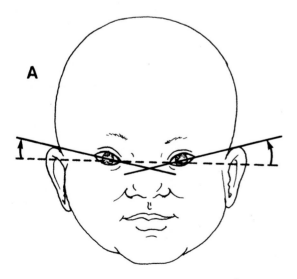
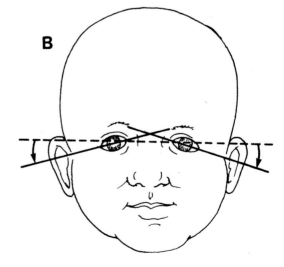

Figure 7. Obliquity of the eye. **A:** Upward slant. **B:** Downward slant.

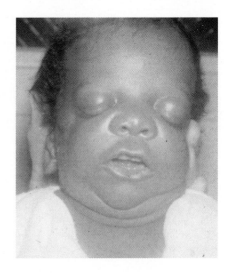

Figure 8. Treacher Collins. Downward slant to eyes is clear, even though the buccal fat pads and the closed, edematous upper lids obscure the canthal landmarks.

Eyelashes and Eyebrows

Abnormalities of the eyelashes and eyebrows:

Absence
  Madarosis
  Localized loss of lashes (especially with coloboma)
  Absent brow hair
Size or number
  Unusually numerous or long lashes
  Distichiasis
Shape of eyebrows
  Synophrys
  Medial flaring
  High arch

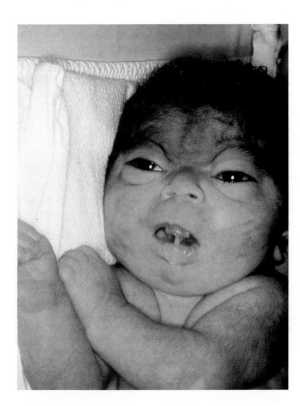

Figure 9. Prominent lashes and brows in de Langes syndrome. The eyes are prominent because of relatively shallow orbits associated with brachycephaly. Associated ocular findings in this syndrome variably include microcornea, coloboma of the optic nerve, astigmatism, myopia, and strabismus. The lashes are long and thick, giving an eyeliner appearance to the lids. The brows extend low to a prominent medial canthus.

The eyebrows are not always well defined at birth and tend to be relatively sparse, particularly in premature infants or if the hair is lightly pigmented. Infants with dark facial hair may seem to have heavy eyebrows, but normal brows should not meet (synophrys) or flare in the mid-line, nor should they have notably high arching (cornelia de lange) (Fig. 9). Normal eyelashes are soft, sparse, and often relatively lightly pigmented but should have a continuous distribution directed away from the globe.

Nasolacrimal Puncta and Duct Pathway

Figure 10 is a diagram of the nasolacrimal system, and Fig. 11 demonstrates an unusually enlarged lacrimal gland.

Disorders of the nasolacrimal drainage system with epiphoria (16):

Atresia of the lacrimal puncta
Congenital mucocele of the lacrimal sac (dacryocele)
Congenital obstruction of the nasolacrimal duct

Term neonates produce normal reflex tears sufficient to keep the eyes lubricated, whereas markedly premature infants may not. Alacrima, or absence of tearing, is almost always a physiologic delay in lacrimation rather than a manifestation of true inability to make tears. Crying rarely produces significant tearing until 2 to 4 months after birth. The initial reaction to silver nitrate for eye prophylaxis temporarily stimulates tearing, often with copious exudate, but this response resolves within 48 hours. Epiphoria after that period is abnormal and represents excess production or, more likely, decreased ability to clear the tears. Look for disorders of the nasolacrimal drainage system as the most likely cause, but also

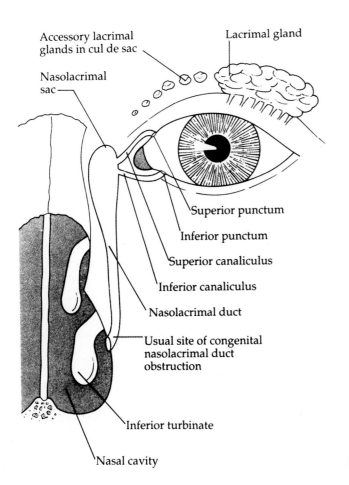

Figure 10. Anatomy of the nasolacrimal system.

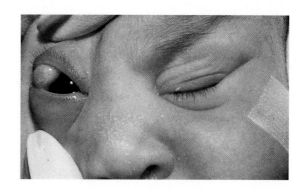

Figure 11. Enlarged lacrimal gland. The swelling in the superior lateral location of the lacrimal gland is apparent. Swelling of this magnitude would indicate dacryoadenitis if inflammatory signs were present. Normal sebaceous hyperplasia of the nose is present.

consider the less common but important causes of infection and glaucoma (16). Excess tearing presents as a moist appearing eye or matting on the eyelids after sleeping. Fluorescein dye placed in the eye should disappear in a few minutes if the nasolacrimal duct is patent (17).

The nasolacrimal duct system is not fully patent right after birth in as many as 73% of term infants but spontaneously opens or remains asymptomatic in all but 6% (18). Atresia of the lacrimal puncta presents with only mild epiphoria compared with more distal obstructions to the duct. The opening of each puncta normally is visible over the medial elevation of the ampulla on both the upper and lower lids. A congenital mucocele, which is an obstruction at both ends of the lacrimal sac, appears as a bluish subcutaneous mass just below the medial palpebral ligament. The blue appearance often leads to their frequent misdiagnoses as a hemangioma. Most dacryoceles are unilateral, with a strong female preponderance (19). Although primarily located outside the nasal passage, more internally located or prolapsed congenital mucoceles are a cause of respiratory distress from airway obstruction (20–24). If the mucocele is within the nasal passage, there may be no visible mass external to the nose, but one would be evident at the level of the internal duct on the inferior turbinate (Table 3) (18).

Obstruction of the nasolacrimal duct is more often at the most distal end at its exit into the nose. Massage of the duct causes regurgitation of tears and mucoid material onto the medial canthal area. Massage also appears to alleviate most obstructions. A recommended technique of massage is initially to exert gentle pressure in the medial canthal area and stroke upward to remove stagnant material (16). Follow this with firm downward pressure over the same medial canthal area and not continuing down the nasal bone. Three to four strokes should be applied several times a day with the purpose of increasing the hydrostatic pressure within the duct to force it open.

Table 3. *Differential diagnosis of dacryocystocele*

Finding	Dacryocystocele	Dacryocystitis	Encephalocele	Hemangioma
Onset	Birth	Neonatal	Birth	Birth
Skin color	Blue–gray	Erythematous	Blue or gray	Violaceous
Palpation	Tense, firm	Warm, indurated	Soft, may be pulsatile	Reducible
Transilluminates	Yes	No	Yes	No
X-ray changes	Rare	No	Yes	No
Aspirate	Serous or mucoid	Mucopurulent	CSF	Blood
Relationship to canthal tendon	Below	Below	Usually above	Varies

Reprinted from Ogawa, ref. 18, with permission.

Conjunctiva and Sclera

Pull the lower lid down and out to inspect its margin and surface for color and smoothness. Evaluate the orbital conjunctiva and sclera for hemorrhage and abnormal color. If it is necessary to examine the upper palpebral conjunctiva and the lid does not evert upon opening, lay the stick of a sterile cotton swab along the upper lid about ¾ to 1 cm from the edge and turn the lid over the stick. Do not press on the globe itself.

The conjunctiva is relatively edematous, hypervascular, and hyperemic in the first few days after birth, but its surface should be smooth. Scleral color is normally white but is bluer with decreasing gestational age because the sclera is thinner. Other causes are listed. Scleral icterus develops more slowly than dermal icterus in the newborn period and indicates higher bilirubin levels than it signals in older patients.

Blue sclera:

Frequent associations
    Extreme prematurity (6)
    Marked myopia (6)
    Hypophosphatasia (25)
    Marshall-Smith syndrome (26)
    Osteogenesis imperfecta syndrome, autosomal recessive (26)
    Robert's syndrome (26)
    Russell-Silver syndrome (26)
Occasional associations
    Ehlers-Danlos syndrome (27)
    Focal dermal hypoplasia (28)
    Hallermann-Streiff syndrome (29)
    Incontinentia pigmenti syndrome (30)
    Marfan's syndrome (31)
    Pseudoxanthoma elasticum (32)
    Trisomy 18 syndrome (33)

Subconjunctival hemorrhages are common, particularly after vaginal delivery, and do not represent ocular trauma unless massive and associated with other findings (13). When present in the limbus, they will resolve more slowly than when in the more peripheral sclera (Fig. 12).

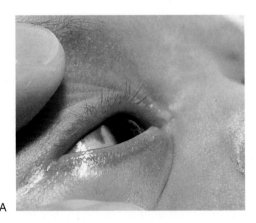
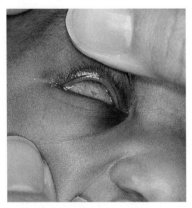

Figure 12. Normal conjunctival findings in newborn eyes. **A:** Small scleral hemorrhage not touching the lateral limbus. There is a double row of upper eyelashes. **B:** Increased vascularity on bulbar conjunctiva normal in the first week and not related to instillation of ophthalmic medication.

Anterior Structures

Use a penlight, ophthalmoscope, or portable slit lamp to illuminate the anterior structures from the side. Look for irregularities in the surface and shape. Assess the color and clarity, size, shape, and position of the individual structures and compare between the eyes. View through the ophthalmoscope at +10 diopters to focus on the anterior structures. In preterm infants assess for the presence and pattern of vessels in the anterior capsule of the lens. (see Chapter 3 Fig. 2).

Elicit the gemini choroidal light reflex (red reflex). Use an ophthalmoscope on its wide beam and hold it at 45 to 50 cm from the infant's face so the circle of light covers both eyes. Adjust the focus wheel to give the most distinct glow in the pupils. Look for symmetry of color, brightness, and position of the reflex. If the pupils are constricted even in a darkened room, dilate the pupils to elicit this response. If the infant will not allow examination of both eyes concurrently, compare the characteristics of the reflex in each eye but recognize that some conditions can be missed when the reflex is not assessed simultaneously.

Abnormalities of the anterior structures:

Shape
  Keratoconus
  Cornea plana
Color of the irides
  Heterochromia of iris
  Nonpigmented iris
  Brushfield's spots
  Pigmented depositions
Color of the pupil
  Leukocoria
Clarity
  Corneal opacity, diffuse or localized
  Sclerocornea
  Presence of vessels in the iris (depends on gestational age)
Absence or malposition
  Aniridia
  Congenital absence of the lens
  Coloboma of iris or lens
  Lens dislocation

The cornea and vitreous are relatively cloudy at birth compared with the appearance a few days later (11). This transient cloudiness affects the whole corneal area and is symmetrical in the two eyes. Additionally, the corneal surface will be smooth (6). Cloudiness may vary within infants of a multiple gestation, with the smaller infants more likely to show the cloudy corneas (6). The corneas of darkly pigmented eyes reflect more light and appear more cloudy than do light eyes. In premature infants of less than 27 weeks gestational age, the corneas and vitreous are especially unclear so that it may be impossible to see through them or to elicit a choroidal light reflex (6). In normal term infants the cloudiness resolves within a few days, and in premature infants it should be resolved by approximately 28 weeks corrected gestational age. Any asymmetric, irregular, or dense cloudiness at term requires further investigation. It is also difficult to elicit the finding in some newborn infants because the pupil is too constricted even in a darkened room. In this case, look for the reflex after mydriasis (11).

A white pupil (leukocoria) is an indication for further evaluation. The white color may be seen either on direct visualization or as an absent red reflex.

Differential diagnosis of leukocoria:

Angiomatosis retinae
Cataracts
Coats disease
Coloboma
Congenital retinal fold
High myopia
Incontinentia pigmenti
Medulloepithelioma
Myelinated nerve fibers
Persistent hyperplastic primary vitreous
Retinal detachment
Retinal dysplasia
Retinoblastoma
Retinopathy of prematurity
Toxocariasis
Uveitis
Vitreous hemorrhage

Iris color is markedly diluted in lightly pigmented infants at birth. Eyes that appear blue should arrive close to their adult color by 6 months, but, if normal, there is always enough pigment to give some color to the iris. In congenital Horner's syndrome, the affected eye remains blue even if the other eye becomes darker. Complete absence of pigmentation allows the choroidal vessels to be seen through the iris, bestowing a red color.

Most conditions characterized by increased pigmentation or deposition of abnormal metabolites in the iris, cornea, or lens are either inapparent or incomplete at the time of birth. Some changes can be seen relatively quickly, such as Brushfield spots in Down's syndrome or Keyser-Fleischer rings in cholestatic jaundice (34). Cataracts of the lens or cornea can also develop within weeks when due to accumulation of metabolic products that deposit only after birth (e.g., in untreated galactosemia). Clearly, repeated examinations to verify clarity of the anterior structures is needed throughout the newborn period and infancy (Figs. 13 and 14).

Differential diagnosis of infantile cataracts:

Infectious: rubella, cytomegalovirus, herpes simplex
Familial: as an isolated family trait, usually autosomal dominant
Metabolic
    Galactosemia: central oil droplet cataract; may be relatively early
    Hypocalcemia: late and prolonged hypocalcemia
Deficiency of Vitamins A and D
Exposure to toxins
Radiation exposure
Trauma
Ocular conditions associated with retinal detachment
Chromosomal defects: trisomies 13, 18, 21

See full list of associations with systemic conditions in the appendix.

Examination of the Fundus

To dilate the pupils, instill one drop of a mild combination mydriatic into the eye. Lift the lower lid to get the drops onto the eye if the fluid accumulates on the lids. Wipe away any excess. Repeat in 30 to 45 minutes if the pupils are not dilated. Provided mydriasis is successful, use local anesthetic drops and a self-retaining lid retractor to effect a good opening if a detailed examination is required. Instill a topical anesthetic such as 0.5% proparacaine hydrochloride (Ophthaine HCl, Squibb Mark, Princeton, NJ).

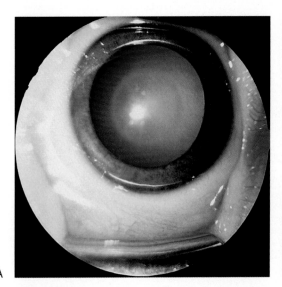
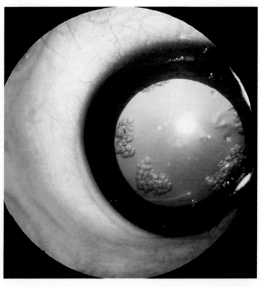

A   B

Figure 13. Cataracts of the lens. **A:** Congenital lamellar cataract. This type of cataract develops late in gestation compared with the nuclear cataracts found in congenital rubella. **B:** The oil droplet cataract of galactosemia is due to accumulation of hyperosmotic dulcitol, which draws water into the lens. This type of change reverses with treatment of the primary metabolic condition.

Assess the fundi for color of the disk, macula, vessels, and peripheral fields. Look at the retinal vessels for direction and extent of development. Note any tortuosity of the vessels, hemorrhages, or exudate.

In the usual examination sequence the function of the eye is assessed before the fundus is examined. It is especially important to assess pupil response and visual attention before mydriasis. When pupil response is abnormal for the gestational age, funduscopy is indicated to assess the ocular media, size and appearance of the optic nerve, and retina. Direct funduscopy does not allow visualization of more than the most posterior segment. For evaluation of retinal vascular development into the periphery, indirect opthalmoscopy is required.

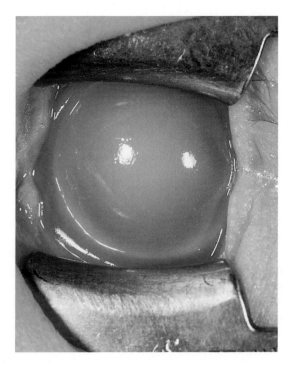

Figure 14. Complete corneal opacity. Immediate evaluation for glaucoma is indicated.

Side effects of funduscopic examination in neonates:

1. Systemic effects of mydriatic agents
   a. Sympathomimetic: hypertension
   b. Parasympatholytic: decreased gastric motility, bowel distention
2. Potential disruption of necessary intensive care equipment
3. Ocular complications
   a. Retinal hemorrhages (especially in retinopathy of prematurity [ROP])
   b. Central artery occlusion (especially during scleral depression)
   c. Conjunctival hemorrhage and chemosis
   d. Oculocardiac reflex (potentially lethal)
4. Increased distress and oxygen consumption from crying, air swallowing, potential for temperature instability

The sympathetic fibers supplying the iris cause dilatation when stimulated. The parasympathetic fibers that are stimulated by light cause constriction. Mydriatic agents need to stimulate the sympathetic function while interfering with the parasympathetic reaction. In neonates it is important to use the lowest effective concentration of agents because the systemic side effects are significant with higher doses. Appropriate solutions would be the parasympatholytic agent 0.2% cyclopentolate (Cyclogyl, Alcon Laboratories, Inc., Fort Worth, TX) and the sympathomimetic agent 1.0% phenylephrine (Neo-Synephrine, Winthrop Consumer Products, New York, NY). These are combined in the proper concentrations as Cyclomydril (Alcon). Higher concentrations of phenylephrine have been reported to increase blood pressure by up to 50% (1). Parasympatholytic agents such as cyclopentolate (0.5%) can inhibit gastric acid volume and concentration and contribute to abdominal distention and slowed motility (2). Infants who are ill and have marginal oxygen saturation may become sufficiently distressed from the examination to require more respiratory support or oxygen. A funduscopic examination with mydriasis should be undertaken in these infants only when there is a strong suspicion of retinal findings that will determine outcome, confirm a suspected diagnosis, or require therapeutic intervention such as multiple system involvement in suspected chronic or opportunistic infections or rapidly progressive ROP.

Droplets of mydriatics on the lashes can make sufficient contact with the tears to be effective. For lightly pigmented infants, one instillation should be enough to cause a dilatation up to 6 mm (11). For darkly pigmented eyes, a second instillation may be necessary. Failure to dilate after appropriate applications of mydriatics is itself a sign of ocular pathology, including advanced ROP and glaucoma.

The color of the optic disk in newborn infants is paler than in adults but is still easily distinguished (6,35). The macula appears as a slightly darker yellow area lateral and below the optic disk. Its color is not as well developed in newborn infants, but there is an expected pattern of development in the last trimester that helps determine its normalcy (36) (Table 4).

It is not possible on direct funduscopy to visualize the more peripheral zones of the retina for the development of the vessels in evaluating maturation or ROP. However, if tortuosity is seen on direct funduscopy, more extensive and immediate evaluation by a pediatric ophthalmologist or retinal specialist is indicated. See Retinopathy of Prematurity below for guidelines in screening and follow-up examinations.

For most examinations on infants after 32 weeks of gestation, a quick view of the fundus enough to see the vessels is possible even without mydriasis if the pupils are sufficiently dilated. The information that can be reliably obtained is similar to that from a properly performed choroidal light reflex, namely, there are no major impediments to sufficient light entering the eye for normal development of vision and the retinal structures.

In some infants it is easier to visualize the fundus directly, albeit briefly, than to elicit a gemini choroidal light reflex. If a more detailed examination is needed or if a choroidal light reflex is not obtained, mydriasis should be used (37).

Retinal hemorrhages occur in 2.5% to 50% of all births, with about one half of these occurring unilaterally. They may be widespread or isolated, are venous in origin, and tend to

Table 4. *Development of the macula in normal preterm infants*

Stage	Gestation (wk)	Observation in macular area
0	31.5 ± 1.5	No pigmentation
1	34.8 ± 1.0	Dark red pigmentation appears
2	34.7 ± 2.4	Annular reflex is partially evident
3	36.3 ± 2.2	Complete annular reflex is present
4	37.6 ± 3.3	Foveolar pit seen with difficulty
5	41.7 ± 4.0	Foveolar light reflex is present

Reprinted from Isenberg, ref. 36, with permission.

resorb within 10 days (38). One study reported the highest frequency after vacuum extraction (50%), only slightly less in spontaneous vaginal deliveries (41%), and the lowest after forceps-assisted deliveries (16%) (39). In a series of eight newborn infants with retinal hemorrhages, there was no demonstrable intracranial pathology on magnetic resonance imaging (38). There is no apparent correlation between the presence of hemorrhages and the umbilical artery pH or Apgar scores (40). Retinal hemorrhages found in association with ROP are not benign but develop after the early newborn period.

Because premature infants have more opportunistic infections than do older children, the incidence of endophthalmitis is high enough to warrant a funduscopic examination in the evaluation of unusual infections. When retinal findings are specific, a presumptive diagnosis can be made (e.g., *Candida* species produce fluffy, white retinal patches). Chronic intrauterine infection involves the retina in variable frequency. The extent and involvement of other ocular structures depend on the timing of infection in relation to oculogenesis as well as to the postnatal age of the infant (41–43) (Table 5).

Table 5. *Retinal findings in congenital infection*

Organism	Typical findings	Expected occurrence
Cytomegalovirus	Necrotizing retinitis with multiple retinal hemorrhages and white exudates Cheese and tomato sauce fundus	23–29%
Herpes simplex	Varies from a few hemorrhages and exudates to massive retinal necrosis with retinal and vitreous exudates	Occurs as only finding or with systemic involvement. True incidence not established
Toxoplasmosis	Necrotizing retinitis that produces large, atrophic retinal scars, especially in the macular area, which may be irregularly pigmented or yellow	80% of cases
Rubella	Unilateral or bilateral presentation of diffuse granular pigmentary changes Salt and pepper fundus	25 to 50% of cases
Syphilis	Chorioretinal atrophy Salt and pepper fundus	Unusual to have significant involvement at birth

Data from Waldstein (41), White (42), and Eller (43).

Table 6. *Functional maturation of the eye*

Age	Description
30 wk gestation	Lid closure in response to bright light
	Pupillary light reaction present
34 wk gestation	Vestibular eye rotations well developed
Birth	Conjugate horizontal gaze well developed
	Cornea 80% of adult diameter
	Eyeball 70% of adult diameter
	Optokinetic nystagmus well developed
	Visual fixation present
1 mo	Ocular alignment stable
	Pupillary light reaction well developed
2 mo	Conjugate vertical gaze well developed
	Fixation well developed
2–5 mo	Blink response to visual threat
3 mo	Visual following well developed
4 mo	Accommodation well developed
	Differentiation of fovea completed
6 mo	Fusional convergence well developed
	Iris stromal pigmentation well developed
	Stereopsis well developed
	Visual evoked potential acuity at adult level
7 mo–2 yr	Myelination of optic nerve completed
1 yr	Cornea 95% of adult diameter

Adapted from Telang, ref. 45 and from Greenwald, ref. 44.

Function

Sensory
  Pupil response
  Optical blink response
  Corneal light reflex
  Visual fixation
  Visual acuity

Extraocular movements
  Rotation
  Doll's eye

It is important to recognize the functional maturation of the eye before looking for certain responses or deciding if there absence is truly abnormal (Table 6) (44,45).

Pupil Response

Elicit the response to light before mydriasis. In a darkened environment, present a bright and sharply focused light from the periphery to avoid reflex closure (optical blink reflex). If there is no response and the pupils are dilated, use a brighter source and repeat the stimulus. Repeat the test to verify that a change in pupil size is a true response and not a random fluctuation. If the pupils are already constricted, delay this evaluation. As an alternative, because the pupillary reactivity to light is poor in the newborn period, partially cover and then uncover one eye to detect a change. Assess the roundness of the pupils, size equality, and amount of constriction to light. If the responses are abnormal, evaluate the ocular media for clarity, the size and appearance of the optic nerve, and the retina.

The direct pupil response demonstrates the intactness of the afferent and efferent pathways of cranial nerve III and implies subcortical visual function. It may remain intact despite cortical blindness. The response may not be present until at least 32 weeks gestational age although it appears as early as 30 weeks (46). Its absence in a more premature infant may correlate with vitreous cloudiness, therefore precluding internal ophthalmoscopic visualization. The extent of pupil response increases with gestational age (47). The diameter of the pupils decreases with advancing gestational age until about 30 weeks (Fig. 15).

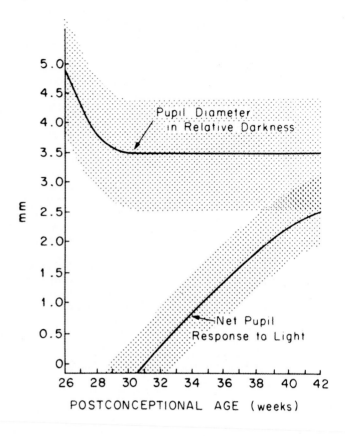

Figure 15. Diameter of pupil (mean ± SD) in term and preterm neonates in relative darkness (<10 foot-candles) and after light stimulation (600 foot-candles). Reprinted with permission (47).

Major pupillary abnormalities and causes in the neonatal period (48):

Bilateral increase in size
    Hypoxic-ischemic encephalopathy (reactive early, unreactive late)
    Intraventricular hemorrhage (unreactive)
    Local anesthetic intoxication (unreactive)
    Infantile botulism (unreactive)
Bilateral decrease in size
    Hypoxic-ischemic encephalopathy
Unilateral decrease in size
    Horner's syndrome (reactive)
Unilateral increase in size
    Convexity subdural hematoma, other unilateral mass (unreactive)
    Congenital third-nerve palsy (± unreactive)
Hypoxic-ischemic encephalopathy (± unreactive)

Optical Blink Reflex

The neonate will demonstrate a brisk optical blink reflex to bright light, indicating at least subcortical function in response to a visual stimulus but will show no protective blink to other stimuli. An absent blink response in an alert infant indicates the need for a more complete evaluation of the ocular media for clarity and of the retina.

Corneal Light Reflex

Stimulate simultaneous fixation of vision on a penlight.

If the reflected light comes from the same point on each cornea, the vision is conjugate and there should be no lens dislocation. The choroidal red reflex can be used in the same way as long as both eyes are opened. The ability of an infant to maintain gaze on even a bright light varies by gestational and chronologic age as well as by level of alertness. The presence of a normal response is reassuring, but the absence of a normal simultaneous corneal light reflex is not abnormal until at least 6 to 8 weeks after birth, or 2 months corrected gestational age in premature infants (49).

Visual Fixation and Maintenance of Gaze

Hold the infant at a distance of approximately 12 inches from your eyes in a plane that allows the infant to view your face without having to elevate his (or her) eyes beyond midline. Alternatively, present a soft light to the infant. Talking softly helps to achieve and maintain visual engagement.

If an infant continues to look at your eyes or the light after blinking, his gaze is maintained. Observing the infant turning his gaze toward a light source such as a window or the overhead lights determines the same supranuclear visual function and is a reassuring observation.

Visual Acuity

The level of visual acuity changes so dramatically during the neonatal period that there is little clinical value in assessing acuity in the first few weeks of life, although there has been extensive clinical research into the subject. It is important to determine that any infant can see, but the finding of a maintained gaze or fixing and following of gaze satisfies that need for the majority of infant examinations. Infants with an increased risk for impaired vision because of congenital or neonatal conditions require a more specific assessment of acuity. There are three methods of estimating acuity: opticokinetic nystagmus (OKN), pattern visual evoked potential (PVEP) (50), and forced choice preferential looking (FCPL) (51). OKN is the easiest and least expensive method that elicits an involuntary response, but a response can be elicited even in the absence of a visual cortex. An estimation of acuity is made by detecting eye movement with progressively smaller stimuli on a rotating drum. PVEP requires expensive equipment and the most technical expertise but minimal patient cooperation because it records and summates electrical responses to rapidly alternating black and white patterns. Acuity is assessed by decreasing the size of each stimulus pattern until no electrical response is measured. There may be some response even in the absence of a normal visual cortex. Expected results throughout infancy have been published (50). FCPL requires full patient cooperation, but the test is easy to administer with well-established norms for term infants for both monocular and binocular vision (51–53). A commercially prepared kit for FCPL is the Teller Acuity Cards set.* In FCPL a grating is presented in one of two sites toward which the infant directs his eyes as long as he detects a pattern. The test administrator who watches the eye movements through a small hole behind the grating is unaware on which side the pattern is and has to detect definite looking in the infant for an objective evaluation. Infant cooperation and a controlled environment are essential in this evaluation.

On each of the tests of visual acuity the results may be abnormal and yet not accurately indicate later vision ability. Similarly, normal acuity and discrimination of grating patterns does not guarantee future normal discrimination of shapes (Table 7) (44,54).

Extraocular Movements

To get an infant to look in a horizontal direction if he (or she) is awake and able to be moved, hold him upright and turn slowly while watching his eye movements. He will look

---

*Teller Acuity Cards is a trademark of the Washington Research Foundation. The systems are distributed by Vistech Consultants, Inc., Dayton, Ohio.

Table 7. *Development of visual acuity in infancy as assessed by various techniques*

Method	Full-term newborn	2 mo	4 mo	6 mo	1 yr	Age at which 20/20 vision is detectable
OKN	20/400	20/400	20/200	20/100	20/60	—
VEP	20/100–20/200	20/80	20/80	20/20–20/40	20/20	6–12 mo
FCPL	20/200–20/400			20/100	20/50	18–24 mo

OKN, opticokinetics; VEP, visual evoked potential; FCPL, forced choice preferential looking.
Reprinted from Traboulsi and Maumenee, ref. 54, with permission.

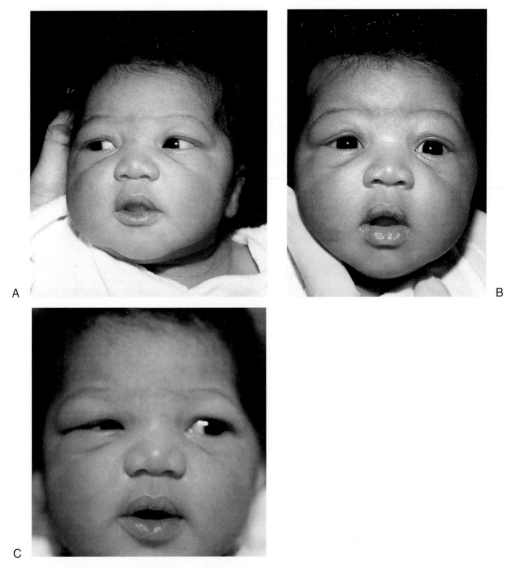

A

B

C

Figure 16. Conjugate eye movements with corneal light reflex in the only cardinal positions likely in the newborn period. **A:** To the right. Right eye moves to the right on contraction of right lateral rectus innervated by the abducens (CN VI) and left eye moves to the right on contraction of the left medial rectus muscles innervated by the oculomotor nerve (CN III, inferior division). **B:** Neutral position, demonstrating a conjugate, maintained gaze. **C:** To the left (left lateral rectus and right medial rectus). Infant is 1 day of age with marked eyelid edema and a difference in palpebral width due to eye prophylaxis with silver nitrate. The edema improved significantly in 24 hours (**A and B**).

CLINICAL EXAMPLES

Neonatal Conjunctivitis (Neonatal Ophthalmia)

Conjunctivitis in the neonatal period is a diffuse conjunctival papillary reaction. Unlike that found in older patients, neonatal conjunctivitis does not include formation of follicles but can involve copious discharge, chemosis, subconjunctival hemorrhages, and eyelid edema, regardless of the pathologic agent (59) (Fig. 17).

Conjunctivitis is the most common neonatal infection, occurring in 1% to 12% of all newborn infants (60). In some developing countries, the incidence is as high as 23% (61). The most common cause of conjunctivitis in developed countries is not infectious, however, with chemical conjunctivitis occurring in at least 90% of infants receiving silver nitrate for prophylaxis. It is thought that the inflammatory reaction incited by silver nitrate is the source of its efficacy (62). A chemical irritation is also seen after prophylaxis with erythromycin or tetracycline as well, although not to the same degree (63). The onset of chemical conjunctivitis should be within 24 hours after instillation and resolve by 48 hours. Conjunctivitis due to chemicals is clinically indistinguishable from that due to infectious agents except for its lack of organisms on Gram stain and culture and spontaneous resolution.

Infectious agents in decreasing order of isolation in the newborn period:

Staphylococcus aureus
Chlamydia trachomatis
Neisseria gonorrhoeae
Haemophilus species
Streptococcus pneumoniae
Enterococcus
Pseudomonas aeruginosa
Herpes simplex

Staphylococcus aureus is the most frequent isolate, but it does not necessarily cause a reaction in all colonized infants. *Chlamydia trachomatis* occurs in approximately 50% of infants born to colonized women with an incidence of 8.2 per 1,000 live births (64,65). Infection is often associated with systemic signs of cough, tachypnea, and respiratory distress due to pneumonia. *Neisseria gonorrhoeae* is associated with the most copious discharge and the greatest risk of corneal perforation and permanent sequelae. The prevalence of chlamydial and gonorrheal conjunctivitis varies widely by country. In Belgium the ratio of gonorrheal to chlamydial ophthalmia approximates 1:1,000; in the United States it is 1:200; in Kenya it is 1:2 (66,67). *Haemophilus* species and *Streptococcus pneumoniae* infections are especially associated with dacryostenosis. *Enterococcus* and *Pseudomonas aeruginosa* occur particularly in premature infants or infants with depressed immunity. Herpes simplex is the most frequent viral agent.

The major complications of neonatal ophthalmia are corneal ulcers, infiltrates, and endophthalmitis (68). A differential diagnosis includes trauma, foreign body, glaucoma, and nasal lacrimal duct obstruction (68).

Retinopathy of Prematurity

Previously called retrolental fibroplasia, ROP is a disease of the retinal blood vessels in which their normal pattern of development is affected by a variety of stimuli, resulting in abnormal proliferation of vessels. In the healing process the findings may completely regress, or permanent and progressive changes may result. The factors that affect the development of ROP are multiple and include high blood oxygen levels, but the essential element is prematurity. The more prematurely born an infant is, the greater the likelihood of developing ROP, even in the absence of supplemental oxygen. Of all infants born at 1,250 g or less, 65.8% develop ROP to some degree; 81.6% of infants weighing less than 1,000 g birth weight develop ROP (69). White infants have a greater likelihood of developing some degree of ROP than do black infants (Fig. 18) (69,70).

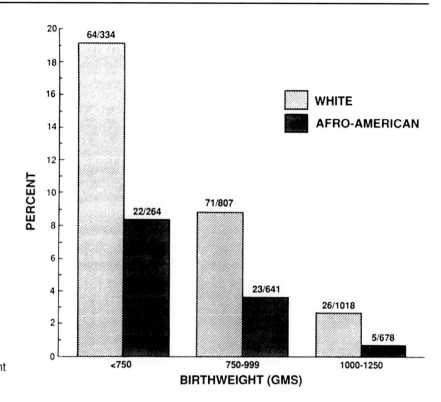

Figure 18. Incidence of ROP by birth weight and race. Reprinted with permission (70).

Pathophysiology

The retinal vessels begin to grow from the region of the optic disk at approximately 16 weeks of gestation and reach the ora serrata in the periphery by 40 to 44 weeks. If development is altered, the vessels are easily obliterated and respond by forming new vessels. The extent of neovascularization defines the severity of the acute process. In due time, as repair progresses, it may be orderly and effect almost complete resolution without sequelae. With disorderly repair, vitreous hemorrhage and scars cause more permanent damage. If these scars retract, detachments and tearing of the retina can develop at any time, especially during the adolescent growth spurt and even into adulthood.

The changes of ROP take several weeks to develop after premature birth so will not be apparent on examination within the actual newborn period. Examining for ROP or normal retinal maturation is an important component of a complete examination in infants at risk for this disease. The criteria for which infants are at risk and when they should be screened as recommended by the American Academy of Pediatrics are listed below, but each infant must be examined until retinal maturity or absent risk of ROP is determined (71).

Criteria for ROP screening examinations (71):

Patient selection
1. Infants born weighing <1,300 g or at <30 weeks' gestation, irrespective of oxygen use.
2. Infants born weighing <1,800 g or at <35 weeks' gestation if they have received oxygen.[†]

Time of first examination
1. 5 to 7 weeks after birth
2. Before discharge home[‡]

[†] It is generally accepted that this means oxygen for a duration longer than that required merely for initial resuscitation.

[‡] When the discharge is before 5 to 7 weeks after birth, a decision has to be made as to the feasibility of an outpatient examination as compared with a predischarge examination that is earlier than recommended. If development of the retinal vessel is complete enough at the time of this examination, later funduscopy may not then be indicated.

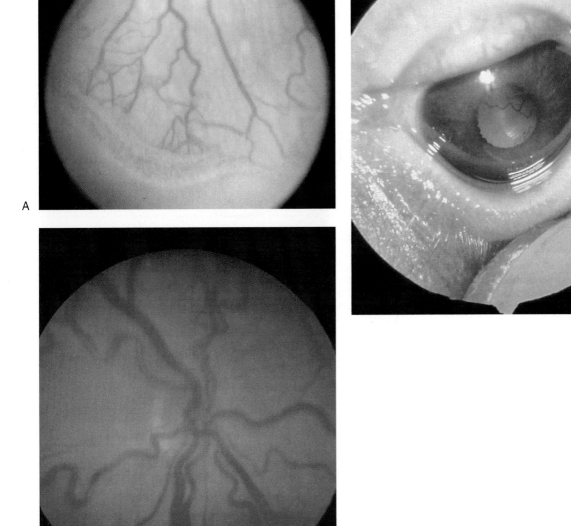

Figure 19. A: ROP on indirect ophthalmoscopy. The dilated and tortuous vessels end in shunts in a ridge of fibrovascular tissue. Beyond the ridge is avascular retina. **B:** Tortuous vessels seen on direct ophthalmoscopy indicating plus disease. **C:** External ocular findings in severe ROP. Dilated and tortuous vessels are visible on the iris. Reprinted with permission (72).

For pediatricians needing an estimation of urgency for retinal evaluation, an examination by direct ophthalmoscopy that detects the presence of vascular tortuosity indicates the need for immediate evaluation by an individual experienced in neonatal ophthalmology and indirect ophthalmoscopy (Fig. 19) (72). If there is no tortuosity seen, there is some leeway in how soon a full eye examination is needed (73).

Guideline for examination of the retina based on initial screening examination (74).

1. If vascularization has proceeded well past the equator of the eye temporally (zone III), if ora can be visualized in the indirect lens field together with the ends of the vessels, and no abnormality is seen at the tips of the developing vessels, there is almost no risk for ROP, so no further examination is needed.
2. If vascularization is at or just beyond the equator (border zones II to III) but without abnormalities visualized at the tips of the vessels, there is only a low risk, but it is prudent to reexamine at 4–6 weeks when vascularization is complete
3. If vascularization has not reached that far, examine biweekly.

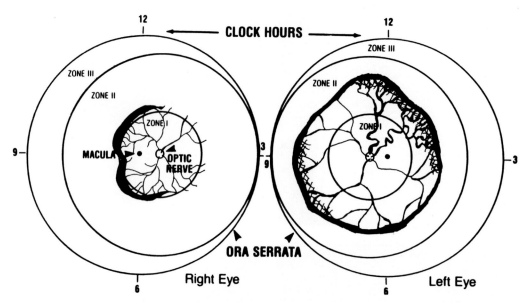

Figure 20. Sketches of ROP of different severity. The right eye demonstrates stage 2 ROP in 6 o'clock hours of zones 1 and 2. The absence of tortuosity indicates no "plus" disease. The left eye shows a mix of stages 2 and 3 over 12 o'clock hours in zone 2. There is "plus" disease in one quadrant indicated by vascular tortuosity. Reprinted with permission (70).

4. If ROP is present, determine location and extent
   a. If changes are anterior to the equator (zone III), plus disease is always absent and an outcome of regression is almost universal.
   b. If disease occupied part or all of the temporal aspect of zone II, examine every 2 to 3 weeks.
   c. If disease is between macula and equator (inner zone II, outer zone I) and for more posterior disease or 12 clock hours in extent, observe weekly.
5. Consult retinal-vitreous specialist for disease posterior to the equator and over more than one half circumference of developing vasculature.

To allow universal communication in describing the changes of ROP, there is a classification that uses a standardized division of the visible retina into zones to denote location and clock hours to code the extent (75). The radii of zones I and II each equal twice the distance from the macula to the optic nerve. Abnormal findings are then divided into stages of progression, so the physical examination would include description of staging in specific zones covering a number of clock hours (Fig. 20).

Definition of retinal zones (73,75):

Zone I: inner zone extending from the optic disk to twice the distance between the disk and the macula or 30° in all directions from the optic disk.

Table 10. *Stages of retinopathy of prematurity*

1	Demarcation line
2	Ridge
3	Ridge with extraretinal fibrovascular proliferation
4	Subtotal retinal detachment
	A. Extrafoveal
	B. Retinal detachment including fovea
5	Total retinal detachment

Funnel:	Anterior	Posterior
	Open	Open
	Narrow	Narrow
	Open	Open
	Narrow	Open

Reprinted with permission, ref. 73.

Table 11. *Ocular findings in regressed retinopathy of prematurity*

Peripheral changes	Posterior changes
Vascular	
1. Failure to vascularize peripheral retina	1. Vascular tortuosity
2. Abnormal, nondichotomous branching of retinal vessels	2. Straightening of blood vessels in temporal arcade
3. Vascular arcades with circumferential interconnection	3. Decrease in angle of insertion of major temporal arcade
4. Telangiectatic vessels	
Retinal	
1. Pigmentary changes	1. Pigmentary changes
2. Thin retina	2. Stretching and folding of retina in macular region leading to periphery
3. Peripheral folds	
4. Vitreous membranes with or without attachmentg to retina	3. Vitreoretinal interface changes
5. Latticelike degeneration	4. Vitreous membrane
6. Retinal breaks	5. Dragging of retina over disk
7. Traction/rhegmatogenous retinal detachment	6. Traction/rhegmatogenous retinal detachment

Data from ref. 73.

Zone II: middle zone extending from the border of zone I to the ora serrata on the nasal side and to the approximate equator on the temporal side.

Zone III: outer zone that extends as a crescent from the outer edge of zone II to the ora serrata on the temporal side.

Table 10 describes the stages of ROP (73,75), and Table 11 lists the ocular findings in regressed ROP (73).

APPENDIX

Eye Findings in Newborn Infants Associated with Multisystem Conditions or Syndromes[§]

Summary findings

Abnormalities in position or size
    Hypotelorism
    Hypertelorism
    Shallow orbits
    Cryptophthalmos
Abnormalities of eyelids
    Telecanthus
    Blepharophimosis
    Upslanting palpebral fissures
    Downslanting palpebral fissures
    Lid colobomas
    Ectropion
Abnormalities of eyebrows and eyelashes
Abnormalities of size of eye parts
    Microphthalmia, colobomatous
    Microphthalmos, noncolobomatous
    Microcornea
    Megalocornea
Glaucoma

[§] Modified with permission (76).

Abnormalities of the iris
    Colobomas of the iris
    Iris, unusual color or structure
    Heterochromia
Lens opacity

Hypotelorism

Frequent associations
    Down's syndrome (33)
    Holoprosencephaly sequence (77)
    Maternal phenylketonuria fetal effects (26)
    Trisomy 13 syndrome (33)
    Trisomy 20p syndrome (78)
    5p+ syndrome (33)

Occasional associations
    Cockayne's syndrome (79)
    Coffin-Siris syndrome (26)
    Goldenhar's syndrome (80)
    Meckel-Gruber syndrome (81)
    Oculodentodigital syndrome (82)
    Williams' syndrome (83)
    Ring 22 syndrome (33)
    18p− syndrome (33)

Hypertelorism

Frequent associations
    Aarskog's syndrome (84)
    Acrocollosal syndrome (85)
    Acrodysostosis syndrome (85)
    Apert's syndrome (26)
    BBB syndrome (86)
    Cat-eye syndrome (33)
    Cleft lip and palate sequence (26)
    Clefting, ectropion, and conical teeth syndrome (85)
    Coffin-Lowry syndrome (87)
    Craniometaphyseal dysplasia (85)
    DiGeorge sequence (26)
    Dubowitz's syndrome (88)
    Fetal aminopterin effects (26)
    Fetal hydantoin effects (26)
    Frontonasal dysplasia sequence (26)
    Larsen's syndrome (26)
    Meckel-Gruber syndrome (81)
    Melnick-Needles syndrome (89)
    Multiple lentigines syndrome (leopard syndrome) (90)
    Noonan's syndrome (91)
    Otopalatatodigital syndrome (Taybi syndrome) (26)
    Pena-Shokeir type 1 syndrome (26)
    Pfeiffer syndrome (26)
    Primary hypertelorism (92)
    Pyle syndrome (26)
    Rieger's syndrome (93)
    Robert's syndrome (pseudothalidomide syndrome) (26)
    Robinow's syndrome (fetal face syndrome) (26)
    Saethre-Chotzen syndrome (acrocephalosyndactyly, type III) (26)
    Sotos' syndrome (26)
    Trimethylaminuria (94)
    Triploidy syndrome (26)

Trisomy 8 syndrome (95)
Trisomy 9p syndrome (33)
Weaver syndrome (26)
Whistling face syndrome (85)
XXXX syndrome (33)
4p− syndrome (Wolf syndrome) (33)
5p− syndrome (cri du chat syndrome) (33)
9p− syndrome (33)
13q− syndrome (33)

Occasional associations
Basal cell nevus syndrome (96)
Camptomelic dysplasia syndrome (26)
Cleidocranial dysostosis syndrome (26)
Conradi-Hünermann syndrome (97)
Crouzon's syndrome (98)
Cryptophthalmos syndrome (26)
Holt-Oram syndrome (26)
Hurler's syndrome (26)
Oculodentodigital syndrome (82)
Sjögren-Larsson syndrome (26)
Williams' syndrome (83)
XXXXX syndrome (33)
XXXXY syndrome (33)
5p− syndrome (cri du chat syndrome) (33)
10q+ syndrome (33)
18p− syndrome (33)
18q− syndrome (33)

Shallow orbits
Frequent associations
Apert's syndrome (26)
Carpenter's syndrome (99)
Crouzon's syndrome (98)
Dubowitz's syndrome (88)
Familial hypoplasia of orbital margin (85)
Fetal aminopterin effects (26)
Marshall-Smith syndrome (26)
Melnick-Needles syndrome (89)
Osteogenesis imperfecta syndrome, autosomal recessive (100)
Robert syndrome (pseudothalidomide syndrome) (26)
Saethre-Chotzen syndrome (26)
Trisomy 18 syndrome (33)
Zellweger's syndrome (26)
9p− syndrome (33)

Occasional associations
Kleeblattschädel syndrome (85)
Trisomy 13 syndrome (33)
6q+ syndrome (33)

Cryptophthalmos
Associated conditions
Ankyloblepharon, cleft lip and palate (26)
CHANDS (curly hair, ankyloblepharon, nail dysplasia) syndrome (85)
Hay-Wells ectodermal dysplasia (26)
Popliteal pterygium syndrome (85)

Telecanthus
Frequent associations
Aarskog's syndrome (84)

Blepharonasofacial syndrome (101)
Camptomelic dysplasia (26)
Carpenter's syndrome (26,99)
Dubowitz's syndrome (88)
Facio-oculoacousticorenal syndrome (FOAR syndrome) (102)
Fetal alcohol effects (26)
Frontonasal dysplasia sequence (26)
KBG syndrome (103)
Oculodentodigital syndrome (82)
Orofaciodigital (OFD) type I and type II (Mohr's syndrome) (104)
Trisomy 18 syndrome (33)
Waardenburg's syndrome (105)
Williams' syndrome (83)
5p− syndrome (33)
Occasional associations
Basal cell nevus syndrome (96)
4p+ syndrome (33)
6p+ syndrome (33)

Blepharophimosis
Associated conditions
Blepharophimosis amenorrhea syndrome (106)
Clefting syndrome with anterior chamber and lid anomalies (107)
Dubowitz's syndrome (88)
Marden-Walker syndrome (85)
Oculopalatoskeletal syndrome (85)
Pena-Shokeir type II syndrome (108)
Schwartz syndrome (109)
10q+ syndrome (33)
3p− syndrome (33)

Upslanting palpebral fissures
Frequent associations
Down's syndrome (33)
Femoral-facial syndrome (26)
Jarcho-Levin syndrome (26)
Miller-Dieker syndrome (lissencephaly syndrome) (110)
Oto-palato-digital syndrome (26)
Pfeiffer's syndrome (26)
Rhizomelic chondrodysplasia punctata syndrome (97)
Trisomy 9 mosaic and 9p− syndromes (33)
Trisomy 20p syndrome (78)
XXXXX syndrome (33)
XXXXY syndrome (33)
4p+ syndrome (33)
5p+ syndrome (33)
Occasional associations
Fetal hydantoin effects (26)
Prader-Willi syndrome (33)
Trisomy 13 syndrome (33)
Trisomy 18 and 18q syndromes (33)

Downslanting palpebral fissures
Frequent associations
Aarskog's syndrome (84)
Apert's syndrome (26)
Coffin-Lowry syndrome (26)
Cohen's syndrome (111)

Conradi-Hünermann syndrome (97)
DiGeorge sequence (26)
Maxillofacial dystocias (85)
Nager's syndrome (112)
Rubenstein-Taybi syndrome (113)
Saethre-Chotzen syndrome (26)
Sotos' syndrome (26)
Treacher Collins syndrome (26)
Trisomy 9p syndrome (33)
Occasional associations
Cat-eye syndrome (33)
Hallermann-Streiff syndrome (29)
Ruvalcaba's syndrome (114)
4q+ syndrome (33)
21q− syndrome (33)

Lid colobomas
Association with lower lid lesion
Crouzon's syndrome (98)
Facial clefting syndrome (Tessier's syndrome, types 3 and 4) (85,115)
Linear sebaceous nevus sequence (116)
Miller's syndrome (112)
Nager's syndrome (112)
Palpebral colobomalipoma syndrome (85)
Treacher Collins syndrome (26)
Frontonasal dysplasia sequence (26)
Associated with upper lid lesion
Amniotic band syndrome (26)
Frontofacionasal dysplasia (85)
Goldenhar's syndrome (80)
Linear sebaceous nevus sequence (116)

Ectropion
Associated conditions
Down's syndrome
Ectropion and distichiasis (85)
Facial clefting syndromes (no. 3 and 4 of Terrier's syndrome) (85,115)
Miller's syndrome (112)
Robinow's syndrome (26)
Sjögren-Larrson syndrome (26)
Harlequin fetus
Colloidin infant

Eyebrow abnormalities
Synophrys (eyebrows extending to mid-line)
Frequent associations
Coffin-Siris syndrome (26)
Congenital hypertrichosis (85)
de Lange's syndrome (26)
Fetal trimethadione effects (26)
Trisomy 4p syndrome (33)
Waardenburg's syndrome (105)
3q+ syndrome (33)
Occasional associations
Basal cell nevus syndrome (96)
Blepharophimosis-amenorrhea syndrome (106)
Trisomy 13 syndrome (33)
4p+ syndrome (33)

Flaring of nasal part of eyebrow

Associated conditions

    Blepharophimosis-amenorrhea syndrome (106)

    Partial trisomy 10q syndrome (33)

    Waardenburg's syndrome (26)

    Williams' syndrome (83)

High arched brow

Associated conditions

    Kabuki makeup syndrome (117)

    Shprintzen-Goldberg syndrome (85)

Absent brow hair

Associated conditions

    Cryptophthalmos

    Pseudoprogeria syndrome (85)

Abnormal eyelashes

    Madarosis

Associated conditions

    Acrodermatitis enteropathica (85)

    Congenital atrichia (118)

    Ectodermal dysplasia (118)

    Ehlers-Danlos syndrome, unspecified type (85)

    Generalized hypotrichosis (118)

    Hypomelia, hypotrichosis, facial hemangioma (118)

    Isolated madarosis (118)

    Keratosis follicularis spinula decalvans (32)

    Pseudoprogeria syndrome (85)

Localized loss of lashes

Associated conditions

    Cryptophthalmos

    Lid colobomas

    Unusual numerous or long lashes

Associated conditions

    Blepharophimosis-amenorrhea syndrome (106)

    de Lange syndrome (85)

    Schwartz syndrome (109)

    Trichomegaly

Extra rows of lashes (see madarosis, above)

Associated conditions

    Anodontia-hypotrichosis syndrome (85)

    Distichiasis, lymphedema syndrome (85)

    Ectropion and distichiasis (85)

    Tristichiasis (85)

Microphthalmia, colobomatous

Frequent associations

    Cat-eye syndrome (26,33)

    CHARGE (coloboma, heart anomaly, choanal atresia, retardation, genital and ear abnormalities) association (85)

    Cohen's syndrome (111)

    Facial clefting syndromes (85,115)

    Focal dermal hypoplasia (Goltz syndrome) (28)

    Hepatic fibrosis, polycystic kidneys, colobomas, and encephalopathy (119)

    Lenz's syndrome (119)

    Meckel-Gruber syndrome (81)

    Sjögren-Larsson syndrome (119)

    Triploidy syndrome (26)

    Trisomy 13 syndrome (33)

Warburg's syndrome (120)
3q+ syndrome (33)
4p− syndrome (33)
4p+ syndrome (33)
13q− syndrome (33)
Occasional associations
Basal cell nevus syndrome (96)
Congenital contractural arachnodactyly (119)
Humeroradial synostosis (119)
Linear sebaceous nevus sequence (116)
Rubinstein-Taybi syndrome (113)
Treacher Collins syndrome (26)
Many chromosomal defects (33)

Microphthalmos noncolobomatous

Frequent associations
Cross syndrome (119)
Fetal rubella effects (26)
Frontonasal dysplasia sequence (26)
Gorlin-Chaudhry-Moss syndrome (118)
Hallermann-Streiff syndrome (29)
Pena-Shokeir type II syndrome (COFS syndrome) (108)
Warburg's syndrome (120)
Occasional associations
Aicardi's syndrome (121)
Fanconi pancytopenia syndrome (26)
Fetal alcohol effects (26)
Fetal varicella effects (26)
Goldenhar's syndrome (80)
Hyperthermia-induced defects (26)
Hypomelanosis of Ito (122)
Maternal phenylketonuria fetal effects (26)
Oculodentodigital syndrome (82)
Ring B syndrome (33)
Treacher Collins syndrome (26)
Trisomy 9 syndrome (33)
10q+ syndrome (33)

Abnormalities in corneal diameter

Microcornea

Associated conditions
Aniridia (123)
Cataract-microcornea syndrome (124)
Deafness, retardation, arched palate syndrome (123)
Microcornea, glaucoma, absent frontal sinuses (85)
Oculodentodigital dysplasia (82)
Oculocerebrofacial syndrome (85)
Ring 7 chromosome (123)
Trisomy 18 syndrome (33)
18q− syndrome (33)

Megalocornea

Associated conditions
Down's syndrome (33)
Facial hemiatrophy (123)
Isolated megalocornea (123)
Marfan's syndrome (31,123)
Megalocornea, mental retardation syndrome (Neuhauser's syndrome) (85)

Glaucoma
Frequent associations
    Aniridia (125)
    Cicatricial ROP (126)
    Lowe's syndrome (125)
    Cataract-microcornea syndrome (85,124,125)
    Microphthalmos
    Nevus of Ota (hyperpigmentation of lids and ocular layers) (125)
    Peters' anomaly
    Rieger's syndrome
    Stickler's syndrome (127)
    Sturge-Weber sequence (128)
    Sulfite oxidase deficiency (125)
    Trisomy 13 syndrome (33)
    Weill-Marchesani syndrome (70)
    3q+ syndrome (33)
    18q− syndrome (33)
Occasional associations
    Basal cell nevus syndrome (96)
    C syndrome (118)
    Down's syndrome
    Ectopia lentis
    Ehlers-Danlos syndrome (27)
    Fetal rubella effects (26)
    Goldenhar syndrome (80)
    Hallermann-Streiff syndrome (29)
    Homocystinuria syndrome (127)
    Klippel-Trenaunay-Weber syndrome (26)
    Marfan's syndrome (31)
    Mucopolysaccharidoses (125)
    Neurofibromatosis syndrome (125)
    Oculodentodigital syndrome (82)
    Robinow's (fetal face) syndrome (26)
    Scheie's syndrome (26)
    Treacher Collins syndrome (26)
    Turner syndrome (125)
    von Hippel-Lindau disease (125)
    Zellweger's syndrome (26)

Abnormalities of the iris

Colobomas of the iris
    Frequent associations (frequent in)
        Acroreno-ocular syndrome (85)
        Biemond's syndrome, type II (85)
        Cat-eye syndrome (26)
        CHARGE association (85)
        Rieger's syndrome(93)
    Occasional associations
        Aniridia (93)
        Langer-Giedion syndrome (85)
        Joubert's syndrome (85)

Iris, unusual color or structure
    Associated conditions
        Albinism (32)
        Aniridia (26,85)
        Anisocoria (85)
        Down's syndrome (33)

Ectopic pupils
Iris cleavage syndrome (85)
Microcoria (85)
Nail-patella syndrome (osteo-onychodysplasia) (129)
Neurofibromatosis (130)
Rieger's syndrome (93)
Spastic ataxia, microcoria (85)
Synechiae
William's syndrome (83)

Heterochromia

Associated conditions

Congenital Horner's syndrome (85)
Hypomelanosis of Ito (122)
Incontinentia pigmenti (30)
Waardenburg's syndrome (85)

Lens opacity

Frequent associations

Alport's syndrome (131)
Aniridia (85)
Cataract and congenital ichthyosis (85)
Cataract-cardiomyopathy syndrome (132)
Cataract-microcephaly, kyphosis (85)
Cataract-microcornea syndrome (85)
Cataract, microphthalmos, nystagmus (85)
Cockayne's syndrome (79)
Conradi-Hünermann syndrome (97)
Crome's syndrome (85)
Fetal rubella effects (26)
Hallermann-Streiff syndrome (29)
Isolated hereditary congenital cataracts (133)
Lowe's syndrome (133)
Mannosidosis (133)
Marinesco-Sjögren syndrome (26)
Marshall's syndrome (26)
Martsolf's syndrome (85)
Pena-Shokeir type II syndrome (108)
Rhizomelic chondrodysplasia punctata syndrome (97)
Rothmund-Thomson syndrome (124)
Schafer'r syndrome (124)
Smith-Lemli-Opitz syndrome (134)
Steinert myotonic dystrophy syndrome (26)
Stickler syndrome (Wagner syndrome) (127)
5p− syndrome (33)

Occasional associations

Abetalipoproteinemia (135)
Albright hereditary osteodystrophy (26)
Basal cell nevus syndrome (96)
Cockayne's syndrome (79)
Down's syndrome (33)
Fetal alcohol effects (26)
Karsch-Neugebauer syndrome (136)
Multiple sulfatase deficiency (137)
Fetal varicella effects (26)
Galactosemia (26)
Homocystinuria (26)
Incontinentia pigmenti (30)

Nail-patella syndrome (129)
Pachyonychia congenita syndrome (26)
Partial trisomy 10q syndrome (33)
Progeria syndrome (26)
Robert's syndrome (26)
Rubinstein-Taybe syndrome (113)
Schwartz's syndrome (109)
Smith-Lemli-Opitz syndrome (134)
Trisomy 13 syndrome (33)
Trisomy 18 syndrome (33)
Trisomy 20p syndrome (78)
Zellweger's syndrome (26)
3q+ syndrome (33)
4-0 syndrome (33)
18p− syndrome (33)
18q− syndrome (33)

GLOSSARY

Absence of the lens, congenital   A condition due either to failure of lens vesicle formation or to degeneration after the vesicle develops. It is associated with microphthalmos and coloboma.

Amblyopia   Loss of vision resulting from an obstruction in the line of sight or from suppression of vision in one eye to avoid diplopia.

Aniridia   Hypoplasia rather than aplasia of the iris. It appears as an absence of a portion of the iris and an enlarged, asymmetric red reflex. Aniridia predisposes to development of secondary congenital glaucoma, congenital cataract, and macular aplasia, and is associated with increased risk of a Wilms' tumor (nephroblastoma). It occurs sporadically or as an autosomal-dominant disorder.

Ankyloblepharon   Adhesion of the ciliary edges of the eyelid to each other. This occurs as single threads of attachment or complete fusion of the lids.

Anophthalmos   Usually a bilateral condition resulting from either failure or optic vesicle development or regression after initiation of vesicle development.

Anterior chamber cleavage syndrome   Incomplete separation between the cornea, lens, and iris, causing distortion of anterior chamber architecture and the filtration angle apparatus.

Axenfeld's anomaly   Refers to persistence of strands or iris processes extending peripherally toward a prominent Schwalbe's line (the peripheral termination of Descemet's membrane; also referred to as posterior embryotoxon). Not usually associated with congenital glaucoma but may develop during infancy (138).

Bell's phenomenon   The normal tendency of the eye to move out and up with forceful retraction of the lid or during sleep.

Blepharitis   Inflammation of the eyelids.

Blepharophimosis   Narrowness of the palpebral fissures in the horizontal direction, generally caused by a lateral displacement of the inner canthi.

Blepharophimosis syndrome   An association of ptosis, inferior epicanthal folds, and blepharoptosis that is autosomally dominant with variable expressivity.

Blepharoptosis   Synonym *Ptosis.* Unilateral or bilateral decrease in the vertical distance between the upper and lower lids, usually due to dysfunction of the levator muscle. It may be transmitted as an autosomal-dominant condition or caused by third-nerve palsy (e.g., congenital Horner's syndrome or myotonia congenita), trauma, or chronic inflammation of the lid or anterior segment of the eye. Congenital blepharoptosis is more often unilateral. Normally, the open lid rests just below the superior limbus during maintained gaze but its position is racially and individually variable.

Blepharospasm   Uncontrollable closure of the eyelids resulting from spasm of the orbicularis oculi muscles.

Brushfield's spots   A speckled appearance due to tiny areas of normal iris surrounded by rings of mild hypoplasia on the surface of the iris just medial to the corneoscleral limbus. Occur in 75% of infants with Down's syndrome but also in normal as well. Not always visible at birth.

Buphthalmos   Enlargement of globe, especially as seen in glaucoma.

Cardinal gaze   Position of eyes from action of single muscle use.

Cataracts   A nonspecific reaction to altered lens metabolism. Diverse conditions can cause similar cataracts. Because the lens is avascular, it depends primarily on anaerobic pathways to generate energy for the constantly dividing epithelial cells of the lens. Any process that interferes with glycolysis or mitosis can produce a cataract. The outer cells (cortex) of the lens are the newest, with the older nuclear lens cells being those laid down in earliest fetal life. Twenty-five percent of congenital cataracts are autosomal dominant. Congenital cataracts may occur in isolation or associated with other intraocular anomalies (e.g., aniridia, persistent hyperplastic primary vitreous, vitreoretinal disease) or with congenital infections and trisomy 21.

Chalazion   Chronic granulomatous inflammation of the eyelid meibomian glands developing away from the lid margins. This is not seen in neonates.

Chemosis   Excessive edema of the ocular conjunctiva.

Coloboma   Cleft-shaped fissure representing incomplete embryologic closure in the eyelid, iris, ciliary body, retina, choroid, or optic nerve, isolated or in combination as part of continuum to anophthalmia. The majority are sporadic, but there is an increased incidence with trisomy 13 or as a result of maternal ingestion of LSD or thalidomide. Familial colobomas are autosomal dominant.

Coloboma, atypical   Cleft-shaped defect occurring in any eye quadrant other than inferior nasal quadrant. It is usually restricted to the iris. Associated with persistence of anterior hyaloid vessels and pupillary membrane.

Coloboma, typical   Persistence of a cleft-shaped fissure on the inferonasal aspect of the eye, resulting from incomplete fusion of the fetal fissure during the 6th week of development. Looks like a keyhole of iris.

Corectopia   Pupil is significantly off center.

Corneal dystrophy, hereditary congenital   Corneal clouding is present from birth due to edema of basal layer of epithelium, subepithelial fibrosis, reduction of the thickness of Bowman's membrane, and central attenuation of the endothelial cell density (138).

Cryptophthalmos   Synonym *Ankyloblepharon totale* (covered eye). Failure of eyelid separation resulting in absence of fissure and eyelashes, with resultant external absence of eye development, uni- or bilateral; frequently associated with other anomalies, particularly in the kidneys. May have a variety of underlying ocular malformations or, more rarely, a normal orbit.

Cyclopia   Consequence of anomalous development of a single optic vesicle. Single orbital fossa, with the globe absent or rudimentary, apparently normal, or duplicated, and the nose absent or present as a tubular appendage located above the orbit.

Dermoid, corneal   Hamartomas arising due to arrested migration of ectoderm at the corneoscleral junction (limbus), most commonly on the temporal aspect. Corneal dermoids are a feature of Goldenhar's syndrome.

Dextroversion   Eye movement to the right.

Districhiasis   Double row of eyelashes with an accessory row along the posterior border of the eyelid. It is a sequela of severe inflammation or is an autosomally dominant condition.

Duane's syndrome   Retraction of the globe on attempted adduction.

Dystopia canthorum   Synonym *Hypertropia*. Widely spaced eyes; increased distance between middle canthi.

Ectopia lentis   Dislocation or subluxation of the lens resulting from zonular rupture. Causes secondary glaucoma. Associated with hyperlysinemia, sulfite oxidase deficiency, homocystinuria, buphthalmos, and Marfan's, Weill-Marchesani, and Ehlers-Danlos syndromes.

Ectropion Eversion of the eyelid margin, which creates a pool of stagnant tears and does not allow protection of the cornea and conjunctiva. The exposed tarsal conjunctiva is susceptible to repeated trauma. This may develop after facial nerve paralysis.

Endophthalmitis Inflammation involving the ocular cavities and their adjacent structures.

Entropion Inversion of eyelid margins, resulting in contact of the eyelashes with the corneal and conjunctival surfaces, with subsequent irritation and scarring. Congenital entropion is uncommon and usually resolves spontaneously without damage because the soft lashes in neonates generally do not cause irritation. Cicatricial entropion results as scarring pulls the lid inward and is common after chronic *Chlamydia trachomatis* conjunctivitis.

Epiblepharon A single row of lashes rotated against the surface of the globe. This is relatively common in especially plump neonates because the facial tissue pushes the medial third of the eyelid upward, rotating the lashes toward the eye. It resolves spontaneously, usually without irritation.

Epicanthal fold Synonyms *Epicanthic fold, palpebronasal fold.* A vertical fold of skin on either side to the nose, sometimes covering the inner canthus.

Epiphoria Excess tearing due to either increased production or decreased tear outflow.

Epiphoria due to decreased drainage Functional or anatomic block in nasolacrimal drainage system between the punctum and the ostium of the nasolacrimal duct under the inferior meatus of the nose.

Epiphoria due to hypersecretion Indicates ocular inflammation or congenital glaucoma.

Eso- and exo- Prefixes used with tropia and phoria to denote horizontal deviations.

Esophoria Deviation of the visual axis of an eye toward that of the other eye in the absence of visual fusional stimulation.

Esotropia Deviation of the visual axis of an eye toward that of the other eye.

Exophoria Deviation of the visual axis of an eye away from that of the other eye after the visual fusional stimuli have been eliminated.

Exophthalmos Synonym *Proptosis.* Denotes abnormal anterior displacement of the eye and requires inspection from above as well as laterally to detect asymmetry. Graves' disease is the most frequent cause in children.

Exotropia Deviation of the visual axis of an eye away from that of the other eye.

Falciform retinal fold, congenital A fold of retina extends from the optic nerve head anteriorly toward the ciliary body, most commonly in the inferior temporal quadrant. This may be associated with remnants of hyaloid vessels.

Fluorescein disappearance test Fluorescein placed in the eye sulcus is cleared through the nasolacrimal duct system. Failure to disappear within a few minutes after instillation suggests obstruction to this system (17).

Glaucoma, primary congenital (PCG) Increased pressure at birth or in neonatal period due to structural abnormalities that impede the flow of aqueous humor. Both eyes are affected, presenting with photophobia, lacrimation, buphthalmos, and eye rubbing. Usually autosomal recessive with male predominance. Incidence is one in 10,000 live births. Structural abnormalities predisposing to PCG include microcornea, abnormal anterior chamber angel cleavage, Barkan's membrane (a mesodermal membrane covering and occluding the drainage angels), and insertion of persistent fetal iris processes above the scleral spur (138).

Glaucoma, secondary congenital Increased pressure presents after the neonatal period. Causes: rubella, aniridia, Lowe's syndrome, Sturge-Weber syndrome, mesodermal dysgenesis syndrome (Peter's anomaly and Reiger's syndrome), persistent hyperplastic primary vitreous, and retinopathy of prematurity (ROP) (138).

Heterochromia Difference in color of the two irides or in different areas on one iris.

Hordeolum An acute infection of eyelid glands and hair follicles. Self-limited, responds to heat and antibiotics.

Hordeolum, external Infection involving the sweat glands and hair follicles (sty); occurs on the surface of the skin at the edge of the lid.

Hordeolum, internal   Infection involving the meibomian (oil) glands; marked by swelling on the conjunctival surface of the lid.

Hyaloid vascular structure   Seen as a gray stalk behind the pupillary membrane. May remain visible until 32 weeks' gestational age.

Hyperopia   Synonym *Hypermetropia.* Farsightedness. Most common refraction error in infants. Marked hyperopia is associated with smaller eyes.

Hypertelorism   Increased separation between the bony orbits.

Hypotelorism   Decreased separation of the orbits as determined by smaller than expected pupillary distance. Most accurately measured by radiograph of orbits or computed tomography.

Incyclo- and excyclo-   Prefixes used with tropia and phoria to denote torsional deviations.

Irideremia   Congenital absence of the iris.

Keratitis   Inflammation of the cornea.

Keratoconus   Noninflammatory, usually bilateral protrusion of the cornea, the apex being displaced downward and nasally.

Leber's congenital amaurosis   An autosomal-dominant disorder. An affected infant has congenital blindness or severe impairment, deafness, and renal tract abnormalities. Other ocular defects may be present, including keratoconus, cataract, and variable degrees of retinal pigmentation.

Lenticonus   Conically shaped anterior or posterior surface of the lens. A posterior protrusion more frequent than an anterior one. This condition is usually unilateral.

Leukocoria   White pupillary reflex caused by reflection of light from a light-colored intraocular mass or structure. It is most commonly caused by cataracts, but also seen in neonates with retinoblastoma, persistent hyperplastic primary vitreous, retinal detachment, vitreous hemorrhage, or intraocular inflammation.

Levoversion   Eye movement to the left.

Macrophthalmia   Enlarged eye. May occur with buphthalmos or without an increase in the normal neonatal corneal diameter of 12 mm.

Macular cherry-red spot   A spot of normally pigmented epithelium visible because of abnormal thinning of the ganglion cell layer in the center of the macula retinae.

Madarosis   Severe diminution or absence of lashes or eyebrows.

Marcus-Gunn "jaw-winking" syndrome   The lid elevates with movement of the pterygoid (jaw) muscles due to anomalous innervation between the trigeminal and oculomotor nerves. Infants show vertical lid retraction and jerking when sucking or chewing.

Megalocornea   Cornea measuring more than 11.5 mm in diameter in a term neonate.

Microcornea   A cornea measuring less than 9 mm diameter at term predisposes to a shallow anterior chamber and angle closure glaucoma. Associated with microphthalmos, abnormalities of corneal curvature, or sclerocornea.

Microphakia   Small lens.

Microphthalmia   (Small eye) Eye measures less than 15 mm maximum diameter at birth. A small cornea and small lids suggest but do not define a small globe. It may be necessary to measure the globe by ultrasound. May show a range of changes from mild size reduction without significant structural distortion (nanophthalmia) through to significant size reduction and structural distortion within the range seen in anophthalmia. Often have coexistent colobomas.

Microspherophakia   Small spherical lens associated with hyperlysinemia and Marfan's and Weill-Marchesani syndrome.

Mydriasis   Extreme dilation of the pupils.

Myopia   Synonym *Nearsightedness.* Usually due to abnormally large eyes causing the light to focus in front of the retina. It is unusual in the first year of life, except in premature infants.

Nanophthalmia   Refers to an eye in which there is proportional decrease in the size of all the internal architectural structures. Predisposes to greater risk for developing glaucoma. Eye is hypermetropic (farsightedness) due to reduction of eye's axial dimension.

Nonattachment of the retina, congenital   Partial or complete failure of fusion of the inner and outer layers of the optic vesicle with an intervening void forming a congenital subretinal space.

Paralytic ectropion   Chronic seventh nerve paralysis that causes eversion of the lower lid margin because of loss of strength in the orbicularis oculi muscle.

Persistent primary vitreous   Primary vitreous is a gelatinous matrix derived from mesoderm and includes the hyaloid vessels that undergo degeneration and resorption during the second trimester. Mesodermal remnants may persist either anteriorly or posteriorly within the posterior compartment. Idiopathic persistence and proliferation of the normally transient primary vitreous vasculature and matrix leading to formation of a retrolental mass with subsequent visual impairment. Usually is sporadic and unilateral. It presents as a small eye with leukocoria and a funnel-shaped retrolental mass with apex attached to optic disk. Contains remnants of hyaloid vessels.

Peter's anomaly   Bilateral condition results in central opacification of the cornea due to a defect in Descemet's membrane with or without adhesion to the iris or lens. Anomaly is secondary to arrested separation of the lens vesicle from the overlying ectoderm and is associated with congenital glaucoma in up to half the individuals affected (138).

Phoria   A latent deviation of the eye held in normal position by sensory fusion. It is demonstrated by occluding the vision and allowing the eye to seek a position of rest. Used with prefixes to describe direction (e.g., eso-, exo-, hyper-, hypo-, incyclo-, excyclo-).

Primary gaze   The eyes are in primary gaze when looking straight ahead.

Proptosis   Exophthalmos but distinct shallow orbits.

Pseudostrabismus   The false impression of ocular deviation because the white of the sclera between the cornea and inner canthus is obscured by prominent medial canthal folds, flat nasal bridges, or closely placed eyes. The corneal light reflex remains symmetric.

Ptosis   Synonym *Blepharoptosis.*

Ptosis, congenital   A lowered upper eyelid from birth due to an intrinsic defect in the levator muscle fibers. Will have diminished or absent horizontal upper lid crease with decreased levator muscle function.

Red reflex   Blood vessels of the transparent retina give a red glow to the eyes when viewed through a lens, i.e., ophthalmoscope or camera. This finding indicates a clarity of the ocular structures between the external surface of the cornea and the retina.

Reiger's syndrome   Usually bilateral with corneal and drainage angle abnormalities, similar to Axenfeld's anomaly, but with additional adhesion of the peripheral portion of the iris and pupillary aperture distortion due to hypoplasia of the iris. Congenital glaucoma is present in up to half the individuals affected (138).

Retinal dysplasia   Occurs in isolation or as part of a syndrome: Norrie's disease, trisomy 13, incontinentia pigmenti, Peter's anomaly, cyclopia, synophthalmia, maternal ingestion of LSD.

Retraction of lid   Visible sclera above the limbus when the eye is in the primary position.

Sclerocornea   Opacification of the cornea that may be complete or peripheral. When complete, the cornea appears as white as the sclera.

Strabismus   Misalignment of the visual axes that is congenital or acquired and occurs in 1–4% of the population. It may be due to poor vision or to cranial nerve palsies or neuromotor disorders that interfere with function of the extraocular muscles.

Synophrys   Eyebrows extending to the mid-line.

Synophthalmus   More common than cyclopia, resulting from varying degrees of fusion of the paired optic vesicles. Both cyclopia and synophthalmia are associated with severe neural tube malformations incompatible with fetal survival; e.g., severe end of spectrum of holoprosencephalic malformations.

Telecanthus   Lateral displacement of the inner canthi.

Transient cataracts   Vacuoles in the three apices of the inverted Y-suture beneath the posterior lens capsule. The etiology is unknown.

Transitory intraocular blood vessels Pupillary membrane: network of blood vessels continuous with iris blood vessels whose function probably is the nourishment of the anterior portion of the developing fetal lens. At its greatest extent, it covers the pupillary aperture. As development progresses, there is a "retraction" of blood vessels away from the central region until there are just remnants around the border. May vary within twin sets. Best seen with the magnification provided by direct ophthalmoscope focused at the pupil plane with the pupil well dilated.

Tropia A constant or intermittently present ocular deviation not affected by gaze. Compare to phoria. Used with prefixes to describe direction (e.g., eso-, exo-, hyper-, hypo-, incyclo-, excyclo-).

Vergence Convergence or divergence of eyes, which should be well established by 6 months of age.

Version Movement of both eyes together in conjugate gaze. This should be present by 4 months of age.

Zone Regions of the retina based on distance from the optic nerve. Used in the International Classification of Retinopathy of Prematurity.

References

1. Isenberg SJ, Everett S. Cardiovascular effects of mydriatics in low-birth weight infants. *J Pediatr* 1984;105: 111–112.
2. Isenberg SJ, Abrams C, Hyman PE. Effects of cyclopentolate eyedrops on gastric secretory function in preterm infants. *Ophthalmology* 1985;92:698–700.
3. Torczynski E. Normal development of the eye and orbit before birth. In: Isenberg SJ, ed. *The Eye in Infancy.* Chicago: Year Book Medical; 1989:27.
4. Moore KL, Persaud TVN, Shiota K. *Color Atlas of Clinical Embryology.* 1st ed. Philadelphia: WB Saunders; 1994.
5. Appel TC. Laryngoscopic ophthalmoscopy. *J Pediatr* 1979;94:847.
6. Isenberg SJ. Examination methods. In: Isenberg SJ, ed. *The Eye in Infancy.* 1st ed. Chicago: Year Book Medical; 1989:57.
7. Thomas IT. Palpebral fissure length from 29 weeks gestation to 14 years. *J Pediatr* 1987;111:267–268.
8. Jones KL, Hanson JW, Smith DW. Palpebral fissure size in newborn infants. *J Pediatr* 1978;92:787–788.
9. Leung A, Ma K, Siu T, Robson W. Palpebral fissure length. In Chinese newborn infants. Comparison with other ethnic groups. *Clin Pediatr (Phila)* 1990;29:172–174.
10. Fuchs M, Iosub S, Bingol N, Gromisch DS. Palpebral fissure size revisited. *J Pediatr* 1980;96:77–78.
11. Adler R, Lappe M, Murphree AL. Pupil dilation at the first well baby examination for documenting choroidal light reflex. *J Pediatr* 1990;118:249.
12. Merlob P, Sivan Y, Reisner SH. Anthropomorphic measurements of the newborn infant. In: Paul NW, ed. *Birth Defects.* Original article series, Vol. 20. White Plains, NY: March of Dimes Birth Defects Foundation; 1984.
13. Katzman GH. Pathophysiology of neonatal subconjunctival hemorrhage. *Clin Pediatr* 1992;31:149–152.
14. Weiss AH. The swollen and droopy eyelid. *Pediatr Clin North Am* 1993;40:789–804.
15. Jones MD. Unilateral epicanthal fold: diagnostic significance. *J Pediatr* 1986;108:702.
16. Lavrich JB, Nelson LB. Disorders of the lacrimal system apparatus. *Pediatr Clin North Am* 1993;40: 767–777.
17. MacEwen CJ, Young JD. The fluorescein disappearance test (FDT): an evaluation of its use in infants. *J Pediatr Ophthalmol Strabismus* 1991;28:302–305.
18. Ogawa GSH, Gonnering RS. Congenital nasolacrimal duct obstruction. *J Pediatr* 1991;119:12.
19. Mansour AM, Cheng KP, Mumma JV, et al. Congenital dacryocele. A collaborative review. *Ophthalmology* 1991;98:1744–1751.
20. Edmond JC, Keech RV. Congenital nasolacrimal sac mucocele associated with respiratory distress. *J Pediatr Ophthalmol Strabismus* 1991;28:287–289.
21. Castillo M, Merten DF, Weissler MC. Bilateral nasolacrimal duct mucocele, a rare cause of respiratory distress: CT findings in two newborns. *Am J Neuroradiol* 1993;14:1011–1013.
22. Mazzara CA, Respler DS, Jahn AF. Neonatal respiratory distress: sequela of bilateral nasolacrimal duct obstruction. *Int J Pediatr Otorhinolaryngol* 1993;25:209–216.
23. Righi PD, Hubbell RN, Lawlor PP Jr. Respiratory distress associated with bilateral nasolacrimal duct cysts. *Int J Pediatr Otorhinolaryngol* 1993;26:199–203.
24. Yee SW, Seibert RW, Bower CM, Glasier CM. Congenital nasolacrimal duct mucocele: a cause of respiratory distress. *Int J Pediatr Otorhinolaryngol* 1994;29:151–158.
25. Brenner RL, Smith JL, Cleveland WW, et al. Eye signs of hypophosphatasia. *Arch Ophthalmol* 1969;81: 614–617.
26. Jones K, ed. *Smith's Recognizable Patterns of Human Malformation.* 4th ed. Philadelphia: WB Saunders; 1988.
27. Judisch GF, Waziri M, Krachmer JH. Ocular Ehlers-Danlos syndrome with normal lysyl hydroxylase activity. *J Pediatr Ophthalmol Strabismus* 1976;19:279–280.
28. Thomas JV, Yoshizumi MO, Beyer CK, et al. Ocular manifestations of focal dermal hypoplasia syndrome. *Arch Ophthalmol* 1977;95:1977–2001.

29. François J. François' dycephalic syndrome. *Birth Defects* 1982;18:595–619.
30. Manthey R, Apple DJ, Kivlin JD. Iris hypoplasia in incontinentia pigmenti. *J Pediatr Ophthalmol Strabismus* 1982;19:279–280.
31. Maumenee IH. The eye in the Marfan syndrome. *Trans Am Ophthalmol Soc* 1981;79:684–733.
32. Worobec-Victor SM, Bain M. Oculocutaneous genetic diseases. In: Renie WA, ed. *Goldber's Genetic and Metabolic Eye Disease.* 2nd ed. Boston: Little, Brown; 1986:489.
33. Gieser S, Carey J, Appel D. Human chromosomal disorders and the eye. In: Renie W, ed. *Goldberg's Genetic and Metabolic Eye Disease.* Boston: Little, Brown; 1986:185–240.
34. Dunn LL, Annable WL, Kliegman RM. Pigmented corneal rings in neonates with liver disease. *J Pediatr* 1987;110:771.
35. Isenberg SJ, ed. *The Eye in Infancy.* 2nd ed. St. Louis: Mosby-Year Book; 1994.
36. Isenberg S. Macular development in the premature infant. *Am J Ophthalmol* 1986;101:74–80.
37. Caputo AR, Schnitzer RE, Lindquist TD, Sun S. Dilation in neonates: a protocol. *Pediatrics* 1982;69:77–80.
38. Smith WL, Alexander RC, Judisch GF, Sata Y, Kao SCS. Magnetic resonance imaging evaluation of neonates with retinal hemorrhages. *Pediatrics* 1992;89:332–333.
39. Egge K, Lyng G, Maltau JM. Effect of instrumental delivery on the frequency and severity of retinal hemorrhages in the newborn. *Acta Obstet Gynecol Scand* 1981;60:153.
40. Svenningsen L, Eidal K. Lack of correlation between umbilical artery pH, retinal hemorrhages and Apgar score in the newborn. *Acta Obstet Gynecol Scand* 1987;66:639.
41. Waldstein G, Keyser R, Stocker JT. The eye. In: Stocker JT, Dehner LP, eds. *Pediatric Pathology.* 1st ed. Vol. 1. Philadelpia: JB Lippincott; 1992:465–489.
42. White VA, Rootman J. Eye. In: Dimmick JE, Kalousek DK, eds. *Developmental pathology of the embryo and fetus.* 1st ed. Vol. 1. Philadelphia: JB Lippincott; 1992:401–423.
43. Eller AW, Brown GC. Retinal disorders of childhood. *Pediatr Clin North Am* 1983;30:1087–1101.
44. Greenwald MJ. Visual development in infancy and childhood. *Pediatr Clin North Am* 1983;30:977–993.
45. Telang V, Dweck H. The eye of the newborn: a neonatologist's perspective. In: Isenberg SJ, ed. *The Eye in Infancy.* Chicago: Year Book Medical; 1989:4.
46. Robinson RJ. Assessment of gestational age by neurological examination. *Arch Dis Child* 1966;41:437.
47. Isenberg SJ. Clinical application of the pupil examination in neonates. *J Pediatr* 1991;118:650.
48. Volpe JJ. *Neurology of the Newborn.* 3rd ed. Philadelphia: WB Saunders; 1995.
49. Repka MX. Common pediatric neuro-ophthalmologic conditions. *Pediatr Clin North Am* 1993;40:777–788.
50. Norcia AM, Tyler CW, Hamer RD. Development of contrast sensitivity in the human infant. *Vision Res* 1990;30:1475–1486.
51. Vital-Durand F. Acuity card procedures and the linearity of grating resolution development during the first year of human infants. *Behav Brain Res* 1992;49:99–106.
52. Dobson V, Schwartz TL, Sandstrom DJ, Michel L. Binocular visual acuity in neonates: the acuity card procedure. *Dev Med Child Neurol* 1987;29:199–206.
53. Teller DY, McDonald MA, Preston K, Sebris SL, Dobson V. Assessment of visual acuity in infants and children: the acuity card procedure. *Dev Med Child Neurol* 1986;28:779–789.
54. Traboulsi EI, Maumenee IH. Eye problems. In: Oski FA, DeAngelis CD, Feigin RD, Warshaw JB, eds. *Principles and Practice of Pediatrics.* 1st ed. Vol. 1. Philadelphia: JB Lippincott; 1990:805–825.
55. Hoyt CS, Mousel DK, Weber AA. Transient supranuclear disturbances of gaze in healthy neonates. *Am J Ophthalmol* 1980;89:708–713.
56. Weiss AH, Biersdorf WR. Visual sensory disorders in congenital nystagmus. *Ophthalmology* 1989;96:517–523.
57. Gelbart SS, Hoyt CS. Congenital nystagmus: a clinical perspective in infancy. *Graefes Arch Clin Exp Ophthalmol* 1988;226:178–180.
58. Hoyt CS. Nystagmus and other abnormal ocular movements in children. *Pediatr Clin North Am* 1987;34:1415–1423.
59. de Toledo AR, Chandler JW. Conjunctivitis of the newborn. *Infect Dis Clin North Am* 1992;6:807–813.
60. Rapoza PA, Quinn TC, Kiessling LA, Green WR, Taylor HR. Assessment of neonatal conjunctivitis with a direct immunofluorescent monoclonal antibody stain for *Chlamydia. JAMA* 1986;255:3369–3373.
61. Whitcher JP. Neonatal ophthalmia: have we advanced in the last 20 years? *Int Ophthalmol Clin* 1990;30:39–41.
62. Nishida H, Risemberg HM. Silver nitrate ophthalmic solution and chemical conjunctivities. *Pediatrics* 1975;56:368–373.
63. Wilson FMd. Adverse external ocular effects of topical ophthalmic medications. *Surv Ophthalmol* 1979;24:57–88.
64. Hammerschlag MR. Conjunctivitis in infancy and childhood. *Pediatr Rev* 1984;5:285–290.
65. Preece PM, Anderson JM, Thompson RG. Chlamydia trachomatis infection in infants: a prospective study [see comments]. *Arch Dis Child* 1989;64:525–529.
66. Fransen L, Nsanze H, Klauss V, et al. Ophthalmia neonatorum in Nairobi, Kenya: the roles of *Neisseria gonorrhoeae* and *Chlamydia trachomatis. J Infect Dis* 1986;153:862–869.
67. Fransen L, Klauss V. Neonatal ophthalmia in the developing world. Epidemiology, etiology, management and control. *Int Ophthalmol* 1988;11:189–196.
68. O'Hara MA. Ophthalmia neonatorum. *Pediatr Clin North Am* 1993;40:715–725.
69. Palmer EA, Flynn JT, Hardy RJ, et al. Incidence and early course of retinopathy of prematurity. The Cryotherapy for Retinopathy of Prematurity Cooperative Group. *Ophthalmology* 1991;98:1628–1640.
70. Phelps DL. Retinopathy of prematurity. *Pediatr Rev* 1995;16:50–56.
71. AAP Committee on Fetus and Newborn and ACOG Committee on Obstetrics: Maternal and Fetal Medicine. *Guidelines for Perinatal Care.* 3rd ed. Elk Grove Village, IL: American Academy of Pediatrics and American College of Obstetricians and Gynecologists; 1992.
72. Fletcher MA, MacDonald MG, eds. *Atlas of Procedures in Neonatology.* 2nd ed. Philadelphia: JB Lippincott; 1993.

73. Prematurity FtICftCotLSoRo. An international classification of retinopathy of prematurity II. The classification of retinal detachment. *Pediatrics* 1988;82:37–43.

74. Flynn JT. Retinopathy of prematurity. In: Nelson LB, Calhoun JH, Harley RD, eds. *Pediatric Ophthalmology.* 3rd ed. Vol. 1. Philadelphia: WB Saunders; 1991:59–77.

75. Prematurity FtICftCoRo. An international classification of retinopathy of prematurity. *Pediatrics* 1984;74: 127–133.

76. Kivlin JD. Systemic disorders and the eye. In: Isenberg SJ, ed. *The Eye in Infancy.* Chicago: Year Book Medical; 1989:459–484.

77. DeMeyer W, Zeman W, Palmer C. The face predicts the brain: diagnostic significance of medial facial anomalies for holoprosencephaly (arhinencephaly). *Pediatrics* 1964;34:256.

78. Francke U. Partial duplication 20p. In: Yunis J, ed. *New Chromosomal Syndromes.* New York: Academic; 1977.

79. Levin P, Green W, Victor D. Histopathology of the eye in Cockayne's syndrome. *Arch Ophthalmol* 1983; 101:1093.

80. Baum J, Feingold M. Ocular aspects of Goldenhar's syndrome. *Am J Ophthalmol* 1973;75:250–257.

81. Salonen R. The Merckel syndrome: clinicopathological findings in 67 patients. *Am J Med Genet* 1984;18: 671–689.

82. Judisch G, Martin-Casals A, Hanson J. Oculodentodigital dysplasia. *Arch Ophthalmol* 1976;97:878–884.

83. Jensen O, Warburg M, Dupont A. Ocular pathology in the elfin face syndrome. *Ophthalmologica* 1976;172: 434–444.

84. Grier R, Farrington F, Kendig R. Autosomal dominant inheritance of the Aarskog syndrome. *Am J Med Genet* 1983;15:39–46.

85. McKusick V. Mendelian Inheritance in Man. 7th ed. Baltimore: The Johns Hopkins University Press; 1986.

86. Cordero J, Holmes L. Phenotypic overlap of the BBB and G syndromes. *Am J Med Genet* 1978;2:145–152.

87. Vles J, Haspeslagh M, Raes M. Early clinical signs in Coffin-Lowry syndrome. *Clin Genet* 1984;26: 448–452.

88. Moller K, Gorlin R. The Dubowitz syndrome: a retrospective. *J Craniofac Genet* 1985;1:283–286.

89. Perry L, Edwards W, Bramson R. Melnick-Needles syndrome. *J Pediatr Ophthalmol Strabismus* 1978;15: 226–230.

90. Seuanez H, Mane-Garzon F, Kolski R. Cardio-cutaneous syndrome (the "Leopard" syndrome). Review of the literature and a new family. *Clin Genet* 1976;9:266–276.

91. Allanson J, Hall J, Hughes H. Noonan syndrome: the changing phenotype. *Am J Med Genet* 1985;21: 507–514.

92. Abernethy D. Hypertelorism in several generations. *Arch Dis Child* 1927;15:361–365.

93. Alkemade P, ed. *Dysgenesis Mesodermalis of the Iris and the Cornea.* Assen, The Netherlands: Charles C Thomas; 1969.

94. Shelley E, Shelley W. The fish odor syndrome. *JAMA* 1984;251:253–256.

95. Weleber R, Magenis R. The importance of chromosomal studies in opthalmology. *Ophthalmol Clin* 1984; 24:15.

96. Feman S, Apt L, Roth A. The basal cell nevus syndrome. *Am J Ophthalmol* 1974;78:222–228.

97. Spranger J, Opitz J, Bidder U. Heterogeneity of chondrodysplasia punctata. *Humangenetik* 1971;11:190.

98. Gorlin R, Pindborg J, Cohen M, eds. *Syndromes of the Head and Neck.* 2nd ed. New York: McGraw-Hill; 1976.

99. Robinson L, James H, Mubarak S. Carpenter syndrome: natural history and clinical spectrum. *Am J Med Genet* 1985;20:461–469.

100. Chan C, Green W, de la Cruz Z. Ocular findings in osteogenesis imperfecta congenita. *Arch Ophthalmol* 1982;100:1459–1463.

101. Pashayan H, Prazansky S, Putterman A. A family with blepharo-naso-facial malformations. *Am J Dis Child* 1973;125:389–393.

102. Holmes L, Schepens C. Syndrome of ocular and facial anomalies, telecanthus and deafness. *J Pediatr* 1972; 81:552–555.

103. Fryns J, Haspeslagh M. Mental retardation, short stature, minor skeletal anomalies, craniofacial dysmorphism and macrodontia in two sisters and their mother. *Clin Genet* 1984;26:178–186.

104. Anneren G, Arvidson B, Gustavson K-H. Oro-facio-digital syndromes I and II: radiological methods for diagnosis and the clinical variations. *Clin Genet* 1984;26:178–186.

105. Delleman J, Hageman M. Opthalmological findings in 34 patients with Waardenburg syndrome. *J Pediatr Ophthalmol Srabismus* 1977;15:341–345.

106. Townes P, Muechler E. Blepharophimosis, ptosis, epicanthus inversus, and primary amenorrhea. *Arch Ophthalmol* 1979;97:1664–1666.

107. Michels V, Hittner H, Beaudet A. A clefting syndrome with ocular anterior chamber defect and lid anomalies. *J Pediatr* 1978;93:444–446.

108. Grizzard W, O'Donnell J, Carey J. The cerebro-oculo-facio-skeletal syndrome. *Am J Ophthalmol* 1980;89: 293–298.

109. Edwards W, Root A. Chondrodystrophic myotonia (Schwartz-Jampel syndrome): report of a new case and follow-up of patients initially reported in 1969. *Am J Med Genet* 1982;13:51–56.

110. Dobyns W, Gilbert E, Opitz J. Further comments on the lissencephaly syndrome. *Am J Med Genet* 1985;22: 197–211.

111. Norio R, Raitta C, Lindahl E. Further delineation of the Cohen syndrome: report on chorioretinal dystrophy, leukopenia and consanguinity. *Clin Genet* 1984;25:1–14.

112. Halal F, Herrmann J, Pallister P. Differential diagnosis of Nager acrofacial dysostosis syndrome: report of four patients with Nager syndrome and discussion of other related syndromes. *Am J Med Genet* 1983;14: 209–224.

113. Roy F, Summitt R, Hiatt R. Ocular manifestations of the Rubinstein-Taybi syndrome: case report and review of the literature. *Arch Ophthalmol* 1968;79:272.

114. Sugio Y, Kajii T. Ruvalcaba syndrome: autosomal dominant inheritance. *Am J Med Genet* 1984;19: 741–753.
115. Tessier P. Anatomical classification of facial, craniofacial and laterofacial clefts. *J Maxillofac Surg* 1976; 4:69.
116. Wilkes S, Campbell R, Waller R. Ocular malformation in association with ipsilateral facial nevus of Jadassohn. *Am J Ophthalmol* 1981;92:344–352.
117. Ohdo S, Madokoro H, Sonoda T. Kabuki make-up syndrome (Niikawa-Kuroki syndrome) associated with congenital heart disease. *J Med Genet* 1985;22:126–127.
118. Bergsma D, ed. *Birth Defects Compendium.* 2nd ed. New York: Alan R Liss; 1979.
119. Bateman J. Microphthalmos. *Int Ophthalmol Clin* 1987;24:87–107.
120. Pagon R, Clarren S, Milam DJ. Autosomal recessive eye and brain anomalies: Warburg syndrome. *J Pediatr* 1983;102:542–546.
121. Del Pero R, Mets M, Tripathi R. Anomalies of retinal architecture in Aicardi Syndrome. *Arch Ophthalmol* 1986;104:1659–1664.
122. Reese P, Judisch G. Hypomelanosis of Ito. *Arch Ophthalmol* 1986;104:1136–1137.
123. Hirst L. Congenital corneal problems. *Int Ophthalmol Clin* 1984;24:87.
124. Salmon J, Wallis C, Murray A. Variable expressivity of autosomal dominant microcornea with cataract. *Arch Ophthalmol* 1988;106:505–510.
125. Nixon R, Phelps C. Glaucoma. In: Renie W, ed. *Goldberg's Genetic and Metabolic Eye Disease.* 2nd ed. Boston: Little, Brown; 1986:275–296.
126. Silverman W. *Retrolental Fibroplasia. A Modern Parable.* New York: Grune & Stratton; 1980.
127. Maumenee I. Vitreoretinal degeneration as a sign of generalized connective tissue disease. *Am J Ophthalmol* 1979;88:432–449.
128. Stevenson R, Morin J. Ocular findings in nevus flammeus. *Can J Ophthalmol* 1975;10:136–139.
129. Fenske H, Spitalny L. Hereditary osteo-onychodysplasia. *Am J Ophthalmol* 1970;70:604–608.
130. Lewis R, Riccardi V. Von Recklinghausen neurofibromatosis: incidence of iris hamartoma. *Ophthalmology* 1981;88:348–354.
131. Govan J. Ocular manifestations of Alport's syndrome: a hereditary disorder of basement membranes? *Br J Ophthalmol* 1983;67:493–503.
132. Cruysberg J, Sengers R, Pinckers A. Features of a syndrome with congenital cataract and hypertrophic cardiomyopathy. *Am J Ophthalmol* 1986;102:740–749.
133. Merin S. Congenital cataracts. In: Renie W, ed. *Golberg's Genetic and Metabolic Eye Disease.* 2nd ed. Boston: Little, Brown; 1986:369.
134. Kretzer F, Hittner H, Mehta R. Ocular manifestations of the Smith-Lemli-Opitz syndrome. *Arch Ophthalmol* 1981;99:2000–2006.
135. Judisch G, Rhead J, Miller D. Abetalipoproteinemia. *Ophthalmologica* 1984;189:73–79.
136. Pilarski R, Pauli R, Bresnick G. Karsch-Neugebauer syndrome: split foot/split hand and congenital nystagmus. *Clin Genet* 1985;27:97–101.
137. Bateman J, Philippart M, Isenberg S. Ocular features of multiple sulfatase deficiency and a new variant of metachromatic leukodystrophy. *J Pediatr Ophthalmol Strabismus* 1984;21:133–138.
138. McDonald B. The special senses. In: Keeling JW, ed. *Fetal and Neonatal Pathology.* 2nd ed. New York: Springer-Verlag; 1993:699/
139. Cheng KP, Biglan AW, Hiles DA. Pediatric ophthalmology. In: Zitelli BJ, Davis HW, eds. *Atlas of pediatric physical diagnosis. 2nd ed.* New York: Gower Medical Publishing, 1992:19.1.

8

The Ears

EMBRYOLOGY OF THE EXTERNAL EAR

The external ear is formed from the six hillocks of His, which develop from the first and second branchial arches surrounding the first branchial cleft. The hillocks begin to grow and fuse while migrating laterally and upward from their original mid-line position below the mandible. Most of the pinna is formed from the second arch. The tragus, antitragus, and anterior wall of the canal come from the first branchial arch (Fig. 1).

ANATOMY OF EXTERNAL EAR

The auricle is a flexible appendage of thin elastic cartilage covered by perichondrium and skin. Anteriorly the skin is firmly attached, whereas posteriorly the skin is separated from the cartilaginous surface by a subcutaneous layer. The tight adherence of the skin results in ridges and concavities of the auricle corresponding to the ridges and concavities of the auricular cartilage (Figs. 2 and 3).

The auricle is connected to the skull and scalp by three major extrinsic muscles: the anterior, superior, and posterior auricular muscles. There are also intrinsic muscles with no functional significance. Even though these auricular muscles are not especially functional in most humans, their presence and correct insertion appear to be integral to a normally folded external ear (1,2).

The arterial supply originates from the superficial temporal and posterior auricular arteries; venous drainage is supplied by the corresponding veins and mastoid emissary vein. Lymphatic drainage is to the anterior, posterior, and inferior auricular nodes.

Branches of the fifth and tenth cranial nerves and the third cranial nerve provide sensory innervation to the auricle. The great auricular nerve, a branch of the second and third cervical nerve, innervates the medial side of the auricle; the upper portion is innervated by the lesser occipital nerve. The lateral side is innervated by twigs of the great auricular nerve coursing over the helix and by a branch of the fifth cranial nerve. The auricular branch of the tenth cranial nerve innervates a small portion of the auricle and meatal floor. Motor nerves are from the facial nerve.

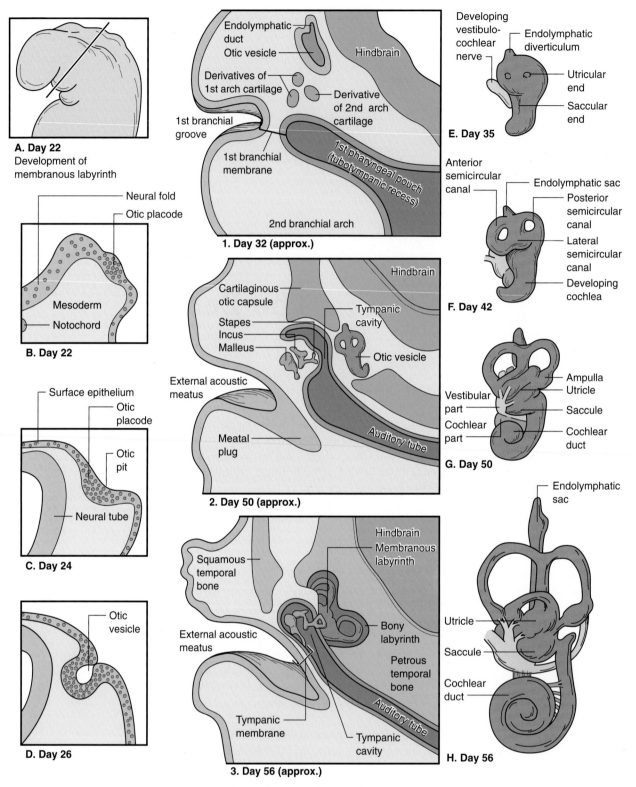

A. Day 22
Development of
membranous labyrinth

B. Day 22

C. Day 24

D. Day 26

1. Day 32 (approx.)

2. Day 50 (approx.)

3. Day 56 (approx.)

E. Day 35

F. Day 42

G. Day 50

H. Day 56

Figure 1. Embryology of the ear.

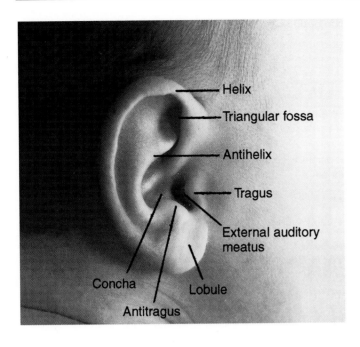

Figure 2. Anatomy of the external ear.

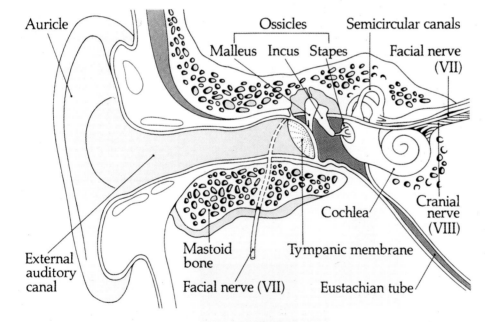

Figure 3. Coronal section of the ear.

TECHNIQUE OF EXAMINATION: EXTERNAL EXAMINATION OF EAR

Steps in examining the external ear:

Inspect both ears
    Preauricular area: skin appendages, fistulae, pits, and skin markings
    Postauricular area: ecchymoses, swelling, fistulae, and skin markings
    Auricle: size, shape, and symmetry; anterior and posterior surface
    Tragus: size in proportion to the size of the ear
    Attachment of ear lobe
    External auditory meatus: patency and size
Determine position and rotation
Palpate the auricle
    Texture
    Firmness of cartilage and recoil
    Masses

Examine and compare each auricle for shape, configuration, size, and position. Palpate the auricle for firmness. Fold it forward and release to estimate recoil. Inspect for ecchymoses, abrasions, or lacerations relating to birth trauma. Look for the presence of a normally sized and directed canal. Palpate the pre- and postauricular areas for induration, edema, masses, or tenderness, and look for any extraneous features.

Evaluate the position of the auricle first by maintaining the infant's head in a neutral resting position with your eyes at the same plane as the infant's. Judge symmetry in the vertical position of the ears by comparing the position of the tragi. Next, determine asymmetries in the horizontal position by comparing the linear distance between each tragus and the facial mid-line. Determine the angle between the long axis of the auricle and the vertical axis of the head. Finally, look at the ears and their protrusion from the head by viewing from the top and back of the head. If the ears appear to be abnormal or unequal in size, measure them in the horizontal and vertical dimensions.

The length of the auricle is roughly the same as the distance from the arch of the eyebrow to base of the ala nasi (Fig. 4). At birth, the width of a normal ear is about two thirds its length. With age, the ear becomes moderately narrower and longer. Final relationship is established by age 15 in boys and age 13 in girls, when width is slightly more than half the length (3,4) (Table 1).

The position of the ears depends on how complete their cephalad migration and anterior rotation are and on how much cranial molding or deformation there may be. The position at term should be similar on both sides, with approximately 30% of the pinna above a line extended through the two inner canthi toward the occiput and tragus (Fig. 5). An appearance of low-set or posteriorly rotated ears may be suggested by a small chin, excessive protruding or folding of the ears, hypoplasia of the nose, mid-face hypoplasia, highly posi-

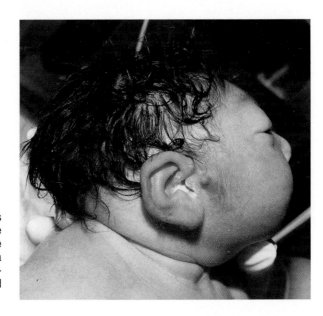

Figure 4. Evaluating ear size. This particularly fleshy ear appears abnormally long because of craniofacial disproportion from severe microencephaly vera but the ear length is within normal limits. The distance between the arch of the eyebrow and the base of the ala nasi allows a visual estimation of expected size. There is a preauricular accessory appendage, and the canal and concha are filled with vernix.

Table 1. *Average minimal and maximal lengths and widths of left ear in 2-week-old white boys*

	Males		Females	
	Minimum (mean −2 SD)	Maximum (mean +2 SD)	Minimum (mean −2 SD)	Maximum (mean +2 SD)
Length	28.1	42.7	28.3	41.3
Width	18.7	28.3	19.6	28.4

Modified from Farkas, ref. 4, with permission.

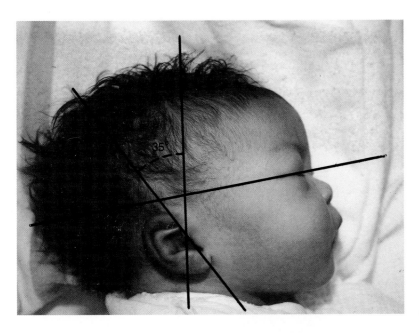

Figure 5. Low-set and posteriorly rotated ear in an infant with Stickler's syndrome.

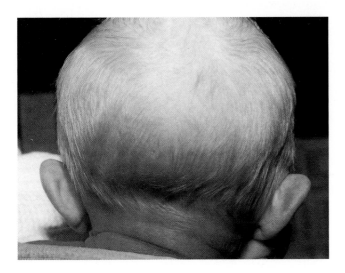

Figure 6. Prominent ear. The angle between the ear and the skull is greater than 20°.

tioned or arched eyebrows, prominent or high forehead, an uptilted head, or, most commonly, intrauterine molding of head. Plagiocephaly with occipital flattening and contralateral prominence is associated with the ear on the flattened side appearing ahead of the ear on the opposite side. The horizontal distance from the ear to the mid-face will be shorter on the side with the plagiocephaly (5).

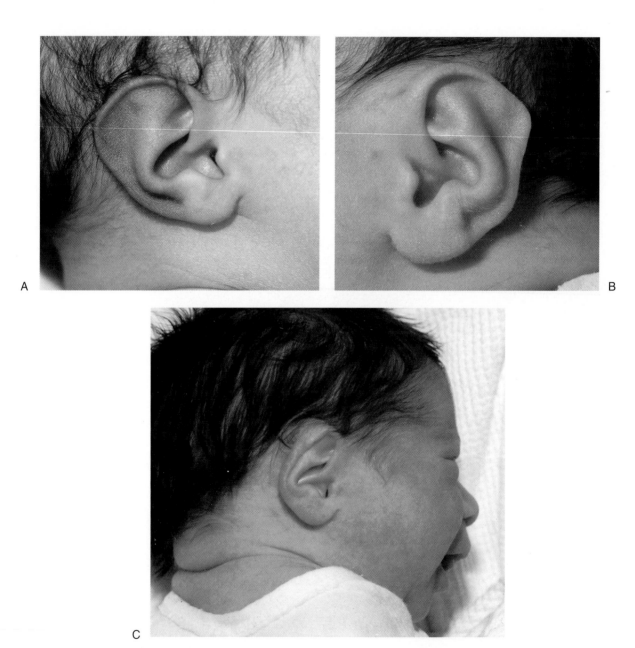

A

B

C

Figure 7. Variations in shape of the helix. **A:** Simple pinna with minimal folding of the helix, posterior rotation, and mildly low set location. This type of ear is especially compliant and cannot be used for gestational age assessment. **B:** Partially folded helix with prominent anthelix in a firm ear. There is a small preauricular tag. **C:** Folded helix due to intrauterine breech position.

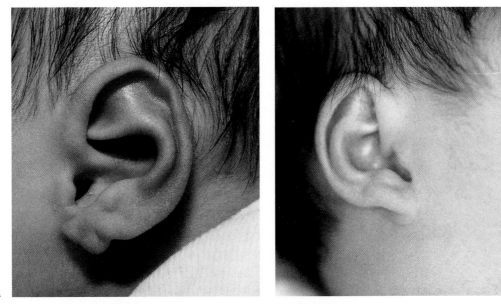

Figure 8. Variations in ear lobe. **A:** Cleft lobe. **B:** Attached lobe at medial margin.

The long axis of the pinna is approximately 15° posterior to the true vertical axis of the head. An angle greater than 20° indicates posterior rotation. Significant molding of the cranium makes it difficult to determine the vertical axis, but a line following the coronal suture provides a good estimate (Fig. 5). In neonates the pinna is most often quite flat against the skull at an angle of less than 10° to 15°. If an angle against the skull is greater than 15°, determine if that ear is prominent, lopped, or cupped (Fig. 6).

The shape of the external ear is determined in part by intrauterine forces and by the activity of extrinsic and intrinsic auricular muscles. Some abnormal forms are signs of generalized neuromuscular weakness or abnormalities in auricular muscle insertions (2). Abnormalities of auricular formation are part of many specific syndromes, but except for a few instances, some of which are discussed herein, the malformations are nonspecific. Additionally, there are many variations of normal, many of which are clinically described by comparison with familial objects (e.g., cat ear, Mr. Spock ear). Although these comparisons may call to mind a visual impression, it is important in the evaluation of the appearance of the ear to use standard descriptors of anatomic landmarks, including size, number, shape, position, color, texture or consistency, continuity, and alignment as described in Chapter 1 Table 7 (Figs. 7 and 8).

TECHNIQUE OF EXAMINATION: OTOSCOPY

Steps in otoscopy:

Clear the canal of obstructive debris.
Examine the canal surface for integrity, color, size, and direction.
Inspect the eardrum for visual characteristics.
Determine the mobility of eardrum by insufflation.

Hold a pneumatic otoscope like a pencil and stabilize the infant's head with the palm of that hand; use the opposite hand to pull the lobule caudally and to hold the pneumatic bulb. Clear the canal with a small curette or, if necessary, low pressure through a soft suction catheter. Following a caudad to cephalad direction, advance a small speculum while applying a light positive pressure to the bulb and visualizing the canal. Continue to apply light pressure on the rubber bulb to give a positive pressure to the drum and canal. Examine the eardrum. Keeping the bulb compressed, move the speculum to break and reapply

the seal momentarily, and then release the bulb to effect a negative pressure. Observe for movements of the tympanic membrane as the pressure changes.
Observations of eardrum:

Color
Luster
Translucence
Light reflex
Vascularity
Contour (bulge or retraction)
Landmarks
Mobility on positive and negative pressure
Other conditions
    Otorrhea
    Hemotympanum
    Amber serous effusion

The direction of the canal differs in young infants compared with adults. In older patients, for visualization of the drum the auricle is pulled away from the chin and the speculum directed toward the face; in neonates, the lobule should be pulled toward the chin with the speculum directed away from the face. It helps to apply a positive pressure through the pneumatic otoscope while advancing the speculum to keep the cartilaginous canal from obscuring the membrane.

The ear canal is filled with amniotic debris, vernix caseosa, or blood during the first few days after a term gestation birth. It may take several days to weeks for this debris to clear spontaneously, but at least 60% of term infants will have spontaneous visibility by 1 week (6). Preterm infants may clear more quickly because of less amniotic debris, although the pliability of their canals makes them collapse and expand more in response to insufflation (7).

The eardrum is less vertical in neonates than in older children, so it will not be viewed perpendicular to its plane (Fig. 9). This more horizontal position, almost parallel to the superior wall of the external canal, gives an appearance of normal width but shorter height to the drum and suggests retraction when none is present. It also makes it difficult to distinguish the pars flaccida from the skin of the superior wall of the canal. By 1 month of age after term, the tympanic membrane is more oblique and presents an appearance more similar to that in the older patient (8).

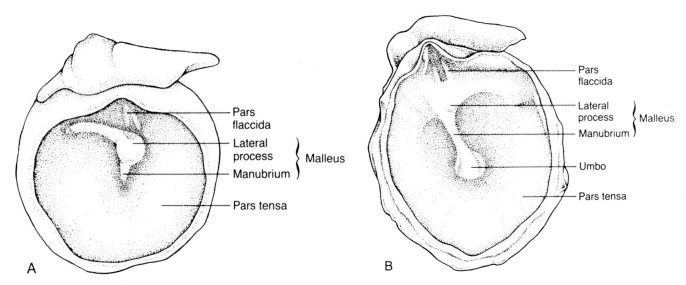

Figure 9. Appearance of tympanic membrane through otoscope. **A:** Neonatal ear. The angle of the membrane makes it appear shorter than it is. **B:** Adult.

It is relatively difficult to detect movement of the eardrum in neonates. Movement of the tympanic membrane relates to the amount of pressure applied during insufflation, the pliability of the drum and canal, and the pressure within the middle ear. On insufflation the skin of the canal moves more freely than does the membrane itself in newborn infants. The inferior canal wall rises over the inferior portion of the tympanic membrane, so it is necessary not to misinterpret its movement during insufflation as that of the drum. When compared with the surface of the canal, the tympanic membrane moves more readily with crying and has more visible blood vessels.

Compared with normally expected findings in older infants or adults, the neonatal tympanic membrane is thicker, grayer, more vascular, and likely to have material behind it (9). The classic findings for otitis media of tympanic membrane dullness, decreased or diffused light reflex, diminished translucence, and decreased motility may be present in healthy newborn and young infants. Progressive resolution of these changes occurs during the first 4 months of age. Space-occupying cellular elements in the middle ear that do not normally exist in older patients include the following:

1. Mesenchyme. This is a loose, connective tissue interposed between the epithelium of the middle ear lumen and the underlying bone. The postgestational length of time that mesenchyme might persist in the middle ear is unclear. The amount of mesenchyme decreases in volume with increased postpartum maturity and nearly disappears by one year of age but persists in some areas of the middle ear for several years (9). There appears to be an inverse relationship between the amount of mesenchyme persisting at and after birth and the amniotic fluid volume. Infants who had extremely low volumes of amniotic fluid tend to have more membrane opacity due to persistent mesenchyme (9).

2. Blood. If present in the amniotic fluid or oropharynx, maternal blood may be found in significant volume in the middle ear, enough to cause a decrease in tympanic membrane mobility and in hearing (9). When accompanied by peripartum temporal bone fracture, neonatal blood should resorb by 3 weeks of age. The presence of the blood in the middle ear cannot confirm a diagnosis of perinatal temporal bone fracture if there is a potential intrapartum history of ingested blood.

3. Congenital otitis media. Well-documented cases of inflammation and purulent cells have been reported within hours after birth (9).

TECHNIQUE OF EXAMINATION: ASSESSMENT OF HEARING BY BEHAVIOR RESPONSE

With the infant in a quiet alert or light sleep state and in a quiet examination area, observe the response to a standardized stimulus applied at the prescribed distance from the ear. Be careful not to direct the noise maker in such a way to elicit a false reaction to air movement or a visual stimulus rather than to the sound itself.

Behavioral observation audiometry is any procedure in which the examiner presents a sound stimulus and observes the reaction of the infant. Involuntary responses that follow sound stimulation include eye blinks, eye widening, startle or Moro reflex, leg kicks, crying, and quieting. The more complex the spectrum of the sound and the greater the intensity, the more likely the infant is to respond. The best state for testing is a quiet or lightly sleeping state; testing in states of deep sleep or loud crying provides no reliable result. If the infant is in an active, awake state even if quiet, he or she may be moving too much for the examiner to distinguish which movements are a specific response to sound.

For a general screening, appropriate stimuli include bicycle horns, musical bells, or even mid-tone tuning forks. Because the stimulus has to be quite loud, a behavioral reaction to a standardized sound excludes only gross bilateral deficits, but its presence is an indicator of probably sufficient hearing for speech development.

Assessment of auditory function by evoked potential is specifically indicated in infants at risk for hearing deficits, particularly those with craniofacial anomalies, a family history of childhood deafness, very low birth weight (1,500 g), severe asphyxia, fetal nonbacterial infection, meningitis, intracranial hemorrhage, potentially toxic levels of bilirubin, prolonged administration or toxic levels of ototoxic drugs, and after hyperventilation therapy. Anomalies associated with hearing deficits include neural crest abnormalities, first or second branchial arch abnormalities, or specific syndromes known to be associated with hearing loss (10–12). The likelihood of hearing loss depends on the type of anomaly present. All infants with aural atresia have deficits. At least 50% of infants with major craniofacial anomalies have hearing loss, but fewer than 20% with isolated external ear anomalies such as tags or mild microtias have loss (10).

Early detection of a deficit is important for hearing augmentation before the critical epoch of speech development. In large part, the concept of general screening in the neonatal period is important for those infants not otherwise identified as needing a more detailed evaluation by evoked potentials. If infants have a particular risk for hearing loss, a normal neonatal screen by behavior response does not give enough information to substitute for further evaluation. The best time for an examination more detailed than the behavior screen described above depends on multiple factors, including reliable access to future medical care, current therapies including a noisy environment from a ventilator or incubator, and clearance of middle ear debris as well as the ideal of early identification. Many of the newborn infants at risk for hearing loss are those that require intervention for other medical problems, precluding reliable testing. In these cases this assessment becomes an important part of the examination at discharge from the intensive care nursery or in early follow-up.

CLINICAL EXAMPLES

Aural atresia
Auricular sinus
Auricular appendage
Microtia
Lop ear
Cup ear

Aural atresia. Figure 10 (13)

Synonyms: Auditory canal atresia, meatal atresia
Description: Atresia of the auditory canal with or without abnormalities of the pinna. The atresia may be either osseous or membranous and is usually associated with varying de-

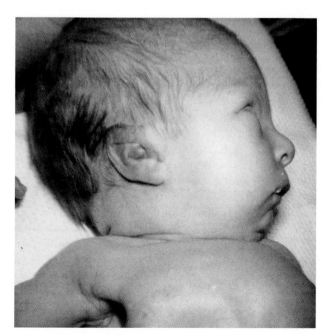

Figure 10. Atresia of the external auditory canal in association with hypoplasia of the mandible and ribs, widely spaced nipples, and blepharophimosis with upslanting of the deeply set eyes. These findings are compatible with trisomy 20p syndrome. A cursory examination that does not include inspecting for an ear canal might miss this defect, particularly in the presence of more striking nonaural defects.

Table 2. *Disorders associated with aural atresia*

Classification	Inheritance	Example
Aural atresia ± microtia	Autosomal dominant	(15, 16)
	Autosomal recessive	(17, 18)
	Sporadic	(16)
Associated with first and second branchial arch defects	Autosomal dominant	Treacher-Collins
	Autosomal recessive	(19)
	Sporadic	Goldenhar syndrome
Associated with organ system involvement not including mental retardation	Autosomal dominant	Acrocephalosyndactyly type III
		Branchio-oto-renal syndrome (BOR)
		Cleidocranial dysostosis
		Oculodentodigital syndrome
		Otopalatodigital syndrome type I
		Townes syndrome
	Autosomal recessive	Acrofacial dysostoses
		Otopalatodigital syndrome type II
	Associations	MURCS
		VATER
Associated with organ system involvement including mental retardation	Autosomal dominant	Velocardiofacial syndrome
	Autosomal recessive	Johanson-Blizzard syndrome
		Cooper-Jabs description (14)
Chromosomal abnormalities		Trisomy 13
		Trisomy 18
		18q-syndrome
		Trisomy 21

Data from Cooper (14).

grees of microtia. The incidence is estimated to be between one and five per 20,000 live births.

Embryology: Results from a failure of the meatal plug to canalize.

Predilection for sex or race: None.

Inheritance pattern: Sporadic, autosomal dominant, autosomal recessive, or associated with chromosomal syndromes. Many sporadic cases are seen without other anomalies. Most familial cases of meatal atresia are associated with malformations, involving the derivatives of the first and second branchial arches (14).

Associations: See Table 2.

Further evaluation: Hearing evaluation required; further evaluation dependent on associated conditions

Auricular sinus. Figure 11

Synonyms: Preauricular pit, preauricular sinus, ear pit, congenital auricular fistula, fistula auris congenita.

Description: A small opening of a narrow tract most often just in front of the ascending limb of the helix. Less commonly, a sinus may be found in the lobule, cavum conchae, or external canal. Rarely, fistulas may extend from the meatal floor to the angle of the mandible or from the tonsillar pillar to the middle ear.

The opening may be bilateral or unilateral but tends to be unilateral without a predilection for one side or the other.

Embryology: The opening may represent incomplete fusion of the first arch hillocks, defective closure of the most dorsal part of the first branchial cleft (21), or ectodermal folds that are sequestered during auricle formation (22).

Predilection for sex: None described.

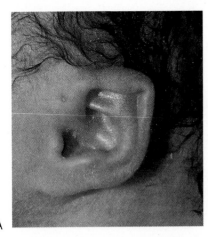
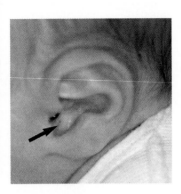
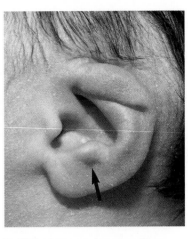

A   B, C

Figure 11. Preauricular and auricular sinus. **A:** Simple preauricular pit. **B:** Pit just at opening of auditory canal (*arrow*). **C:** Congenitally pierced ear. The dimple on the lateral surface of the ear lobe has a similar indentation on the medial surface. The helix is folded from intrauterine position.

Predilection for race: White, 0.9%; black, 5.2%; Asian 10%.

Inheritance pattern: Most likely not a single gene or single inheritance pattern, so not a predictable occurrence in nonsyndromic cases.

Associations:

> May accompany microtia, auricular appendage, branchial cysts or fistulas, facial cleft syndromes, and some syndromic anomalies of the external ear.
>
> Branchio-oto-renal syndrome (16)
>
> Isolated hereditary renal disease and preauricular pits (23)
>
> Suggested higher incidence of renal disease detectable on ultrasonography but not necessarily in the neonatal period (24)
>
> Rare association with deafness (25,26)

Further evaluation: Consider evaluation of renal status in follow-up, sooner if part of syndromic pattern.

Expected course or treatment: Occasionally the sinus may become infected or form retention cysts when the opening is blocked.

Auricular appendage. Figure 12

Synonyms: Preauricular tag, accessory tragus, supernumerary ear, supernumerary auricle, accessory external ear, accessory auricle, rudimentary auricle, preauricular appendage, cartilaginous nevus, cutaneous cervical tag, cervical auricle, wattle.

Description: Accessory tragi appear most commonly in the pretragal area but may occur within or behind the ear, on the lobule, or anywhere along the mandible, as well as in the sternoclavicular areas and even on the glabella. Accessory tragi may be single or multiple. They are most often unilateral without a predilection for right or left. They vary in size from minimal protuberances to pedunculated polyps up to 2 cm in length and usually have hair arising from the papule. Accessory tragi are often misnamed as skin tags, but because they contain cartilage, they are not truly skin tags (27).

Etiology: Histologically, the lesions have numerous hair follicles, sebaceous glands, eccrine sweat glands, dermal connective tissue, adipose tissue, and most often a central core of elastic cartilage. They probably represent anomalous branchial arch development of accessory hillocks because they usually occur in the line of fusion of the mandibular and hyoid arches and less frequently in the fusion line of the maxillary process and mandibular arch.

Predilection for sex: None for nonsyndromic occurrence.

Predilection for race: This is one of the most frequently encountered malformations. For nonsyndromic cases (16), the general rate is 17 per 10,000 births; 13.66/10,000 in whites and 19.10/10,000 in blacks.

Inheritance pattern: In familial cases, inheritance is autosomal dominant (28).

Nonsyndromic frequency is >90% sporadic and nonfamilial (16).

Associations: Unless there are other diffuse malformations, their primary significance is cosmetic. They may be associated with other first branchial arch abnormalities, including cleft lip, cleft palate, and hypoplasia of the mandible. The association with other defects is greater when they occur further away from the pretragus region. They are seen consistently in Goldenhar's syndrome (oculo-auriculo-vertebral dysplasia or facio-auriculo-vertebral spectrum) but also occur in Treacher-Collins syndrome, Nager's syndrome, the chromosome 4 short arm deletion syndrome (4p-syndrome), oculocerebrocutaneous syndrome, and Townes' syndrome.

Further evaluation: When nonsyndromic, they are rarely associated with ipsilateral conductive or sensorineural hearing loss (16). When associated with other anomalies, especially craniofacial anomalies, there is direct indication for hearing assessment.

Expected course or treatment: Rarely, auricular appendages become infected or twist and strangulate (29).

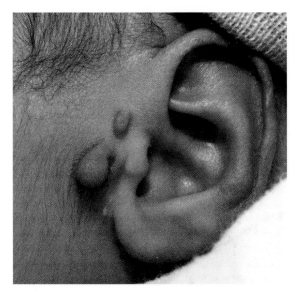

Figure 12. Accessory tragi. Note the variable shape, with the smallest appendages likely simple skin tags. The larger appendages have well-developed hair and cartilage within, as well as glandular openings.

Figure 13. Microtia (13,16,17,19,30–33)

Synonyms: Not synonymous with small auricle (microear). Some investigators refer to this disorder as lop ear, cup ear, and cryptotia, although the embryology likely differs.

Description: A severely dysplastic or disorganized external ear. Typically, the rudimentary auricle forms a longitudinal skin-fold that includes misshapen remnants of cartilage. The skin-fold is positioned vertically. The preserved lobule is displaced, most often superiorly to the level of the opposite, normal side unless incomplete migration leaves it inferior. When the term is applied restrictively, microtia is divided into three degrees, with type III the most severe, including external canal atresia and a small vestige of external ear.

Type I: small auricle that is deformed but possesses the essential structures

Type II: existence of a curving elevation representing a deformed helix

Type III: presence of only primordial hillocks

Embryology: The origin of true microtia appears to be a decreased proliferation of the auricular hillocks or a defect in their fusion.

Predilection for sex: The overall occurrence of nonsyndromic cases is 1.69 per 10,000

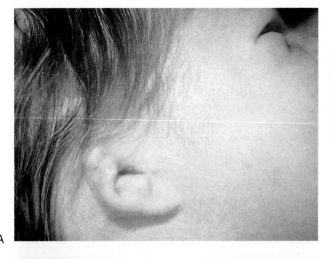

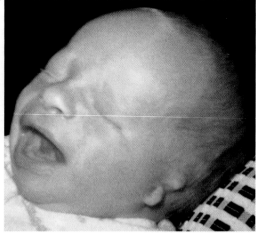

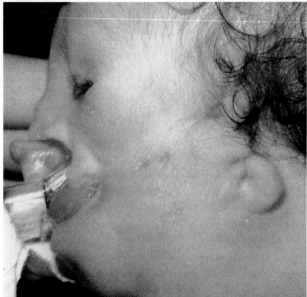

Figure 13. Microtia of increasing difficulty relating to ease of repair. **A:** Cryptotia. The upper portion of the helix is covered by the skin, and the rest of the auricle is tightly adherent. **B:** Microtia with microphthalmia. **C:** Microtia associated with cleft upper lip and palate, lateral cleft lip, hypoplasia of the mandible, microphthalmia, blepharophimosis and coloboma of the eyelids, midfacial hypoplasia, and blind pits between the angle of the mouth and the ear (Treacher-Collins syndrome).

births (16) with no significant racial difference or familial recurrence. Males, 68%; females, 32% (31).

Predilection for race: See Table 3

Inheritance pattern: Familial autosomal dominant, autosomal recessive, or as isolated cases. The probable recurrence risk in the absence of affected family members is 3% to 8% based on a multifactorial pattern of occurrence. Recurrent malformation may be in variable degree of effect (31).

Associations: Microtia is usually found in association with other malformations, including atresia of the external auditory meatus and abnormalities of the middle ear, resulting in conductive hearing loss. In general, but only roughly predictably, the more severe the degree of microtia, the more likely there will be middle ear malformation and hearing loss. In unilateral microtia, hearing loss may be present on the contralateral side even with a normal external ear. More often than not, microtia is associated with ipsilateral craniofacial microsomia. The right-to-left-to-bilateral ratio is 5:3:1.

Further evaluation: Evaluate for associated anomalies as well as for hearing loss.

Table 3. *Prevalence of nonsyndromic microtia*

Racial group	Rate/100,000	Reference
American Indian	53.8	(30)
Spanish-American	11.1	(30)
White	6.3	(30)
Japanese	19	(13)
National Collaborative Perinatal Project (approximately equal white and black)	16.9	(16)

Expected course or treatment: The success of full surgical correction depends in part on how much residual cartilage is present; hence, the surgical classification of types I, II, III, representing the gradations of severity but without clear anatomic demarcations.

Comments: Some epidemiologic studies appear to combine microtia, small auricle, and the various partial defects, giving a higher incidence of occurrence than those studies that limit the definition to the more anatomically restrictive definitions (13,16,30).

Lop ear. Figure 14 (1,16,31,34,35)

Description: Downward folding of the helix and scapha due to inadequate development of the superior crus of the anthelix. This needs to be distinguished from a folded ear that is temporarily deformed from intrauterine compression or from a resting position in premature infants with softer cartilage.

Embryology: Represents some degree of dysplasia of the second branchial arch hillocks, so it may be considered a mild form of microtia. Smith et al. have considered this malformation indicative of a deficiency in the superior auricular muscle (1).

Inheritance pattern: Nonsyndromic occurrence most often isolated.

Associations: Seen in association with anencephaly, micrencephaly vera, and severe congenital neuromotor deficiencies (1). May be only feature present at birth in fragile X syndrome but not diagnostic. Many of the conditions associated with microtia occur with lop ear. Ossicular malformation leading to deafness (34).

Further evaluation: Conductive hearing assessment and cranial motor nerve evaluation.

Expected course or treatment: May respond to early splinting therapy (36–38), although there is no controlled study on efficacy using strict diagnostic criteria. Many of the good responders reported in the literature may have been less severe or temporary deformations and would have undergone spontaneous resolution.

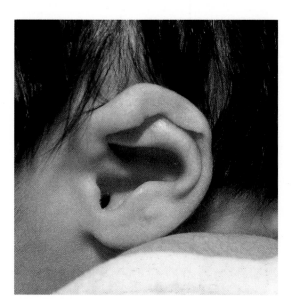

Figure 14. Mild lop ear.

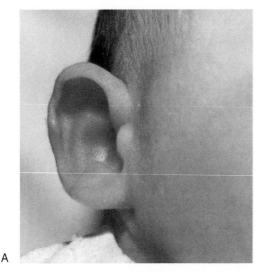
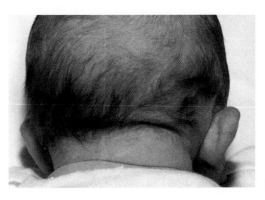

Figure 15. Mild unilateral cup ear, anterior (**A**) and posterior (**B**) views.

Cup ear. Figure 15 (35)

Description: The overall ear size is relatively smaller, with the pinna appearing as if there had been a purse string suture applied along the helix to the lobule. There is an excessively concave concha causing the cup shape.

Embryology: Represents abnormal proliferation and fusion of the auricular hillocks. This is often in association with microtia.

Predilection for sex or race: None.

Inheritance pattern: Sporadic in nonsyndromic cases.

Associations: Many of the same associations as lop ear and microtia.

Further evaluation: Hearing assessment and further evaluation as required by associated anomalies.

Expected course or treatment: Defining an ear as being lop versus protruding or cupped is important, but as a predictor of what type of surgical correction may be required, does not have clinical relevance in the absence of other findings.

GLOSSARY

Adherent lobule   The ear lobe is attached anteriorly. A frequent variant found in otherwise normal individuals that may have a familial pattern (see Fig. 8B).

Anotia   Complete absence of any identifiable auricular structures where the skin passes smoothly over the aural region, with no elevation or depression suggesting even a rudimentary development. This is exceedingly rare because there is more often some remnant even in extreme malformations. This is most often associated with major malformations of the face and head.

Battle's sign   Ecchymotic discoloration overlying the mastoid tip, immediately posterior to the pinna that usually represents a basal skull fracture in older patients. Ecchymosis behind the ear in neonates commonly occurs in association with subgaleal hemorrhage and application of forceps.

Cat ear   Ear has prominent upper and posterior segment of the helix.

Cryptotia   Denotes abnormal adherence of the upper segment of the pinna to the head. The cartilaginous framework adheres to the mastoid bone. The external auditory meatus may appear to lie at the base of a pocket of skin. Normally, the upper part of the auricle becomes detached in the 4th month of gestation. Cryptotia is attributed to a failure of programmed cell death or to secondary reattachment (39).

Darwinian tubercles   Synonym *Darwinian point.* Small thickening or projection of the descending segment of the helix most often at the junction of the superior and middle thirds. The projections may be posterior, anterior, or lateral. Not a consistent indicator of malformation syndromes.

Goldenhar syndrome The more severe form of the facio-auriculo-vertebral spectrum or oculoauricular vertebral dysplasia, including, at the least, epibulbar dermoids, vertebral anomalies, and accessory auricles.

Hemotympanum Discoloration of the tympanic membrane due to blood in the middle ear; usually due to a basilar skull fracture. In neonates, hemotypanum may represent only ingestion of bloody amnionic fluid without associated cranial fractures.

Melotia Synonym *Otocephaly.* An uncommon malformation. In association with micrognathia, the pinna is located on the cheek, and the lobule may be located at the angle of the mouth. The external auditory meatus may be normal despite the abnormal external ear.

Micro-ear An ear with normal architecture but smaller than normal size. It likely represents true hypoplasia with undergrowth of all six auricular hillocks or undergrowth after initial formation. See Appendix Fig. 20 (ear length) for expected normal sizes.

Microtia A severely dysplastic or disorganized external ear, not synonymous with small auricle.

Otorrhea Discharge from the ear, which may be serous, mucoid, purulent, bloody, or clear.

Satyr ear Pinna with a sharp superior tip of the auricle. Not a consistent indicator of malformation syndromes.

Synotia In extreme cases of agnathus or absence of the mandible, the ears are near the mid-line below the mouth.

Wattle Synonym *Cervical auricle.* A cutaneous cervical tag that is the cervical version of accessory tragus and contains cartilage embedded in dense collage (40).

References

1. Smith DW, Takashima H. Ear muscles and ear form. *Birth Defects* 1980;16:299–302.
2. Zerin M, Van Allen MI, Smith DW. Intrinsic auricular muscles and auricular form. *Pediatrics* 1982;69:91–93.
3. Stool SE, Marasovich WA. Postnatal craniofacial growth and development. In: Bluestone C, Stool S, Scheetz M, eds. *Pediatric Otolaryngology.* 2nd ed. Vol. 1. Philadelphia: WB Saunders; 1990:17–31.
4. Farkas LG. Anthropometry of normal and anomalous ears. *Clin Plast Surg* 1978;5:401–418.
5. Jones MD. Unilateral epicanthal fold: diagnostic significance. *J Pediatr* 1986;108:702.
6. McLellan MS, Webb CH. Ear studies in the newborn infant. II. Age of spontaneous visibility of the auditory canal and tympanic membrane and the appearance of these structures in healthy newborn infants. *J Pediatr* 1961;58:523–527.
7. Warren WS, Stool SE. Otitis media in low-birth-weight infants. *J Pediatr* 1971;79:740–743.
8. Bluestone CD, Klein JO. Methods of examination: clinical examination. In: Bluestone C, Stool S, Scheetz M, eds. *Pediatric Otolaryngology.* 2nd ed. Vol. 1. Philadelphia: WB Saunders; 1990:111–124.
9. Eavey RD. Abnormalities of the neonatal ear: otoscopic observations, histologic observations, and a model for contamination of the middle ear by cellular contents of amniotic fluid. *Laryngoscope* 1993;103:1–31.
10. Hayes D. Hearing loss in infants with craniofacial anomalies. *Otolaryngol Head Neck Surg* 1994;110:39–45.
11. Roizen NJ, Wolters C, Nicol T, Blondis TA. Hearing loss in children with Down syndrome. *J Pediatr* 1993;123 (suppl):9–12.
12. Gellis S, Feingold M, Fikar CR, Lee MA. Picture of the month: Ota's nevus. *Am J Dis Child* 1980;134:1083–1084.
13. Ohmori S. Congenital atresia of the ear. A review of the surgical findings in 83 cases. *Clin Plast Surg* 1974;1:3–25.
14. Cooper LF, Jabs E. Aural atresia associated with multiple congenital anomalies and mental retardation: a new syndrome. *J Pediatr* 1987;110:747–750.
15. Zankl M, Zang KD. Inheritance of microtia and aural atresia in a family with five affected members. *Clin Genet* 1979;16:331–334.
16. Melnick M, Myrianthopoulos NC. External ear malformations: epidemiology, genetics, and natural history. In: Bergsma D, Paul NW, eds. *Birth Defects:* Original Article Series. Vol. XV, No. 9. New York: Alan R. Liss; 1979:1–138.
17. Ellwood LC, Winter ST, Dar H. Familial microtia with meatal atresia in two sibships. *J Med Genet* 1968;5:289–291.
18. Konigsmark BW, Nager GT, Haskins HL. Recessive microtia, meatal atresia and hearing loss. *Arch Otolaryngol* 1972;96:105–109.
19. Schmid M, Schroeder M, Langenbeck U. Familial microtia, meatal atresia and conductive deafness in three siblings. *Am J Med Genet* 1985;22:327–332.
20. Feingold M, Baum J. Goldenhar's syndrome. *Am J Dis Child* 1978;132:136–138.

21. Moore KL. *The Developing Human. Clinically Oriented Embryology.* Philadelphia: WB Saunders; 1973.

22. Aronsohn RS, Batsakis JG, Rice DH, Work WP. Anomalies of the first branchial cleft. *Arch Otolaryngol* 1976;102:737–740.

23. Lachiewicz AM, Sibley R, Michael AF. Hereditary renal disease and preauricular pits: report of a kindred. *J Pediatr* 1985;106:948–950.

24. Leung AKC, Robson WLM. Association of preauricular sinuses and renal anomalies. *Urology* 1992;40: 259–261.

25. Fourman P, Fourman J. Hereditary deafness in family with ear-pits (fistula auris congenita). *Br Med J* 1955; 2:1354–1356.

26. McLaurin JW, Kloepfer HW, Laguaite JK, Stallcup TA. Hereditary branchial anomalies and associated hearing impairment. *Laryngoscope* 1966;76:1277–1288.

27. Sebben JE. The accessory tragus: no ordinary skin tag. *J Dermatol Surg Oncol* 1989;15:304–307.

28. Gao J, Chen Y, Gao Y. A survey of accessory auricle anomaly. *Arch Otolaryngol Head Neck Surg* 1990;116: 1194–1196.

29. Brownstein MH, Wanger N, Helwig EB. Accessory tragi. *Arch Dermatol* 1971;104:625–631.

30. Aase JM, Tegtmeier RE. Microtia in New Mexico: evidence for multifactorial causation. *Birth Defects* 1977; 13:113–116.

31. Aase JM. Microtia—clinical observations. Morphogenesis and malformation of the ear. *Birth Defects* 1980; 16:289–297.

32. deSa DJ. Ear. In: Dimmock JE, Kalousek DK, eds. *Developmental Pathology of the Embryo and Fetus.* 1st ed. Philadelphia: JB Lippincott; 1992:424–436.

33. Sánchez-Corona J, Garcí-Cruz D, Ruenes R, Cantú JM. A distinct dominant form of microtia and conductive hearing loss. *Birth Defects* 1982;18:211–216.

34. Jaffe BF. Pinna anomalies associated with congenital conductive hearing loss. *Pediatrics* 1976;57:332–341.

35. Tanzer RC. The constricted (cup and lop) ear. *Plast Reconstr Surg* 1975;55:406–415.

36. Brown FE, Colen LB, Addante RR, Graham JMJ. Correction of congenital auricular deformities by splinting in the neonatal period. *Pediatrics* 1986;78:406–411.

37. Millay DJ, Larrabee WF, Dion FR. Nonsurgical correction of auricular deformities. *Laryngoscope* 1990;100: 910–913.

38. Matsuo K, Hayashi R, Kiyono M, Hirose T, Netsu Y. Nonsurgical correction of congenital auricular deformities. *Clin Plast Surg* 1990;17:383–95.

39. Warkany J. *Congenital Malformation.* Chicago: Year Book Medical; 1971.

40. Christensen P, Barr RJ. Wattle: an unusual congenital abnormality [Letter]. *Arch Dermatol* 1985;121:22–23.

The Trunk Region

9

The Chest, Abdomen, Genitalia, Perineum, and Back

Compared with assessments of the head and neck and of the extremities, inspection of the trunk during an initial regional screening examination is least likely to show the presence of anomalies. With notable exceptions, the difference comes from their being fewer visible anomalies in the trunk so that finding those malformations or disease processes hidden within requires more emphasis on palpation and auscultation than on simple inspection. In contrast, after screening examinations the trunk is the region of emphasis in reassessments because pathophysiologic conditions in newborn patients most frequently involve the thoracic and abdominal viscera. The skills of palpation and auscultation assume more importance in all the later examinations, with the possible exception of assessments of neurodevelopment.

For purposes of discussion, the examination of the trunk is described in a progression that suggests an operative sequence. As in other regional assessments, this examination often has to be in nonsequential parcels to take full advantage of optimal patient state and position. Auscultation and palpation require an undisturbed, quiet infant. Therefore, to a large extent it is the patient who determines just when to examine the heart and abdomen. Regardless of the actual order in completing each portion, every component is necessary in the final synthesis. In practice, because of the infant's small size, the front of the chest, abdomen, and genitalia are inspected and palpated as a unit before the back is inspected unless the infant is already lying on the stomach. Furthermore, aside from a cursory inspection upon approach to the bedside, auscultation may be the first step in the process if the infant is quiet.

The suggested steps follow a practical sequence that varies according to infant state and the detail of information needed in each examination.

STEPS IN EXAMINATION OF THE TRUNK

Count respiratory rate
Inspect anterior trunk for
    contour and size of chest and abdomen
    bilateral symmetry
    retractions or bulging
    depth and ease of respiratory movements
    precordial activity
    character of skin and dermal structures
        size, number, and position of nipples
        presence of breast hypertrophy and nipple discharge
    umbilical cord location and anatomy
    abnormal swelling from hernia of umbilicus, abdominal wall, or inguinal canal
Auscultate region for
    cardiac rate and rhythm
    character and location of
        cardiac sounds
        pulmonary sounds
        bowel sounds
Assess the character of the cry and all extrinsic sounds
Palpate
    chest wall for compliance and subcutaneous definition
    precordium for character and location of cardiac impulses and extraneous cardiac
        vibrations
    abdomen
        wall for muscle mass and tone
        location and size of viscera
        tenderness
        abnormal masses
    male: scrotum for location, size, and character of contents
    female: vulva for masses
    femoral and axillary pulses
    for lymph nodes in axillae, inguinal region, and proximal to any area of suspected
        infection
Percuss abdomen for location and size of organs and character of resonance
Percuss anterior chest for location of upper margin of liver
Inspect genitalia
    determine sex
    locate anus relative to genital landmarks
    in female: presence of vaginal opening and discharge; sizes of clitoris, labia majora, and
        labia minora
    in male: size and shape of penis and scrotum; location of urethral opening
Perform a rectal examination when indicated
Inspect back
    symmetry between the two sides
    position and symmetry of scapulae
    length, shape, and integrity of spine
    presence of dermal lesions overlying or adjacent to vertebral column
Palpate spine for integrity of vertebral bodies or small masses
Transilluminate chest, abdomen, or genitalia for definition of abnormal fluid or air accu-
    mulations when indicated

Section I: The Upper Trunk

TECHNIQUE OF EXAMINATION OF THE CHEST

Review history pertinent to pulmonary and cardiovascular systems
Count respiratory rate
Inspect anterior trunk for
    contour and size of chest and abdomen
    bilateral symmetry
    depth and ease of respiratory movements
    coordination of chest and abdominal movements during breathing
    retractions or bulging
    precordial activity
    character of skin and dermal structures
        size, number, and position of nipples
        presence of breast hypertrophy and nipple discharge
Auscultate region for
    cardiac rate and rhythm
    character and location of
        cardiac sounds
        pulmonary sounds
Assess the character of the cry and all extrinsic sounds
Palpate
    chest wall for compliance and subcutaneous definition
    precordium for character and location of cardiac impulses and extraneous cardiac
        vibrations
    peripheral pulses
Percuss anterior chest for location of upper margin of liver
Transilluminate chest for definition of abnormal fluid or air accumulations when indicated

Pertinent History for Pulmonary Assessment

In the initial newborn screening examination, scrutiny for congenital anomalies and success in physiologic transition is paramount. After the initial examination, respiratory symptoms are the most frequent indications for reassessment of young infants, both for those who remain in intensive care for prolonged periods and for those who are seen as outpatients. Accordingly, each reevaluation requires some historical information equivalent to a chief complaint as well as description of events in the period from birth to presentation. Furthermore, if the family history is not well known, specific items should be readdressed when respiratory symptoms develop as a new problem in the newborn period.

Questions in assessing for pulmonary disease (1):

Is the disorder immediately or potentially life-threatening?
Is the disorder new, chronic, or recurrent?
What are the symptoms?
When did the symptoms begin?
Are the respiratory symptoms constant or episodic?
What factors affect the severity of symptoms?
Are other nonpulmonary symptoms present?
Are any environmental factors involved?
Have any tests been performed?
Have any treatments been given?
Is there a family history of pulmonary disease?

Is the disorder immediately or potentially life-threatening? A first impression about the severity of illness is made upon approach to the patient's bedside through an immediate assessment of degree of respiratory distress. If an infant is cyanotic, gasping, choking, or apneic, the threat is clear. If feeding comfortably, the disorder is either periodic and currently silent or mild enough not to interfere with the basic necessity of nursing.

Is the disorder new, chronic, or recurrent? Chronic means persistence of symptoms beyond a designated time period. The principal chronic lung disease affecting patients in intensive care nurseries is bronchopulmonary dysplasia (BPD), the diagnosis of which requires the persistence of respiratory symptoms in infants requiring oxygen with abnormal radiographic findings beyond 36 weeks corrected gestational age or 1 month, whichever is longer (2–4). Within BPD, symptoms can reflect an exacerbation of the primary condition or superimposed respiratory diseases such as pneumonia. Recurrent disorders are those that have disease free intervals between episodes. Aspiration pneumonia, pulmonary hemorrhage, or lobar atelectases are examples of the types of recurrent chest disorders encountered in neonatology.

What are the signs and symptoms? In young infants the most reliable indicator of pulmonary function is the sleeping respiratory rate (1). Waking rates vary widely with patient activity, feeding, and environmental stimulation, but changes in sleeping rate are more indicative of changes in minute ventilation. In general, an increase in sleeping rate is a sign of worsening lung disease until eventually there is respiratory failure and exhaustion when decreased rates supervene. Pulmonary disease is not the only reason for changes in respiratory rate, but, barring a new condition, changes in rate help define progression or resolution of a pulmonary condition. Other signs of respiratory distress include cyanosis, labored or noisy breathing with nasal flaring, retractions, grunting, stridor, wheezing, snoring, cough, inability to take oral feeds, and apnea. Few of these signs are specific for respiratory illness because metabolic, neuromotor, and cardiovascular conditions may manifest each of these. It is the combined pattern of signs that would suggest a pulmonary etiology.

When did the symptoms begin? The time of onset of symptoms is one of the best historical assistants for physical diagnosis. Symptoms such as stridor or noisy breathing that start at birth suggest a congenital anomaly. Those that develop as the volume of feeds increases suggest gastroesophageal reflux and aspiration. Those that develop only after intubation suggest mechanical complications from tube placement, obstruction, or air leaks, but those with an onset only after extubation suggest trauma from the endotracheal tube or atelectasis.

Are the respiratory symptoms constant or episodic? A troublesome neonatal respiratory condition that presents with a history of periodic or clustered symptoms is apnea of prematurity (5). Apnea can be an indicator of illness in virtually any body system in the newborn infant, but its long differential diagnosis is narrowed considerably by its history of presentation.

Conditions associated with apnea in newborn period (5,6):

Immaturity (7)
Gastroesophageal reflux
Respiratory exhaustion from increased work of breathing
Pulmonary hemorrhage
Patent ductus arteriosus
Hiccups (8)
Sighing (9)
Gavage feeding (10)
Bowel disease (localized perforation or necrotizing enterocolitis) (11)
Laryngomalacia (12)
Craniofacial anomalies and upper airway obstruction (13)
Vascular anomalies and airway obstruction (14)
Structural lesions of the central nervous system (15)
Intraventricular hemorrhage
Seizure disorder (16)
Infantile botulism (17)
Spinal cord injury (18)

Inborn errors of metabolism (19)
Hypoxic brain damage
Severe infections
Maternal drug abuse: cocaine (20)
Maternal sedation (magnesium or narcotics)
Hypothermia, hyperthermia
Hypoglycemia
Hyponatremia, hypernatremia
Hypocalcemia
Hyperammonemia
Hypoxia
Anemia

What factors affect the severity or timing of symptoms? Important factors for very young infants are the relationship of symptoms to crying, feeding, sleeping, and resting positions (21,22). For example, stridor from a unilaterally paralyzed vocal cord tends to worsen when the infant lies on the back or the unaffected side but improves when the paralyzed side is down (23). The symptoms associated with gastroesophageal reflux tend to worsen as the volume increases and in the period after a feeding.

Are other nonpulmonary symptoms present? Although symptoms might seem to indicate a pulmonary etiology, it is always prudent to inquire about symptoms outside the lungs, including signs of systemic illness from sepsis, hypoglycemia, heart failure, anemia, or hydrocephalus as well as symptoms from the upper airway. For example, an infant who has BPD can deteriorate in pulmonary status from a cause outside the lungs such as upper airway narrowing from traumatic stenosis or obstructive nasal secretions. Tachypnea associated with sweating is more likely to represent cardiac failure than a pulmonary condition, but it also can signal an abnormally hot and humid environment. Respiratory symptoms have causes other than pulmonary disease.

Are any environmental factors involved? In the early newborn period an important environmental factor affecting pulmonary symptoms in hospitalized infants is ambient humidity. The sudden loss at birth of bathing from amnionic fluid is associated with dry nasal mucosa to which a healthy infant often responds with sneezing. The thickness of secretions in sick infants depends heavily on added humidity, be it through an endotracheal tube, oxygen cannula, or in the environment. Ambient temperature also greatly affects symptoms, especially tachypnea or apnea and tachycardia, with rapid changes in body temperature in response to the environment. The entire nursery environment impacts on infant stability and reactions, so factors range from sound and light to painful stimulation. Certainly a major environmnetal factor affecting respiratory symptoms such as wheezing in young infants after discharge home is passive exposure to smoking (24,25).

Have any tests been performed? Tests of pulmonary status range from transcutaneous monitoring of oxygen saturation, blood gases, or chest radiographs to complete pulmonary function testing. Many mechanical ventilators have built in airway monitoring devices that continuously measure airflow and assess some pulmonary mechanics in intubated infants. This information augments but does not supplant the chest examination.

An important piece of historical information is what airway procedures have been performed. Intubation in the delivery room for tracheal removal of meconium or blood suggests that respiratory symptoms may be due to an aspiration, but potential local trauma from the procedure itself causes distress.

Have any treatments been given? Information about the timing and response to treatment includes use of respiratory and nonpulmonary medications. For instance, sedative medications easily decrease the respiratory drive. Prenatal maternal medication with sedatives including magnesium sulfate will not completely suppress a newborn infant's respiratory drive but may lessen responsiveness. Clinically, these infants have elevated carbon dioxide levels but do not have appropriately elevated respiratory rates because of mild depression from maternal sedatives. They do not appear to care that their pCO_2 is too high and are more comfortable than they should be were they appropriately responding.

Is there a family history of pulmonary disease? Important information about family members is a history of asthma, congenital anomalies, or cystic fibrosis, for which the recurrence risks are significant (25). It is helpful to know if family members smoke, especially when evaluating respiratory symptoms after hospital discharge (24).

Inspection and Palpation of the Chest

Observe the chest and abdomen with the infant undressed, lying supine and undisturbed on the bed. Count the respiratory rate before touching the infant by watching the movement of the chest and abdomen. Observe for periodicity of breathing and the frequency of respiratory pauses or true apnea. Look at the infant's overall color for evidence of cyanosis or pallor. If questionable, inspect the mucous membranes to verify a pink color.

Palpate the chest wall for compliance and subcutaneous consistency including edema. Note any irregularities along the ribs and sternum. Identify any areas of tenderness in the ribs, clavicles, or subcutaneous tissues. If the clavicles were not examined as part of the head and neck region, feel and compare their outlines, noting any tenderness, or swelling. Note the presence of lymph nodes or other swellings in the axilla or supraclavicular regions.

With both hands flat on the chest, feel for transmitted vibrations or rattling. Find the point of maximum cardiac impulse and note its character, including intensity, duration, rate, rhythm, crispness, and any extra impulses or thrill. Turn the infant to inspect and palpate the posterior chest.

Shape and Size of the Chest

To describe the shape of the chest, view it in all profiles. Note any lateral asymmetry or sternal prominence. If there is asymmetry, determine which side is the more likely abnormal. Compare diameters of the upper and lower rib cage, noting the angle of flare in the lower chest. Assess the thoracic index by comparing the anterior-posterior diameter to the mid-horizontal diameter. Estimate if the chest size is appropriate by comparing the circumference at the level of the breasts with those of the abdomen and head. If there is a significant discrepancy for gestational age, determine whether it is the head, chest, or abdomen that is aberrant.

The normal neonatal thorax narrows at the top and flares at the bottom and is slightly wider than deep, so its overall shape is that of an elliptical cone. Until approximately 2 years of age, but especially in the newborn period, the ribs are more horizontal and the shape of the chest is more rounded than in older children or adults (26). The anterior-posterior diameter of the thorax is between 0.87 to 1.04 times that of the horizontal diameter (27). This thoracic index decreases as the trunk lengthens and the ribs slope more caudally (26). Increases in the index to greater than one in neonates are primarily caused by intrathoracic air trapping due to aspiration pneumonitis, pneumothorax, or emphysema, but also by abnormal chest masses, notably herniated abdominal contents in congenital diaphragmatic hernia. At all gestational ages the chest circumference normally is less than the head circumference.

The shape of the chest is affected by a combination of intrinsic and extrinsic forces as well as the stiffness of the chest wall itself. Internal forces expanding the chest include the location and volume of thoracic contents and, most specifically, the lung volume, but these structures are relatively compressible by stronger external forces. Abdominal contents, especially the liver, also affect the shape of the lower chest. External forces compressing the fetal chest may be exceptional when there is an abnormal uterine shape, large maternal fibroids, severe oligohydramnios, or a co-twin. Sometimes impressions on the chest wall at birth conform with the resting arm position when there has been prolonged restriction to free fetal movement. How easily the shape is altered depends on the strength of the internal and external forces as well as the stiffness of the chest wall between them. The chest

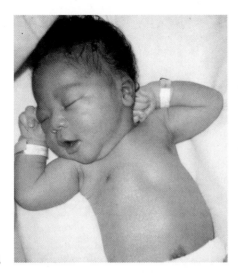 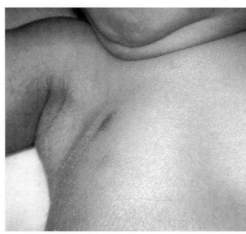

Figure 1. Aplasia of the right pectoralis major as a cause of thoracic asymmetry. **A and B:** There is a concavity above the right breast and loss of the anterior axillary fold. With this anomaly, there also may be absence of the ribs (Poland anomaly) and therefore a very thin chest wall. Despite the major chest wall anomaly, these infants do not have respiratory distress as a consequence or any limitation in arm movement.

wall is quite flexible in newborn infants because of its thinness and the relative paucity of calcification in the rib cage and sternum. Some of the thoracic stiffness comes from muscle tone, which increases with vigorous activity like crying or seizures and decreases with sleep (28–30). Congenital absence of chest muscles or bones changes chest shape but rarely causes clinical symptoms (Fig. 1). Conditions under which growth of the rib cage was insufficient because of disordered growth in the bones lead to undergrowth of the thorax; many of the severe skeletal dysplasias demonstrate abnormal thoracic size and shape as important features (31,32). In most of these conditions when the thorax is too small, the abdomen appears relatively large and distended. If the thoracic cage is significantly undergrown or severely compressed during gestation, the lungs are secondarily hypoplastic as well (31).

Causes of precordial prominence:

Noncardiac conditions in left chest
   emphysema
      aspiration syndrome
      congenital lobar emphysema
   pneumothorax
   diaphragmatic hernia
Fetal compression or deformation
Cardiac conditions*
   large arteriovenous malformations
   acardiac twin
   Ebstein anomaly with severe tricuspid regurgitation
   tetralogy of Fallot with absent pulmonary valve
   fetal arrhythmia
      complete heart block
      supraventricular tachycardia
   myocarditis

The length of the trunk in neonates is a greater proportion of total length than in older children and adults. Although a large contributor to length at birth is head height, which is

---

*In order for cardiac conditions to cause precordial prominence in the newborn period, there must be alteration in the fetal hemodynamics not corrected by placental–fetal circulation. Noncardiac causes are more likely.

disproportionately large, the trunk is also relatively longer (33). Within gestational age groups, length of the trunk does not vary as much as weight does (34).

When the chest appears too large, it is likely either asymmetrical or barreled with an increase in thoracic index. Because the neonatal chest is already somewhat rounded, further increases in thoracic volume are subtle, but most increases also cause abdominal distention that is more obvious. When thoracic contents are under enough pressure to flatten the diaphragm, there is generally an accompanying increase in abdominal diameter and tension. Chest and abdominal size increase in response to trapping of air in the pleural space (pneumothorax, pneumomediastinum), at the distal airways (aspirations, emphysema), from space-occupying processes, or overdistention from mechanical ventilation. Increase in mediastinal contents, be it from masses or from a large pneumomediastinum, specifically causes the sternum to bulge with a distancing of heart sounds and decrease in precordial impulse. An abrupt increase in abdominal size suggests either intrathoracic or abdominal pathology. The notable exception to this association of increased intrathoracic volume causing abdominal distention is prenatal herniation of abdominal contents through an incomplete diaphragm. In this case a scaphoid abdomen accompanies thoracic distention.

The chest wall itself is subject to deformations, the most common of which relate to the sternum as being too protuberant (pectus carinatum) or depressed (funnel chest or pectus excavatum). These deformities are not present at birth but can develop in response to conditions that do present in the newborn period, particularly pectus excavatum associated with laryngomalacia (35,36). Short sternum is a regular feature of trisomy 18, making the anterior chest look short (32). Flail chest deformations due to unilateral, multiple rib fractures would be extraordinarily unusual in the absence of pathologic bone fragility, but a similar phenomenon results from prolonged compression of one side of the rib cage (Fig. 2).

In premature infants the rib margins are readily apparent because of thinner layers of fat and muscle, and if not so visible, they may signal the presence of edema. Term infants whose ribs are easily seen are too thin and have insufficient subcutaneous fat.

Respiratory Pattern and Chest Movements

Look for retractions or protrusions of the soft tissues adjacent to the bony rib cage and of the ribs themselves. Lift the chin and arms if necessary to expose the areas. Time any retractions or bulging with the respiratory or cardiac cycles.

Describe the ease and coordination of respiratory effort by noting the depth of retractions and the timing of the chest and abdominal components during each respiratory cycle. Observe that movements of both sides of the chest are simultaneous and equal in excursions. Estimate the average tidal volume as low, normal, or high by noting if the respiratory excursions are shallow, normal, or deep. Evaluate the presence and degree

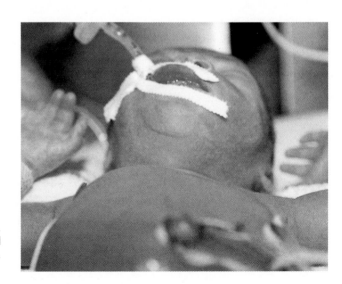

Figure 2. Chest asymmetry due to intrauterine compression. This fraternal twin had the physiologic equivalent of a left flail chest because of chronic compression from his sister's head. The anterior cartilage was palpably softer on the left.

of nasal flaring. Notice if each respiratory cycle is fluid and regular or stuttered and irregular. Determine if the infant is able to interrupt breathing long enough to cry or to suck effectively. Determine if air flow is nasal, oral, or both when the infant is not crying. If nasal, confirm equal flow on both sides by listening with a stethoscope bell in front of each nostril or by holding a thin filament of cotton and watching the deflections on inspiration and expiration.

Nasal air flow should be quiet and bilaterally equal on clinical assessment. Neonates are preferential nasal breathers, although term infants can learn to switch to oral breathing if the nasal airway is insufficient (37). For most newborn infants, nasal obstruction causes significant distress with absent or diminished airflow, retractions, and cyanosis that abates with crying. Because the nasal mucosa is relatively redundant and swollen in already narrowed passages at birth, mild trauma from intubations, feeding tubes, suctioning, or dry air easily increases resistance enough to cause distress from partial nasal obstruction (37–39). Positional changes accentuate unilateral obstruction. When the head is positioned laterally, the percentage of the tidal volume through the dependent nasal passage normally increases and that through the upper nasal passage decreases (22). The presence of a nasogastric tube significantly inhibits flow through the nares, with the greatest decreases seen when the tube is in the upper side (22). If one side is anatomically compromised, respiratory symptoms will increase with positional changes unless the other side compensates. Expected physical findings include broader nasal flaring and tachypnea, a decrease in nasal flow detected by poor movement of a simple filament, and auscultatory changes of softening or whistling on the affected side. Difficulty in oral feeding is noted.

Respiratory Rate

The respiratory rate factored with tidal volume determines minute ventilation so, to the extent that an infant's level of maturation and physiologic state allow, the rate adjusts in response to factors affecting the control of spontaneous ventilation. Rates vary widely in the first hours after birth and, in healthy term infants, the sleeping rate generally slows to about 35 breaths per minute after postnatal transition is completed (40). Smaller premature infants without lung disease normally breathe faster at 40 to 60 breaths per minute.

A sleeping infant breathes about one third more slowly than when awake and active but not crying (41). Sleeping breathing rates vary according to the sleep state in an individual and among individuals in any state. There is a high correlation between breathing rate found in different sleep states for given individuals such that some infants breathe more rapidly and others more slowly in all sleep states (42). This variability makes comparisons among infants or against an average standard less meaningful than repeated counts of an individual's rate in the same sleep state each time.

Vigorous crying is associated with a rate slower than in quiet awake infants but is still faster than during sleep (41). Some infants will have a resting respiratory rate of greater than 60 to 80 breaths per minute but still appear comfortable and able to feed effectively. It is likely that the majority of infants who breathe this rapidly while remaining capable of feeding well are taking relatively shallow breaths rather than needing to have a higher than normal minute ventilation. The ability to feed well despite tachypnea is somewhat reassuring in the absence of other significant findings, but isolated tachypnea is a presenting symptom in acidosis, sepsis, and cardiac disease as well.

Breathing Rhythm and Periodicity

Besides a fluctuating average rate, the rhythm of breathing varies in the different sleep or activity states. In rapid eye movement (REM) sleep, breathing is generally more irregular than in quiet sleep, but irregular breathing occurs in all infant states (7,43). Breathing is periodic when a regular cycle of 10 to 18 seconds is interrupted by pauses of at least 3 seconds (5). In clinical neonatology, periodic breathing associated with hemoglobin desaturations or bradycardia is called apnea even when a pause is just 10 seconds. Periodic breathing is the predominant pattern in newborn infants, who spend a greater portion of their sleep-wake cycles asleep (44). As gestational age decreases, the proportion of REM sleep increases, contributing to even more epochs of periodic breathing (44). Hiccuping, sighing, general body movements, and physical contact also affect the respiratory rate and periodicity (8,9).

Work of Breathing

One of the important impressions made from the chest examination is whether or not an infant is having to work hard or is breathing comfortably. Similarly one decides if the subject is working as hard as he or she should; i.e., is there enough effort being exerted to match the physiologic state? Work of breathing is simply how much effort is being expended. It is a subjective clinical evaluation that includes assessing nasal flaring, retractions, head bobbing, and depth of breathing as well as respiratory rate.

In the first half hour after birth, signs of increased work of breathing, including nasal flaring, grunting, and tachypnea, along with retractions and tachycardia, are common even in

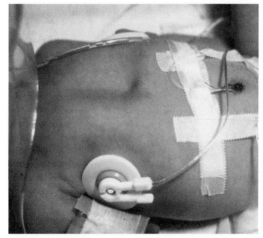
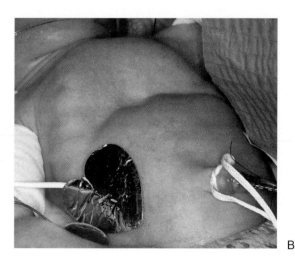
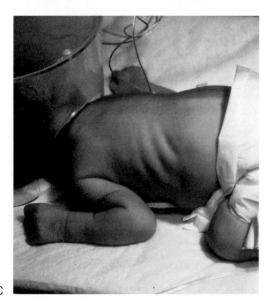
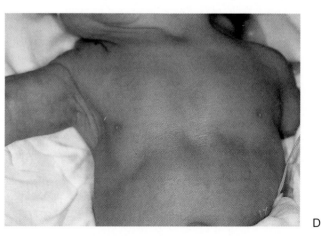

Figure 3. Retractions. **A:** Sternal. **B:** Subcostal and intercostal. **C:** Deep intercostal retractions. **D:** Subcostal and suprasternal without intercostal retraction from proximal airway obstruction.

Table 1. *Retractions and the clinical correlates*

Site of retraction	Probable region affected	Likely clinical association
Intercostal (see Fig. 3C)	Pulmonary parenchyma or distal airway	Conditions of decreased parenchymal compliance Hyaline membrane disease, retained lung fluid, pneumonia Infant likely to be tachypneic
Subcostal (see Fig. 3B and D)	Insertion of diaphragm	Mild degrees of retraction are normal in neonates; depth of retraction reflects diaphragm activity Airway obstruction or parenchymal disease; in the absence of intercostal retractions, indicates proximal airway obstruction
Unilateral subcostal (see Fig. 4B)	Decreased movement of opposite diaphragm	Isolated phrenic nerve weakness Brachial palsy Massive pleural effusion Tension pneumothorax Congenital diaphragmatic hernia
Suprasternal (see Fig. 3D)	Obstruction in the upper airway	Choanal atresia or stenosis Laryngeal stenosis or malacia Paralysis or web of vocal cords Obstruction of upper airway due to secretions, edema Obstruction of oropharynx by tongue, retrognathia
Sternal (see Fig. 3A)	Sternal compliance greater than pulmonary compliance	Proximal airway obstruction Immaturity with pliable cartilage

perfectly healthy infants (45). These findings are more notable in infants born after a short labor or by cesarean section without labor. As physiologic transition progresses normally, work of breathing decreases. Persistence or worsening of symptoms can signal delayed transition or illness.

Nasal Flaring. Visible flaring of the alae nasi is normal in newborn infants, especially during active sleep, when one third to one half of breaths include some degree of nasal flaring (46). Flaring increases when there is a need to decrease airway resistance so that it is present in most breaths in infants trying to increase their minute ventilation. Flaring can be present even in the absence of nasal air flow (46).

Retractions. Neonates demonstrate retractions more readily than do adults, and their thin chest walls make even mild intercostal retractions readily apparent (Fig. 3). The pattern of moderate to deep retractions suggests the region of abnormal compliance relationships (Table 1).

Head Bobbing. When breathing efforts are labored enough to recruit accessory muscles in the upper thorax, contractions of the sternocleidomastoids cause head bobbing with each respiratory cycle (1). Use of accessory muscles is not as common in newborn infants as in older patients, so the presence of head bobbing indicates significant distress when accompanied by other respiratory symptoms.

Hiccup. Infants hiccup before birth and continue a similar pattern after birth. An expectant mother is often able to report that her fetus has hiccuping episodes. Neonates are basically silent in their hiccuping and tend to hiccup briefly only after feeding with an average duration of approximately 8 to 9 minutes (8). In some infants, episodes of hiccups precede apneic events (8). Frequent hiccuping may be an individual variation or indicate low pCO_2, irritability to the diaphragm, seizures, drug withdrawal, or encephalopathy (Sarnat or Amiel-Tison postasphyxia stage 1) (47,48).

Paradoxical Breathing

In a normal, mature breathing pattern the chest expands during inspiration as the diaphragm pushes against the abdominal contents and generates a negative intrathoracic pressure, allowing the lungs to fill (49). In paradoxical breathing, the chest wall collapses when the abdomen distends on inspiration. A paradoxical pattern is typical for newborn infants, particularly during sleep when chest wall compliance increases. Breathing out of phase is characteristic of active sleep, with more variability in individual pattern during quiet sleep (28). In premature infants without lung disease the initial approximate one third of the inspiratory cycle involves paradoxical movement of the chest wall (50). If their lungs are stiff, the pliable chest wall collapses even more deeply and for a longer portion of the inspiratory cycle, resulting in a see-saw appearance to the respirations. Paradoxical or out-of-phase breathing is not as efficient as in-phase breathing. Observing an increase in the amount and severity of the out-of-phase pattern suggests less efficiency and potential respiratory fatigue. Pathologic conditions that change the visible relationship of the chest and abdomen during the breathing cycle can arise in either area, so the pattern of breathing movements must include consideration of the entire trunk region as well as neurologic maturity and integrity.

Causes of disruption of normal relationship of abdomen to chest during breathing cycle:

Absence of primary muscle of respiration
    Diaphragmatic paralysis or paresis
    Diaphragmatic hernia
Decreased pulmonary compliance in infant with pliable chest wall
    Respiratory distress syndrome (hyaline membrane disease)
    Pulmonary hypoplasia
    Sleep cycle and immaturity
Abnormally increased chest wall compliance: flail chest
Restriction to elevation of diaphragm
    Excessive ventilator pressure: PEEP intended or inadvertent, or overdistention
    Intrathoracic mass effect
        Tension pneumothorax
        Severe pulmonary interstitial emphysema
        Congenital lobar emphysema
        Massive pleural effusion
        Herniated abdominal contents
Restriction to depression of diaphragm: abdominal distention
    Gaseous distention of stomach
    Bowel perforation and peritonitis
    Massive organomegaly
    Ascites
    Congenitally small abdominal cavity (omphalocele)

Asymmetric Chest Movement

The two sides of the chest should move equally during respiratory excursions. Using both inspection and palpation, one can assess the fullness and equality of respiratory excursions. If there is an apparent difference, the differential diagnosis includes factors that inhibit movement of the chest, such as space-occupying conditions like tension pneumothorax; those that represent failure of neuromotor activity such as paralysis or absence of a diaphragm; or those that change the thoracic compliance such as unilateral flail chest or pulmonary interstitial emphysema.

Paralysis of the Diaphragm. Noting that chest movements are unequal in spontaneous breathing suggests a diagnosis of unilateral paralysis of the diaphragm (Fig. 4). The side

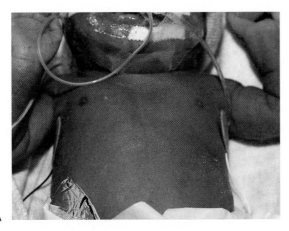
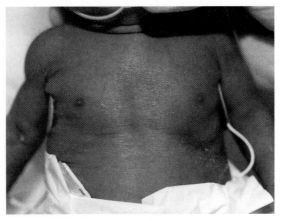

A B

Figure 4. Paralysis of right diaphragm. **A:** At rest or on exhalation there is symmetry to the anterior and lateral thorax. **B:** With deep inspiration there is marked retraction of the left subcostal region with minimal retraction on the right. Additionally, the right lower ribs flare out and up. These changes will not be observed unless the infant is breathing spontaneously and deeply enough.

with a functioning diaphragm shows the expected mild subcostal retractions with inspiration, whereas the other side has none. There is also asymmetry in chest wall excursions, with the affected side collapsing more on inspiration. The umbilicus moves upward and toward the affected side, the belly dancer's sign (51). This is best demonstrated by holding a straight edge over the umbilicus at full expiration and observing its shift with each inspiration. Shifting in the umbilicus is much less notable in neonates than in adults with diaphragmatic paralysis. To detect diaphragmatic asymmetry in ventilated infants, the spontaneous breathing efforts have to be visually separated from the mechanical breaths because the diaphragm will depress more normally with mechanical tidal ventilation. On radiography, elevation of a paralyzed diaphragm may not be immediately apparent if the infant is mechanically ventilated, but on fluoroscopy or sonography there will be differential movements between the sides with the spontaneous breaths (52). Unilateral paralysis occurs spontaneously, associated with other brachial plexus or spinal injuries, or after surgery near the mediastinum or neck. If recovery is to occur, it requires from days to 6 to 12 weeks.

Bilateral paralysis of the diaphragm is rare but an immediate cause of respiratory failure (53). It is ordinarily associated with other nerve injuries or may occur as congenital absence of the phrenic nerves (53).

Diaphragmatic Hernia. Complete or partial absence of the diaphragm presents with progressive, severe respiratory distress, thoracic distention, and a scaphoid abdomen when much of the abdominal contents have herniated into the thorax. Differential movements of the subcostal area similar to the findings in phrenic nerve paralysis are apparent.

Hernias or eventrations of the diaphragm are associated with extrapulmonary malformations often enough to warrant careful evaluation of all regions. These associations can be single additional defects, including, most commonly, cardiac defects, omphalocele, cryptorchidism, polydactyly, hip dislocation, or bowel complications, but they are also found in genetic disorders such as trisomy 18 syndrome, Turner's syndrome, Fryns syndrome, Brachmann-de Lange, and in other combinations of multiple organ involvement, notably cardiac, renal, and gastrointestinal (54).

Cyanosis

The presence of cyanosis should be considered with evaluation of each body region. It is clinically difficult to detect the mild hypoxemia that may be associated with respiratory ill-

Table 2. *Diagnostic evaluation of severe neonatal hypoxemia*

Test	Method	Result	Suggested diagnosis
Hyperoxia	Expose to 100% F_IO_2 for 5–10 min	P_aO_2 increases to >100 torr	Pulmonary parenchymal disease
		P_aO_2 increases by <20 torr	Persistent pulmonary hypertension or cyanotic congenital heart disease
Hyperventilation-hyperoxia	Mechanical ventilation with 1.0 F_IO_2 and respiratory rate 100–150 breaths/min	P_aO_2 increases to >100 torr without hyperventilation	Pulmonary parenchymal disease
		P_aO_2 increases at a critical P_{CO_2}, often to <25 torr	Persistent pulmonary hypertension
		No increase in P_aO_2 despite hyperventilation	Cyanotic congenital heart disease or severe, fixed pulmonary hypertension
Simultaneous preductal-postductal P_{O_2}	Compare P_{O_2} of right arm or shoulder to that of lower abdomen or extremities	Preductal P_{O_2} ≥15 + postductal P_{O_2}	Patent ductus arteriosus with right-to-left shunt
Echocardiography	M-Mode	Increased RVPEP and RVET	Right ventricular systolic time interval ratio >0.5 predicts PPHN (RVSTI = RVPEP/RVET)
	Venous contrast injection	Simultaneously appears in PA and LA	Patent foramen ovale
	Two-dimensional echocardiography	Deviation of intraatrial septum to left; rule out congenital heart defect	Increased pulmonary arterial pressure
	Doppler	Failure of acceleration of systolic blood flow between large main pulmonary artery and small peripheral pulmonary artery	Suggests right-to-left PDA or intracardiac shunt

LA, left atrium; PA, pulmonary artery; PDA, patent ductus arteriosus; PPHN, persistent pulmonary hypertension of the newborn; RVET, right ventricular ejection time; RVPEP, right ventricular ejection period; RVSTI, right ventricular systolic time interval.

Reprinted from Whitsett, ref. 108 with permission.

ness (55). Combinations of physical findings that include behavior changes such as loss of attentiveness, quality of cry, or irritability, or respiratory effort and auscultatory findings are more likely to lead to a diagnosis of hypoxemia than color changes alone (55). The evaluation of cyanosis includes determining if its cause is primarily pulmonary or cardiovascular (Table 2). Other sources such as hypoglycemia or neurologic factors may be present, especially when apnea is associated with the cyanosis, but the major diagnoses for causes of cyanosis primarily involve the lungs and heart.

Findings on Chest Palpation

The chest wall feels softer and more pliable with decreasing gestational age. The softness should be equal between the two sides. Any areas where there are unequal patterns of retractions or flaring should be palpated for difference in chest wall compliance. Rib fractures are unusual in neonates because of rib flexibility; their occurrence suggests abnormal bone structure from conditions such as osteogenesis imperfecta or rickets or from unusual trauma.

The finding of small knobs or beads at the chondrocostal junctions is typical of severe rickets, the so-called rachitic rosary. Physical evidence of rickets will not be present at birth but can develop in susceptible infants in the first few months if their nutritional status is inadequate.

Fremitus is a palpable vibration on the chest wall, generally caused by air passing through fluid-filled tubes. Rattling in the chest is one of the more common findings observed by parents, with the usual source being an accumulation of secretions just above the vocal cords but clearing easily. Another source of palpable vibrations in intubated infants is the water hammer effect of fluid oscillations accumulated in ventilator tubing, potentially strong enough to effect a measure of ventilation with each fluid oscillation. Newly born infants who have not yet cleared their fetal lung fluid have marked, but temporary, fremitus. Areas of consolidation have increased tactile fremitus; pneumothorax or pleural effusions have decreased fremitus.

Auscultation

Auscultation of the thorax is used to assess sounds of breathing, added pulmonary sounds, transmitted ventilator sounds, and vocalizations. In newborn infants, there are no opportunities to assess the voice sounds of whispered pectoriloquy or egophony, two wonderful physical diagnosis terms lost in neonatology.

Vocalizations

Listen to the cry and note its intensity, volume, pitch, and variability. Note how readily the infant cries and how easily he or she quiets when an annoyance eases. Listen for extrinsic sounds such as a grunt, whine, or stridor. If hiccups are present, weigh their effect on the respiratory cycles.

Cry

The infant's cry is his or her only verbal communication until more mature skills are learned, the first of which is cooing. Interpreting the cry has been a mainstay of physical diagnosis and has evolved into refined techniques of spectral analysis. A full chapter in a pediatric textbook from 1908 was devoted to the cry and described how to diagnose a variety of conditions by a characteristic pattern of crying (56). More recent studies have analyzed the components of a cry and have tried to use the analyses to predict future conditions of infants, including neurologic outcome and sudden infant death, or to diagnose specific levels of involvement in airway disease (57–60). The use of sound spectography for cry analysis provides interesting information about something heard in almost every newborn assessment but does not have practical clinical application. From these studies we have learned that individual infants have identifiable crying characteristics and that infants with some specific conditions do have typical cries, most of which are detectable by simply listening carefully. Some of the conditions associated with characteristic cry include Down's syndrome, kernicterus, infectious encephalopathy, asphyxial encephalopathy, cri du chat (5p− syndrome), and cretinism (61–67).

The pitch of a cry depends in part on the size of the infant, so that small, premature infants have higher pitched, less resonant cries with shorter cycles than bigger infants. Infants who have respiratory compromise will not be able to cry in cycles as long as other infants.

The experienced clinician senses characteristics in the neonatal cry that contribute to the physical examination, even though it may not be possible to define exactly what it is about a cry that is significant. There are features about the cry that should be considered in each assessment, some of which reflect behavior or general condition and some of which reflect the anatomy and physiology of the airway. Just like other aspects of physical diagnosis, the finding should be carefully described using standard terms rather than merely labeled as abnormal.

Questions to answer when assessing a cry:

How loud is it?

Is the pitch low, normal, or high? Is it shrill or well modulated?

Is there stridor or hoarseness associated?

Does the intensity match the effort? Is the infant crying hard but only generating a muffled sound?

How does crying affect the infant's well-being or associated conditions?

Does the infant change color with the cry? Does it make him or her pinker or bluer?

Is the infant able to cry only in short spurts because of respiratory distress? Is there breath holding with expiration?

What does it take to stimulate or to suppress crying? Is it spontaneous or stimulated with mere handling, or does it take a strong noxious stimulus? Does it lessen in intensity as soon as the noxious stimulus is removed?

How strong is the effort used to generate it? Is the infant crying hard or is he or she whimpering or whining even with a strong stimulus?

Hoarseness

Hoarseness indicates lesions affecting the length, mass, or tension of the vibrating portion of the vocal cords or their shape at the margins. When present, it helps identify the site of airway pathology as specifically involving the cords or their neurologic control. Hoarseness may be present with or without stridor.

In the first day of life, a temporary cause of mild hoarseness is trauma from intubation or suctioning of meconium. Infants who are hoarse from suctioning usually also demonstrate discomfort on swallowing and refuse to feed despite apparent hunger, but the symptoms quickly resolve. Inconsolable infants with strenuous crying become hoarse if their crying persists.

Differential diagnosis of hoarseness in newborn period (23,68):

Neurogenic vocal cord paralysis

Trauma

    postintubation

        acute edema or hematoma

        granuloma

        stenosis

    dislocation of arytenoid cartilage during intubation

    foreign body

Congenital anomalies of larynx

    web of vocal cord

    laryngeal cyst

    thyroglossal duct cyst

    laryngotracheoesophageal cleft or fissure

    vocal cord sulcus

    subglottic stenosis

Miscellaneous

    gastroesophageal reflux

    hypothyroidism

    lingual thyroid

    de Lange's syndrome

    cri-du-chat syndrome

    maternal thiamin deficiency

    congenital syphilis

    hemangioma

    lymphangioma (cystic hygroma)

Cooing

Infants start to make social sounds within 1 to 2 weeks after they learn to smile socially, so some term infants initiate cooing as early as 3 weeks of age (69). Achieving this easily enjoyed milestone is a reassuring sign of cortical maturation because it will not develop in infants with severely damaged or malformed neurologic systems.

Other Spontaneous Sounds

Grunt and Whine

Grunting is the sound produced when the first part of expiration is forced against a closed glottis. The process generates a higher pressure in the airways than would be seen if there were no resistance during expiration. Newborn infants grunt in an effort to hold open distal airways and prevent or reverse the collapse occurring in conditions such as hyaline membrane disease (HMD) or pulmonary edema. Grunting is not specific to HMD and is common in infants with sepsis and acidosis, as well as other pulmonary conditions. It also occurs in infants with nonpulmonary distress, including abdominal pathology (70).

The process of grunting prolongs expiration, so the potential respiratory rate is limited. In most distressed infants, epochs of grunting with rates of 40 to 60 breaths per minute alternate with periods of tachypnea with rates of 80 to 100 breaths per minute as the infant seeks the most effective means of ventilation.

The effort of grunting often continues even after artificial continuous airway pressure is started. Absent an endotracheal tube, the infant's own grunt is still audible and signals that he or she is trying to generate even higher expiratory pressures. With a tube through the glottis, the infant may continue to attempt to accomplish the same physiologic result by consistently exhaling against the machine's inspiratory cycle or out of phase with the mechanical breaths.

Whining is similar to grunting but with less complete closure of the glottis during exhalation. Whining may be normal, a sign of pain, or the equivalent of mild grunting.

Cough

Spontaneous cough is always abnormal in the neonatal period and requires evaluation. The cough reflex involves three sites variably developed at birth: (a) the cough receptors in the nose, pharynx, trachea, ear canal, and pleura; (b) the cough center in the brain stem, which processes the efferent stimuli; and (c) effectors to the muscles of respiration and the glottis. An effective cough is a series of coordinated actions in sequence: glottic closure, forceful contraction of the diaphragm, and sudden opening of the glottis for exhalation. How much stimulus it takes to generate a cough response depends in part on maturity so the absence of cough is not a reassuring finding in premature or sick infants.

The mnemonic CRADLE is suggested for causes of cough in the neonatal period (71). Of these possibilities, aspiration and respiratory infections, notably infection with respiratory syncytial virus or chlamydia, are most likely.

C cystic fibrosis
R respiratory infection
A aspiration (reflux, swallowing dysfunction, tracheoesophageal fistula)
D dyskinesia of cilia
L lung, airway, vascular malformation
E edema (heart failure, bronchopulmonary dysplasia)

"Snurgles"

The term "snurgles" has been used to describe a common sound heard especially in premature infants and others with high arched palates and narrow nasal passages (72). The sound is produced by inhalation through loose mucus in the nasopharynx so is not present at birth because of limited production of mucus until the end of the first month. Although noisy, it has little if any effect on breathing.

Snoring

Noisy breathing while sleeping may be simple nasal congestion or, if true snoring, indicate more serious obstruction to airflow. In young children, adenoid hyperplasia is the most commonly found airway problem associated with chronic snoring (73). This is unlikely in the neonatal period because the tonsils and adenoids are very small, but it is a common finding later on for infants who have had indwelling nasal tubes in intensive care nurseries. Snoring represents a form of upper airway obstruction and can be severe enough to cause sleep apnea (74). Infants with micrognathia and craniofacial anomalies appear particularly prone to snore and demonstrate sleep apnea, particularly when on their backs (13,74,75).

Sounds on Auscultation of the Chest

If the infant is crying, console him or her until quiet. Use the small diaphragm of a stethoscope to listen on alternating sides over at least four anterior quadrants, under each axilla, and four back quadrants. Compare the sounds on each side and front to back. Determine how well air is moving and if it seems to be filling the alveoli. If there is sufficient air movement, listen for extra sounds. If breath sounds are asymmetric, soft, distant, or insufficient in the presence of good respiratory effort, evaluate for the factors interfering with transmission of sound, including pleural air or fluid. Make certain that breath sounds are not replaced by bowel sounds, indicating a diaphragmatic hernia.

For the infant on a ventilator, separate and compare the sounds made by the machine to those made by the infant. Assess the duration of inspiration compared with expiration. Determine if there is a pause in the cycle at the end of expiration before beginning the next inspiration or if inspiration seems to begin just as soon as expiration slows. In the sounds generated by ventilator breaths, determine if there continues to be inspiratory filling throughout the positive pressure breath or if it stops before the end of each mechanical breath.

Recommended techniques for examination of the adult chest involve listening in 18 to 36 sites (76,77). For a small chest, it is necessary in screening to listen only over the major quadrants and under the arms because sounds are so well transmitted through the thin chest wall. If abnormal sounds are present, more sites of auscultation help localize the source so the stethoscope head should be inched over the entire chest surface (Table 3).

The first step for assessing pulmonary status through auscultation is establishing the presence of air movement. Air entry can be described as normal, fair, or poor. There must be sufficient air flow to generate extrapulmonary sounds so the absence of crackles, wheezes, or rhonchi is not reassuring if air entry is insufficient in the first place.

Table 3. *Sites for auscultation of lobes*

Lobe	Chest site
Right upper	Anterior above nipple; posterior above midpoint of scapula
Right middle	Anterior in triangle from nipple to sternum and to xiphoid
Right lower	Axilla onto back below midpoint of scapula
Left upper	Anterior chest where not occupied by heart
Left lower	Axilla onto back below tip of scapula

Table 4. *Normal breath sounds heard on auscultation in adults*

Sound	Quality	Location
Bronchial	Loud, pitch high, dominant in expiration	Trachea, anterior
Bronchovesicular	Medium volume and pitch, heard equally in inspiration and expiration	Main bronchi, anterior and some interscapular
Vesicular	Soft to medium, pitch lower, dominant in inspiration	Over remainder of lung fields

Reprinted from Willms, ref. 321, with permission.

Normal Breath Sounds

Compared with larger patients, breath sounds in neonates are high pitched and, over the upper lobes, even higher pitched in premature infants (78). The median frequencies of normal lung sounds in both premature and term infants are significantly higher than in adults (78). Additionally, there is less difference in the sound intensity between inspiration and expiration (79). The expiratory breath sounds are more similar to inspiratory sounds the smaller the infant, with more appreciable differences in larger infants. Using comparable nomenclature, normal breath sounds in neonates would be classified as bronchovesicular, particularly in small premature infants (Table 4). They are comparable to the sounds made when air is blown and sucked through straws of different diameters. Bronchovesicular sounds are heard over much of the small chest with little difference in the periphery compared with the anterior chest.

Adventitious Sounds

Additional pulmonary sounds occurring with the respiratory cycle are timed and characterized (Table 5). The nomenclature now accepted by international consensus divides sounds into three general categories: crackles, wheezes, and rhonchi (80,81).

Crackles. Crackles are the tiny explosions heard at the chest wall during inspiration that are discontinuous and timed as early or late in the first or second half of the inspiratory cycle, respectively. They also can be described as fine or coarse. Early, fine crackles emanate from small distal airways, having collapsed on expiration, that snap open on inspiration. Early, coarse crackles are associated with pneumonia and hyaline membrane disease but are heard in normal transition of the lungs after birth. Late crackles, especially when sounding like Velcro separating, cutting across styrofoam, or walking on dry snow, are typically found in infants with pulmonary interstitial emphysema. The approach to treating an infant in whom early, fine crackles predominate differs from that used in one in whom late crackles predominate. In the former, the early crackles suggest a need for higher tidal ventilation or end-expiratory pressure to expand the alveoli, whereas in the latter, late crackles suggest a need to shorten inspiration or lower tidal ventilation to relieve alveolar air trapping.

Table 5. *Adventital lung sounds*

Description	Term
Discontinuous	
Fine (high pitch, low amplitude, short duration)	Fine crackles
Coarse (low pitch, high amplitude, long duration)	Coarse crackles
Continuous	
High-pitched	Wheezes
Low-pitched	Rhonchus

Based on International Symposium on Lung Sounds (322).

Wheezes. Wheezes are continuous sounds in the sense that their duration is longer than crackles but not necessarily throughout the respiratory cycle. A wheeze is musical and high but its pitch depends on the rate of gas flow because a more rapid flow produces a higher tone. The sounds are generated by air passing at high velocity through an airway narrowed to the point of closure. If airflow is not high enough, no wheeze is generated, even if the airway is very constricted; loss of wheezing can signal either recovery if the air flow is improving or respiratory failure if it is decreasing. When flow is extraordinarily high, wheezing occurs even if the airway size is normal. Wheezing is heard most often on exhalation because the airways inside the chest normally get smaller on exhalation. It is heard on both phases of a respiratory cycle if the diameter of the airway is restricted and fixed.

Wheezing is described as heterophonous or homophonous depending on its variability throughout the lung fields (82). If only the most distal airways are constricted, the loudness and quality of the wheezing is not uniform over all the lung fields, so it would be heterophonous. Wheezing is homophonous if the quality is consistent through the lung fields even though it might soften at some distance from a more central source. Conditions such as tracheal compression or bronchomalacia that cause wheezing from constriction of large airways are likely to have homophonous wheezing.

Most of the causes of wheezing in children, including foreign bodies, can appear in the newborn period (72,82) (Table 6).

Rhonchi. Rhonchi are also continuous but not musical, are low pitched, and occur on inspiration and expiration. They arise in larger airways from partial obstruction by mucus, secretions, or stricture. Rhonchi clear or improve with coughing, suctioning, and postural drainage if secretions can be removed.

Other Sounds. Because newborn infants do not develop significant pleural inflammatory reactions even with strong stimuli, they rarely develop pleural or pericardial friction rubs. Extraneous sounds with the periodicity of the respiratory or cardiac cycles more likely represents air leaks in the pleural, mediastinal, or pericardial spaces rather than friction rubs.

When infants are on mechanical ventilatory support, be it by mechanical ventilation, nasal continuous positive airway pressure, or nasal cannula, assessing the artificially generated sounds is an important part of an examination both for the information it can add di-

Table 6. *Causes of wheezing in children*

Homophonous	Heterophonous
Acute	
Foreign body aspiration	Bronchiolitis
	Asthma
Persistent or recurrent	
Nonstructural	
Gastroesophageal reflux	Asthma
Retained foreign body	Cystic fibrosis
Chronic bacterial bronchitis	Bronchopulmonary dysplasia
	Immotile cilia syndrome
	Gastroesophageal reflux
Structural	
Tracheomalacia/bronchomalacia	
Vascular compression/rings	
Tracheal stenosis/webs	
Cystic lesions/masses	
Tumors	

Reprinted from Panitch, ref. 82, with permission.

rectly and because of their interference in listening to the breath sounds generated by the infant. For example, when an infant is being treated with continuous positive airway pressure through a device that stops above the glottis, an absence of the sounds of continuous air flow on chest auscultation suggests that the therapy is not being effectively delivered. The device may be dislodged or occluded, or the infant may be closing his or her own glottis against the air flow. Similarly, when an infant is intubated, the examination assesses efficacy and complications, including location of the endotracheal tube and air leaks into the pleural space or out of the tracheal tube. Because cuffed tubes are not used and some tracheal leak may be desirable to help prevent air trapping, auscultation over the trachea into the neck helps localize and quantitate the characteristic high-pitched, coarse, inspiratory wheezing associated with air escaping through the glottis with each mechanical breath.

Stridor. Stridor is a rough, harsh sound emanating from a narrowing in upper airways proximal to the thoracic inlet. In contrast to wheezing, stridor is worse during inspiration because the diameter of the extrathoracic airways decreases during inspiration and increases during exhalation. Stridor is present in both phases of the respiratory cycle if the narrowing is fixed or severe as long as there is enough air flow to generate the turbulence heard as stridor. As a narrowing increases, the pitch of stridor elevates, then becomes biphasic, and, eventually after a critical point of decreased air flow, softens.

The characteristics of the stridor and accompanying physical findings help localize the site of narrowing. Laryngomalacia generates a low-pitched, vibrating quality in comparison with subglottic stenosis, which generates a higher-pitched, more fixed, but softer noise. A tracheal vascular ring typically causes both inspiratory and expiratory stridor but may be difficult to distinguish from a very loud wheeze (83). If a lesion is extrathoracic, the inspiratory phase is more pronounced, but if it is intrathoracic, the expiratory phase is louder (83). When two conditions such as laryngomalacia and a vascular ring occur together, as is often the case, it may be impossible to separate the findings.

Stridor accompanies hoarseness or aphonia when the narrowing involves the glottis; if subglottic, the cry is softened but not hoarse. If the narrowing is above the glottis, the cry takes on a nasal or muffled character. The causes of stridor in infants are numerous and include everything that can impact on the diameter of the upper airway. Such causes can originate either inside or outside the respiratory tract (84) (Table 7).

Percussion of Chest

Chest percussion is not as useful in the physical assessment in small patients as it is when the thoracic cage is larger because bimanual percussion is technically difficult on the small surface and significant changes in pulmonary density such as lobar consolidation or complete atelectasis may be too small to detect. These limitations should not lead to complete neglect of its potential value. A modification of this technique, auscultatory topographic percussion, is more feasible and provides information on major changes in intrathoracic density and the location of solid viscera such as the liver.

Auscultatory Percussion

Lay the diaphragm of a stethoscope over the area assumed to have the highest density such as the liver or collapsed lung. Lightly scratch the chest or abdominal wall and listen for a change in pitch as the stroking is brought closer to the stethoscope. Start the scratching several centimeters away from the suspected liver margin and progress toward the margin in 0.5- to 1-cm advances. The pitch elevates and seems closer when the scratching overlies the higher density structures.

Table 7. *Conditions associated with stridor*

Condition	Physical or historical finding	Associated conditions	References
Laryngomalacia (most frequent cause)	Stridor increased by crying or exertion Stridor improved by prone position or neck extension	Gastroesophageal reflux Obstructive sleep apnea Failure to thrive Pectus excavatum Sporadic or autosomal dominant	12, 35, 323–326
Vocal cord paralysis or paresis, congenital or acquired at birth	Unilateral abductor cord paralysis: hoarse cry that lessens in severity with time but generally with little stridor. Symptoms lessen when affected side is in a dependent position. Bilateral paralysis: aphonia and stridor of varying severity with obstructive respiratory distress	Incidence is higher when other anomalies are present Arnold-Chiari malformation associated with myelomeningocele Intracranial hemorrhage Familial vocal cord paralysis Brachial palsy Postoperative: particularly after procedures involving mediastinum (ligation of PDA), neck or neurosurgery	327–330
Congenital laryngotracheal stenosis	Severe stenosis: stridor from birth Less severe: presents as recurrent croup when overlying airway narrows with infection		331
Acquired laryngotracheal (subglottic) stenosis	History of intubation but not necessarily related to duration or repetition of intubation Inability to tolerate extubation	Bronchopulmonary dysplasia	332, 333
Laryngeal cysts, saccular or ductal (branchial cyst, bronchogenic cyst)	Stridor accompanied by dyspnea and feeding difficulty	25% have more than one cyst with the aryepiglottic folds and vallecula the most common sites; subglottic less common	134, 334–336
Vascular ring, double aortic arch (most common), right arch and persistent ductus arteriosus or ligamentum; anomalous subclavian artery; aberrant innominate artery; or pulmonary sling	Stridor present in inspiration and expiration with a fixed pitch in both phases	Respiratory symptoms may increase with feeding	14, 337–339

Thyroid
  Goiter
  Lingual thyroid
	Enlargement of anterior neck or tongue	Symptoms of hypothyroidism with goiter	340, 341

Postextubation laryngeal edema	Stridor present or increasing after extubation associated with hoarseness and hypophonia	Peak time of symptoms in 12–48 h after extubation	324

Infection
  candidiasis
  herpes simplex
  acute epiglottitis with *Staphylococcus aureus*
		Feeding difficulty
		Systemic symptoms
			342–344

Dislocated arytenoid cartilage	Onset of stridor after intubation		
Gastroesophageal reflux	Periodic stridor relating to feeding	Arching, emesis, feeding refusal, bradycardia, apnea	345, 346
Glottic web	Aphonia or hypophonia	Isolated finding	347
Laryngeal fibromatosis	Progressive increase in stridor	Isolated finding	348
Laryngeal foreign body	Acute onset of stridor after invasive procedure	Isolated finding	68
Lymphangioma	Stridor related to size	Isolated or with other sites	349

By auscultating through the diaphragm of a stethoscope for pitch modulation, one can outline the borders of larger objects that are denser than normal lungs or bowel. This technique is unlikely to detect changes in pulmonary density from partial segmental atelectasis, but it is useful for defining the upper and lower margins of the liver, the left cardiac border, complete lobar atelectasis, or massive effusion.

Transillumination of the Chest

If there are physical signs of an intrathoracic air leak, transilluminate the chest wall by holding a fiberoptic light source tightly against the chest wall. Rather than holding the light directly over an area suspected to contain the air, start at a distance so the light shines across the collected air and advance the light source until all areas have been transilluminated or a diagnosis made. Use transillumination findings to determine efficacy of therapy and resolution of air leaks as well.

A light source has to be bright, yet cool, and with a tip that seals closely to the skin. The transilluminator will produce a corona around its tip with the width of the glow depending on light intensity and the amount of subcutaneous fat and edema. A contained air leak will glow in the shape of its compartment and change in shape accordingly with respiratory or cardiac excursions (Fig. 5). Breathing movements of the lung or contractions of the heart may be apparent in the abnormal areas of increased light transmission.

Causes of Respiratory Distress

The causes of respiratory distress in the newborn and young infant may lie in the pulmonary system but also can be well outside that system. Almost any disruption or pathologic process causes apnea in premature infants (5,10,11,13–15,17–20). Increased work of breathing indicates pulmonary involvement but not necessarily a pulmonary origin. It is also important to remember that the pulmonary system includes far more than the lungs alone and that it has both intra- and extrathoracic components. It is the complex of physical findings that aid in localizing the source of distress (Tables 8 and 9).

A frequent cause of illness and respiratory distress in neonates and young infants is pneumonia. Recognizing the distinguishing features of specific etiologic agents is helpful, although none are pathognomonic (Table 10).

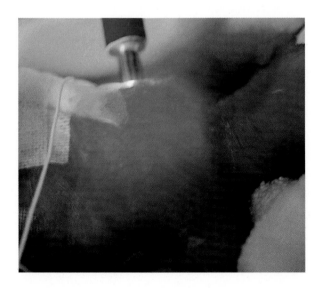

Figure 5. Transillumination of the chest in tension pneumothorax. The bright red glow follows the shape of the right thoracic cavity.

Breasts

Inspect the breasts for definition of each nipple, areolar stippling, width of areola, and breast bud. Determine if their distance from the mid-line is appropriate for age in relation to chest circumference. Palpate the breast tissue for consistency without compressing the tissue enough to express fluid. Look along the mammary lines for accessory nipples that may range in development from well-formed accessory breasts to just slightly pigmented dimples.

Breast size varies according to birth weight and gestational age. Infants who are large for gestational age have larger breast nodules than those who are normal or undergrown for gestational age. There is little appreciable difference is breast size between female and male infants of the same weights, although measured diameters in female infants are larger (8.5 ± 2.0 mm in females compared with 7.8 ± 2.1 mm in males) (85).

As the fetal breast develops, both the mass of the breast bud and the definition of the nipple and areola progress. The stage of development is useful as one of the parameters for assessing gestational age. The areola becomes more stippled and pigmented in addition to increasing in diameter as the nipple becomes more erectile. Inversion of the nipple is present in some infants at birth, but the relationship to this condition in adults in unknown (Fig. 6).

The internipple distance varies with gestational age and chest circumference (See Appendix Fig. 22). A ratio of internipple distance to chest circumference is more constant throughout gestation and should be less than 0.28 (86). Widely spaced nipples have an index greater than 0.28 and are seen in a variety of conditions, including fetal hydantoin effects, trisomies of 4, 8, 18, and 20, monosomy XO (Turner's syndrome), and deletion of 9p,18q (32) (Fig. 7).

Witch's Milk

In response to maternal hormones, the newborn breasts hypertrophy and produce a milky discharge called witch's milk that appears by the end of first week and lasts for a few weeks

Table 8. *Differential diagnosis of respiratory distress in the newborn period*

Respiratory		Extrapulmonary				
Parenchymal	Extraparenchymal	Heart	Metabolic	Brain	Blood	Abdominal
Respiratory distress syndrome (hyaline membrane disease)	Upper airway obstruction, choanal atresia, stenosis, hemangioma, goiter	Congestive heart failure	Metabolic acidosis	Hemorrhage	Acute blood loss	Necrotizing enterocolitis
Transient tachypnea	Pneumothorax	Patent ductus arteriosus	Hypoglycemia	Edema	Hypovolemia	Tension pneumoperitoneum
Amnionic fluid aspiration syndrome (meconium, blood, or clear fluid)	Intrathoracic space-occupying lesion, e.g., diaphragmatic hernia, pleural effusion	Cyanotic congenital heart disease	Hypothermia	Drugs	Twin-to-twin transfusion	Large mass
Primary pulmonary hypertension	Bilateral vocal cord paralysis	Vascular ring	Hyperthermia	Trauma	Hyperviscosity	
Pneumonia	Diaphragmatic paralysis		Septicemia	Obstructed hydrocephalus		
Pulmonary hemorrhage, edema			Hyperammonemia	Pain		
Interstitial emphysema						
Immature lung syndrome						
Pulmonary hypoplasia						

Table 9. *Clinical findings in contained pulmonary air leaks*

Site	Findings on observation	Findings on auscultation	Other findings
Pneumothorax, unilateral under tension	Unilateral decrease in chest wall movement Abdominal distention Flaring of anterior, inferior rib cage Bulging of intercostal spaces	Decrease in breath sounds Sometimes air bubbling into the pleural space may be heard	Shift in EKG Decrease in excursion (tidal volume) on impedence pneumogram
Pulmonary interstitial emphysema, bilateral	Decrease in chest wall movement	Dry crunching (walking on dry snow or cutting styrofoam) Crepitation (350)	Poor pulmonary compliance
Lobar emphysema	Increase in thoracic volume limited to affected area (rib flaring, diameter)	Decrease in breath sounds over affected area	
Pneumomediastinum	Increase in anterior-posterior dimension of chest at the sternum; may appear to be a loss of the normal curvature inward at the sternum	Distancing of heart sounds but without a shift Rarely get a classical mediastinal crunch in neonates	Decrease in heart sounds similar to change in pneumopericardium but generally without severe restriction in cardiac output so arterial pulse pressure is not affected
Pneumopericardium with tamponade	Dampening in peripheral pulses	Decrease in heart sounds	Decrease in voltage on EKG Dampening in amplitude on arterial wave patterns Decrease in palpable pulses
Pneumoperitoneum	Abdominal distention with tension	No findings on auscultation. Even when due to severely diseased bowel and perforation, there may still be audible bowel sounds.	Transillumination that can be distinguished from normal bowel or bladder by its seeking the highest point upon shift in patient position When the air leak is from dissection of mediastinal air, there are few accompanying abdominal signs of peritonitis
Subcutaneous emphysema, (nuchal emphysema)	Crepitance and bumpy appearance under the skin of the anterior neck due to dissection of gas along mediastinal structures. If the air leak is high in oxygen content, the area may be paradoxically pink in an infant who is otherwise cyanotic.	Crunching with movement of the stethoscope over the affected area.	

to several months (Fig. 8). All newborn infants of either sex have rudimentary milk production with the quantity produced directly proportionate to the size of the breast nodule and increasing if the breasts are massaged to express the milk (87). Clinical galactorrhea develops in less than 5% of infants but can persist for at least 2 months (88). Rarely, nipple discharge becomes bloody or purulent, usually indicating mastitis. Bloody nipple discharge not related to mastitis, although rare, can persist for months until it spontaneously resolves (89). Extramedullary hematopoiesis is found microscopically in all neonatal breast tissue but is not clinically significant (90). A relationship to bloody discharge is not described. Although rare, purulent discharge indicates mastitis or abscess, most commonly

Table 10. *Clinical features of pneumonia in infants less than 3 months of age*

	Respiratory syncytial virus	Other respiratory viruses	Chlamydia	Cytomegalovirus	Pertussis
Symptoms and signs					
Season	Winter	Unique to each virus	Any	Any	Any
Onset	Acute, days	Acute, days	Insidious	Insidious	Progressive, days
Fever	One-half	Majority	No	Unusual	No
Cough	Yes	Yes	Staccato	Yes	Paroxysmal
Associated features	Apnea, URI	URI, croup, conjunctivitis, rash	Conjunctivitis, failure to thrive	Failure to thrive, hepatosplenomegaly, petechial rash	Apnea, cyanosis posttussive vomiting
General appearance	Not toxic	Not toxic, stridor	Well, tachypnea	Chronically ill	Well between paroxysms
Auscultation	Wheezes, sonorous rales	Rales, wheezes	Diffuse rales	Rales, wheezes	Clear
Cardinal feature	Respiratory distress	Respiratory distress	Cough	Failure to thrive	Cough
Degree of Illness	Severity comparable with findings	Severity comparable to findings	Findings greater than severity	General appearance worse than respiratory symptoms	Limited to a cough
Laboratory tests					
Chest radiograph	Hyperinflation, peribronchial thickening, subsegmental atelectasis	Hyperinflation, ± peribronchial thickening, ± diffuse interstitial infiltrates	Hyperinflation, diffuse alveolar and interstitial infiltrates	Diffuse interstitial infiltrates	Normal or perihilar infiltrate
White blood cell count	Normal or lymphocytosis	Normal or lymphocytosis or neutropenia	Eosinophilia	Normal or eosinophilia or lymphocytosis	Lymphocytosis eosinophilia
Other findings	Hypoxemia		Increase in IgG, IgA, IgM	Increase in IgG, IgA, IgM, thrombocytopenia	
Diagnostic test	Nasal wash FA, culture	Nasal wash FA, culture, throat culture	Conjunctival scraping FA, Leuken's FA	Leuken's, urine culture	NP FA, culture
Treatment	Ribavirin for some	None, or possibly ribavirin	Erythromycin or sulfisoxazole	None	Erythromycin

URI, upper respiratory infection; FA, fluorescent antibody test; NP, nasopharyngeal.
Modified from Long, ref. 350, with permission.

due to infection from *Staphylococcus aureus* and without other systemic symptoms (91). Abscesses cause loss of enough breast tissue to affect adult breast size (91). The breast enlargement in mastitis may be uniform, but the presence of other symptoms of inflammation, including erythema and warmth, help distinguish it from noninflammatory hypertrophy. In either condition the breast is tender (Figs. 9 and 10).

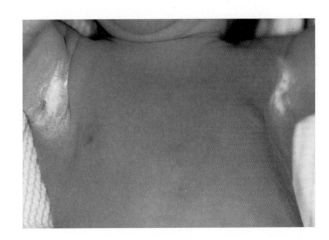

Figure 6. Unilateral inverted nipple on the right with normal protrusion on the left. The axillae are coated with vernix.

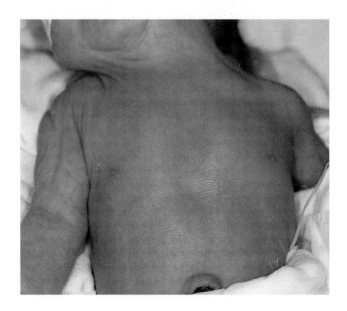

Figure 7. Widely spaced nipples in infant with Noonan's syndrome. Note also the redundant skin in the neck.

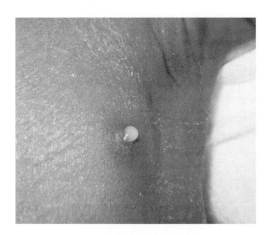

Figure 8. Witches milk expressed from mild hypertrophied left breast.

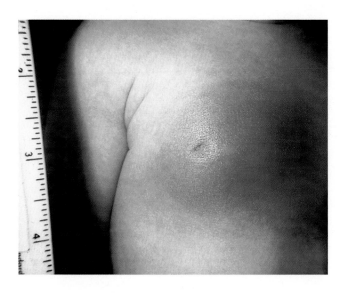

Figure 9. Mastitis. Breast is swollen, erythematous, warm and tender.

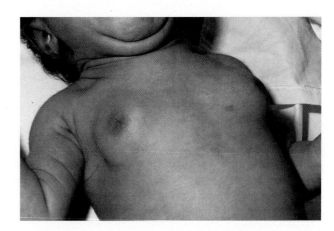

Figure 10. Breast hypertrophy at 1 month of age.

Supernumerary Nipples

Polythelia, or the presence of supernumerary nipples, is a common variation of normal with an incidence relating to race and family (92,93) (Fig. 11). In some instances it appears to be autosomal dominant (94). Extra nipples may be rudimentary, appearing as little more than slightly pigmented linear dimples of 1 to 2 mm in the mammary lines, or they may be more defined, with palpable breast nodules. There is at least a 1% incidence in darkly pigmented newborns with the lowest frequency reported in Asians (93). Some studies have suggested an association with renal anomalies, but other prospective studies have refuted this association and confirm that there is no indication for further evaluation based on polythelia alone (95,96).

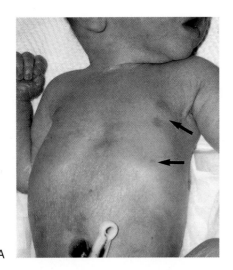

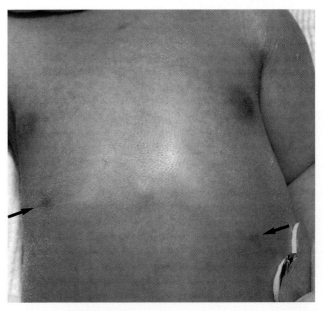

Figure 11. Supernumerary nipples. **A:** Two extra rudimentary nipples on left along mammary line. **B:** Extra nipple on each side at different levels along the mammary line. There is a small skin tag at medial margin of the left areola that should not be confused with polythelia.

TECHNIQUE OF EXAMINATION OF THE CARDIOVASCULAR SYSTEM

Review history pertinent to cardiovascular system
Assess growth
Determine what phase of cardiopulmonary transition the infant has completed
Count respiratory rate and assess work of breathing
Inspect
    anterior trunk for
        shape and symmetry of anterior chest
        precordial activity
    forehead for sweating
    visible pulsations in the neck
    presence of associated noncardiac anomalies
Palpate
    precordium for
        location, timing, character, and intensity of cardiac impulses
        extraneous cardiac vibrations
    peripheral pulses for
        intensity
        comparison of preductal and postductal pulses
    abdomen for liver size and pulsations
Auscultate
    precordium for
        cardiac rate and rhythm
        character and location of
            first and second heart sounds
            other systolic and diastolic sounds
    other areas for cardiac auscultation
        thoracic periphery
        neck, head, abdomen, back, and any areas of dermal swelling or apparent vascular
            malformations
Measure blood pressure
Select appropriate laboratory tests
    blood gases, oxygen saturation monitoring
    chest x-ray
    electrocardiogram
    cardiology consultation

Pertinent History for Cardiovascular Assessment

Many of the pertinent questions in the evaluation of pulmonary conditions also apply to the cardiovascular assessment. Because pulmonary and cardiac symptoms compare, the time course and family history are especially important in determining which of these two systems is more likely the primary site of pathology. Additionally, the time of presentation suggests the type of cardiac condition (Table 11) (97). The frequency with which any condition presents in the first month of life does not directly indicate its overall prevalence. How likely the condition is to be diagnosed by cardiologists after referral for symptoms relates more to the severity of those symptoms than to the prevalence of the condition. Tertiary centers reporting on their admissions will have prevalence rates skewed toward more serious diagnoses compared with what a general clinician will see. Conditions likely to require referral as urgent cardiac crises are far less common than conditions having cardiac signs for the primary caregiver to interpret. In premature infants by far the most frequent cardiac diagnoses are patent ductus arteriosus in the first month and peripheral pulmonary stenosis, problems relatively infrequent in term infants without other anomalies or syndromic findings. In infants weighing less than 1,500 g undergoing mechanical ventilation,

Table 11. *Top five diagnoses presenting at different ages*

Diagnosis	Percentage of patients
Age on admission: 0–6 days (n = 537)	
ᴅ-Transposition of great vessels	19
Hypoplastic left ventricle	14
Tetralogy of Fallot	8
Coarctation of aorta	7
Ventricular septal defect	3
Others	49
Age on admission: 7–13 days (n = 195)	
Coarctation of aorta	16
Ventricular septal defect	14
Hypoplastic left ventricle	8
ᴅ-Transposition of great vessels	7
Tetralogy of Fallot	7
Others	48
Age on admission: 14–28 days (n = 177)	
Ventricular septal defect	16
Tetralogy of Fallot	7
Coarctation of aorta	12
ᴅ-Transposition of great vessels	7
Patent ductus arteriosus	5
Others	53

Reprinted from Flanagan and Fyler, ref. 97, with permission

significant patent ductus arteriosus is found by echocardiography in some 36% (98). Some cardiac conditions present prenatally, notably those associated with congestive heart failure and hydrops, including cardiomyopathies, premature closure of the foramen ovale, and arrhythmias. For this reason, a cardiac history includes pregnancy information as well as intrauterine growth assessment.

Infants with congenital heart disease may have a relatively low weight for length at birth, especially when compared with the birth weights of their siblings. Postnatal growth may be affected by either excessive weight gain from fluid retention or poor growth from an inability to consume sufficient calories.

Questions included in assessing for possible cardiac disease:

Was oxygen needed for any time beyond the first few minutes of life?

Has cyanosis ever been observed, and, if so, what seemed to precipitate it?

Did the infant require assisted ventilation? If so, did his time course match one generally expected for primary lung disease process or was it prolonged or atypical?

Is the pattern of intrauterine and postnatal growth appropriate and comparable with siblings and other infants of similar demographic and racial background?

Can the infant take feedings well by mouth or does he (or she) need frequent periods of rest even though he seems hungry?

Does the infant sweat in a cool environment?

Is there a family history of congenital heart disease?

Were there any pregnancy factors associated with fetal heart disease?

Are there extracardiac anomalies suggesting multisystem organ involvement, especially skeletal, ear, or oral-facial anomalies?

Are there any dysmorphic findings suggesting a syndrome commonly associated with cardiac disease?

Were the symptoms present from birth or was there a gradual increase or an acute onset of symptoms after an initially normal period?

Pregnancy factors associated with congenital heart disease:

Maternal autoimmune disease: lupus erythematosus
Maternal diabetes mellitus, phenylketonuria
Prenatal infection: rubella, mumps, cytomegalovirus
Drug ingestion: alcohol, hydantoin, valproic acid, trimethadione, primidone, carba-
    mazepine, lithium, thalidomide, retinoic acid, amphetamine, cocaine, antineoplastic
    drugs
Environmental teratogens: altitude, trichloroethylene, irradiation

Cardiac Transition

In the first postnatal hours for a healthy term infant, the pulmonary vascular resistance and pulmonary arterial pressures are elevated, but below levels present in the fetus. The pulmonary vascular resistance normally falls precipitously in the first day (99). Some measure of pulmonary resistance remains, but in the absence of lung disease, the greatest decline is over the first 8 hours and is well underway by just 4 hours of age (100). Lung disease delays the lowering of pulmonary resistance, causing a relative pulmonary hypertension, the level of which correlates with the severity of the respiratory condition (100,101). With the decrease in pulmonary resistance and consequent increase in pulmonary blood flow, the volume returned to the left atrium increases. Removal of placental circulation causes a decrease in volume through the umbilical vein and inferior vena cava to the right atrium. The combined effect of the volume differences in the two atria forces functional closure of the foramen ovale. Anatomical closure follows in most infants several weeks later (102).

Removal of the low-resistance placental circulation also causes the second important change in circulatory transition, i.e., an increase in systemic resistance. Until pulmonary and systemic pressures reach levels normal for extrauterine physiology, the direction and volume of blood flow throughout the system will be affected. How completely an infant has adjusted the pressures and circulatory pathways determines in what phase of cardiac transition he or she is and what the physical findings will be.

Premature infants can be expected to be more delayed in effecting transition with longer intervals before closing the ductus arteriosus and foramen ovale (103). The more immature the infant and the more severe any lung disease associated with prematurity, the more incomplete and delayed the transition will be (103). Some premature infants appear to complete the process quickly, but others take much longer. Besides unpredictable timing and pattern in completing transition, the thin chest wall and higher heart rates of premature infants makes their physical findings even more different from those in healthy term infants who more predictably complete transition in the first day of life.

In the earliest stages of transition, both the first and second heart sounds are somewhat accentuated (104,105). The second heart sound will be single and especially loud and may be accompanied by a pulmonary systolic ejection sound or click (105). With a drop in pulmonary vascular resistance, the second heart sound begins to split appreciably and becomes less accentuated. For a variable time after birth, the ductus arteriosus remains anatomically and functionally open and shunts bidirectionally, but the velocity across the shunt is low enough that it produces no murmur. As ductal resistance increases, shunt velocity increases and becomes turbulent enough to transmit a murmur until the duct functionally closes. For most infants, the ductus is functionally closed on the first day, but in some healthy term infants, a murmur or accentuation of S_2 persists for several days.

An aid in evaluating a neonate's cardiac status is to estimate at what point an infant is in his or her postnatal transition. This means assessing how effective has been the decrease in pulmonary resistance with its increase in pulmonary blood flow, increase in systemic resistance, and closing of prenatal shunts. A best friend in this evaluation process is simply time, i.e., being able to observe an infant over a period of several hours to days while the transition progresses without having to intervene or make a definitive diagnoses. Obviously, delay is only possible when the infant is otherwise well and remains accessible for evaluation. With early discharges after routine deliveries, the need for rapid assessment is more of an issue than it used to be. Unfortunately, for an infant who is relatively asymptomatic only because persistence of his fetal pathways maintains his circulatory integrity, delay in diagnosis leads to rapid decompensation when his ductus closes. Physical findings along with pertinent laboratory findings help in discerning these infants who depend on a shunt from those who are either harmed or asymptomatic from theirs, but making the diagnosis presents a significant challenge.

For the primary caregiver the purpose of the cardiac examination is to supplement information about the overall well-being and to detect the presence of significant heart disease. When there is evidence of heart disease, the goal becomes one of assessing the current physiologic impact and the likelihood of decompensation more than one of making a precise diagnosis of what the defect is. For example, it is essential to determine if there is congestive heart failure, if pulmonary blood flow is increased or decreased, whether or not there is a shunt present, and, if present, is the shunt helping or hurting the overall status. By determining these factors, one can then make a reasonable assessment of the infant and decide how urgently there needs to be involvement by a pediatric cardiologist for more precise definition of the defect and a plan of therapy.

Murmurs or their absence are especially problematic in the newborn examination for several reasons. In the neonate a murmur does not always signify the presence of heart disease nor does its absence provide complete reassurance of normalcy. A murmur will be heard in most newborn infants if one listens at just the right time (105). Conversely, it may take days or weeks until cardiovascular transition is completed for an infant with a major cardiac anomaly to develop a murmur or one that fits the classical description for the lesions. McNamara reports that of patients who will develop a heart murmur from congenital heart disease by 2 years of age, only 20% have an audible murmur in the first weeks of life (106). If a diagnosis of a congenital heart condition relies on the presence of a murmur, most will be missed in the early newborn period. Detecting congenital heart disease requires using more than just listening for a murmur in the physical evaluation.

Inspection

Count respiratory rate and assess work of breathing
Assess growth
Inspect
   skin and mucous membranes for color and perfusion
   anterior trunk for
     shape and symmetry
     precordial activity
   forehead for sweating
   visible pulsations in the neck
   presence of associated noncardiac anomalies

Look at the breathing pattern of the infant and assess the work of breathing. Inspect the inside of the mouth for cyanosis or plethora. Estimate the general perfusion by timing capillary refill over the precordium. Compare color over the face, abdomen, and extremities. Look for sweating over the forehead or chest.

Inspect the precordial area for contour and symmetry. View from several angles for perceptible cardiac pulsations.

Look at the neck for venous pulsations. Expose the anterior neck structures by elevating the head of the bed and putting the infant in supine with his (or her) neck extended and head turned aside, facilitated with a roll under his shoulders. While feeling the precordial systolic impulse, look for more than one pulse per heart beat in an undulatory pattern. If venous pulsations are seen, palpate the liver for similar pulsations.

Inspect the facies and extremities to detect noncardiac anomalies and genetic syndromes.

Color

Cyanosis or pallor is one of the more frequent signs for suspecting congenital heart disease and prompts an immediate evaluation, but heart disease is only one of many possible factors in a newborn infant (107). The classical means of evaluating cyanosis include measuring blood gases and oxygen saturation and noting the response to oxygen and to hyperventilation (Table 2) (108). Interpreting the response requires including important caveats.

Caveats in relating cyanosis to heart disease:

Absence of cyanosis does not rule out serious congenital heart disease.

Acyanotic heart disease may be associated with cyanosis when there is pulmonary edema.

Some congenital cyanotic heart lesions may not present with cyanosis in the early newborn period, e.g., TAPVR or tetralogy of Fallot.

Sampling sites must take into consideration pre- and postductal flow and mixing.

Hyperventilation may mask some types of cyanotic heart disease, notably anomalous pulmonary venous return.

Cyanosis does not always indicate insufficient arterial oxygen tension.

Shunting across a patent ductus arteriosus confounds an evaluation of cyanosis and, when the shunted volume is large enough, causes differential cyanosis between the upper and lower body (Table 12). The most dramatic differential cyanosis occurs when shunting is so complete that there is complete separation of unsaturated blood and saturated blood in the systemic distributions. More commonly, differences are not apparent but are demonstrable on simultaneous monitoring of transcutaneous oxygen saturation in the right arm and lower limbs. A transient but obvious differential is sometimes remarkable in the seconds immediately after birth when the face, right arm, and chest are pink, and the lower body is brightly cyanosed. Other than this physiologic phenomenon, differentials in regions of cyanosis or measured saturation indicate pathologic shunting.

Precordial Contour

Newborn infants may have thoracic asymmetry from a number of reasons (see list previously), but precordial prominence from cardiomegaly is unusual (109). If precordial prominence is due to cardiomegaly, the cardiac condition affected fetal circulation, and placental circulation did not compensate for this effect. Cardiovascular conditions that can lead to neonatal precordial bulges include large arteriovenous malformations, including acardiac twinning and placental chorangioma, Ebstein's anomaly, pulmonary valve atresia, and tachy- or bradyarrhythmias.

Table 12. *Differential cyanosis associated with patent ductus arteriosus*

Color change	Lesions or hemodynamic state
Pink upper body, blue or pale lower body	Early transitional circulation with elevated pulmonary vascular resistance
	Persistent pulmonary hypertension
	Left heart obstruction or hypoplasia (early)
	Coarctation of the aorta
	Interrupted aortic arch
Blue upper body, pink lower body	Transposition of the great arteries with intact septum and with right to left shunt across the PDA (with or without aortic arch anomalies)

Venous Pulsations

In plump young infants the anterior neck structures are obscured when the infant is in normal repose with the chin lying close to the chest. Even when a baby's neck is inspected, the rapid heart rate makes timing of any visible waves difficult. When venous pulsations are apparent and separable from arterial pulses or the precordial systolic impulse, they are important findings because they indicate an increase in the venous volume or obstruction to emptying of the right atrium. If venous pulsations are visible in association with right atrial obstruction, hepatic pulsations should be palpable.

Table 13. *Congenital disorders associated with cardiac disease*

Disorder	Percentage of patients with cardiac disease	Types of cardiac abnormalities
Primary isolated cardiac disorders		
Hypertrophic cardiomyopathy	100	Hypertrophic cardiomyopathy
Romano-Ward Syndrome	100	Prolonged QT interval, VT, sudden death
Autosomal-dominant syndromes		
de Lange	30	VSD, ASD, PDA, AS, EFE
Holt-Oram cardiac-limb syndrome	100	ASD
Marfan syndrome	67–100	Aortic aneurysm, AR, MR, TR, prolapse, dysrhythmias
Noonan syndrome	67	PS, ASD, hypertrophic cardiomyopathy, VSD, PDA, LAD
Osler-Weber-Rendu hemorrhagic telangiectasis	15–25	Pulmonary and systemic arteriovenous malformations
Shprintzen velocardiofacial syndrome	80	VSD, TF, right aortic arch, aberrant left subclavian artery
Treacher Collins mandibulofacial dysostosis	Uncommon	ASD, VSD, PDA
Tuberous sclerosis	30	Cardiac rhabdomyomas
Autosomal-recessive syndromes		
Carpenter syndrome	33	PDA, PS, VSD, TF, TGA
Ellis-van Creveld chondroectodermal dysplasia	50–60	Single atrium, primum ASD, COARC, small LV, CHF
Mycopolysaccharidosis	>50	Myocardial hypertrophy, coronary disease, AR, MR, TR, CHF
Pompe glycogenolysis type II	100	Myocardial hypertrophy, EFE, short PR, CHF
Smith-Lemli-Opitz syndrome, types I and II	20/100	VSD, PDA, ASD, TF
Thrombocytopenia with absent radii	33	ASD, TF
X-linked syndromes		
Duchenne muscular dystrophy	Common	Cardiomyopathy
Trisomy 21 (Down's syndrome)	40–50	AV canal, VSD, PDA, ASD primum, TF
Trisomy 18 (Edward syndrome)	90–100	VSD, polyvalvular disease, ASD, PDA
Trisomy 13 (Patau syndrome)	80	PDA, VSD, ASD, detrocardia, COARC, AS, PS
XO (Turner syndrome)	45	COARC, bicuspid aortic valve, aortic aneurysm
Syndromes with unknown etiology		
Beckwith-Wiedemann syndrome	16–92	Cardiomegaly, ASD, VSD, PDA, TF
Cardiofacial (asymmetric crying facies) syndrome	5–10	VSD
CHARGE association	65–75	TF, DORV, ASD, VSD, PDA, COARC, AV canal
DiGeorge syndrome	50 –	Interrupted aortic arch, truncus arteriosus, TF
Goldenhar facioauriculovertebral spectrum	5–80	VSD, PDA, TF, CAORC
Rubinstein-Taybi syndrome	35	VSD, PDA, ASD, COARC, PS
VACTERL association	10	VSD, ASD, TF
Williams syndrome	50–80	Supravalvar AS, branch PS, VSD, hypoplastic aorta

AR, aortic valve regurgitation; AS, aortic stenosis; ASD, atrial septal defect; AV, atrioventricular; CHF, congestive heart failure; COARC, coarctation of the aorta; DORV, double-outlet right ventricle; EFE, endocardial fibroelastosis; LAD, left axis deviation; LV, left ventricle; MR, mitral valve regurgitation; PDA, patent ductus arteriosus; PS, pulmonary stenosis; TF, tetralogy of Fallot; TGA, transposition of the great arteries; TR, tricuspid valve regurgitation; VSD, ventricular septal defect; VT, ventricular tachycardia.
Reprinted from Flanagan and Fyler, ref. 97, with permission.

Table 14. *Incidence of severe noncardiac anomalies associated with specific cardiac lesions*

Cardiac diagnosis	Incidence (%)
Endocardial cushion defect	43
Patent ductus arteriosus	31
Ventricular septal defect	24
Malpositiions	13
Tetralogy of Fallot	10
Coarctation of aorta	9
Pulmonary atresia with intact septum	1
D-transposition of the great arteries	1

Data from 2,220 infants with heart disease (97).

Breathing Pattern

Infants with heart disease, even in the presence of cyanosis, tend to demonstrate less anxiety and work of breathing than do infants who have primary lung disease. A classical early presentation of congenital heart disease is a deeply cyanosed infant who is tachypneic but not distressed. Significant respiratory effort is seen when heart disease causes pulmonary edema that is severe enough to decrease pulmonary compliance. Cardiac conditions associated with pulmonary edema such as obstructed pulmonary venous return are often thought to be pulmonary disease before the correct diagnosis is made.

Association with Noncardiac Anomalies

A number of genetic syndromes or associations have congenital heart disease as part of their symptom complex. For some the relationship is so strong that full evaluation is a part of their diagnostic assessment. For example, evaluation of infants with trisomy 21 or monosomy X requires cardiac evaluation even in the absence of symptoms at birth. Other combinations of anomalies come by their classifications as associations because of the presence of heart disease: e.g., CHARGE or VACTERL associations (Table 13) (97). Conversely, some types of cardiac malformations, notably endocardial cushion defect, have such a strong coincidence with noncardiac malformations or syndromes that their presence should direct an evaluation for possible syndrome or genetic association if it has not already been considered. Others have no greater relationship than that in the general population (Table 14) (97).

Palpation

Palpate the anterior chest for impulses. Start by laying a flat hand across the sternum and left hemithorax to assess the general pattern of cardiac activity. Then with the finger tips localize the point of maximal impulse (PMI). If not clearly located on the left sternal border, palpate the right side of the hemithorax as well. Assess the character of the PMI, including intensity, rate, crispness, extra impulses, or thrill.

The heart position changes during infancy. As the left ventricle becomes more prominent after birth, its point of impulse shifts further from the sternal border. The heart also descends within the chest as the thorax elongates. Its center lies beneath the mid-sternum during the first 6 months of life and beneath the lower sternum after infancy. This position does not vary with age in relation to the internipple line, but in approximately three fourths of all infants, the cardiac center is below the internipple line (110).

In the first days after birth, the apical impulse will be primarily under the lower sternum and during cardiopulmonary transition causes a sternal heave. There is a slow progression of the apical impulse toward the left chest so that during the first week the apical impulse will be parasternal on the left. Displacement toward the right occurs in dextrocardia, or loss of right lung volume from complete atelectasis or hypoplasia, as well as in conditions with major space-occupying lesions on the left, such as tension pneumothorax, diaphragmatic hernia, and congenital lobar emphysema.

It helps to assess the cardiac activity by observing the movement of a light-weight object overlying the precordium. This object can be the head of the stethoscope or simply a small dot of paper with its rocking movement timed with the heart rate rather than with respiratory excursions. In infants with thin chest walls, cardiac impulses are apparent even with normal cardiac activity, but the chest markers are not hyperactive. For premature infants at particular risk to develop circulatory overload from a patent ductus arteriosus, changes in precordial impulses are sometimes noticeable even from a distance. Comparison observations are helpful in following status when the precordial impulse remains visible in infants likely to develop overload with patent ductus arteriosus or fluid management.

A precordial impulse along the left sternal border is often visible in the first several hours after birth, but most disappear by 6 hours of age. Those that persist beyond 12 hours are generally associated with volume overload and in cardiac conditions that lead to early failure including aortopulmonary shunts. A visibly prominent impulse is characteristic of transposition of the great arteries (109).

Absence of a palpably increased precordial impulse in the presence of cyanosis suggests lesions associated with obstruction of the right side such as pulmonary atresia, tetralogy of Fallot, or tricuspid atresia and helps to distinguish these lesions from transposition of the great vessels in which a parasternal lift is expected.

Thrill

Palpable thrills are unusual in the early neonatal period. There is rarely enough flow across a patent ductus or ventricular septal defect to cause the turbulence and vibrations necessary to produce a thrill until pulmonary vascular resistance has decreased sufficiently, but neonates with thin chest walls and large shunts can develop thrills after the first few weeks of life. Systolic thrills develop in newborn infants with gross tricuspid valve regurgitation or severe pulmonary stenosis. Systolic and diastolic thrills accompany tetralogy of Fallot with absent pulmonary valve.

Liver

Determine the overall span and location of the liver lobes. Assess the liver edge for firmness and sharp definition. Feel for hepatic pulsations, taking care to separate any movement due to rapid breathing.

Hepatomegaly secondary to congestive heart failure is a relatively late physical finding, albeit an important one. The rapidly increasing liver size that develops from birth in conditions of severe right-sided obstruction such as tricuspid atresia with restrictive interatrial communication is a dramatic exception. In this case pulsations would also be palpable over the enlarged liver. Hepatic pulsations are a feature of severe obstruction to the right atrium or right ventricle and, rarely, large arteriovenous malformations of the liver.

Hepatosplenomegaly associated with cardiomyopathy suggests intrauterine viral infections or storage disease, although cardiac presentation within the newborn period for most storage diseases is unlikely. Hepatosplenomegaly associated with cardiac malformations and low birth weight suggests rubella, mumps, or cytomegalovirus as probable infectious agents in the first trimester.

A centrally placed liver points to asplenia or polysplenia syndromes, whereas a left-sided liver suggests situs inversus with the associated cardiac conditions.

Pulses

Assess the pulses for strength, shape of their impulse curve, and synchrony. First find both brachial pulses and compare their timing and intensity. Next compare both femoral pulses. Then feel pre- and postductal pulses simultaneously; feel the right brachial or axial artery with the left hand and the left femoral pulse with the right hand. If there is any decrease in palpable pressure in one area, evaluate the pulses in the carotid arteries as well.

To find the femoral pulses, put the infant in a relaxed, supine position with the hips slightly abducted and flexed. Standing at the infant's feet, hold an index finger along the long axis of each femur with the tip of the finger resting just below the inguinal crease. If a pulse is not felt with a light touch, advance the fingertip a few millimeters toward the abdomen. Keeping the finger flat, palpate the structures of the femoral triangle.

Elevate the arm above the head to look for arterial pulsations in the axilla.

Finding the femoral pulses takes some patience, especially if the infant is active. It is easier to locate a pulse when the touching finger lies along the artery rather than crossing it. Over the femoral artery there is so often a soft lymph node 3 to 5 mm in length that it serves as a consistent signal of the femoral pulse lying just beneath it. When the nodule is first felt superficially, advancing the finger tip toward the abdomen reliably leads to the pulse.

The character of the peripheral pulse is influenced by multiple factors. Because the normal pulse pressure is relatively low, almost any increase is palpable. For example, palmar pulses in a premature infant that are difficult to feel might become quite evident after a feeding, blood transfusion, crying, and over-heating in an incubator.

Pulses that are bounding or collapsing with a peaked impulse curve indicate a low diastolic resistance, generally from aortic run off. In premature infants, most commonly collapsing pulses indicate a patent ductus arteriosus with aortic runoff into low pulmonary vascular resistance. Bounding pulses also occur in arteriovenous fistula, truncus arteriosus, or any other cardiac lesion with aortic run-off. For patent ductus arteriosus to be associated with bounding pulses, the pulmonary vascular resistance has to be significantly lower than the systemic resistance. Bounding pulses are not found in the presence of significant pulmonary hypertension or in situations of low systemic volume and pressure, even though the ductal pathway is still open. Infants who have significant systemic hypertension have pulses that are stronger although not necessarily bounding in nature. Pulses are accentuated in thyrotoxicosis, anemia, and fever.

The opposite clinical situation of weak pulses throughout signals conditions of vascular collapse such as septic or hypovolemic shock or severe congestive heart failure. Decreased pulse pressures are also present in left ventricular outflow obstruction when the ductus arteriosus closes, but unlike the other conditions of vascular collapse, there will be a right ventricular heave and increased precordial activity from the overloaded right heart. Differences in pulses between those in the upper extremities and those in the lower extremities develop when there is obstruction to the flow to one area or an increase to the other. Decreased pulses in the lower extremities with normal pulses in the upper extremities results from obstruction to aortic flow, so the differential diagnosis starts with coarctation but must include aortic or femoral thrombosis or spasm. If a coarctation occurs above either normal or aberrant origins of the subclavian arteries, the pulses in all four extremities are diminished, but the carotid pulses are increased and the precordium hyperactive.

Before a patent ductus arteriosus closes in an infant with critical coarctation, there is a subtle difference in the character of the pulses, but it is this difference that is critical to the physical diagnosis. The regions supplied only through the ductus arteriosus (the lower extremities) will have pulse pressures that are slightly delayed with a broader curve than those supplied by the left ventricle, where the pulses are more forceful (the right arm or carotid pulses). As the ductus closes, differences in the pulses will be detectable before there are any demonstrable changes in the blood pressures of the four extremities.

One helpful observation is the presence of visible arterial pulsation in the axilla when the arm is held away from the side. Pulses that are clearly visible correlate with palpable bounding.

Measure Blood Pressure

Measure the blood pressure by whatever route is appropriate to the situation. If there is an indwelling arterial line, use direct continuous measurement by transducer.

For hospitalized patients without arterial lines, a technique using the Doppler method is preferred, but if electronic monitoring is not available, particularly in an outpatient setting, the indirect methods of oscillometry, peripheral pulse palpation, or the flush technique provide at least a screening tool.

Flush Blood Pressure

To take a mean blood pressure by the flush method, wrap or squeeze the hand or foot firmly enough to blanch the skin (111). Inflate the cuff and remove the wrapping. Lower the pressure slowly until there is a flush of color and document the pressure at that point. Repeat until there are two consistent readings.

The values obtained by the blanching and flush method are mean pressures and are lower than those registered by direct intravascular or Doppler monitoring (112). The flush method for mean pressure is easier to obtain in an active infant and requires only a sphigmomanometer and appropriately sized cuff. The Doppler methods, although providing both diastolic and systolic pressures, require electronic equipment and a quieter patient. Two important elements for obtaining accurate blood pressures are a quiet infant and a properly sized cuff with a width 50% to 67% of the length of the arm or 0.4 to 0.5 times the circumference of the extremity (113,114). Other techniques suggest that cuff size should be the widest possible that will encircle the arm (115). Clearly, regardless of what values are used for comparison, the technique should be identical, although the differences among techniques are slight compared with the variations caused by infant factors such as activity and size.

In deciding if pressures are appropriate for any patient, one has to consider gestational age, age in hours and days, method of obtaining pressures, and whether a cuff pressure is from an arm or leg (111–113,116–123). Blood pressure tends to increase with both gestational and chronologic age, so what is considered within normal limits for a very low birth weight infant in the first hours may be well below adequate perfusion pressure for older and bigger infants.

Pulse pressure is the difference between the systolic and diastolic blood pressure and averages 25 to 30 mmHg in term infants and 15 to 25 mmHg in preterm infants. Narrow pulse pressures are seen in infants with low circulating blood volumes, myocardial failure, peripheral vasoconstriction, or generalized vascular collapse. Widened pulse pressure occurs in infants who have just eaten or in conditions where there is vascular run-off: patent ductus arteriosus with low pulmonary vascular resistance, arteriovenous fistula, aorticopulmonary window, and truncus arteriosus.

Normal Values for Blood Pressure

The normal ranges depend on the method used as well as on the gestational and chronologic ages and are strongly affected by the activity, body temperature, and posture of the infant (113,119,124) (see Appendix, Fig. 35 and Tables 1–3). Readings taken in extremities that are lower than the heart may be falsely elevated, although the differences are normally clinically insignificant (121). Pressures obtained in the calf essentially equal those in the arm or are within one standard deviation or 6 to 9 mmHg lower than in the arm (113). The increase in calf compared with arm measurements that are typical of older children and adults are not reliably found until 6 months of age (122). Infants who are awake have levels of both systolic and diastolic pressures that average 6 to 10 mmHg higher than infants who are sleeping (113). Pressure is lower in the first 3 to 4 hours after birth but is strongly influenced by the extent of placental transfusion (117,120). In premature infants, the values are proportional to their size and gestational age (120).

Auscultation

Examine the patient in the quietest possible environment. If practicable, examine after a feeding while the infant is in a quiet state, preferably sleeping. If the infant is crying or fussing, take the time to calm him or her first. When the patient is on assisted ventilation, decrease all extraneous noises as much as possible. It may even be necessary to stop endotracheal air flow for a few seconds if the patient can tolerate this.

Listen to the right and left second intercostal spaces at the sternal edge (aortic and pulmonary valve areas, respectively); at the right and left fourth intercostal space (tricuspid and mitral valve areas, respectively). Listen over the apex, generally in the fifth intercostal space medial to the mid-clavicular line (mitral area). Listen to both the right and left axilla in the fifth intercostal space and to the back medial to the tip of the scapulae. If there is a need to localize and characterize the heart sounds more precisely, inch the stethoscope along the sternal margins in progressions of approximately half the diameter of the diaphragm.

Listen to the cardiac sounds by dissection of each component in all locations. Listen to the first heart sound, second heart sound, for extra sounds or clicks, and systole and diastole as separate entities. Count the rate and assess the rhythm.

Start with proper equipment that is cleaned for each patient. Listen first with the diaphragm and repeat each precordial area with the bell.

Remember that lesions that are dependent on low pulmonary resistance can be influenced by the presence of background airway pressures that are high enough to impede systemic venous return or to increase pulmonary capillary resistance so it may be necessary to decrease the mechanical pressure temporarily in order to have enough shunt to generate an audible murmur. Additionally, the noise from the mechanical device will easily distort or obscure most heart sounds. Briefly stopping the mechanical noises helps in the process because soft heart sounds are easily obscured by the sounds of mechanical air flow. Clearly, an infant must not be compromised by the process. Before disconnecting any device, identify the sounds caused by the machine and characterize the heart sounds as much as possible. While continuing to listen, briefly disconnect the flow for a few beats. The same principle applies if the infant is exerting a Valsalva maneuver or grunting. Listen with the infant's airway as relaxed as possible.

Many of the stethoscopes designed for use in neonatology make listening for the sounds far more of a challenge than it need be. Requirements for single use disposable equipment or sterilization between patients means a loss of quality. Lengthening the tubing to make it reach into closed incubators decreases the intensity. There are some advantages to having a bell and diaphragm correlate with the size of the infant, but smaller end pieces decrease the intensity of sound so much that many designs marketed for use in newborn and premature infants are ineffective for anything more than counting heart rate. For most circumstances, a moderately sized but good quality diaphragm suffices, but when a bell is indicated to listen to low-pitched sounds, it is necessary to have a good seal with the chest wall. Especially in thin premature infants this means that the sealing surface should be soft enough to conform to the chest shape so it may be necessary to modify the rigid bell commercially supplied on most stethoscopes. If a bell is too tightly applied in order to effect a seal, the stretched skin acts as a diaphragm and loses the bell's advantage in hearing low tones. The trimmed base of a soft, infant feeding nipple that is drawn over the metal bell works remarkably well in making an effective sealing surface.

The intensity of the heart sounds are modified by both intracardiac and extracardiac factors. If both sounds are affected, the factor is more likely extracardiac, but if only one is, the cause is likely to be intracardiac. Extracardiac factors include chest wall thickness, pulmonary air leaks, and pericardial fluid or air collections. A thin chest wall means the neonatal heart sounds should be relatively loud, but rapid rates makes discriminating the components challenging. Changes in intensity among individual infants or in the same infant who is subject to any of the above conditions is a pertinent finding.

Heart Rate and Rhythm

The heart rate varies widely depending on infant state, so for comparative assessments, a resting heart rate is the most consistent (Table 15) (125). The rate can be taken by palpation of the precordium or peripheral pulses, but auscultation is easier in a quiet infant. The rhythm has beat-to-beat variability unless the infant is quite distressed, but because of the rapid heart and respiratory rates, fluctuations with respirations are not easily perceived.

First Heart Sound

The first heart sound, S_1, emanates from closure of the atrioventricular valves at the beginning of systole. It is slightly lower pitched or duller than the second heart sound and is heard best over the apex of the heart. The first part of the sound arises on closure of the mitral valve and the second part on closure of the tricuspid valve, but the interval between closure of the two valves is normally so small that S_1 is perceived as single. If splitting is present, it suggests delayed closure of the tricuspid valve, especially in Ebstein anomaly, right bundle branch block, or complete heart block with a very slow heart rate (Table 16) (126).

Cardiac factors that affect the intensity of S_1 are those that affect the position of the valve leaflets at the time of closure. If the valves are widely open at the beginning of systole, the sound is louder than if they are more closely opposed. The two important conditions associated with softened S_1 are prolonged atrioventricular conduction and congestive heart failure. In prolongation of the P-R interval, the mitral valve leaflets are almost closed passively before systole actively begins so their contributions to the first heart sound is softened. Conditions with P-R prolongation and softening of S_1 include hypothyroidism, cardiomyopathy, shock, and first-degree heart block (127).

The first heart sound is normally accentuated at birth (109). An increase in intensity of the first heart sound occurs when the left ventricular contraction is more forceful, there is increased flow across an atrioventricular valve, or the P-R interval is shortened. Pathologic accentuation of S_1 occurs in conditions where there is increased flow across the mitral valve such as in patent ductus arteriosus, ventricular septal defect, and mitral insufficiency (105). Accentuation from increased flow across the tricuspid valve occurs in total anomalous pulmonary venous return or arteriovenous malformations (109). In tetralogy of Fallot, the first heart sound is accentuated more specifically at the lower left sternal border (109). The intracardiac cause of increased intensity of S_1 in young infants after the newborn period is most commonly atrial septal defect; other conditions affecting S_1, such as mitral stenosis (increased intensity and delayed) or aortic insufficiency (decreased intensity), are rare in infants (127,128). Extracardiac conditions leading to an increase in the intensity of the first heart sound include anemia, hyperthermia, hyperthyroidism, and arteriovenous fistula (127).

Clicks

What is often thought to be a split in the first heart sound is more commonly an aortic or pulmonic ejection click or, rarely, a fourth heart sound preceding S_1 (127). A click is a short, snappy sound of high frequency following the first sound and is best heard with the

Table 15. *Heart rate in first week of life in term infants (beats/min)*

	5th percentile	50th percentile	95th percentile
0–24 h	99	123	148
1–3 days	97	123	149
3–7 days	100	128	160

Data from Davignon (125).

Table 16. *Heart sound comparisons*

Sound	Resembles
Normal heart sounds (S_1–S_2)	lub-*dub*
Split first heart sound	t-r-up-*dub*
Split second heart sound	lub-*du-bu*
Mid-systolic click	lud-ip-*dub*
	with rhythm of tenn-es-*see*
Third heart sound	lub-*dub*-huh
	with rhythm of ken-*tuck*-y

Data from McNamara (126).

diaphragm. Clicks are caused by opening of aortic or pulmonic heart valves (127). If an apparent split is better heard away from the sternal border than adjacent to it, the second vibration is more likely an aortic ejection click. If louder at the base well above the tricuspid region, it is more likely a pulmonic ejection click (127). Differentiating the origin in neonates is difficult at best. Pathologic clicks indicate dilation of a great vessel or deformity of a valve. Transient nonejection clicks are detectable in the first hours after birth, especially along the left lower sternal border in infants who have had relatively brief insults such as birth asphyxia or fluid overload (105,109).

Second Heart Sound

The second heart sound represents the end of systole and is produced by vibration of the closed aortic (A_2) and pulmonary valves (P_2). Closure of the valves is actually silent, but vibration of the compliant valve tissue immediately after closure causes the sound (127). Aortic valve closure (A_2) is coincident with the end of left ventricular ejection, and pulmonary valve closure (P_2) coincides with the end of the right ventricular ejection period. After a neonate has completed circulatory transition to low pulmonary vascular resistance, P_2 normally occurs after A_2 because right ventricular ejection ends after left ventricular ejection. Immediately after birth this relationship may be reversed so that the P_2 arises first. The most common finding is almost simultaneous closure of the two valves so that there is no discernible splitting in the second heart sound. Instead of a distinct splitting of S_2, one may appreciate a slurring or prolongation of the second sound rather than the discrete sound made by a single valve closure. Absence of splitting of S_2 is an important finding in a number of the congenital heart conditions important to diagnose as early as possible: aortic atresia, pulmonary atresia, truncus arteriosus, and transposition of the great arteries.

S_2 is loudest at the upper left sternal border. It is accentuated when there is high resistance in either the pulmonic or systemic vascular systems. More commonly a loud S_2 with narrow splitting indicates pulmonary hypertension in neonates (109). The widening of splitting heard during inspiration in adults is not perceptible in most very young infants. Wide splitting of S_2 is heard with anomalous pulmonary venous return or delay in right ventricular ejection because of either a conduction delay or an obstruction to right ventricular ejection. The wide splitting of S_2 associated with ASD is not heard until later in the newborn period. The presence of a widely split second heart sound in an infant with cyanotic congenital heart disease suggests Ebstein's anomaly. The pulmonic component of S_2 is accentuated in pulmonary hypertension but is softened in pulmonic stenosis. Because there may be a systolic ejection click with pulmonic stenosis, the S_2 may sound widely split but with a variable interval.

Third and Fourth Heart Sounds

Third heart sounds are caused by sudden, intrinsic limitation of longitudinal expansion of the ventricular wall, producing a low-frequency vibration. They reflect increased flow across an atrioventricular valve, most commonly in patent ductus arteriosus. They are also heard in congestive heart failure but are generally perceived as summation gallops when S_3 and S_4 are heard together.

Third heart sounds are best heard over the lower sternal borders at the cardiac apex with the infant lying on the left side (127).

Fourth heart sounds are dull, low-frequency, indistinct soft thuds that precede S_1. They are produced by vibrations in the expanding ventricles during rapid diastolic filling when the atria contract. They are best heard with a bell, whereas S_1 is best heard with a diaphragm. Fourth heart sounds are rare in neonates but indicate primary myocardial disease and low left ventricular compliance (109).

Murmurs

Murmurs are generated by turbulence in blood flow. As cardiovascular pathways and pressure gradients change in adaptation to extrauterine existence, various sources of turbulence in anatomically normal systems cause transient murmurs (Table 17) (105,109). The description of the murmurs found in textbooks as typical for various anatomic conditions are not necessarily applicable in newborn infants. Some murmurs may not become audible until cardiovascular transition is complete.

Murmurs in the newborn nursery and when first heard (107):

Early (first day)
    Transient tricuspid valve dysfunction
    Patent ductus arteriosus
    At least moderate-to-severe obstruction of left or right ventricular outflow
Late (after first 24–48 hours)
    Ventricular septal defect
    Turbulence in proximal pulmonary arteries (L>R) secondary to obstruction
Later
    Severe outflow tract obstruction clinically unmasked by closing ductus arteriosus and
        possibly by associated atrioventricular valve insufficiency
    Ventricular septal defects unmasked by decrease in pulmonary vascular resistance

Because murmurs can change as the postnatal adaptation progresses, it is probably better to use clear descriptions of findings rather than characterization that directly involves interpretation. One approach in defining murmurs is to classify murmurs as either ejection or regurgitant. Ejection murmurs arise from narrowing at a valve either because of true narrowing or irregularity in the valve or from a relative stenosis in the face of increased flow. The murmur of VSD is a relative stenosis from increased flow across a normal mitral valve. Regurgitant murmurs arise when a valve allows back flow either because the valve is deformed as in endocardial cushion defect or is stretched from ventricular dilation.

Another approach in describing murmurs is to classify them by their specific characteristics including timing, duration, intensity, pitch, and quality. Timing relates to the murmur's place within the cardiac cycle. A first step in the process is to determine if the murmur is systolic or diastolic. With rapid neonatal heart rates, it is sometimes difficult to determine where a murmur falls within the cycle. Simultaneously feeling a peripheral pulse or the precordium for the ventricular impulse of systole while listening is helpful.

The next step is to determine if the murmur is early, middle, or late in the cycle in relation to the first and second heart sounds. Because of the rapid heart rates, this is the most difficult characterization to make in newborn infants when the diastolic and systolic cycles are only a small fraction of a second. Holosystolic murmurs continue to the second heart sound and continuous murmurs go through the second heart sound.

The intensity of a murmur or its loudness depends on how strong the turbulence and vibrations are and on how close their source is to the point of examination. The relatively thin chest wall of newborn infants puts cardiac sounds in proximity to the stethoscope. The pitch of a murmur also affects how easily it is heard, with higher pitches more easily perceived than low-pitched vibrations. The standard classification of intensity as proposed originally by Freeman and Levine is traditionally applied (129).

Grade I: audible only very faintly; not audible except in a quiet environment
Grade II: louder than I but still faint
Grade III: intermediate intensity, with or without a thrill
Grade IV: louder and with a thrill

Grade V: very loud
Grade VI: heard with stethoscope not even touching chest

Other characterizations for murmur quality are harsh, blowing, rough, rumbling, and musical.

A helpful rule to follow in examining the cardiovascular system is to listen for murmurs last after assessing all other aspects so that their presence will not distract the clinician. When a murmur is heard as the first finding on auscultation, it is easy to forget to listen over the entire chest to locate its areas of radiation or origin or to characterize the first and second heart sounds carefully. It is the combination of physical findings that suggest the diagnosis, so the total examination is important.

Select Appropriate Laboratory Information

Even before an examination begins there may be suspicion of cardiac disease; throughout an assessment, findings help direct our final impressions about the cardiovascular system. When the suspicion of heart disease is high enough, a basic evaluation beyond the physical examination includes blood gases, hemoglobin and hematocrit values, oxygen saturation comparisons, chest radiograph, and an electrocardiogram. Armed with this information, the necessary decisions about immediacy of cardiology intervention can be determined. The signs and symptoms may suggest congestive heart failure or cyanotic heart disease, either of which require immediate intervention.

Findings suggesting cardiac disease:

Presence of other organ system anomalies
Genetic syndrome associated with cardiac anomalies
Cyanosis or decreased saturation
Tachypnea especially in the absence of increased work of breathing
Change in clinical behavior
    alert appearance but decreased activity
    whining
Precordial changes
    increased precordial activity
    thrill
    abnormally placed apical impulse
    diffuse apical pulse
Other system involvement
    poor perfusion
    decreased urine output
    hepatic pulsation
Murmur
Bruit
Abnormal heart tones

Table 18 lists the causes of congestive heart failure (97); Table 19 lists the findings in acyanotic 0- to 2-week-old neonates with congestive heart failure; Table 20 lists the findings in acyanotic 2- to 8-week-old neonates with congestive heart failure (97); and Table 21 provides the differential diagnoses of cyanotic heart disease (97).

Evaluate chest radiograph for:

Major bony and structural malformations
Lung volumes and parenchymal changes
Extrinsic compression of lung parenchyma: pleural, thoracic, abdominal, pneumothorax,
    hydrothorax, tumor
Pulmonary vascular markings,
Heart size
Heart contour
Aortic arch side
Position of the stomach and liver

Interpret pulmonary blood flow, pulmonary vascular markings, and pulmonary edema.

Table 17. *Characteristics of physiologic murmurs found in the neonatal period*

Physiologic condition	Character	Location	Time of presence	Incidence
Ductus arteriosus left-to-right flow	Systolic crescendo continuous (occasionally)	Cardiac base, left scapula	5–6 h of age	15% of term infants
Mild bilateral peripheral pulmonary artery stenosis	High-pitched, short, crescendo–decrescendo Sometimes blowing	Cardiac base into the lung fields	Any time after first 48 h Disappears by 6–8 mo	Common, particularly in premature infants
Increased blood flow across pulmonary valve associated with rapidly decreasing pulmonary vascular resistance	Early systolic ejection, grade 1 to 2	Along mid and upper left sternal border Left back but with wide radiation to the right	Appears within first 48 h; disappears by end of second week	Up to 56% of term infants
Arise from chordae tendineae cordis	Systolic, vibrating, grade 1–2 or louder	Between mid left sternal border and apex	Persists Difficult to distinguish from pathologic murmur	Uncommon

Data from Johnson (109) and Braudo and Rowe (105).

Lymph Nodes

Lymph nodes are palpable in a significant number of normal infants and during the first month of life (130) (Table 22). Nodes are most common in the inguinal region but can be found in any of the expected locations except the supraclavicular areas. The nodes tend to be single, discrete, nontender, and freely mobile with normal skin overlying them, but less commonly up to three nodes will be together (130). Node sizes range from 3 to 12 mm in width and length in the first month (130). In my experience at least one inguinal lymph node is palpable in a majority of newborn infants and serves as a convenient locator for the femoral pulse that lies just beneath the node.

Table 18. *Causes of heart failure in newborn infants*

In utero	In neonatal period
Anemia	Myocardial dysfunction
Immune-mediated hemolysis	Asphyxia
Fetal-to-maternal transfusion	Sepsis
Fetal-to-fetal transfusion	Hypoglycemia
Hypoplastic anemia	Myocarditis
Volume overload	Pressure overload
Atrioventricular valve regurgitation in AV canal	Aortic stenosis
Tricuspid regurgitation in Ebstein's disease	Coarctation of the aorta
Arteriovenous fistula	Hypoplastic left heart syndrome
Chorioangioma of placenta	Arterial hypertension (pulmonary or systemic)
Donor twin in twin-to-twin, particularly with an acardiac recipient	Volume overload
Premature closure of foramen ovale	Great vessel level shunts
Myocarditis	Patent ductus arteriosus
Arrhythmias	Truncus arteriosus
Supraventricular tachycardia	Aortopulmonary window
Atrial flutter	Ventricular level shunts
Atrial fibrillation	Ventricular septal defect
Ventricular tachycardia	Single ventricle without pulmonic stenosis
Complete heart block	Atrioventricular canal
	Arrhythmias
	Supraventricular tachycardia
	Atrial flutter
	Atrial fibrillation
	Congenital complete heart block
	Hematologic abnormalities
	Anemia
	Polycythemia with hyperviscosity syndrome

Table 19. *Findings in acyanotic 0- to 2-week-old neonates with congestive heart failure*

Diagnosis	Physical examination	Radiographic findings	Electrocardiographic findings
Coarctation	# Leg pulses and leg BP, soft SEM in back, ± SRM, ± click, S_3, ± differential cyanosis, shocklike sepsis picture	" Heart size, pulmonary edema	± RVH, develops LVH, BVH
Critical aortic stenosis	Shock, # pulses and perfusion, SEM, click, S_3, single S_2	" Heart size, pulmonary edema	LVH, T-wave abnormalities
Patent ductus arteriosus in premature infant	Heave, " pulses, " pulse pressure, continuous or SRM	" Heart size (LV, LA), " pulmonary arterial markings	Develops RVH, LVH, BVH
Cardiomyopathy	# Pulses, # perfusion, # pulse pressure, " HR, SRM	Large globular heart, pulmonary edema	# or " voltage, T-wave changes, Q waves in ALCA
Critical pulmonary stenosis	SEM, click, single S_2, most have cyanosis	Normal or # pulmonary arterial markings,	QRS axis 0°–90°, ± LVH, develops RVH
Systemic arteriovenous fistula	Heave, " pulses, wide pulse pressure, soft SEM or SRM, bruit, shock, ± cyanosis	RAE " heart size, " pulmonary arterial markings	Develops RVH, LVH, BVH

Congestive heart failure with cyanosis may be due to hypoplastic left heart syndrome, transposition of the great arteries, truncus arteriosus, total anomalous pulmonary venous connection, pulmonary atresia with tetralogy, tricuspid atresia, Ebstein malformation, or persistent pulmonary hypertension.

±, may or may not be present; #, decreased; ", increased; ALCA, anomalous left coronary artery; BVH, biventricular hypertrophy; HR, heart rate; LA, left atrium; LV, left ventricle; LVH, left ventricular hypertrophy; RAE, right atrial enlargement; RVH, right ventricular hypertrophy; S_2, second heart sound; S_3, third heart sound; SEM, systolic ejection murmur; SRM, systolic regurgitant murmur.

Reprinted from Flanagan and Fyler, ref. 97, with permission.

Table 20. *Findings in acyanotic 2- to 8-week-old neonates with congestive heart failure*

Diagnosis	Physical examination	Radiographic findings	Electrocardiographic findings
Ventricular septal defect[a]	Heave, harsh SRM, ± S_3, ± diastolic rumble, normal pulses	" Heart size (RV, LV, LA), " pulmonary arterial markings	Develops RAE, RVH, LVH, BVH
Endocardial cushion defect	Same as ventricular septal defect, fixed split S_2	Same as ventricular septal defect	Left axis deviation, develops RAE, RVH, LVH, BVH
Atrial septal defect	Hyperdynamic precordium, soft SEM, fixed split S_2, ± diastolic rumble	" Heart size (RV, normal LA and LV), " pulmonary arterial markings	Develops RAD, RVH
Patent ductus arteriosus in full-term infants	Same as presentation at 0–2 weeks of age		
Cardiomyopathy	Same as presentation at 0–2 weeks of age		

±, may or may not be present; #, decreased; ", increased; BVH, biventricular hypertrophy; LA, left atrium; LV, left ventricle; LVH, left ventricular hypertrophy; RAD, right axis deviation; RAE, right atrial enlargement; RV, right ventricle; RVH, right ventricular hypertrophy; S_2, second heart sound; S_3, third heart sound; SRM, systolic regurgitant murmur.

[a] Murmur may be present earlier than 2 weeks of age, and congestive heart failure may occur earlier in premature infants.

Reprinted from Flanagan and Fyler, ref. 97, with permission.

Table 21. *Findings in cyanotic heart disease*

Diagnosis	Physical examination	Radiographic findings	Electrocardiographic findings
Hypoplastic left heart syndrome	Single S_2, " respiratory work, # pulse amplitude, # perfusion, ± SRM	" Pulmonary arterial markings, cardiomegaly	# LV force usually, develops RAE, RAD, RVH
Transposition of great arteries (IVS, VSD)[a]	Split S_2, ± murmur, ± " respiratory work (i.e., peaceful cyanosis)	" Pulmonary arterial markings, ± cardiomegaly with narrow mediastinum (i.e., egg on a string)	Develops RAE, RAD, RVH
Truncus arteriosus	Split S_2, multiple clicks, soft to loud SEM, ± DRM, " respiratory work	" Pulmonary arterial markings, cardiomegaly	Develops RAE, RAD, BVH
Total anomalous pulmonary venous connection	Narrow S_2 split, ± murmur, " respiratory work	" Pulmonary venous markings, " diffuse interstitial markings	Develops RAE, RAD, RVH
Tricuspid atresia			
Without PS	Split S_2, heave, SRM	" Pulmonary arterial markings, cardiomegaly	Left axis deviation
With PS	Single S_2, SEM	# Pulmonary arterial markings, ± cardiomegaly	
Tetralogy of Fallot			
With PS	Single S_2, SEM	± # Pulmonary arterial markings, ± boot-shaped heart	Develops RAE, RAD, RVH
With PA	Single S_2, continuous murmur, LSB back, axillae	", # Pulmonary arterial markings and heart size	
Pulmonary stenosis (IVS or SV)	Single S_2, click, SEM	# Pulmonary arterial markings	In IVS QRS axis 0–100°, develops RAE, RAD, RVH
Pulmonary atresia (IVS or SV)	Single S_2, soft SRM	# Pulmonary arterial markings	In IVS QRS axis 0–80°, # RV forces, ± develops Q waves
Persistent pulmonary hypertension	Narrow split or single S_2, " S_2 loudness, ± SRM	# Pulmonary arterial markings, ± parenchymal infiltrates, ± cardiomegaly	Develops RAE, RAD, RVH

± may or may not be present; #, decreased; ", increased; BVH, biventricular hypertrophy; DRM, diastolic regurgitant murmur; IVS, intact ventricular septum; LSB, left sternal border; LV, left ventricle; PA, pulmonary atresia; PS, pulmonary stenosis; RAD, right axis deviation; RAE, right atrial enlargement; RV, right ventricle; RVH, right ventricular hypertrophy; SEM, systolic ejection murmur; SRM, systolic regurgitant murmur; SV, single ventricle; VSD, ventricular septal defect.

[a] Single ventricle is usually associated with transposition of the great arteries, and in the absence of PS or PA, it presents similar to transposition with ventricular septal defects.

Reprinted from Flanagan and Fyler, ref. 97, with permission.

Table 22. *Prevalence of palpable lymph nodes at various sites from birth to 4 weeks of age*

	0–72 h	72 h–1 wk	1–4 wk	Total
No. of neonates	58	74	82	214
No. of neonates with palpable nodes	14 (24%)	26 (35%)	33 (40%)	73 (34%)
Inguinal	11 (18%)	20 (26%)	21 (25%)	52 (24%)
Cervical	7 (12%)	14 (19%)	18 (22%)	39 (17%)
Axillary	1 (1%)	5 (6%)	8 (10%)	14 (6.5%)

Reprinted from Bamji, ref. 130, with permission.

Section II: The Lower Trunk and Back

THE ABDOMEN

Steps in Examination

Review history pertinent to abdomen
Inspect abdomen for
   contour and size
   bilateral symmetry
   character of skin and dermal structures
   umbilical cord location and anatomy
Auscultate bowel sounds
Palpate for
   muscle mass and tone in abdominal wall
   location and size of viscera
   tenderness
   masses
   femoral pulses
Percuss for location and size of organs, tympanites, or dullness
Percuss anterior chest for location of upper margin of liver
Transilluminate abdomen for definition of abnormal fluid or air accumulations when indicated

Examination of the abdomen in healthy infants involves primarily inspection and palpation, but in those with suspected pathology it entails auscultation and percussion as well. Auscultation is used to follow bowel activity or to evaluate possible arteriovenous shunts but is not otherwise routine. Percussion is used to define organ size and outline as well as to demonstrate tympanites or pathologic areas of dullness. As with other regions, history regarding function of the relevant systems is a first step.

Pertinent History for Abdominal Conditions

Questions to include in assessing the abdomen:

Feeding intake
   signs of hunger
   type of nutrient and route
   quantity consumed over what duration
   intervals between feedings
Emesis or regurgitation
Bowel elimination
   time of first stool
   character and frequency of stooling, including odor
Urine output
   time to first urination
   frequency, quantity, character of urine stream
Maternal medications potentially affecting bowel function
   prenatal
   while breast feeding
Jaundice
   onset and duration
Family history of conditions associated with abdominal organomegaly
   hematologic conditions including maternal blood type
   storage diseases
   thyroid insufficiency
   diabetes
   chronic intrauterine infections

Inspection

Describe the contour of the abdomen and compare it with the thoracic shape and size. Note the color of the abdominal wall and examine the skin for color, moisture and turgor, temperature, texture, and any congenital or developmental lesions, including scars, dimples, or rashes. Look for the visibility of vessels across the wall to estimate epidermal thickness and maturity and note any distention or tortuosity and the direction of venous blood flow. Look for peristalsis and visible masses. Examine the umbilicus.

Inspection is the principal tool for physical diagnosis of the abdomen in the newborn infant; its ease does not detract from its potential yield. This tool is particularly helpful because the relatively thin abdominal wall of neonates suggests the outline of its internal contents and readily reflects changes within. It is not only possible but very effective to be able to see changes in the abdomen without disturbing infants who lie in incubators. For example, acute changes in color, contour, tension, or visible masses signal important changes of the condition in infants under observation for necrotizing enterocolitis (NEC). Points to remember in inspecting the abdomen include having a good light source shining across the abdomen to highlight contour and viewing the region in both horizontal and perpendicular profiles before touching any area. Augmenting inspection is transillumination, which is particularly applicable to thin infants or those premature infants most likely to develop a pneumoperitoneum with NEC or pulmonary air leaks.

Most clinicians divide abdominal topography into four quadrants: right and left combined with upper and lower. Supplementary regional localizations include suprapubic, epigastric, umbilical, or flank.

Abdominal Contour and Size

At birth and before feeding, the abdominal circumference is normally less than the head circumference until 30 to 32 weeks gestation. Between 32 and 36 weeks, the two circumferences are equivalent, and after 36 weeks the abdominal circumference normally is greater even with its wide variations from crying, feeding, and elimination (136). The greatest measurement is at or just above the umbilicus unless organomegaly or distention distort the contour.

In the description of the adult abdomen in *DeGowin & DeGowin's Diagnostic Examination* (137), the abdominal cavity is compared with an oval basin "with a rigid bottom of vertebral column and back muscles. The brim is formed by the intercostal angle at one end, the pubes and ilii at the other. Heavy muscles constitute the long sides. The cover is formed by the flat muscles and fascia of the anterior wall, reinforced and thickened by two parallel bands of rectus muscles suspended from the ends of the basin" (137). The image this description conjures requires some modification to depict the newborn abdomen; the basin would be more rounded and the side walls and lid constructed of far more pliable materials. The ratio of length to width of the abdominal cavity is relatively lower, resulting in a shape more round than oval. Instead of thick or firm muscles, the cover and side walls are thinner and more compliant with fullness in the flanks. Although more compliant, the abdominal musculature is not flaccid unless there is paralysis, abnormally low tone, or defective muscle development. Absent or underdeveloped musculature leads to an appearance of thin skin laying directly over the abdominal viscera so that bowel loops seem covered by only a thin towel.

At birth the volume and, therefore, shape quickly increase in relation to the amount of air swallowed with crying, sucking, or artificial ventilation, particularly through a face mask. Failure to change in size and contour suggests lack of communication to the stomach, failure to swallow, or herniation of abdominal contents through the diaphragm. Later the circumference continues to follow the relative volume of bowel content: increase after feeding, crying, or delayed stooling, and decrease with inadequate intake or excess stooling. The abdomen may be scaphoid, or abnormally flat, and if the chest seems full in comparison, suggests the possibility of a herniation of abdominal contents into the thorax through a partially or completely absent diaphragm, most often into the left chest.

Abdominal profiles as clues to pathology:

Generalized distention of abdomen
> *Pathologic causes*
> Ascites, hemoperitoneum, pneumoperitoneum
> Meconium peritonitis (Fig. 12)
> Lower bowel obstruction
>> ileus
>> distal bowel atresia, lower jejunum, ileum, colon
>> distal bowel stenosis, microcolon
>> imperforate anus (Fig. 13)
> *Benign or extraabdominal causes*
> Postprandial
> Crying, air swallowing
> Mechanical airway leak: mask, endotracheal tube, nasopharyngeal CPAP
> Depression of the diaphragm under tension
>> tension pneumothorax
>> emphysema
>> overdistention from mechanical ventilation

Distention predominantly in upper half of abdomen
> *Pathologic causes*
> Obstruction of upper intestine
>> duodenal atresia (Fig. 14B)
>> choledochal cyst
> Organomegaly
>> hepatomegaly (Fig. 15)
>> hepatic tumor
>> extreme splenomegaly (Fig. 16)
>> pancreatic mass
> *Benign causes*
> Benign gastric bubble
> Resuscitation insufflation
> Postprandial (Fig. 14A)

Distention predominantly in lower half of abdomen
> Distended bladder (Fig. 17)
> Distended uterus, hydrometrocolpos or hematometrocolpos
> Ovarian cyst
> Teratoma

Unilateral distention
> Hydronephrosis
> Wilms' tumor
> Neuroblastomateratoma

Widened flanks
> Ascites (Fig. 18)
> Poor muscle tone (prune belly syndrome) (Fig. 19)

Scaphoid
> Diaphragmatic hernia (Fig. 20)
> Esophageal atresia without distal tracheal fistula
> Severe malnutrition
> Poor muscle tone

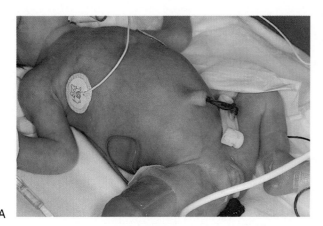
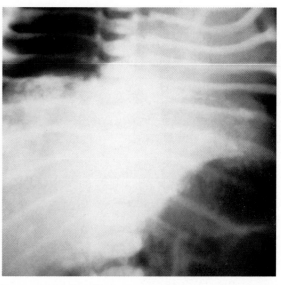

A   B

Figure 12. Generalized abdominal distention. Meconium peritonitis. **A:** Distention with abdominal wall darkening (see Chapter 5, Fig. 3E). In this case a localized bowel perforation was associated with maternal vascular disease and congenital lupus, but the differential diagnosis includes cystic fibrosis and aganglionosis (319). **B:** Diffuse speckling of calcification on radiograph.

Abdominal Distention

Abdominal distention occurs in response to increase in the volume of the intraperitoneal contents, but also from increased size of the thoracic or pelvic contents. For example, an important sign of tension pneumothorax is acute increase in abdominal distension due to depression of the diaphragm.

Measuring abdominal girth to detect or confirm apparent distention in premature infants is suggested as a parameter of feeding tolerance (138). The abdominal girth normally increases after gastric feedings, so what increment is abnormal for any given infant depends on a number of factors, including the baseline girth, quantity of feed, swallowing of air, and measurement technique. Increases of at least 2 cm have been suggested as abnormal, indicating feeding intolerance and significant gastric residuals (138). Taken into consideration with other factors, a 2-cm change in a low birth weight infant may be a reasonable value to warrant further evaluation but by itself is certainly not diagnostic or applicable to all size babies.

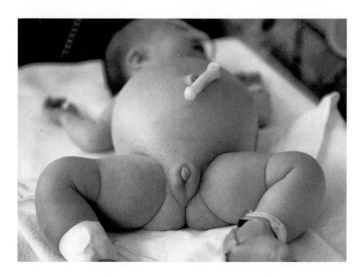

Figure 13. Generalized abdominal distention. Imperforate anus. Infant has ambiguous genitalia with masses in the labioscrotal folds.

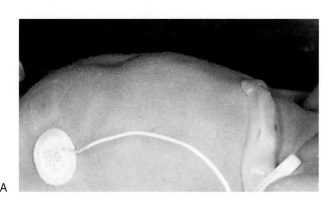 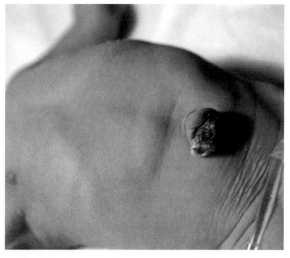

A   B

Figure 14. Distention more prominent in the upper abdomen. **A:** Iatrogenic distention shortly after birth and CPAP in delivery room. The point of maximum distention is just below the rib cage on the baby's left and across the mid-line in the gastric region. Although initially similar to the location of a double bubble of duodenal atresia, the air could be seen to move lower into the abdomen within an hour. If there were a high gastrointestinal obstruction, exogenously caused distention could lead to gastric perforation. **B:** Double bubble of duodenal obstruction. There is one bubble overlying the stomach on the left upper quadrant and one overlying the first portion of the duodenum in the right upper quadrant. The rest of the abdomen is soft and flat. This pattern persisted until decompression from an oral-gastric tube decreased the volume (Part B contributed by A.B. Fletcher).

Causes of abdominal distension in the newborn:

Pathologic distension
   Intestinal obstruction
      functional
      anatomic
   Ascites
   Pneumoperitoneum
   Hemoperitoneum
   Meconium peritonitis
   Abdominal mass
   Organomegaly

   Depression of the diaphragm under tension
      pneumothorax
      emphysema
      overdistention from mechanical ventilation
   Gastric distention associated with tracheoesophageal fistula, esophageal atresia, and artificial ventilation
Benign distension
   Postprandial
   Crying
   Air swallowing with feeding (gulping)
   Airway leak (overflow from mechanical ventilator, CPAP)

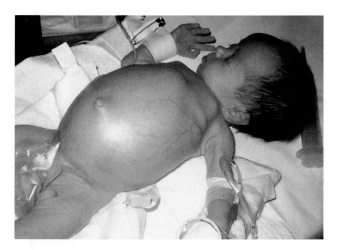

Figure 15. Distention more prominent in the upper abdomen. Massive hepatomegaly with especial distention just below the costal margin. Infant is jaundiced with breast hypertrophy and failure to thrive from untreated classic galactosemia. The vascular markings over the upper abdomen, suggesting liver pathology, are prominent, but the direction of blood flow is normal (contributed by M.C. Edwards).

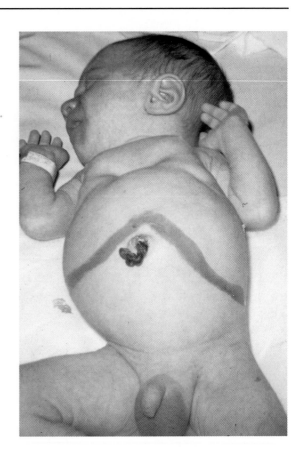

Figure 16. Distention more prominent in the upper abdomen. Massive hepatosplenomegaly in infant with congenital cytomegalovirus (contributed by A.B. Fletcher).

Dermal Markings

As in all regions, the skin over the abdominal wall should be carefully inspected for evidence of congenital or acquired markings. The color of the abdominal wall itself suggests processes within. Jaundice reaching to the lower abdomen in term infants suggests a level of at least 10 mg/dl. Peritonitis quickly causes a cellulitic reaction in the wall with visible induration and erythema. The dark green of meconium, free within the peritoneal cavity, shows through the thin walls if there is enough free material (see Chapter 5 Fig. 3E). Absence of these color changes does not rule out bowel rupture. Ecchymotic changes develop from direct skin trauma but, if limited to the mid-line below the umbilicus, suggest bleeding from umbilical arteries. Edema limited or starting in the same area indicates urine leakage from a patent urachus.

Skin Turgor

Pinching a fold of abdominal skin and estimating how readily it unfolds is a traditional method of assessing skin turgor, which in turn reflects a general state of hydration (139).

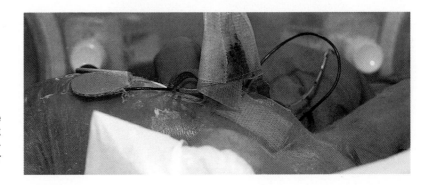

Figure 17. Distention more prominent in the lower abdomen. Bladder distention in 24-week gestation infant. Dotted lines outline the abdominal profile partially obscured by tape over the umbilical vascular lines.

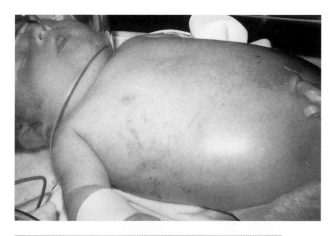

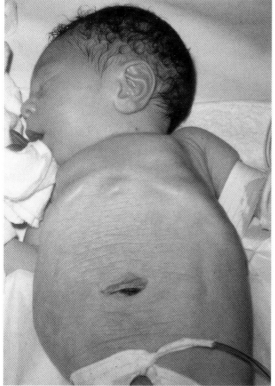

Figure 18. Distention more prominent in the flanks. Anasarca from an intrauterine tachyarrhythmia. The widening of the abdomen is greater than any increase in anteroposterior diameter, typical of free fluid sinking into the flanks with a compliant abdominal wall (contributed by A.B. Fletcher).

Figure 19. Distention more prominent in the flanks. Prune belly syndrome (Eagle-Barrett triad). Enlarged ureters with flaccid abdominal muscles causes widening of the flanks without increasing the anteroposterior diameter of the abdomen. The triad, which occurs almost exclusively in males, includes abnormal abdominal musculature with variable degrees of muscular laxity, abdominal cryptorchidism, and redundant, floppy urinary tracts with vesicoureteric reflux. Associated but inconstant findings include prostatic hypoplasia, dimples on the lateral aspects of the knees, and gastrointestinal and cardiac anomalies. Prognosis depends on the degree of renal dysplasia (contributed by A.B. Fletcher).

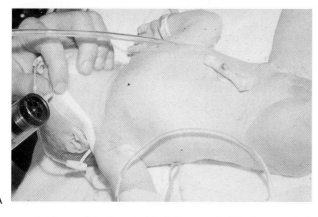

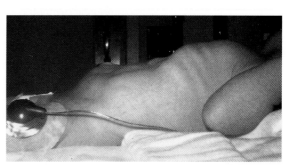

A

B

Figure 20. Scaphoid abdomen. **A:** Diaphragmatic hernia with a scaphoid abdomen because of shifting of abdominal contents into the thorax, causing an increase in anteroposterior diameter there (from M.C. Edwards). **B:** In prune belly syndrome the abdominal contents are well outlined, indicating their presence, unlike the diaphragmatic herniation in **A**. The abdomen will be scaphoid as long as the contents of the bowel are limited. In this case the abdomen below the umbilicus is fuller because of urinary tract obstruction (contributed by M.C. Edwards).

Significant loss of body water of more than 10% is said to result in loss of skin elasticity (139). Skin elasticity is dependent on a number of factors, including water and electrolyte content and nutritional status, so it is a gross and delayed estimate at best. One study in infants over 2 months of age found capillary filling time in the fingernail bed to be more reproducible than abdominal folding and correlated it with volumes required to rehydrate these infants (140). Newborn infants were not included in this study. Capillary refill is so affected by ambient temperature that it is also unlikely to be a valid indicator of hydration state (141). Although assessing skin turgor is only a rough method of determining state of hydration without enough reliability to direct clinical management, a change in turgor should not be overlooked.

Venous Markings

The veins in the abdominal wall are more visible in newborn infants than in older patients, but their visibility depends on the thickness of the dermal and subcutaneous layers, so it correlates to both nutrition and gestational age: the thinner or more premature the infant, the more visible are the veins. Some systems for establishing gestational age use visibility of abdominal wall veins as one factor (142).

Although discernible, the abdominal veins should not be distended and should flow in the expected directions of drainage. Above the umbilicus, venous blood normally flows toward the heart; below the umbilicus, venous blood flows away from the heart. If there is obstruction in the inferior vena cava, the flow in the lower half is reversed, that is, toward the heart. If there is obstruction in the superior vena cava, the flow in the upper half is reversed, away from the heart. Portal hypertension is not associated with reversed flow but will cause venous distention (137) (Fig. 15).

In the Cruveilhier-Baumgarten syndrome, prominent collateral circulation surrounds the umbilicus and is associated with a venous hum, as well as thrill, portal hypertension, and splenomegaly (143). Because this represents failure of obliteration of umbilical vein with development of collateral circulation and portal hypertension, its appearance within the newborn period is unlikely.

Visible Peristalsis

With the first few breaths after birth, the upper abdomen will appear slightly more distended than the lower abdomen. It is not at all unusual to be able to see multiple bowel loops through the abdominal wall (ladder sign), particularly in infants with little subcutaneous fat or low abdominal muscle tone (Figs. 14A and 21). Peristaltic waves should be seen to carry the air along in these loops. If there is a persistence of the visibly distended loops in the same area, particularly in the upper quadrant after the first hour of life, one has to consider that there may be an obstruction to normal bowel transit. When two distinct bowel loop bubbles are seen to persist beyond the first hour, particularly when the rest of the abdomen is relatively less distended, an obstruction of the duodenum is likely (Fig. 14B).

Diastasis Recti

Separation of rectus abdominis muscles away from the mid-line is a common finding in newborn infants. Apparent as a bulge from the umbilicus to the xiphoid process when abdominal muscles are flexed, it has no clinical significance but it does have a role in physical diagnosis. The separation of the muscles allows easier palpation of structures beneath the diastasis, notably in the region of the pylorus (Fig. 22).

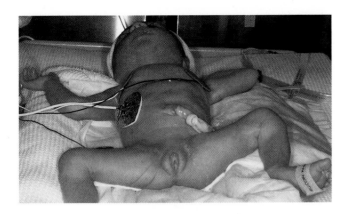

Figure 21. Visible bowel loops in upper abdomen after resuscitation and CPAP. Although there is benign distention of the loops, their visibility is enhanced because of the extremely compliant and thin abdominal wall in this premature infant.

Umbilicus

Note the location and size of the umbilicus. In the first examination after birth, count the number of umbilical vessels and note the character of Wharton's jelly in the cord, looking for average width of the cord, calcifications, hematoma, or herniation. In later examinations but before cord separation, look for normal drying or the presence of abnormal moisture or odor. After separation, look for evidence of complete healing and absence of umbilical granuloma. Examine the base of the cord and the surrounding area for erythema and induration, suggesting omphalitis. Palpate the base of the umbilical cord for a hernia and estimate the diameter of the fascial opening. Note the length of the umbilical skin.

Umbilical cord structures include the umbilical vein, two umbilical arteries, Wharton's jelly, and, variably, remnants of the vitelline vessels and urachus. The umbilical insertion is on the abdominal wall at the level of the top of the iliac crests, opposite the third or fourth lumbar vertebrae or at roughly half the distance from the xiphoid process to the pubic symphysis. In Robinow syndrome the umbilicus is superiorly located and poorly epithelialized (144).

At the insertion of the umbilical cord the skin should extend a few millimeters onto the cord. If the base is not well epithelialized, there may be a defect in formation of the body stalk or an exomphalocele or a residual sign of incomplete fusion of the body wall

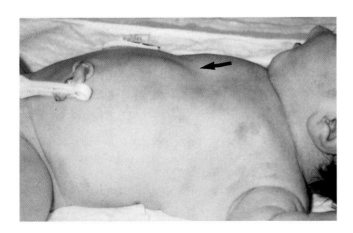

Figure 22. Diastasis rectus (*arrow*). The mid-line bulge becomes apparent only when the adjacent muscles contract.

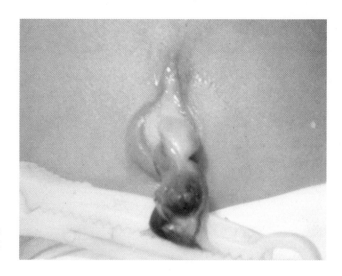

Figure 23. Supraumbilical closure defect in infant of diabetic mother that represents incomplete formation of the body stalk (contributed by A.B. Fletcher).

(Fig. 23). The length of skin onto the cord is variable, but excessive length is seen in infants with Rieger's syndrome. Umbilical skin extends along the cranial aspect of cord farther than along the caudal aspect (mean 11.54 ± 3.58 mm versus 8.71 ± 2.89 mm). The skin lengthens with age but is not related to birth weight, gestational age, or sex (145).

After detachment, the umbilicus is a consolidated scar in the linea alba. Persistence of fetal structures of the cord cause unusual but important clinical problems, including sinus, fistula, cyst, or internal diverticula of the vitelline structure leading to the bowel or of the urachus leading to the bladder (146) (Fig. 24). If a urachal remnant remains patent, either at the umbilical surface as a sinus or all the way to the bladder, its drainage leads to umbilical granuloma, redness, or local swelling, especially below the umbilicus (147). Patients with persistent patent urachus should be evaluated for lower urinary obstruction (146,147). Retraction of the umbilical cord during urination is a sign of persistence of a urachal cord (148).

Any vestige of the vitelline duct similarly forms a sinus, fistula, cyst, band, or Meckel's diverticulum, depending on what segment of duct remains (146). The vitelline duct connects the ileum a short distance above the cecum to the umbilicus. Rarely is this duct patent as a true fistula to the umbilical surface at birth, but internally this blind pouch remnant is Meckel's diverticulum (147,149). An external vitelline remnant is an umbilical polyp that appears as a cherry-red nodule, with poor response to cauterization with silver nitrate (146).

Umbilical Hernia and Exomphalos

The base of the umbilical cord is broader at birth and narrows as the internal structures dehydrate and regress. The umbilical ring is formed by the contracting muscle and fascia around the umbilical structures. The diameter of this ring approximates the cord diameter and decreases with age. Persistence of a small opening through the fascia that allows protrusion of bowel or omentum through the abdominal wall under intact umbilical skin is an infantile umbilical hernia. When the defect is larger, intestines herniate into an intact cord or into a sac without skin, an omphalocele.

Infantile umbilical hernias occur in black infants far more often than in white children, with a prevalence of 40% to 60% in the first year of life (150) (Fig. 25). Most close by 5 years, and others continue to close throughout childhood (150). These hernias do rarely incarcerate and strangulate and are a source of discomfort for some children (151). In infancy the incidence in males and females is equal, but in older patients females predominate (150–152). Large umbilical hernias that develop after the newborn period are associated

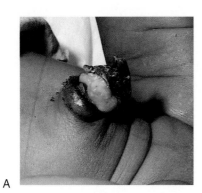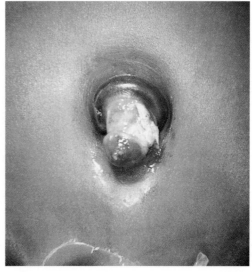

A   B

Figure 24. Abnormal pattern of cord drying due to persistent fetal ducts, either urachal or vitelline. Evaluation should include looking for Meckel's diverticulum if vitelline or urinary obstruction if urachal. **A:** Copious granulation tissue before delayed cord separation. **B:** Leakage of fluid irritates skin below umbilicus (Part B contributed by M.C. Edwards).

with many genetic syndromes, metabolic or storage diseases (including hypothyroid and mucopolysaccharidoses), and conditions of poor connective tissue strength (153).

An omphalocele is an avascular, translucent sac at the base of the umbilicus that consists of peritoneum and amnionic membrane. The sac varies from a few centimeters in diameter and containing a few loops of bowel (exomphalos minor) to a large sac with a defect greater than 5 cm containing the midgut, stomach, and liver (exomphalos major) (Fig. 26). The abdominal muscles are intact although interrupted in all sizes of omphalocele, but when the liver is in the sac, the anterior portion of the diaphragm is missing and the abdominal cavity is extremely small (154). An important distinguishing feature of omphalocele is that the umbilical cord always inserts into the sac. This finding points to the probable etiology as a persistence of body stalk in an area where there should be somatopleure (155). The defect occurs in the first trimester of pregnancy before the fusion of the abdominal wall. Large defects are formed before 56 days after ovulation. Small defects can develop until 10 weeks after ovulation (155).

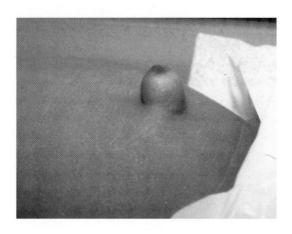

Figure 25. Small umbilical hernia at 2 months of age.

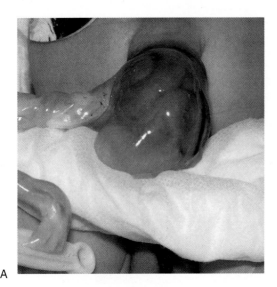
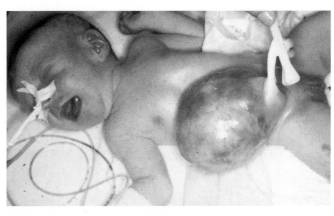

A   B

Figure 26. Omphalocele. **A:** Exomphalos minor. Small defect with diameter of 3 cm herniated loops of bowel only at the base of the cord. Close to one fourth of small omphaloceles are associated with Meckel's diverticulum. **B:** Exomphalos major. Herniated contents include liver, so the repair is much more complicated because of the smaller abdominal cavity and associated defects. Bilious drainage is present in the nasogastric tube (contributed by A.B. Fletcher).

In the smaller omphaloceles there is coexisting Meckel's diverticulum in close to one fourth of cases (156). The membrane covering a large sac is thin and can rupture in utero, at birth, or before surgical correction. Avulsion of the umbilical cord at delivery is another serious association.

A similar defect of the abdominal wall that is confused with omphalocele is gastroschisis (Fig. 27, Table 23) (157). Unlike omphalocele, the defect arises outside the umbilical ring so the umbilical cord does not insert on the defect and the herniated bowel is not covered by peritoneum or amnion. The defect is almost always to the infant's right of the umbilicus. When rupture occurs well before birth, the bowel is matted and covered with amnionic debris and fibrous tissue.

The etiology and timing of gastroschisis is still controversial. The event is found to occur in all trimesters. The earlier the rupture, the more matted the bowel. In most cases, the

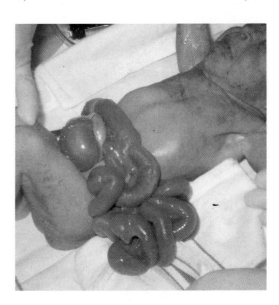

Figure 27. Gastroschisis.

Table 23. *Clinical distinction between gastroschisis and omphalocele*

Characteristic	Gastroschisis	Omphalocele
Size defect (diameter)	Usually <4 cm	Usually >4 cm
Organs extruded, other than bowel	Stomach, urinary bladder, uterus, and adnexa	Liver
Appearance of bowel	Usually matted, bowel atresia and necrosis more common	Usually normal appearance
Presence of sac	Never	Always, either intact or ruptured
Location of defect	Extraumbilical, usually to right of umbilicus	Within umbilical ring
Surgery	Often multistaged	Often one stage
Fatality rate	Higher, short-term; lower, long-term	Lower, short-term; higher, long-term related to multiple anomalies
Proportion with additional birth defects (other than intestinal defects)	21%	75%
Type of additional defects	Structural defects include vascular disruptions; renal and gallbladder agenesis	Trisomies Beckwith-Wiedemann syndrome Mid-line malformations
Birth weight <2,500 g	38% with isolated defect, 50% with multiple defects	21% with isolated defect, 50% with multiple defects
Prematurity (<37 wk)	22% with isolated defect, 43% with multiple defects	11% with isolated defect, 42% with multiple defects
Bowel function after surgery	Often slow recovery	Usually fast recovery, isolated defect

Reprinted from Torfs et al., ref. 157, with permission.

etiology is likely vascular disruption because of the location and associated findings (155,158).

Prenatal diagnosis is possible for both gastroschisis and omphalocele through screening with maternal alpha-fetoprotein and sonography (159,162). The total prevalence rates were 2.52 per 10,000 for omphalocele and 0.94 per 10,000 for gastroschisis in a survey of 3 million European births. Gastroschisis is more prevalent in younger mothers, whereas omphalocele has a more bimodal age distribution (157,162). Interruption of pregnancies found to have either malformation now follows in one fourth to one third of cases (162).

Information about long-term survival and outcome for the two conditions shows significant differences, with more long-term consequences as a result of accompanying malformations in omphalocele (157,162–164). Both conditions have been reported to recur in families, although the likelihood is much greater with omphalocele (157,162,165,166).

Umbilical Infections

Omphalitis appears with the classical signs of inflammation spreading at the base of the umbilical cord. Clinical regimens of cord care attempt to prevent infection at this site. Some of the care procedures have potentially harmful side effects, and others may actually delay natural mechanisms of cord separation and drying (167). Umbilical cord care varies in different cultures and countries. In the United States, regular applications of isopropyl alcohol are recommended. Isopropyl alcohol is sufficiently absorbed through the skin to elevate blood levels in premature infants or, in rare cases of chronic application, to cause systemic toxicity (168,169). Local applications of alcohol can burn sensitive skin (170). In Asian countries where application of ghee, or clarified butter, is a practice, there is a high risk of neonatal tetanus directly related to this practice (171).

The types of organisms found in the umbilical region in hospitalized infants are those of general skin contaminants, including coagulase-negative staphylococci and *Staphylococ-*

cus aureus, but this area is more likely to be colonized with aerobic Gram-negative rods, *Enterococcus* species, and yeast (172). Omphalitis results from any of these organisms, with *Staphylococcus aureus* the major pathogen after hospital birth (167,173). In areas where more home births occur, *Klebsiella* and *Escherichia coli* predominate (173,174). Untreated, omphalitis progresses into overwhelming sepsis or necrotizing fasciitis, a rapidly devastating cellulitis of the abdominal wall (175–180).

Cord Separation

The time of cord separation varies widely, with ranges from 3 days to 11 weeks reported (mean 7–14 days) (181–185). The timing appears to relate in part to the type of cord care given, with the shortest separations occurring when no material is applied (167). Delayed cord separation has been associated with defects in white blood cell function (186,187), but the mean time of separation is also later in premature or low birth weight infants and in infants born by cesarean section (181,185).

After separation, the umbilical cord stump is moist and easily forms a granuloma, appearing as a pink, friable knob. Treatment of granulomas with silver nitrate without drying the cord exudate can stain and even burn the surrounding skin if the silver nitrate remains moist (188).

Palpation and Percussion of the Abdomen

Standing at the infant's right side, use the left hand to hold the feet and lift the pelvis slightly off the mattress. Using the right hand, palpate the muscles of the abdominal wall for tone and tenderness. Palpate the abdomen more deeply to define the location, size, shape, texture, and consistency of the viscera. Outline the margins of the liver and characterize the consistency and thickness of the inferior liver edge. Bring the deep structures close to the palpating hand by lifting the lower extremities. Evaluate the kidneys for location, size, long axis, consistency, and surface texture.

To facilitate palpating deep structures, turn the infant prone so that the mobile structures fall forward closer to the palpating hand. If there is any thinning of the muscles at the base of the umbilicus or in a diastasis rectus, palpate through this area for a less impeded feeling. Keep the finger flat, using the flat of the finger pads to palpate rather than the fingertips. Use the long finger to sense the underlying changes in consistency or texture and the index and ring fingers to press.

Feel for transmitted aortic pulsations, particularly if there is abdominal distention. Free fluid or air will not transmit aortic pulsations, but large solid or fluid-filled cysts may (137).

Percuss the margins of the liver using bimanual finger percussion starting at the level of the umbilicus and moving cephalad. Place the long finger of one hand (the plessimeter) perpendicular to the mid-clavicular line and strike it sharply with the incident finger (the plexor) while listening for a change in dullness. Move the plessimeter one finger breadth at a time until dullness appears and again disappears at the upper margin. Repeat along several points across the right and left upper quadrants to outline the curved margins of the right and left liver lobes.

Note any areas of tympany over the abdomen.

Mild tympany to percussion is expected, but the finding should be correlated with abnormal distension. The most frequent reason for tympany and mild distention in the left upper quadrant is probably simple air swallowing during feeding and before burping in a normal infant.

Use auscultatory percussion to outline the upper and lower margins of the liver and any palpable masses. Place the diaphragm of a stethoscope over the presumed location of the solid mass or just below the right costal margin of the liver. Starting a few centimeters away, scratch the skin surface lightly in series of short motions advancing to-

ward the stethoscope head while listening to the character and pitch of the generated sound. Note the site at which the sound changes in pitch as the margin of the liver or other solid mass. Outline the upper margins over the rib spaces as well.

Note the presence and location of tenderness or abnormal masses. Transilluminate any large masses or generally distended abdomen.

Auscultatory percussion is particularly helpful in newborn infants to define the margins of solid structures. After a margin is outlined by auscultation, direct palpation can more precisely locate an edge unless the abdomen is too tense or palpation is contraindicated. The technique identifies areas of differing densities so it can be used in the same manner as indirect or bimanual percussion but it is technically much easier and remains effective when the abdomen cannot be sufficiently relaxed.

Care should be taken in palpating the abdomen because of potential harmful side effects in susceptible infants. An engorged liver is susceptible to rupture in a thin premature infant, where there is little buffer between the liver surface and the palpating fingers. Palpation of the abdomen elevates the systemic blood pressure up to 25% above baseline levels (189). The risk of these side effects may be significant enough to warrant avoiding deep palpation.

Normal Size of Abdominal Viscera

The shape of the lower thorax in newborn infants is such that the upper abdominal viscera are not as thoroughly covered by the anterior rib cage and are easily felt on examination. Most abdominal viscera are attached to mesenteries or ligaments that move with the diaphragm so those located in the upper abdomen descend caudally with inspiration and move cephalad with expiration. Retroperitoneal masses or those attached to the abdominal wall will not. The solid viscera, the liver, spleen, kidneys, adrenals, pancreas, ovaries, and uterus, tend to enlarge while maintaining much of their same shape and position. The hollow viscera, the stomach, the intestines, colon, gallbladder, urinary bladder, and ureters are not visually outlined or felt unless they are distended with air, fluid, or more solid material (Fig. 17). The notable exception to this is when a normally solid kidney enlarges so greatly with massive hydronephrosis that it assumes some of the characteristics of a hollow viscus.

Liver

Because of the relatively large left lobe, the liver occupies a wider area of the upper abdomen and extends well into the left upper quadrant, often to the left mid-clavicular line immediately after birth. Additionally much of the liver sits below the traditional point of marking in the mid-clavicular line so it is important to assess total area rather than just the distance below a single landmark. Estimated liver size differs by technique but relates to gestational age and body weight (190,191). The size of the palpable liver edge below the costal margin at the mid-clavicular line in normal, healthy term infants ranges from 1.6 to 4.4 cm, so an edge should always be palpable (192). Clinical measurements by palpation and percussion are similar to those found by hepatic ultrasonography (190,193,194). The mean vertical diameter on ultrasound of Mexican term infants was 6.0 ± 0.75 cm with a transverse diameter of 8.26 ± 0.72 cm (193). Brion determined a similar mean value of 6 cm for Belgian infants who were more than 34 weeks and approximately sized for gestational age (AGA), with infants who were small for gestational age having a span of only slightly less at term (194). The liver span reported by ultrasound for Chinese infants at term was smaller (4.58 ± 0.56 cm) but correlated with clinical methods of total span but not distance below the right costal margin (190,191) (Table 24). Liver volume (LV) compared with body weight is higher in the newborn infant than at any time in life (195). There is a directly proportional relationship between the estimated liver volume and body surface area such that LV (mL) = $706.2 \times$ BSA (m^2) + 2.4. A similar estimate comes in using body weight and length LV (ml) = $2.223 \times$ BW (kg) 0.426 $\times$ body length (cm) 0.682 (195).

Table 24. *Measured liver size in healthy newborn infants*

Measurement (cm)	Entire sample, 35–44 wk (n = 100)	Full-term, 38–42 wk (n = 82)	Preterm, 35–37 wk (n = 16)
Percussion/palpation	5.9 ± 0.8	5.9 ± 0.7	5.4 ± 1.1
Percussion	5.6 ± 0.9	5.7 ± 0.8	4.9 ± 1.1
Projection below costal margin	2.4 ± 1.0	2.5 ± 1.0	2.2 ± 1.7

Reprinted from Reiff and Osborn, ref. 190, with permission.

Spleen

The spleen is easily felt in newborn infants without splenomegaly. One clinical study of full-term AGA infants within the first 24 hours of life found that the spleen was palpable in 17.9%. It was palpated less than 1 cm below the costal margin in 11.7%, between 1 and 2 cm in 3.6%, and 2 cm or more in 2.6% (196). Splenic size varies depending on circulating blood volume, day of life, method of delivery, and therapy, so interpreting the significance of mild enlargement includes considering these factors. When studied by serial fetal and neonatal ultrasounds, the normal spleen is seen to decrease in size on the first day of life and then return to near fetal size the next day. Splenic measurements just after vaginal delivery are significantly lower than those in infants delivered by cesarean section (197). Infants undergoing extracorporeal membrane oxygenation (ECMO) demonstrate rapid increase in splenic volume to almost double pretreatment values (from 8.3 ± 1.7 cm^3 to 16.4 ± 4.4 cm^3) (198). Measurements by ultrasound indicate a total length of no more than 6 cm in normal infants less than 3 months of age (199).

Splenomegaly is an important finding associated primarily with hematologic or infectious diseases and less likely with metabolic conditions. In the early newborn period, the most common reasons for splenomegaly are immune-mediated hemolytic disease or chronic intrauterine infection. Splenomegaly associated with portal hypertension is unlikely within the newborn period.

Kidneys

The normal location of the kidneys is in the flanks, with the long axis cephalocaudad. If the lower pole is closer to the mid-line, it suggests a horseshoe kidney. The kidney should feel firm and smooth and not depressible or too irregular. Fetal lobulations are sometimes detectable but have the same firmness throughout. By ultrasound the kidneys measure 4–5 × 2–3 cm at term gestational age (200).

The dome of the bladder is easily felt if it is distended with urine. Its outline will glow when transilluminated. Massively enlarged ureters secondary to ureteropelvic obstruction are felt as remarkably mobile, redundant, and compressible tubular structures. They are easily confused with meconium-filled loops of bowel.

First Elimination

The time to the first passage of urine reflects infant hydration and general perfusion as well as renal function. Current practices of improved maternal hydration during labor and early initiation of feedings suggest that a delay of more than 24 hours is significant. Studies before 1960 suggested that only 92% of infants voided within 24 hours, but more recent studies indicate that 96% of infants have urinated by the first 24 hours (201).

The first passage of stool is more related to gestational age and birth weight (202,203). Ninety-eight percent of infants weighing more than 2,500 g pass stool in the first 24 hours (201). Eighty percent of infants weighing less than 1,500 g pass stool by 48 hours, but only 90% of very low birth weight infants (<1,000 g) pass stool by 12 days after birth (202,203). Initiation of feeding is not related to the first stool, and three quarters of very low birth weight infants pass stool before being fed (202) (see Chapter 1 Fig. 2).

Abdominal Masses

If a mass is felt, the examiner must decide the most likely abdominal structure involved based on its consistency, surface texture, mobility, transillumination, associated findings, and history. By far the majority of abdominal masses in the newborn infant are nonmalignant, with most involving the kidneys or urologic tract (204,205). Abdominal ultrasound and plain radiographs allow the diagnosis of most causes.

Abdominal masses in the newborn (154,204–206):

Renal
 Hydronephrosis, congenital or acquired
 Multicystic renal dysplasia
 Renal vein thrombosis
 Nephromegaly
 Renal polycystic disease
 Wilms' tumor
 Mesoblastic nephroma
 Neurogenic bladder
Adrenal
 Adrenal hemorrhage
 Abscess
 Neuroblastoma
 Teratoma
Retroperitoneal
 Lymphangioma
 Neuroblastoma
 Sacrococcygeal teratoma
 Ganglioneuroma
 Leiomyosarcoma
 Pancreatic cyst
Gastrointestinal
 Intestinal duplication
 Segmental intestinal dilatation
 Mesenteric cyst
 Lymphangioma
 Intraperitoneal meconium cyst

Hepatic
 Hepatomegaly
 Infantile hemangioendothelioma
 Hepatoblastoma
 Mesenchymal hamartoma
 Subcapsular hematoma
 Epidermoid cyst
 Benign teratoma
 Focal nodular hyperplasia
 Angiosarcoma, undifferentiated sarcoma
 Metastatic disease (neuroblastoma)
Biliary
 Hydropic gallbladder
 Acalculous cholecystitis
 Choledochal cyst
 Spontaneous perforation of the common
  bile duct
Genital tract
 Hydrometrocolpos, hydrocolpos
 Ovarian cyst
 Ovarian teratoma
 Urachal cyst
 Inguinal masses: hernia, hydrocele,
  calcified meconium

Infantile Hypertrophic Pyloric Stenosis

Pyloric stenosis is hypertrophy of the circular and longitudinal muscular layers of the pylorus that causes lengthening of the pyloric canal and thickening of the entire pylorus (207). The result is a narrowed lumen restricting gastric emptying. Clinically, infantile hypertrophic pyloric stenosis (IHPS) presents on average at 3 weeks of age with symptoms appearing earlier, occasionally at birth. It affects males five times more frequently than females and is 15 times more likely to recur in siblings of affected infants (207). Presentation in premature infants is more delayed than in term infants, but before 40 weeks corrected gestational age (208). IHPS occasionally presents in premature infants as failure to advance transpyloric tubes or intolerance to gastric feedings but is far less common than gastroesophageal reflux in these infants. In typical pyloric stenosis, vomiting of bile-free feeding begins as occasional emesis and progresses to more complete and frequent episodes as the stricture increases. When the stomach muscles have hypertrophied enough to develop forceful vomiting, the classic projectile pattern develops. Despite recurrent emeses, these infants initially appear healthy and hungry but develop poor weight gain or weight loss and dehydration. Hematemesis associated with gastritis or gastric hypertrophy occurs in some infants (207,208). Jaundice due to unconjugated hyperbilirubinemia is seen in less than 10% of infants with pyloric stenosis (207,209).

The diagnosis of IHPS is suspected on clinical grounds with the definitive diagnosis made on palpation of the olive, which indicates a hypertrophied pylorus. Many surgeons do not feel diagnostic imaging is necessary to confirm a palpable olive, but in its absence or with an atypical history they will use either ultrasonographic measurements of the pylorus or contrast studies (207,210–212).

Palpating the Olive of IHPS

Techniques for palpating the olive are varied, but the prerequisite for each is having an infant with completely relaxed abdominal muscles and an empty stomach (154,207,213, 214).

The infant may be supine, decubitus, or prone. If the stomach is not empty, pass an oral gastric tube and remove all contents including extra air. Allow the infant to suck on clear fluids or a pacifier. For supine examination, sit or stand at the infant's right and hold the head, neck, and shoulder with the left hand to elevate the trunk slightly and assist in relaxing the abdomen. With the right hand, palpate with the middle finger while using the index and ring fingers to depress the rectus muscle. As an alternative, elevate the pelvis off the table by lifting the legs a few centimeters with the left hand and palpate with the right. The pyloric olive is a smooth, firm, oblong, and mobile mass of approximately 1 to 2 cm just above the umbilicus in the mid-line or just into the right upper quadrant. The mass may be superficial or deep. When the mass is found, roll it under the fingers to distinguish it from a liver edge, tense muscle, kidney, or stool. Interrupt the palpation for a few minutes and repeat the process to confirm the finding.

If examining the infant in the prone position, rest the upper abdomen over the palpating hand. The pylorus should fall against the examining fingers after the abdominal wall is flicked gently upward.

Auscultate the Abdomen

Listen in all four quadrants of the abdomen until enough sounds are heard to evaluate for frequency, pitch, and character. If sounds are infrequent, listen for at least 5 minutes before diagnosing absent sounds.

When this is a section of a complete examination, auscultation of the abdomen generally follows listening to the heart. When the reevaluations are directed at an abdominal process, auscultation may be the first step after inspection but preceding palpation.

Bowel sounds are relatively quiet but not absent in newborn infants until feeding is well established. Premature infants have notably less active bowel sounds than do term infants. It may take several minutes of listening to hear any sounds in very premature infants. Infants on artificial ventilation, particularly under sedation, may have very quiet sounds without bowel pathology. Similarly, infants with major bowel pathology, including ileus and perforation, may continue to have some bowel sounds. Changes in bowel sounds over time are clinically more useful findings than isolated assessments.

Transillumination of the Abdomen

One tool available for application in small infants with thin enough abdominal walls is transillumination. This tool augments inspection because it allows further characterization of abdominal contents that would otherwise be defined only by percussion. Masses filled with low-density fluid or air, such as massive hydronephrosis, distended bladder or stomach, and pneumoperitoneum, will transmit light if they are close enough to the surface of the abdominal wall. Factors affecting how well a mass will transilluminate include thickness of the abdominal wall as determined by gestational age, fat, or edema; darkness of skin pigmentation or lesions; proximity to abdominal wall; transparency and size of the mass; and proximity to other air or fluid-containing structures such as the bowel or bladder. Transillumination of the bladder is helpful as a preliminary step to catheterization or suprapubic taps to assure that urine is present (215).

A positive transillumination in the most elevated portion of the abdomen may represent free air within the peritoneum or air risen within a distended viscus. Turning and repositioning the infant is more likely to cause a shift in free air and its point of maximum transillumination than contained air even though bowel is relatively mobile.

Finding: Pneumoperitoneum

Pneumoperitoneum or free air within the abdominal cavity is one cause of abdominal distention, generally associated with an infant acutely ill with intestinal or respiratory disease (Fig. 28). Air gets into the cavity from either a perforation of the intestines or by dissection from the pleural space under tension from a pneumomediastinum or pneumothorax. An important cause of bowel perforation is necrotizing enterocolitis (NEC), which occurs primarily in premature infants weighing less than 1,500 g. In one study comparing perforations in infants with NEC or spontaneous events, the spontaneous perforations were more related to the presence of umbilical artery catheters and indomethacin. Those cases associated with NEC had a closer association with feedings (216). The physical findings in pneumoperitoneum due to bowel perforation are similar unless peritoneal signs of widespread NEC precede the perforation. Spontaneous gastric perforation, acute duodenal ulceration, spontaneous ileal perforation, ileal atresia, meconium plug, or Hirschsprung's disease are causes of regional intestinal perforation. An unusual regional defect in intestinal musculature that may lead to perforation recurs in families (217).

Two important caveats to remember are that bowel perforations are not uniformly associated with free air and that free air does not always mean bowel perforation, so the presence or absence of pneumoperitoneum can only supplement other information in making a physical diagnosis. If air is not located within the bowel in the region of perforation, there will be no air leakage. Especially when muscle relaxants are used to assist in controlling mechanical ventilation, a paucity of bowel gas may preclude pneumoperitoneum after bowel perforation. Infants with congenital meconium peritonitis will not demonstrate pneumoperitoneum at birth. Similarly, all instances of free air in the abdomen do not equate with bowel perforation. Infants who are on high pressure support on a ventilator are at risk for developing dissecting air leaks and pneumoperitoneum. These same infants may also be at risk for bowel perforations due either to NEC or to isolated bowel necrosis, especially after therapy with indomethacin (216).

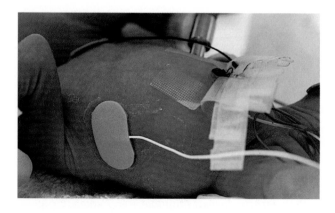

Figure 28. Transillumination of pneumoperitoneum. The shifts in free air to the uppermost region with position changes is demonstrable on transillumination. Contained air does not shift.

THE PERINEUM AND GENITALIA

Steps in examining the perineum and genitalia:

Review history pertinent for the area
Inspect genitalia
    determine sex
    locate anus relative to genital landmarks
    determine patency and tone of anus
In female
    inspect for presence of vaginal opening and discharge
    inspect sizes of clitoris, labia majora, and labia minora
    palpate labia majora for masses
In male
    inspect and palpate for size and shape of penis and scrotum
    inspect location of urethral opening
    inspect force of urine stream
    palpate scrotum for size of testes
    transilluminate any scrotal enlargements
Palpate inguinal region
    compare femoral pulses
    assess for presence of hernia

Pertinent History for Perineum and Genitourinary System

Information to include in assessing this region:

Gestational age
Urinary output
    characteristics of urinary stream
    color on diapers
        red of blood (hemoglobin, myoglobin)
        orange-red of urate crystals
        green of meconium or urobilinogen
        yellow-brown of bilirubin
        brown-yellow of concentrated urine
    frequency of urination
    assessment of reducing substances, pH, specific gravity
Bowel elimination
    time to first stool
    frequency
    site of elimination
    character: color, consistency, presence of hemoglobin, reducing substances
Genitalia
    Female: discharge
    Male: scrotal swelling, discoloration
Presence of visible inguinal mass
Family history of genitourinary conditions

Examination of the Female Genitalia

Examine this area with the infant's hips fully abducted and knees flexed in a supine frog-leg position for full visibility of the genitalia. Simultaneously palpate and inspect the region from front to back. Depress the labia majora laterally and downward to see the vaginal opening and locate the urethral meatus. Alternatively, pull the labia lateral to the orifice and forward. Inspect the clitoris for size. Inspect for pubic hair. Palpate the labia majora, the mons veneris, and groin for masses.

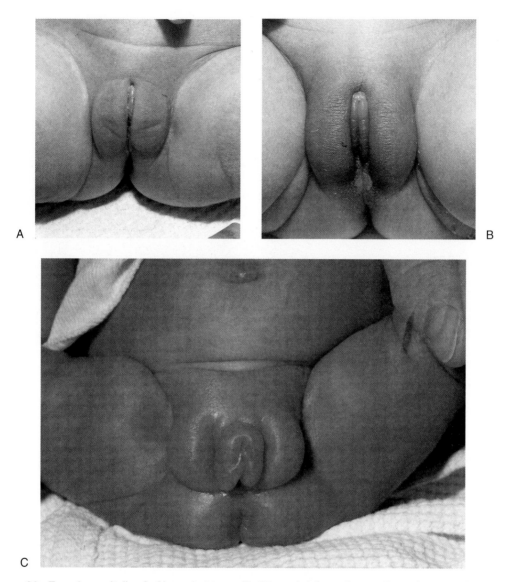

Figure 29. Female genitalia. **A:** Normal at term. **B:** 37-week infant who was large for gestational age with mild edema of the labia. **C:** Extraordinary edema localized to the genitalia in premature infant. Results of evaluation were otherwise normal, and the swelling resolved spontaneously.

Inspect the rectum and urethra for location and appearance. Note if the anal opening is at least 1 cm from the posterior fourchette. When indicated to verify the presence of a uterus and for evaluation of lower abdominal or inguinal masses, perform a rectal-abdominal examination using a lubricated little finger for insertion. Slowly insert the little finger with a constant pressure until the anal sphincter relaxes. Advance as far as possible and note the tension of the anal sphincter. With this finger and the other hand on the lower abdomen, use ballottement to assess the uterus and cervix.

The fullness of the labia majora correlates with body weight and gestational age (see Chapter 3 Fig. 12). The labia majora and minora should be smooth and edematous and the hymen somewhat prominent, reflecting effects of maternal gestational progesterone levels (Fig. 29). Mild wrinkling of the labia majora occurs with weight loss, but there are never true rugae. The urethral meatus is just ventral to the vaginal introitus and often hidden by the relatively protuberant and edematous hymen.

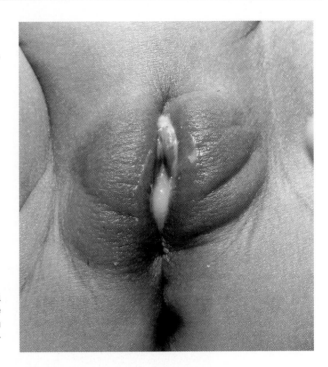

Figure 30. Normal term female genitalia on day 2. There is a tenacious mucous vaginal discharge. In some 10% of infants the discharge becomes bloody in the first week. The pigmentation and labial roughness will decrease as the effect of maternal hormones abates.

Sudden withdrawal of maternal hormones causes vaginal secretions that are bloody in an estimated 10% of infants, causing a pseudomenses, but the bleeding lasts no more than a few days and is limited in amount. More commonly there are just thick, milky secretions that indicate a normal, perforated hymen (Fig. 30).

Variations in Uterine Size

Organ Size

A neonatal vagina is approximately 2.5 to 3.5 cm long and 1.5 cm wide, with only a potential cavity present but greatly hypertrophied vaginal epithelium; the cervix is several times the size of the body of the uterus, with a total length of 2.5 to 5.0 cm, a width of 2.0 cm, and thickness of 1.3 cm (218,219). The long axis is cephalocaudal (220). At this age the ovaries are abdominal rather than pelvic organs so they must be included in the differential diagnosis of abdominal masses (221). The expected size of the ovary is 1.5 to 3.0 cm long, 4.0 to 8.0 mm wide, and weighs 0.3 to 0.6 g (218,219).

Hydrometrocolpos

Uterine enlargement from hydrometrocolpos presents as either a suprapubic mass or as a protruding perineal mass. It is an accumulation of secretions in the vagina and uterus caused by excessive intrauterine stimulation by maternal estrogens with obstruction of the newborn infant's genital tract by an intact hymen, hymenal bands, almost imperforate hymen, vaginal membrane, or vaginal atresia (222,223). If fluid accumulates in the vagina only, the condition is a hydrocolpos. When the mass effect is large enough, the presentation is an abdominal mass with urinary or bowel obstruction or even lower extremity lymphedema with obstructed venous return from the lower extremities (222). Some interference with free vaginal discharge because of an incomplete hymenal opening is possible in up to 14% of newborn infants, but complete blockage is unusual (222,223).

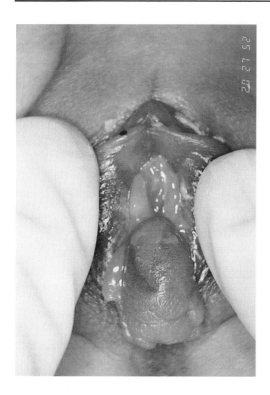

Figure 31. Genital prolapse. The mass protrudes through the hymenal ring. Simple inspection would not determine the makeup of this mass. Reprinted with permission (225). (Contributed by M. Bayatpour.)

Genital prolapse in the neonate is another rare cause of a protuberant mass on the female perineum (224,225) (Fig. 31). Most cases occur in infants with associated congenital spinal defects or neuromuscular abnormalities (224,225).

Hymen

Hymenal tissue is present in virtually all female infants at birth but normally not fully intact and with many variations (223,226) (Fig. 32). A glossary of terms describing these morphologic and anatomical variations is useful in documenting the physical examination (Table 25) (227). Berenson et al. have carefully documented with color photography hymenal variations found in newborn infants (227). In some 468 female newborns, they found abundant hymenal tissue in all infants that appeared redundant. In 80% of the infants the hymenal configurations were annular with a smooth edge. Clefts were present in 35% of

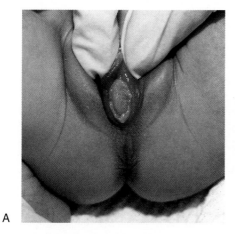

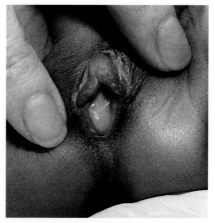

Figure 32. Normal anatomic variations of hymen. **A:** Fimbriated. **B:** Crescentic.

Table 25. *Descriptions of hymenal findings*

Term	Definition
Morphology	
Annular	Circumferential; a hymen that surrounds the vaginal opening 360°
Crescentic	Posterior rim of hymen with attachments at 11 and 1 o'clock positions
Fimbriated	Redundant and folded with ruffled and/or fringed edge
Septated	Two hymenal openings with band of tissue between
Cribriform	Multiple hymenal openings
Imperforate	No hymenal opening
Anatomical variations	
Cleft	Division or split of the rim
External ridge	Longitudinal ridge of the vestibular hymen from the rim to the fossa navicularis or urethra
Longitudinal intravaginal ridge	Longitudinal intravaginal ridge extending to or beyond the rim
Tag	Flap or appendage extending ≥1 mm from the rim
Bump	Solid elevation of tissue
Cyst	Fluid-filled elevation of tissue
Periurethral bands	Symmetrical bands lateral to urethra and connected to the vestibular wall; sometimes called support bands or ligaments

Reprinted from Berenson et al., ref. 227, with permission.

the annular hymens. Approximately 20% had fimbriated hymen with several clefts in the rim, resulting in a fringed or ruffled edge (227). By 1 year of age, most of these configurations change to a more crescentic shape (228,229). Hymenal tags ranging from 1 to 15 mm were present in 13% of newborns and cysts in 1% (228). Hymenal tags tended to disappear within the first year, but some persisted or new ones appeared (228).

A normal finding in approximately 25% of neonates, which should not be confused with scarring from trauma, is a linea vestibularis, which appears as a white streak or spots in the posterior vestibule, extending internally from the posterior commissure to the posterior hymenal border (230). This is best seen when the labia are fully retracted. This area represents mid-line avascularity or a posterior fourchette raphe (231).

Clitoris

The clitoris of the newborn appears relatively prominent, especially if the labia are not fully developed or the infant is premature. The clitoral size does not vary that greatly during the last trimester of gestation or early infancy so that a premature female appears to have a relatively large clitoris (232). Because clitoral hypertrophy is a sign of masculinization from exposure to excess androgens after the third month of gestation, it requires differentiation from penile hypoplasia with hypospadias resulting from feminization (232) (Fig. 33). Hypoplasia of the clitoris is reported in females with syndromes that cause hypogonadism and microgenitalia in males, including Prader-Willi syndrome and growth hormone deficiency (153,232).

There have been several attempts to establish normal values for clitoral measurements in neonates (232–234). The most clinically feasible method is to measure clitoral width because it closely correlates to clitoral length, which is more subject to technique variability. The width ranges from 2 to 6 mm, with a mean of 3.22 mm (± 1 SD of 0.78 mm) (233). Clitoral size does not correlate with birth weight or gestational age (232). The more premature the infant, the greater the clitoral breadth-to-weight ratio (232). At 27 to 28 weeks' gestation the ratio obtained by dividing the clitoral breadth in millimeters by the weight in kilograms is close to 4, but at term this ratio is 1 (232). Oberfield et al. found ranges for clitoral length of 2.0 to 8.5 mm, with a mean length of 4.0 mm (± 1 SD of 1.24 mm).

Clitoromegaly

True clitoral hypertrophy is reasonably obvious with significant increases of eight- to 10-fold in a clitoral index derived as the product of the width and length (235). In a study of young girls and infants with congenital adrenal hyperplasia, the index was grossly larger in the virilized infants in the first year of life (mean of 138 mm^2 compared with 15 mm^2) (235).

Causes of clitoromegaly (234):

Fetal causes
    Congenital adrenal hyperplasia
    Virilizing adrenal tumors
    Virilizing ovarian tumors
    Tumors of the clitoris
        Neurofibroma (236)
        Hemangioma (237)
        Lymphangioma
    Cyst of clitoris (238)
Maternal conditions
    Increased androgen production
        Luteoma of pregnancy
        Arrhenoblastoma
        Adrenal adenoma
    Drug-induced
        Synthetic progestogens
        Stilbestrol
        Vitamins containing methyltestosterone
        Medroxyprogesterone acetate
        Danazol
Syndromic
    Beckwith-Wiedemann syndrome
    Fraser's syndrome (cryptophthalmos)
    Leprechaunism
    Popliteal pterygium syndrome
    Roberts syndrome
    Zellweger's syndrome
    Chromosomal (trisomy 14 mosaicism)
    True hermaphroditism

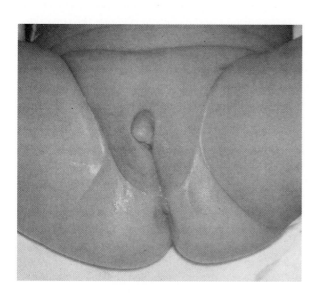

Figure 33. Clitoral hypertrophy (contributed by A.B. Fletcher).

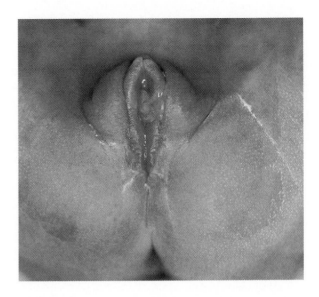

Figure 34. Benign perineal fissure extending from posterior fourchette.

Another suggested variation for measurement to detect virilization and the often accompanying labioscrotal fusion, particularly in the absence of clitoromegaly, is to compare an anogenital ratio (239). In this instance the measurements are made with the infant's hips and knees flexed against the abdomen. The infant must be relaxed and not pushing against the examiner. Measured are the distance from the center of the anus to the anterior base of the clitoris (AC); distance from the center of the anus to the posterior commissure of the fourchette, where the mucosa begins (AF); and the distance from the fourchette to the base of the clitoris (FC). The AF, FC, and AC distances increase with body size and gestational age, but a ratio of AF:AC does not change with age or growth and remains a relatively constant 0.37 (239). Labioscrotal fusion would result in an elevation of this ratio to more than 0.5 (239). Labial adhesions, acquired commonly in older infants, do not develop in neonates. Incomplete fusion from the posterior fourchette to the anus is a variation that should not be confused with trauma (Fig. 34).

Examination of Male Genitalia

Note the formation of the foreskin. If the ventral foreskin is incomplete, locate the urethral opening by pulling outward on the ventral skin to differentiate the more proximal, functioning meatus from a commonly present, more distal, blind-ending pit (240). In the case of a well-formed foreskin, palpate the corpora of the penis to evaluate the size of the penis in relation to gestational age and birth weight. Should the penis appear retracted, without stretching it, compare the ventral and dorsal lengths, determining a scrotal insertion ratio (see below). Determine the specific length and width of the penis by first stretching the skin and then measuring from the root of the shaft to the edge of the glans, excluding the foreskin. Measure the width of the stretched penis at its mid-point.

Inspect the skin overlying the scrotum for color, rugae, edema, or ecchymoses. Palpate each sac for its testis and cord. If the scrotum or testis is enlarged or discolored, transilluminate the scrotum. Should the testis not be in the scrotum, inspect and palpate along the canal. If not located in the canal or high scrotum, apply gentle pressure on the abdomen just medial to the iliac crest at the level of the internal inguinal ring. Gently sweep the examining hand down the inguinal crease while palpating the ipsilateral scrotum with the other hand. Bring the testis to the most dependent portion of the hemiscrotum. Take care not to mistake a low, cryptorchid testis as descended by bringing scrotal tissue up around the testis instead of lowering the testis into the scrotum. Note the position as being palpable or nonpalpable. If palpable, note the location at the internal or external rings, the scrotal inlet, or as ectopic if outside the normal path of descent.

The urethral meatus is a cleft or slit of 2 to 3 mm at the tip or on the ventral surface of the glans penis (240,241). A round, nonelastic meatus suggests meatal stenosis. Because abnormally positioned urethral openings that are clinically significant are associated with incomplete foreskins, it is not necessary to retract the foreskin to visualize the urethral opening for routine examination (240).

Variations in Appearance of the Newborn Penis

Variations in penile appearance most often represent variations of normal (Fig. 35). To describe the characteristic variations in normal appearance and their frequencies, Ben-Ari et al. examined all male newborns during a 2-month period (241). Of the 274 neonates examined, three were excluded because of hypospadias with chordee. The spontaneous direction of the shaft was in the mid-line in 76.8%, to the left side in 15.5%, and to the right side in 7.7%. Partial absence of the prepuce was observed in 10%; an unretractable foreskin was seen in 23.2%. The mean meatal aperture was 2.6 ± 0.8 mm. Deviation of the median raphe was present in 10% of the newborns and was associated with deviation of the meatus in 2.2%. Mild torsion of the penis was noted in 1.5%; isolated torsion of 90° was seen in 0.7% of the patients (241).

Penile Size

The prenatal growth of the penis occurs at an almost linear rate after 14 weeks' gestation, and the length relates statistically to fetal body length, body weight, and gestational age (see Chapter 3 Fig. 11) (242). Penile length in the term infant is a mean of 3.5 cm (±0.7 cm); the mean diameter is 1.1 cm (±0.2 cm) (243). Identical means but with less deviation were found in a larger series of term infants, with ranges from 2.9 to 4.5 cm in length, and 0.9 to 1.2 cm in diameter (242). At term a measurement of less than 2 cm is more than 2.5 SD from the mean. Some investigators suggest that anything less than 2.5 cm (−2 SD) at term is abnormal, whereas others suggest 1.9 cm (−2.5 SD) as a lower limit (240,244,245).

Micropenis is an abnormally small penis with an otherwise normal appearance (245). A micropenis may or may not have erectile tissue, depending on the presence of corpora cavernosa and corpora spongiosum. The scrotum is present but may be underdeveloped with cryptorchidism, either unilateral or bilateral. True micropenis is a sign of incomplete or inadequate virilization from either end-organ unresponsiveness or inadequate production, so its presence predicates further evaluation. More than 30 clinical syndromes or chromosomal aberrations are associated with micropenis, most of which are apparent in the neonatal

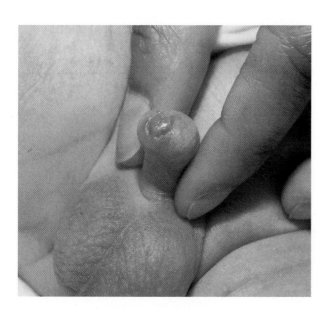

Figure 35. Variation of normal penis. Meatus is exposed with partially retracted, tightly adherent foreskin. The median raphe is slightly deviated.

period, but in the majority of cases, the primary fault lies in the hypothalamus with hypogonadotropic hypogonadism (153,244–246). Less commonly, the fault is in the testes themselves with hypergonadotropic hypogonadism (244). Micropenis associated with hypopituitarism and cortisol deficiency is the most life threatening in the newborn period and prompts early evaluation to determine normal adrenal function (244). A review of this condition and its evaluation is available (244). If there are any associated abnormal findings such as severe hypospadias, or epispadias with exstrophy, the terms "diminutive penis" and "microphallus" are applied (245,247). Microphallus is more etymologically correct than micropenis, but common usage is with the latter term indicating small size.

Inconspicuous penis refers to a phallus that either appears or is too small (Fig. 36). There are a number of urologic entities that fall under this general term, including buried penis, webbed penis, trapped penis, concealed penis, diminutive penis, micropenis, and poor penile suspension (247,248). Except for the conditions of diminutive penis and micropenis, the penile size in these entities is normal. Buried penis is one covered within an overabundance of prepubic fat and may be seen in the newborn period in plump infants. Applying pressure at the base of the penis to retract the fat pad easily exposes the normal phallus. Trapped penis is a potential complication of routine neonatal circumcision and results after cicatricial scarring or phimosis binds down the penis so it is embedded in the scrotum and prepubic fat. Trapping occurs after neonatal circumcision if too much skin is removed, if an enlarged fat pad pushes the remaining skin over the glans, or if too little inner preputial skin is removed. Webbed penis has a mid-line skin web or dartos band at the penoscrotal angle that binds the ventrum of the penis to the scrotum, obscuring the penoscrotal angle. Webbed penis occurs commonly in conjunction with a hypospadias, chordee, or micropenis. The concealed penis is covered by an overlapping abdominal fat pad and is unlikely in the newborn period. Circumcision in infants with webbed penis is contraindicated before urologic evaluation; in a buried penis healing may be complicated by trapping (248).

Some investigators suggest that a guideline for determining if circumcision should be deferred until after urologic evaluation is a ratio of the ventral and dorsal penile length in the unstretched penis: the scrotal insertion ratio (249). In one series only 2.7% of prospectively measured newborn infants had a scrotal insertion ratio of less than 0.48, which suggested a high insertion of the scrotum that would carry a greater likelihood of postcircumcision trapping (249).

Hypospadias

The normal location of the urethral opening is at the tip of the glans, but it may be proximally displaced as a hypospadias (Fig. 37). Depending on the population studied, the re-

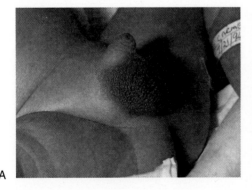
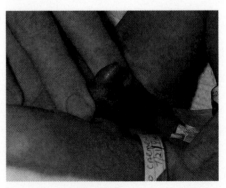

A   B

Figure 36. Inconspicuous penis. **A:** At rest the tip of the glans inside the foreskin lies well below the level of the scrotal margin, suggesting a short phallus. **B:** When gentle pressure was applied at the base of the penis, normal length and diameter could be measured. The results of circumcision are likely to be unsatisfactory at this age.

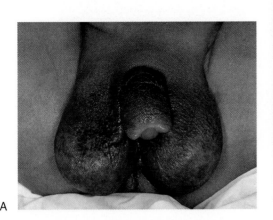
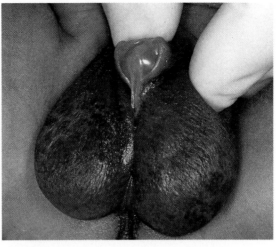

Figure 37. Hypospadias, bifid scrotum. **A:** This appears to be merely a very pendulous scrotum until closer examination. **B:** With elevation of the penis, the presence of chordee (tethering) and the absence of a glandular meatus is apparent. There appear to be as many as three meatal openings along the median of the scrotum, but urine comes only from the upper one.

ported incidence of hypospadias ranges from less than one per 1,000 to 8.2 per 1,000 male births (250–252). The classification of hypospadias is based on meatal position. Systems that use degrees of hypospadias are potentially confusing, so identifying the site of the opening is more specific: glanular; coronal; distal, mid-, and proximal shaft; penoscrotal; scrotal; or perineal (253). More than 80% are coronoglanular, with far fewer in the most proximal location (250–254).

There is a strong familial relationship in the occurrence of hypospadias. In one series, 21% of affected infants had family members with hypospadias: 14% with a brother and 7% with a father (255). The risk for a second child is 12%, but if another family member is affected, the recurrence risk is 19%. If the father also has hypospadias, the risk for the next son is 26% (255). Isolated hypospadias also may occur as a sex-linked autosomal-dominant inheritance (256).

Other findings associated with hypospadias include chordae, meatal stenosis, inguinal hernia, and undescended testes (257). The more proximal the hypospadias, the more likely there are associated findings; close to one third of the more proximal cases have cryptorchidism (257). Some studies report an association with reflux or other urinary tract anomalies, but the incidence of clinically important conditions may not justify evaluating every infant for these conditions (240,258). If both testes are nonpalpable at term in an infant with hypospadias, gender determination and evaluation of masculinization with the adrenogenital syndrome is indicated (240). Chromosomal abnormalities are unusual in simple hypospadias but should be suspected in the presence of other dysmorphic features or in those with unilateral cryptorchidism (240).

Scrotum

Testicular Size

The testis is ovoid and lies with its long axis in a cephalocaudal plane. It is normally quite mobile. Posterior and lateral to the testis lies the epididymis, which is closely applied to the body of the testis, although it may be more loosely attached by a mesoepididymis. The appendix testis and appendix epididymis are rudimentary structures not always present and not palpable unless obstructed. The volume of the testis increases after birth for the first 2 to 3 months in parallel with increases in plasma testosterone concentration and then decreases to the size maintained through infancy. At birth the estimated volume is 1.1 ml (60.14 ml) increasing to a peak of 2 ml by 3 months (259,260).

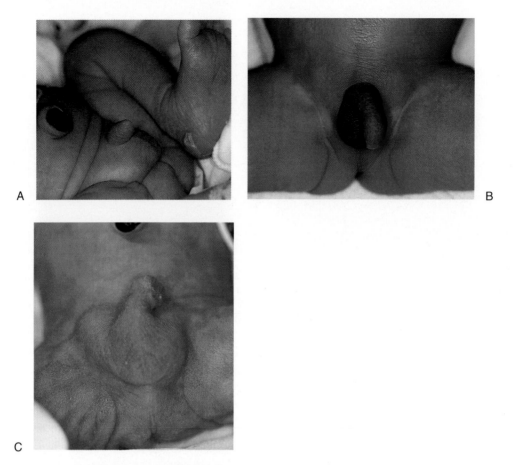

Figure 38. Cryptorchidism. **A:** Complete cryptorchidism with micropenis. The extremely small size of the scrotum indicates that the testes have never been descended. There were no testes in the canal. Infant had other stigmata of Noonan's syndrome. Total length of the stretched phallus was 2 cm (>2 SD less than expected for age). **B:** Incompletely descended testes in term infant. The testes are apparent in the canal. **C:** Incomplete descent in 28-week gestation infant.

Abnormally small testes may be part of a rudimentary testes, hypogonadism syndrome or represent atrophic testes due to prenatal infarction or torsion of the spermatic cord. In the absence of other manifestations of hypogonadism or anomalies, atrophy is likely with intrauterine infarction or torsion a probable cause (261). On examination, normal cord and epididymis may be palpable, but the testis itself is nonpalpable or well below the expected volume at birth.

Causes of small scrotum:

Undescended testis (262–264)
Rudimentary testis syndrome (265)
Atrophic testis (266–269)
Prenatal infarction
Torsion of the spermatic cord (261)

Cryptorchidism

A cryptorchid testis is one that is in an extrascrotal position (270) (Fig. 38). If a palpable testis is not found in a normal position within the scrotum, its location should be described as being at the internal ring, external ring, scrotal inlet, or ectopic. Ultrasonography may demonstrate the position of a nonpalpable testis, but a negative finding does not exclude the presence of testicular tissue. In the presence of other genital anomalies or ambiguous genitalia, the evaluation of undescended testes includes karyotyping and imaging studies of the genital system (264). There is variability over the approach to treatment because of potential loss of fertility and malignancy, so if there are no other apparent malformations that increase the urgency, consultation after the early newborn period is indicated. An exception would be extremely low birth weight infants where cryptorchidism is the norm (262, 270–275).

Cryptorchidism is one of the more common urologic conditions in pediatric practice and the most common problem of male sexual differentiation (263,264,276). In one large series of consecutive male births, 3.7% were found to be cryptorchid at birth, with higher rates for infants who were premature, low birth weight, small for gestational age, or twins. For infants born at less than 37 weeks, the prevalence rate was 17%; for those weighing less than 2,500 g, it was almost 20% (263). This study confirmed the findings of a smaller study that related the incidence to birth weight but with the higher frequencies in those born weighing less than 1,400 g (277). Infants with neural tube defects, abnormalities of testosterone biosynthesis or gonadotropin deficiency, and several dysmorphic syndromes have a higher incidence of cryptorchidism. If present in the father, the incidence is 6%. By 3 months corrected gestational age, the majority of the testes that will do so have descended so that the prevalence in later infancy to adulthood approaches 1% (276).

Although some investigators report the cremasteric reflex as not being present until 3 months after birth, some newborn infants have a strong enough reflex to elevate the testes (262).

Causes of scrotal swelling in the newborn infant:

Hydrocele
Stasis edema after breech presentation
Inguinal hernia
Torsion of the spermatic cord, testis, appendix of testis, or epididymis
Hematocele
Epididymo-orchitis
Syphilitic orchitis
Idiopathic infarction
Ectopic splenic or adrenal rests
Meconium peritonitis
Benign or malignant tumors of testes and epididymis

Hydrocele

Hydrocele results when the proximal processus vaginalis incompletely obliterates, allowing peritoneal fluid into the distal sac in a communicating hydrocele (Figs. 39 and 40).

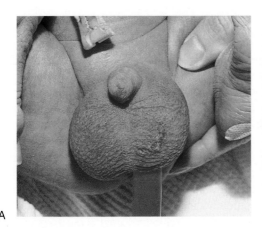
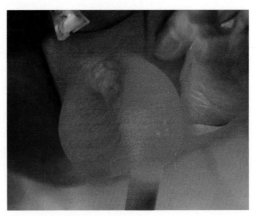

A
B

Figure 39. Scrotal enlargement. **A:** After breech delivery the enlargement may be due to direct trauma, as suggested by the blistered abrasion on the left side; the skin was not edematous. **B:** A positive transillumination indicates hydroceles as probable cause of scrotal enlargement.

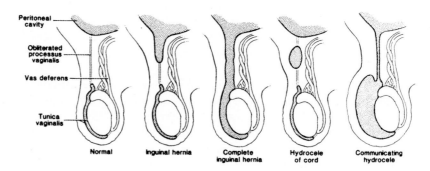

Figure 40. Findings resulting from incomplete obliteration of the processus vaginalis: inguinal hernias and hydroceles. Reprinted with permission (146).

The fluid accumulation may be anywhere along the course of the spermatic cord but most commonly envelopes the testicle, where it appears as a soft, fluid-filled sac in an enlarged scrotum that brightly transilluminates. If the sac is localized to the spermatic cord, a hydrocele appears as a firm, movable lump up to several centimeters in diameter. Hydrocele appears prenatally on ultrasound or shortly after birth (278). The prevalence of all degrees of hydrocele in male newborn infants is relatively high, with as many as 57.9% having some type of hydrocele (249). Most congenital hydroceles rapidly decrease in size, although fluid may reaccumulate periodically. During the first year of life, no treatment is needed unless there is an associated inguinal hernia. Because of the potential communication of peritoneal fluid into the scrotum through a hydrocele, any free material in the abdominal cavity can enter the scrotum and provide an unusual presentation of acute perforated appendicitis, meconium peritonitis, or intraperitoneal hemorrhage (279–281).

Torsion of the Spermatic Cord

Perinatal torsion of the spermatic cord differs from torsion of the testis, presenting in later childhood and adolescence (282). Neonatal torsion is almost exclusively extravaginal or supravaginal torsion of the spermatic cord in contrast to the intravaginal torsion most common in older boys (Fig. 40). Most cases of neonatal torsion are present with few if any symptoms at the time of birth and involve nonviable testes even when immediately surgically explored because the process occurs at some time well before birth (269,282–285). Occasionally, the presentation is an atrophic testicle at the end of a fibrous vas deferens when the clinical diagnosis is undescended testis (154). The most commonly recognized physical findings are discoloration of a nontransilluminating hemiscrotum with variable swelling. There are generally no associated systemic symptoms. Color Doppler ultrasound studies show absence of flow to the affected side or sides (286,287). Both sides are affected equally often and, although unilateral involvement is more common, bilateral torsion occurs (282,285). There is no relationship to prematurity, low birth weight, mode of delivery, or perinatal trauma (268). Although some investigators contend that emergency surgical intervention is indicated, most now appear to indicate that an elective procedure to fix the other side to prevent its torsion and to remove necrotic material is more appropriate only after the risk of anesthesia in a stabilized newborn is lowest (266,267,282,283). The use of color Doppler studies to distinguish which testes still have blood flow may help detect the few that could benefit from aggressive intervention (269,286). When the examination is normal at birth and signs and symptoms develop only after about 10 days of age, the process should be treated in the same emergency manner as torsion occurring in older patients (282) (Fig. 41).

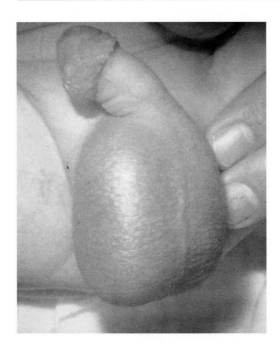

Figure 41. Torsion of the right testis. The scrotum is swollen, tense, and tender, without positive transillumination or discoloration. Torsion occurring after the first 10 days of life, as this was, should be treated as an emergency (contributed by A.B. Fletcher).

Other Scrotal Findings

Scrotal ecchymosis is most commonly due to local trauma, particularly after breech presentation, but it also may be a sign of intraperitoneal hemorrhage, with ruptured subscapular hematoma of the liver being most probable (281) (Fig. 42). Ultrasound examination, with color Doppler flow, defines the causes of scrotal discoloration (286,287).

Scrotal hair is reported in young male infants although outside the true newborn period and is presumed to be in response to the normal transient elevations of testosterone that peak between 1 and 3 months of age (288). Scrotal hairs are long, coarse strands, numbering from two to 15, and disappear spontaneously as serum testosterone levels return to prepubertal levels (288).

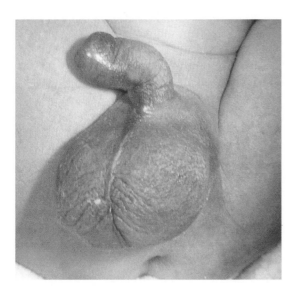

Figure 42. Scrotal ecchymosis after breech presentation. This transient and benign finding on the left scrotal surface should not be confused with scrotal hemorrhage, testicular torsion, or peritoneal leakage of blood or meconium. There is a typical epidermal inclusion cyst adjacent to raphe.

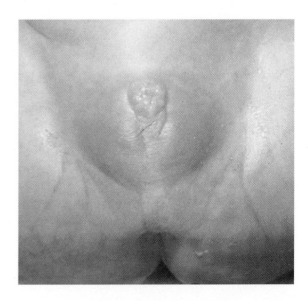

Figure 43. Ambiguous genitalia (contributed by A.B. Fletcher).

Ambiguous Genitalia

Although it would seem relatively easy to determine that there is clitoral hypertrophy when both the width and length of the organ are increased, it is still not possible to determine by examination alone if the structure is a masculinized clitoris or a severely feminized penis, even in the presence of apparent scrotal masses or vaginal openings. When ambiguity is detected at birth, careful evaluation is required before declaring the genetic sex. The parents should be immediately informed of the sexual ambiguity with a careful explanation of the type of evaluation that will be needed before sex assignment is determined (Fig. 43). The most medically emergent evaluation includes assessment of adrenal and pituitary integrity before there is catastrophic collapse from adrenal insufficiency. Other conditions requiring emergency treatment and evaluation are exstrophy of the cloaca or bladder (Figs. 44 and 45).

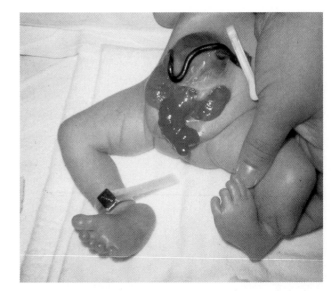

Figure 44. Caudal regression, which manifests in this infant with an omphalocele, exstrophy of the cloaca, imperforate anus, and severe but asymmetric hypoplastic abnormalities of the lower extremities. Cloacal exstrophy is extremely rare but more severe than bladder exstrophy because of associated malformations and the severity of the embryologic mishap. Occurring more often in females, rupture of the cloacal membrane occurs before the urorectal septum separates the hindgut from the bladder. Note lack of creasing on right sole of the foot, indicating poor fetal movement of these defective limbs. There are associated spinal anomalies and sacral agenesis (contributed by A.B. Fletcher).

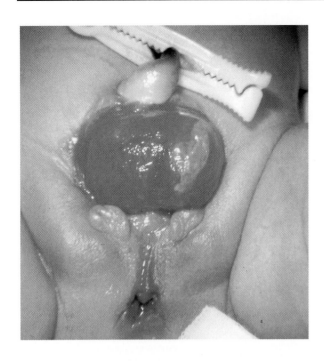

Figure 45. Bladder exstrophy probably results from premature rupture of the cloacal membrane. It occurs in approximately one in 35,000 live births and five to six times more frequently in males. This defect usually occurs in the absence of other system anomalies, but the penis is epispadiac or rudimentary (240,320) (contributed by M.C. Edwards).

Reviews for evaluations of ambiguous genitalia are readily available in all major pediatric textbooks, but initial steps involve sonography to determine if there are müllerian structures and karyotyping (289–292) (Figs. 46 and 47).

Etiology of ambiguous genitalia (292):

Virilization of females
  Congenital adrenal hyperplasia
    21-Hydroxylase deficiency
    11-Hydroxylase deficiency
    3β-Hydroxysteroid dehydrogenase deficiency
  Chromosomal aberrations
    XO/XY
    XX/XY
    Variants
  Maternal virilization
    Drug-induced
    Excess androgen production by mother
  True hermaphroditism
  Idiopathic
    Isolated
    Associated with mid-line congenital anomalies
Inadequate masculinization of males
  Congenital adrenal hyperplasia
    3β-Hydroxysteroid dehydrogenase deficiency
  Partial androgen resistance syndrome
    5α-Reductase deficiency
    Partial androgen receptor defects
  Testicular dysgenesis
  True hermaphroditism

Idiopathic
  Isolated
  Associated with mid-line congenital anomalies

Studies to evaluate ambiguous genitalia (292):

Immediate studies
  Chromosomal analysis
    Bone marrow
    Blood
  Pelvic ultrasonography
  Serum
    17-Hydroxyprogesterone
    17-OH pregnenolone
    Testosterone
    11-Deoxycortisol
    Dihydrotestosterone
Later studies
  Vaginogram
  Exploratory laparotomy and gonadal biopsy
  Radiologic studies, intravenous pyelography, barium enema
  Skin biopsy to evaluate testosterone metabolism

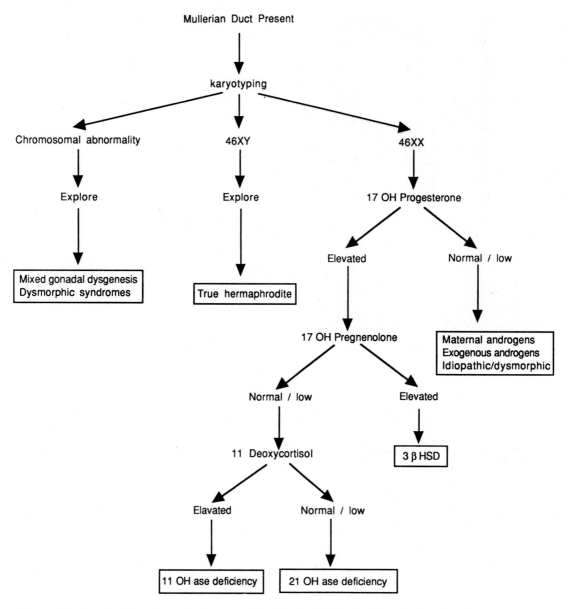

Figure 46. An algorithm for evaluating sexual ambiguity in infants with müllerian structures on sonography. Reprinted with permission (292).

Anus

In the initial assessment of the newborn infant, determining anal patency is one of the routine procedures. However, it is not always possible from simple inspection alone. The passage of meconium assures that there is some degree of communication, but its passage may be through a rectovaginal or rectovestibular fistula in a female or a rectoperineal or rectourethral fistula in a male infant (Fig. 48). In females a fistulous opening is generally sufficient to prevent bowel obstruction, but in males there is more likely to be bowel obstruction.

When the small finger is used to probe the anal sphincter, there should be enough elasticity to allow all but the larger sized examining fingers to enter. With patience most infants can be examined without any crying or apparent discomfort. A stenotic anal sphincter feels tight and ungiving, even when the infant is otherwise relaxed, and leaves an im-

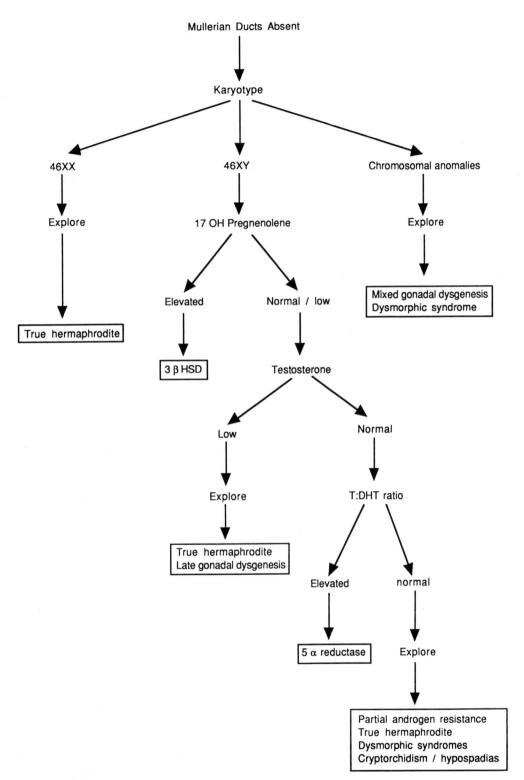

Figure 47. An algorithm for evaluating sexual ambiguity in infants with no müllerian structures identified on sonography. Reprnted with permission (292).

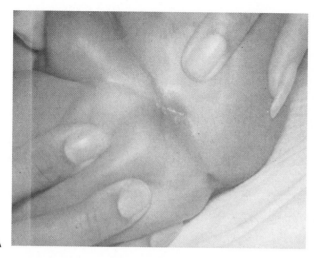
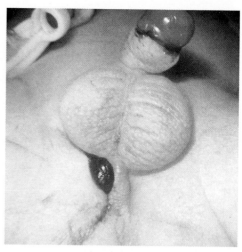

A   B

Figure 48. Imperforate anus. **A:** Imperforate anus without fistulous opening. **B:** Meconium is coming from a fistula at the base of the scrotum. Although there is a fistulous tract, bowel obstruction forces prompt intervention in most male infants (154). Circumcision had been performed at the time of delivery before a pediatric physical examination. High imperforate anus in female infants is commonly associated with ambiguous genitalia and uterine anomalies (contributed by M.C. Edwards).

print of a tight band around the finger. The anal diameter relates linearly to birth weight (293). For practical purposes, if a specific measurement is needed to diagnose severe anal stenosis, one can use the formula: normal anal diameter in mm = 7 + (1.3 × weight in kg) (293).

Anterior displacement of the anus is associated with chronic constipation (294) (Fig. 49). The otherwise normal anal opening in females is closer to the genitalia and is anterior to the mid-point between the fourchette and the coccyx. A ratio of anus-fourchette (AF) distance to coccyx-fourchette (CF) distance for females and anus-scrotum (AS) distance to coccyx-scrotum (CS) distance for males is more reliable than simple distances because it does not change with age (294). The techniques recommended for measuring involves laying a tape along the axis of the inferior border of the coccyx, the middle of the anus, and the fourchette or first fold of the scrotum and then measuring this tape when laid flat against a tape measure (294). In males the mean AS : CS ± 1 SD is 0.58 ± 0.06. In the female the

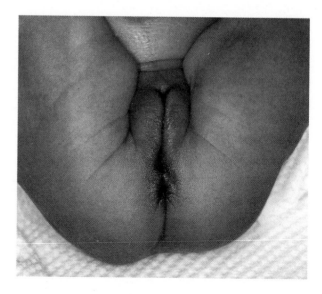

Figure 49. Mild anterior placement of anus in female.

AF:CF is 0.44 ± 0.05 (294). Anterior displacement in males is a ratio of less than 0.46 and in females of less than 0.34.

Inguinal Region

Femoral Pulses

Palpate along the inguinal canal. If any mass is present, note the texture, consistency, and dimensions. Palpate for intestinal peristalsis and listen for bowel sounds if a mass feels compressible.

Feel the femoral pulses by standing at the foot of the infant and placing an index finger along the axis of the femur in the femoral triangle. Very often there is a small lymph node at the fingertip in this triangle that points to the pulse palpable just cephalad to that node. Compare a femoral pulse (usually the left) with the axillary pulse (preferably the right) for intensity and timing.

Not only should the femoral pulses be equal in intensity and timing on both lower extremities, but they should be simultaneous with a pulse in a preductal distribution. The shape and volume of the pressure curve is essentially equal unless there is hypertension in one and low pressure in the other distributions.

Inguinal Hernia

Inguinal hernia presents as a swelling above the inguinal area that may extend well into the scrotum and cause swelling there (Fig. 50). The bulge increases with crying and elevation of intraperitoneal pressure. The swelling may transilluminate within the canal or scrotum. In the fifth week of gestation the mesonephros begins to develop into the gonads in the retroperitoneum. At 12 weeks the mesonephros degenerates and the gubernaculum testes form. At 28 weeks, each testis follows the gubernaculum through the internal ring to descend through the inguinal canal and the external ring into the scrotum. During descent, the processus vaginalis, which is a diverticulum of peritoneum, attaches to the testis and thus, is carried into the scrotum. The portion attached to the testis forms the tunica vaginalis. The remainder of the processus vaginalis involutes by fusing together, obliterating the entrance of the peritoneal cavity into the inguinal canal. Failure of the obliteration to occur allows for the formation of inguinal hernia or hydrocele (Fig. 40).

The incidence of inguinal hernia is four to 10 times more frequent in males than in females except when there are factors that influence the early appearance of hernia, primarily extreme prematurity. Although the right side is involved about twice as often as the left, bilateral involvement is far more likely if the left side is the presenting side (295). In the neonatal period, the most frequent factor associated with inguinal hernia is prematurity: 7% of males born at less than 36 weeks' gestation develop hernias, but only 0.6% of males born after 36 weeks' gestation develop hernias (296). The incidence increases as the gestational age decreases so that a reported 30% of infants weighing less than 1,000 g have hernias (297,298) (Table 26). Inguinal hernia does not appear until several weeks of age in premature infants, generally after the infant has become stronger with more vigorous crying and larger volumes of feedings. It is one of the findings that should probably be explained to parents as a possible occurrence even after discharge from an intensive care nursery.

Other less frequent conditions associated with the development of inguinal hernia in early infancy are a family history, congenital dislocation of the hip, undescended testis, ambiguous genitalia, hypospadias, ascites, the presence of a ventriculoperitoneal shunt, congenital abdominal wall defects, congenital hypothyroidism, and Beckwith-Wiedemann syndrome (146,153). Other associations, including cystic fibrosis, connective tissue disorders, and the mucopolysaccharidoses, are unlikely to cause hernias in the newborn period.

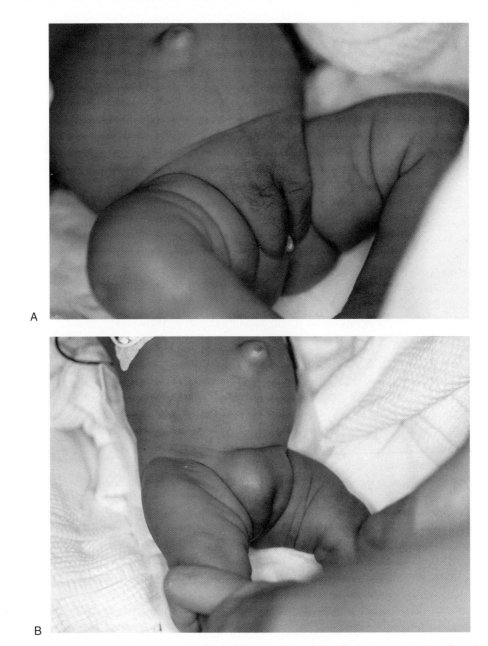

Figure 50. Inguinal hernias before and after reduction (**A and B**). Their occurrence in a female is more frequent with extreme prematurity. Besides herniation of bowel, the uterus, fallopian tubes, and ovaries may herniate. A hymenal tag is apparent after reduction in **B**.

THE BACK

Steps in examining the back

Inspect back
    symmetry between the two sides
    position and symmetry of scapulae
    length, shape, and integrity of spine
    presence of dermal lesions overlying or adjacent to vertebral column
Palpate spine for integrity of vertebral bodies or small masses
Auscultate the posterior chest and the flanks

Table 26. *Relative incidence of inguinal hernia in neonates grouped according to 250-g birth-weight categories*

Birth wt (g)	% of infants with hernia	Relative incidence	p
1,751–2,000	1	1.0	
1,501–1,750	6	6.7	NS
1,251–1,500	5	5.4	NS
1,001–1,250	14	16.6	<0.002
751–1,000	27	28.3	<0.001
501–750	39	65.5	<0.001

Data from Peevy et al. (298).

The examination of the back is easily effected but just as easily overlooked, particularly when an infant is in distress and requiring mechanical assistance. Palpating the spine and the paraspinal structures is a natural part of a thorough neurologic examination, but those infants most neurologically depressed are the ones in whom inspecting the back may be neglected.

Most of the major malformations affecting the spine are readily apparent at the time of birth and are diagnosed well before delivery by sonography and elevations of maternal alpha-fetoprotein levels if they involve open neural tube defects. These defects in formation of the neural tube range in severity from complete failure of formation of most of the neural structures; craniorrhachischisis totalis and anencephaly, which is incompatible with life; to spina bifida occulta, which is asymptomatic (see Chapter 6 Figs. 23 and 26) (Fig. 51). Meningomyeloceles that are completely skin covered appear similar to other lumbosacral masses, most of which have some neurologic involvement, even though their embryologic development differs from that of spina bifida (Fig. 52).

Sacrococcygeal teratomas are varied in size, location, and the tissues involved, with most congenital masses being benign tumors (299–314) (Fig. 53). These tumors develop four times more often in females than in males (313). Even though the tumor is more likely to be benign in early presentations, recurrences occur (313). Extension into the spinal cord occurs, albeit rarely, but the massive resection needed for removal of large tumors, particularly those with presacral involvement, can lead to loss of function in the bowel, bladder, or lower extremities (311,315).

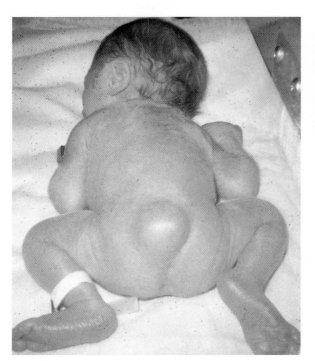

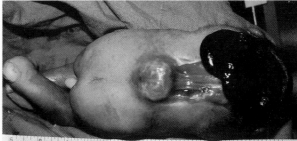

Figure 51. Neural tube defects affecting the back. **A:** Completely covered meningocele (contributed by M.C. Edwards). **B:** Craniorrhachischisis totalis representing complete failure of neuralation with the spinal cord lying splayed apart and a mass of neural tissue at the caudal end. There is anencephaly.

A

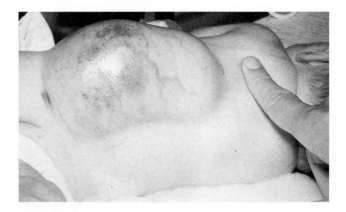

Figure 52. Paraspinal tumor. Although large with dilated vessels in the overlying skin, this was a benign lipoma that was removed without difficulty. Because of the large area involved, residual loss of muscle function and secondary skeletal deformity would be anticipated.

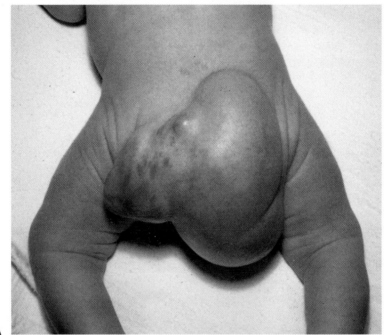

A

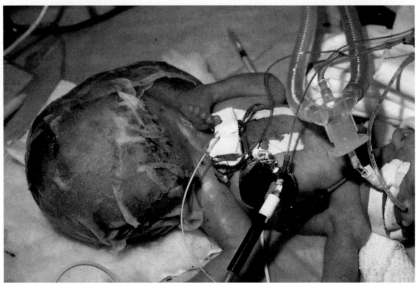

B

Figure 53. Sacrococcygeal teratomas. **A:** Although large, there was no loss of neurologic function, and it was completely covered by skin (contributed by A.B. Fletcher). **B:** Very large teratoma. The tumor made up approximately half the total body weight in this 28-week infant and caused significant prenatal cardiac stress but was resected with relative ease. Note the displacement of the anus.

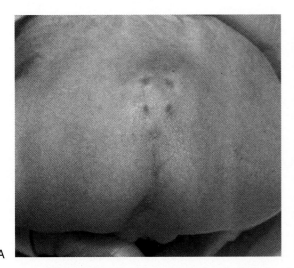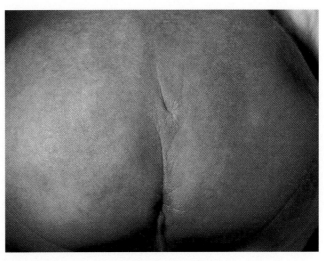

A   B

Figure 54. Dimples on back. **A:** Multiple dimples but with easily visualized base and no abnormal hair (contributed by A.B. Fletcher). **B:** Deep but with visible end located at tip of the coccyx.

More subtle findings on the skin may be signs of internally silent conditions: e.g., hairy tufts, dimples, or hemangiomas signaling spinal defects (Fig. 54). In most cases it is not necessary to embark on an aggressive diagnostic workup of dermal markings overlying the spinal canal in the newborn period if there are no other signs of neurologic involvement or malformations.

GLOSSARY

Arnold-Chiari syndrome Congenital combination of brain herniation and exposed spinal cord in the lower back.

Belly dancer's sign In unilateral diaphragmatic paralysis during inspiration, the umbilicus shifts upward and toward the side of the paralyzed diaphragm (133).

Bronchogenic cyst A congenital lesion of the mediastinum that results from abnormal budding of the ventral segment of the primitive foregut (134). This may be associated with obstructive symptoms, notably stridor.

Chordee Ventral curvature of the penis, most apparent on erection, due to congenital shortness of the ventral skin. The chordee tissue fans out on the ventrum of the penis and likely represents a rudimentary vestige of the urethral plate (318).

Dextroversion, cardiac Location of the heart in the right hemithorax, the left ventricle remaining on the left as in the normal position, but lying anterior to the right ventricle.

Diastematomyelia Congenital defect associated with spina bifida in which the spinal cord is split in half by bony spicules or fibrous bands, each half being surrounded by a dual sac.

Failure of segmentation Failure of a portion or all of two or more adjoining vertebrae to separate into normal units.

Heave A diffuse, gradually rising impulse in the anterior chest overlying the ventricular areas that usually indicates a volume overload (135).

Hematomyelia Effusion of blood (hemorrhage) into the substance of the spinal cord.

Hematorrhachis Spinal apoplexy; hemorrhage into vertebral canal.

Hemivertebra Missing lateral portion of vertebral body, resulting in a wedge shape. If two hemivertebrae are near each other, they may be balanced, i.e., the two wedges point in opposite directions, and a lesser curve or no curve results. Unbalanced means that there is no opposing wedge for one or more hemivertebrae, and the net result is an abnormal curve.

Hoover sign   Paradoxical inward motion (retraction) of the costal margins with inspiration. This finding in older children suggests marked peripheral airway obstruction with overinflated lungs that have pushed the diaphragm down and flattened it. Because the diaphragm is flat, its contraction with inspiration causes a constriction of the costal margin (131,132).

Kyphosis   Round shoulder deformity; humpback; dorsal kyphotic curvature; may refer to any forward-bending area or deformity in the spine.

Mediastinal crunch   Synonym *Hamman's sign.* A series of precordial crackles synchronous with the heart beat, not respiration, but due to pneumomediastinum. A crunch is best heard in the left lateral position but is rarely heard in neonates.

Meningocele   Local cystic protrusion of meninges through a cranial fissure; may be congenital or acquired.

Myelocele   Herniation and protrusion of a substance of spinal cord through defect in the bony spinal canal.

Myelodisplasia   Defective development of any part of the spinal cord.

Myelomeningocele   Cystic protrusion of substance of the spinal cord, with meninges, through a defect in the spinal canal.

Myelorrhagia   Spinal hemorrhage.

Pleural friction rub   Creaking, grating sounds that relate to the respiratory cycle. These sounds may be intermittent and confined to inspiration or heard almost continuously. They are localized over the areas of friction, generally caused by inflammation of the pleural surfaces. Because neonates rarely form any significant pleural reaction even in the presence of infection or significant irritants, pleural friction rubs are not heard.

Pseudohermaphrodite   Rather than a specific diagnosis, this descriptive term is applied when the constitutional karyotype is known but differs from the external genitalia. Causes of pseudohermaphroditism are widely varied, including androgen receptor disorders or disorders of testosterone synthesis in males or virilization syndromes in females.

Rachischisis   Congenital fissure of the spinal cord leaving the incompletely folded cord exposed along the back.

Scoliosis   A general term that applies to any side-to-side curve in the back, i.e., a lateral and rotational deviation of the spine from the mid-line. Such a curve may be termed "fixed," which means that any attempt to eliminate the curve by motion is not successful. Curves may be C-shaped or S-shaped. The apex of a curve is called the convex side, e.g., a right lumbar scoliosis is a lateral deviation of the spine in the lumbar region, with the apex of the curve to the right; the concave side of the curve is the opposite side. Scoliosis may be associated with vertebral anomalies (missing parts of the vertebrae) and with forward bending (round back); the latter is called kyphoscoliosis. Scoliosis may occur at birth (congenital), occur from unknown causes or diseases (acquired), or occur from unknown cause (idiopathic).

Spina bifida   Congenital absence of a large portion of the posterior spine, usually in the lumbosacral region. The severest form is myelomeningocele.

Spina bifida occulta   Congenital defect consisting of the absence of a vertebral arch of the spinal column; normally, there are no symptoms.

Tap   A sharply localized, quickly rising cardiac impulse that usually implies a pressure overload (135).

True hermaphrodite   An individual in whom both ovarian and testicular tissue are histologically demonstrable. The external genitalia are usually ambiguous and may include microphalus, hypospadius, chorda, partial labioscrotal fusion, with or without a vaginal opening. The gonads are partially descended and there are rudiments of uterus and fallopian tubes. Approximately 60% have 46,XX karyotype without Y DNA (316,317).

References

1. Cloutier MM. History and physical examination. In: Schidlow DV, Smith DS, eds. *A Practical Guide to Pediatric Respiratory Diseases.* 1st ed. Philadelphia: Hanley & Belfus; 1994:1–8.

2. Tooley WH. Epidemiology of bronchopulmonary dysplasia. *J Pediatr* 1979;95(5 Pt 2):851–858.
3. Sinkin RA, Cox C, Phelps DL. Predicting risk for bronchopulmonary dysplasia: selection criteria for clinical trials [see comments]. *Pediatrics* 1990;86:728–736.
4. Shennan AT, Dunn MS, Ohlsson A, Lennox K, Hoskins EM. Abnormal pulmonary outcomes in premature infants: prediction from oxygen requirement in the neonatal period. *Pediatrics* 1988;82:527–532.
5. Miller MJ, Martin RJ. Pathophysiology of apnea of prematurity. In: Polin RA, Fox WW, eds. *Fetal and Neonatal Physiology.* Vol. 1. Philadelphia: WB Saunders; 1992:872–885.
6. Green M. *Pediatric Diagnosis. Interpretation of Symptoms and Signs in Infants, Children, and Adolescents.* 5th ed. Philadelphi: WB Saunders; 1992.
7. Rigatto H, Kalapesi Z, Leahy FN, Durand M, MacCallum M, Cates D. Ventilatory response to 100% and 15% O_2 during wakefulness and sleep in preterm infants. *Early Hum Dev* 1982;7:1–10.
8. Brouillette RT, Thach BT, Abu-Osba YK, Wilson SL. Hiccups in infants: characteristics and effects on ventilation. *J Pediatr* 1980;96:219–225.
9. Alvarez JE, Bodani J, Fajardo CA, Kwiatkowski K, Cates DB, Rigatto H. Sighs and their relationship to apnea in the newborn infant. *Biol Neonate* 1993;63:139–146.
10. Heldt GP. The effect of gavage feeding on the mechanics of the lung, chest wall, and diaphragm of preterm infants. *Pediatr Res* 1988;24:55–58.
11. Buchheit JQ, Stewart DL. Clinical comparison of localized intestinal perforation and necrotizing enterocolitis in neonates. *Pediatrics* 1994;93:32–36.
12. Belmont JR, Grundfast K. Congenital laryngeal stridor (laryngomalacia): etiologic factors and associated disorders. *Ann Otol Rhinol Laryngol* 1984;93(5 Pt 1):430–437.
13. Handler SD. Upper airway obstruction in craniofacial anomalies: diagnosis and management. *Birth Defects* 1985;21:15–31.
14. Filston HC, Ferguson TB Jr, Oldham HN. Airway obstruction by vascular anomalies. Importance of telescopic bronchoscopy. *Ann Surg* 1987;205:541–549.
15. Brazy JE, Kinney HC, Oakes WJ. Central nervous system structural lesions causing apnea at birth. *J Pediatr* 1987;111:163–175.
16. Volpe JJ. *Neurology of the Newborn.* 3rd ed. Philadelphia: WB Saunders; 1995.
17. Hurst DL, Marsh WW. Early severe infantile botulism. *J Pediatr* 1993;122:909–911.
18. MacKinnon JA, Perlman M, Kerpalani H, Rehan V, Sauve R, Kovacs L. Spinal cord injury at birth: diagnostic and prognostic data in twenty-two patients. *J Pediatr* 1993;122:431–437.
19. Arens R, Gozal D, Williams JC, Davidson Ward SL, Keens TG. Recurrent apparent life-threatening events during infancy: a manifestation of inborn errors of metabolism. *J Pediatr* 1993;123:415–418.
20. Okoruwa E, Shah R, Gerdes K. Apnea and vomiting in an infant due to cocaine exposure. *Iowa Med* 1995; 85:449–450.
21. Flores-Guevara R, Plouin P, Curzi-Dascalova L, et al. Sleep apneas in normal neonates and infants during the first 3 months of life. *Neuropediatrics* 1982;13(suppl):21–28.
22. Martin RJ, Siner B, Carlo WA, Lough M, Miller MJ. Effect of head position on distribution of nasal airflow in preterm infants. *J Pediatr* 1988;112:99–103.
23. Smith DS. Hoarseness. In: Schidlow D, Smith D, eds. *A Practical Guide to Pediatric Respiratory Diseases.* Philadelphia: Hanley & Belfus; 1994:27–29.
24. Halken S, Host A, Husby S, Hansen LG, Osterballe O, Nyboe J. Recurrent wheezing in relation to environmental risk factors in infancy. A prospective study of 276 infants. *Allergy* 1991;46:507–514.
25. Hilman BC. Evaluation of the wheezing infant. *Allergy Proc* 1994;15:1–5.
26. Openshaw P, Edwards S, Helms P. Changes in rib cage geometry during childhood. *Thorax* 1984; 39(8):624–7.
27. Feingold M, Bossert WH. Normal values for selected physical parameters: an aid to syndrome delineation. *Birth Defects* 1974;10(13):1–16.
28. Curzi-Dascalova L. Thoracico-abdominal respiratory correlations in infants: constancy and variability in different sleep states. *Early Human Dev* 1978;2(1):25–38.
29. Henderson-Smart DJ, Reed DJC. Depression of intercostal and abdominal muscle activity and vulnerability to asphyxia during active sleep in the newborn. In: Guillemiinault C, Dement W, eds. *Kroc Foundation Series: Sleep Apnea Syndromes.* New York: Alan R Liss; 1978:93–117.
30. Davi M, Sankaran K, Maccallum M, Cates D, Rigatto H. Effects of sleep state on chest distortion and on the ventilatory response to CO_2 in neonates. *Pediatr Res* 1979;13(9):982–6.
31. Oberklaid F, Danks DM, V M, Campbell P. Asphyxiating thoracic dysplasia: clinical, radiological and pathological information in 10 patients. *Arch Dis Child* 1977;52:758–65.
32. Jones K, ed. Smith's Recognizable Patterns of Human Malformation. 4th ed. Philadelphia: W B Saunders; 1988.
33. Hall JG, Froster-Iskenius UG, Allanson JE. *Handbook of Normal Physical Measurements.* Oxford: Oxford University Press; 1989.
34. Merlob P, Sivan Y, Reisner SH. Ratio of crown–rump distance to total length in preterm and term infants. *J Med Genet* 1986;23:338–340.
35. McClurg FL, Evans DA. Laser laryngoplasty for laryngomalacia. *Laryngoscope* 1994;104(3 Pt 1):81–85.
36. Ellis DG. Chest wall deformities. *Pediatr Rev* 1989;11(5):147–51.
37. Miller MJ, Martin RJ, Carlo WA, Fanaroff AA. Oral breathing in response to nasal trauma in term infants. *J Pediatrics* 1987;111(6):899–901.
38. Jung AL, Thomas GK. Stricture of the nasal vestibule: a complication of nasotracheal intubation in newborn infants. *J Pediatrics* 1974;85(3):412–14.
39. Loftus BC, Ahn J, Haddad JJ. Neonatal nasal deformities secondary to nasal continuous positive airway pressure. *Laryngoscope* 1994;104:1019–22.
40. Doershuk CF, Fisher BJ, Matthews LW. Pulmonary physiology of the young child. In: Scarpelli EM, Auld PAM, eds. *Pulmonary Physiology of the Fetus, Newborn and Child.* Philadelphia: Lea & Febiger;1975: 166–82.

41. Morley CJ, Thornton AJ, Fowler MA, Cole TJ, Hewson PH. Respiratory rate and severity of illness in babies under 6 months old. *Arch Dis Child* 1990;65(8):834–7.
42. Curzi-Dascalova. L, Gaudebout C, Dreyfus-Brisac C. Respiratory frequencies of sleeping infants during the first months of life: correlations between values in different sleep states. *Early Hum Dev* 1981;5(1):39–54.
43. Hathorn MK. The rate and depth of breathing in new-born infants in different sleep states. J Physiol (Lond) 1974;243:101–113.
44. Stern E, Parmelee AH, Harris MA. Sleep state periodicity in prematures and young infants. Dev Psychobiol 1973;6:357–365.
45. Desmond MM, Rudolph AJ, Phitaksphraiwan P. The transitional care nursery. A mechanism for preventive medicine in the newborn. *Pediatr Clin North Am* 1966;13:651–668.
46. Carlo WA, Martin RJ, Bruce EN, Strohl KP, Fanaroff AA. Alae nasi activation (nasal flaring) decreases nasal resistance in preterm infants. *Pediatrics* 1983;72:338–343
47. Sarnat HB, Sarnat MS. Neonatal encephalopathy following fetal distress. A clinical and electroencephalographic study. *Arch Neurol* 1976;33:696–705.
48. Amiel-Tison C, Grenier A. *Neurologial Assessment During the First Year of Life.* (1st ed.) New York: Oxford University Press; 1986.
49. Woodrum D. Respiratory muscles. In: Polin RA, Fox WW, eds. *Fetal and Neonatal Physiology.* Vol. 1. Philadelphia: WB Saunders Company; 1992:829–841.
50. Heldt GP, McIlroy MB. Distortion of chest wall and work of diaphragm in preterm infants. *J. Apply Physiol* 1987;62:164–169.
51. Nichols MN. Belly dancer's sign. *Clinical Pediatrics* 1976 (April):342–343.
52. Balaji S, Kunovsky P, Sullivan I. Ultrasound in the diagnosis of diaphragmatic paralysis after operation for congenital heart disease. *Br Heart J* 1990;64:20–22.
53. Aldrich TK, H HJ, Rochester DF. Bilateral diaphragmatic paralysis in the newborn infant. *J Pediatr* 1980;97:987–991.
54. Cunniff C, Jones KL, Jones MC. Patterns of malformation in children with congenital diaphragmatic defects. *J Pediatr* 1990;116:258–261.
55. Margolis PA, Ferkol TW, Marsocci S, et al. Accuracy of the clinical examination in detecting hypoxemia in infants with respiratory illness. *J Pediatr* 1994;124:552–560.
56. Kerr LG. The cry and the voice. *Diagnostics of the Diseases of Children.* Philadelphia: WB Saunders; 1907:176–179.
57. Golub HL, Corwin MJ. Infant cry: a clue to diagnosis. *Pediatrics* 1982;69:197–201.
58. Gopal HS, Gerber SE. Why and how should we study infant cry? *Int J Pediatr Otorhinolaryngol* 1992;24: 145–159.
59. Pearce S, Taylor B. Energy distribution in the spectrograms of the cries of normal and birth asphyxiated infants. *Physiol Meas* 1993;14:263–268.
60. Raes J, Michelsson K, Dehaen F, Despontin M. Cry analysis in infants with infectious and congenital disorders of the larynx. *Int J. Pediatr Otorhinolaryngol* 1982;4:157–169.
61. Michelsson K, Sirvio P, Koivisto M, Sovijarvi A, Wasz-Hockert O. Spectrographic analysis of pain cry in neonates with cleft palate. *Biol Neonate* 1975;26:353–358.
62. Michelsson K, Sirvio P. Cry analysis in congenital hypothyroidism. *Folia Phoniatr* (Basel) 1976;28:40–47.
63. Michelsson K, Sirvio P, Wasz-Hockert O. Pain cry in full-term asphyxiated newborn infants correlated with late findings. *Acta Paediatr Scand* 1977;66:611–616.
64. Juntunen K, Sirvio P, Michelsson K. Cry analysis in infants with severe malnutrition. *Eur J Pediatr* 1978;128:241–246.
65. Thoden CJ, Michelsson K. Sound spectrographic cry analysis in Krabbe's disease [letter]. *Dev Med Child Neurol* 1979;21:400–402.
66. Michelsson K, Sirvio P, Wasz-Hockert O. Sound spectrographic cry analysis of infants with bacterial meningitis. *Dev Med Child Neurol* 1977;19:309–315.
67. Sirvio P, Michelsson K. Sound-spectrographic cry analysis of normal and abnormal newborn infants. A review and a recommendation for standardization of the cry characteristics. *Folia Phoniatr* (Basel) 1976;28:161–173.
68. Sheth KR, Patel LR, Mehta AA. Laryngeal foreign body in a neonate. *Ind J Pediatr* 1987;54:601–604.
69. Egan DF, Illingworth RS, MacKeith RC. Developmental screening 0–5 years. *Clinics in Developmental Medicine* 1969;30:1–63.
70. Singer JI, Losek JD. Grunting respirations: chest or abdominal pathology? *Pediatr Emerg Care* 1992; 8:354–358.
71. Schidlow DV. Cough. In: Schidlow DV, Smith DS, eds. *A Practical Guide to Pediatric Respiratory Diseases.* Philadelphia: Hanley & Belfus; 1994:49–51.
72. Fruthaler GJ. Snurgles and gurgles: respiratory sounds that worry parents. *Contemporary Pediatrics* 1988; July:42–46.
73. Wang D, Clement P, Kaufman L, Derde MP. Fiberoptic evaluation of the nasal and nasopharyngeal anatomy in children with snorring. *J Otolaryngol* 1994;23:57–60.
74. Kahn A, Groswasser J, Sottiaux M, et al. Clinical symptoms associated with brief obstructive sleep apnea in normal infants. *Sleep* 1993;16:409–413.
75. Roberts JL, Reed WR, Mathew OP, Menon AA, Thach BT. Assessment of paryngeal airway stability in normal and micrognathic infants. *J Appl Physiol* 1985;58:290–299.
76. Bates B. The thorax and lungs. In: Bates B, ed. *A Guide to Physical Examination and History Taking.* 5th ed. Philadelphia: JB Lippincott; 1991:231–261.
77. Wilkins RL, Hodgkin JE. History and physical examination of the respiratory patient. In: Burton GG, Hodgkin JE, Ward JJ, eds. *Respiratory Care. A Guide to Clinical Practics.* Philadelphia: JB Lippincott; 1991:211–232.
78. Kanga JF, Kraman SS. Comparison of the lung sound frequency spectra of infants and adults. *Pediatr Pulmonol* 1986;2:292–295.

79. Pasterkamp H, Fenton R, Leahy F, Chernick V. Spectral analysis of breath sounds in normal newborn infants. *Med Instrum* 1983;17:355–357.
80. Cugell DW. Lung sound nomenclature. *Am Rev Respir Dis* 1987;136(4):1016.
81. Mikami R, Murao M, Cugell DW, et al. International symposium on lung sounds. Synopsis of proceedings. *Chest* 1987;92:342–345.
82. Panitch HB. Wheezing and lower airway obstruction. In: Schidlow D, Smith D, eds. *A Practical Guide to Pediatric Respiratory Diseases.* Philadelphia: Hanley & Belfus; 1994:39–45.
83. Schidlow DV, Smith DS. Stridor and upper airway obstruction. In: Schidlow D, Smith D, eds. *A Practical Guide to Pediatric Respiratory Diseases.* Philadelphia: Hanley & Belfus; 1994:31–37.
84. Cotton RT, Reilly JS. Stridor and airway obstruction. In: Bluestone C, Stool S, Sheetz M, eds. *Pediatric Otolaryngology.* 2nd ed. Philadelphia: WB Saunders; 1990:1098–1111.
85. Francis GL, Hoffman WH, Gala RR, McPherson JCd, Zadinsky J. A relationship between neonatal breast size and cord blood testosterone level. *Ann Clin Lab Sci* 1990;20:239–244.
86. Sivan Y, Merlob P, Resiner SH. Sternum length, torso length, and internipple distance in newborn infants. *Pediatrics* 2983;72:523–525.
87. Buehring GC. Short communication. Witch's milk: potential for neonatal diagnosis. *Pediatr Res* 1982;16:460–462.
88. Madlon-Kay DJ 'Witch's milk.' Galactorrhea in the newborn. *Am J Dis Child* 1986;150:252–253.
89. Berkowitz CD, Inkelis SH. Bloody nipple discharge in infancy. *J Pediatr* 1983;103:755–756.
90. Anbazhagan R, Bartek J, Monaghan P, Gusterson BA. Growth and development of the human infant breast. *Am J Anat* 1991;192:407–417.
91. Rudoy RC, Nelson JD. Breast abscess during the neonatal period: a review. *Amer J Dis Child* 1975;129:1031–1034.
92. Jaber L, Merlob P. The prevalence of supernumerary nipples in Arab infants and children [letter]. *Eur J Pediatr* 1988;147:443.
93. Robertson A, Sale P, Sathyanarayan. Lack of association of supernumerary nipples with renal anomalies in black infants. *J Pediatr* 1986;109:502–503.
94. Leung A. Familiar supernumerary nipples. *Am J Med Genet* 1988;31:631–635.
95. Varsano IB, Lutfi J, Ben-Zion G, Mukamel MM, Grünebaum M. Urinary tract abnormalities in children with supernumerary nipples. *Pediatrics* 1984;73:102–204.
96. Armoni M, Filk D, Schlesinger M, Pollak S, Metzker A. Accessory nipples: any relationship to urinary tract malformation? [see comments]. *Pediatr Dermatol* 1992;9:239–240.
97. Flanagan MF, Fyler DC. Cardiac disease. In: Avery GB, Fletcher MA, MacDonald MG, eds. *Neonatology. Pathophysiology and Management of the Newborn.* Philadelphia: JB Lippincott; 1994:516–559.
98. Kluckow M, Evans N. Early echocardiographic prediction of symptomatic patent ductus arteriosus in preterm infants undergoing mechanical ventilation. *J Pediatr* 1995;127:774–749.
99. Skinner JR, Boys RJ, Hunter S, Hey EN. Noninvasive assessment of pulmonary arterial pressure in healthy neonates. *Arch Dis Child* 1991;66:386–390.
100. Walther FJ, Benders MJ, Leighton JO. Early changes in the neonatal circulatory transition. *J Pediatr* 1993;123:625–632.
101. Walther FJ, Benders MJ, Leighton JO. Persistent pulmonary hypertension in premature neonates with severe respiratory distress syndrome. *Pediatrics* 1992;90:899.
102. Christie A. Normal closing time of the foramen ovale and the ductus arteriosus: an anatomic and statistical study. *Am J Dis Child* 1930;40:323–326.
103. Skinner JR, Boys RJ, Hunter S, Hey EN. Pulmonary and systemic arterial pressure in hyaline membrane disease. *Arch Dis Child* 1992;67(4 Spec No):366–373.
104. Craige E, Harned HS. Phonocardiographic and electrocardiographic studies in normal newborn infants. *Am Heart J* 1963;65:180–189.
105. Braudo M, Rowe RD. Auscultation of the heart—early neonatal period. *Am J Dis Child* 1961;101:575.
106. McNamara DG. Value and limitations of auscultation in the management of congenital heart disease. *Pediatr Clin North Am* 1990;37:93–113.
107. Santulli TVJ. An approach to the newborn with heart disease. In: Pomerance JJ, Richardson CJ, eds. *Neonatology for the Clinician.* Norwalk, CT: Appleton & Lange; 1993:586.
108. Whitsett JA, Pryhuber GS, Rice WR, Warner BB, Wert SE. Acute respiratory disorders. In: Avery GB, Fletcher MA, MacDonald MG, eds. *Neonatology. Pathophysiology and Management of the Newborn.* 4th ed. Philadelphia: JB Lippincott; 1994:429–452.
109. Johnson GL. Clinical examination. In: Long WA, ed. *Fetal and Neonatal Cardiology.* Philadelphia: WB Saunders; 1990:223–235.
110. Shah NM, Gaur HK. Position of heart in relation to sternum and nipple line at various ages. *Ind Pediatr* 1992;29:49–53.
111. Goldring D, Wohltmann HJ. "Flush" method for blood pressure determinations in newborn infants. *J Pediatr* 1952;40:285.
112. Park MK, Menard SM. Accuracy of blood pressure measurement by the Dinamap monitor in infants and children. *Pediatrics* 1987;79:907–914.
113. Park MK, Lee DH. Normative arm and calf blood pressure values in the newborn. *Pediatrics* 1989;83:240–243.
114. Blumenthal S, Epps RP, Heavenrich R, et al. Report of the task force on blood pressure control in children. *Pediatrics* 1977;59(suppl):797–820.
115. Steinfeld L, Dimich I, Reder R, Cohen M, Alexander H. Sphygmomanometry in the pediatric patient. *J Pediatr* 1978;92:934–938.
116. Zachman RD, Bauer CR, Boehm J, Korones SB, Rigatto H, Gustafson NF. Neonatal blood pressure at birth by the Doppler method. *Am Heart J* 1986;111:189–190.
117. Versmold HT, Kitterman JA, Phibbs RH, Gregory GA, Tooley WH. Aortic blood pressure during the first 12 hours of life in infants with birth weight of 610 to 4220 grams. *Pediatrics* 1981;67:607–613.
118. Shortland DB, Evans DH, Levene MI. Blood pressure measurements in very low birth weight infants over the first week of life. *J Perinatol Med* 1988;16:93–97.

119. Earley A, Fayers P, Ng S, Shinebourne EA, de Swiet M. Blood pressure in the first 6 weeks of life. *Arch Dis Child* 1980;55:755–757.
120. Hegyi T, Carbone MT, Anwar J, et al. Blood pressure ranges in premature infants. 1. The first hours of life. *J Pediatr* 1994;124:627–733.
121. Dellagrammaticas HD, Kapetanakis J, Papadimitriou M, Kourakis G. Effect of body tilting on physiological functions in stable very low birthweight neonates. *Arch Dis Child* 1991;66(4 Spec No):429–432.
122. Crapanzano MS, Strong WB, Newman IR, Hixon RL, Casal D, Linder CW. Calf blood pressure: clinical implications and correlations with arm blood pressure in infants and young children. *Pediatrics* 1996;97: 220–224.
123. Bada HS, Korones SB, Perry EH, et al. Mean arterial blood pressure changes in premature infants and those at risk for intraventricular hemorrhage. *J Pediatr* 1990;117:607–614.
124. Sinkin RA, Phillips BL, Adelman RD. Elevation in systemic blood pressure in the neonate during abdominal examination. *Pediatrics* 1985;76:970–972.
125. Davignon A, Rautaharju P, Boiselle E, Soumis F, Megelas M, Choquette A. Normal ECG standards for infants and children. *Pediatr Cardiol* 1980;1:123–131.
126. McNamara DG. Idiopathic benign mitral leaflet prolapse. The pediatrician's view. *Am J Dis Child* 1982; 136:152–156.
127. Lehrer S. *Understanding Pediatric Heart Sounds.* Philadelphia: WB Saunders; 1992.
128. Fyler DC, Nadas AS. Tools of diagnosis. In: Fyler DC, ed. *Nadas' Pediatric Cardiology.* Philadelphia: Hanley & Belfus; 1992:101–116.
129. Freeman AR, Levine SA. The clinical significance of the systolic murmur. A study of 1000 consecutive "non-cardiac" cases. *Ann Intern Med* 1933;6:1371.
130. Bamji M, Stone RK, Kaul A, Usmani G, Schacter FF, Wasserman E. Palpable lymph nodes in healthy newborns and infants. *Pediatrics* 1986;78:573–575.
131. Nichols DG. Respiratory muscle performance in infants and children. *J Pediatr* 1991;118:493–502.
132. Klein M. Hoover sign and peripheral airways obstruction (letter). *J Pediatr* 1992;119:495.
133. Nichols MN. Belly dancer's sign. *Clin Pediatr* 1976;April:342–343.
134. Lazar RH, Younis RT, Bassila MN. Bronchogenic cysts: a cause of stridor in the neonate. *Am J Otolaryngol* 1991;12:117–121.
135. Belknap WM. Distended abdomen. In: Oski FA, DeAngelis CD, Feigin RD, McMillan JA, Warshaw JB, eds. *Principles and Practice of Pediatrics.* 2nd ed. Philadelphia: JB Lippincott; 1994:430–436
136. Tongsong T, Wanapirak C, Takapijitra A. Ultrasonic measurement of the fetal head to abdominal circumference ratio in normal pregnancy. *J Med Assoc Thai* 1993;76:153–158.
137. DeGowin RL. *DeGowin & DeGowin's Diagnostic Examination.* 6th ed. New York: McGraw-Hill; 1994.
138. Malhotra AK, Deorari AK, Paul VK, Bagga A, Singh M. Gastric residuals in preterm babies. *J Trop Pediatr* 1992;38:262–264.
139. Green M. *Pediatric Diagnosis. Interpretation of Symptoms and Signs in Infants, Children, and Adolescents.* 5th ed. Philadelphia: WB Saunders; 1992.
140. Saavedra JM, Harris GD, Li S, Finberg L. Capillary refilling (skin turgor) in the assessment of dehydration. *Am J Dis Child* 1991;145:296–298.
141. Gorelick MH, Shaw KN, Baker MD. Effect of ambient temperature on capillary refill in healthy children. *Pediatrics* 1993;92:699–702.
142. Ballard JL, Khoury JC, Wedig K, Wang L, Eilers-Walsman BL, Lipp R. New Ballard Score, expanded to include extremely premature infants. *J Pediatr* 1991;119:417–423.
143. Magalini SI, Magalini SC, de Francisci G. *Dictionary of Medical Syndromes.* 3rd ed. Philadelphia: JB Lippincott; 1990.
144. Friedman JM. Umbilical dysmorphology: the importance of contemplating the belly button. *Clin Genet* 1985;28:343–347.
145. O'Marcaigh AS, Folz LB, Michels VV. Umbilical morphology: normal values for neonatal periumbilical skin length. *Pediatrics* 1992;90:47–49.
146. Scherer LR, Grosfeld JL. Inguinal hernia and umbilical anomalies. *Pediatr Clin North Am* 1993;40: 1121–1131.
147. Alessandrini P, Derlon S. [Congenital umbilical fistulas. A report of 12 cases]. *Pediatrie (Bucur)* 1992;47: 67–71.
148. Rowe PC, Gearhart JP. Retraction of the umbilicus during voiding as an initial sign of a urachal anomaly. *Pediatrics* 1993;91:153–154.
149. Kamii Y, Zaki AM, Honna T, Tsuchida Y. Spontaneous regression of patient omphalomesenteric duct: from a fistula to Meckel's diverticulum. *J Pediatr Surg* 1992;27:115–116.
150. Hall DE, Roberts KB, Charney E. Umbilical hernia: what happens after age 5 years? *J Pediatr* 1981;98: 415–417.
151. Mawera G, Muguti GI. Umbilical hernia in Bulawayo: some observations from a hospital based study. *Cent Afr J Med* 1994;40:319–323.
152. Blumberg NA. Infantile umbilical hernia. *Surg Gynecol Obstet* 1980;150:187–192.
153. Jones K, ed. *Smith's Recognizable Patterns of Human Malformation.* 4th ed. Philadelphia: WB Saunders; 1988.
154. Raffensperger JG, ed. *Swenson's Pediatric Surgery.* 5th ed. Norwalk, CT: Appleton & Lange; 1990.
155. deVries PA. The pathogenesis of gastroschisis and omphalocele. *J Pediatr Surg* 1980;15:245–251.
156. Nicol JW, MacKinlay GA. Meckel's diverticulum in exomphalos minor. *J R Coll Surg Edinb* 1994;39:6–7.
157. Torfs C, Curry C, Roeper P. Gastroschisis. *J Pediatr* 1990;116:1–6.
158. Hoyme HE, Higginbottom MD, Jones KL. The vascular pathogenesis of gastroschisis: intrauterine interruption of the omphalomesenteric artery. *J Pediatr* 1981;98:228–231.
159. Morrow RJ, Whittle MJ, McNay MB, Raine PA, Gibson AA, Crossley J. Prenatal diagnosis and management of anterior abdominal wall defects in the west of Scotland. *Prenat Diagn* 1993;13:111–115.
160. Saller DN Jr, Canick JA, Palomaki GE, Knight GJ, Haddow JE. Second-trimester maternal serum alpha-fetoprotein, unconjugated estriol, and hCG levels in pregnancies with ventral wall defects. *Obstet Gynecol* 1994;84:852–825.

161. Sipes SL, Weiner CP, Sipes DRI, Grant SS, Williamson RA. Gastroschisis and omphalocele: does either antenatal diagnosis or route of delivery make a difference in perinatal outcome? *Obstet Gynecol* 1990;76: 195–199.

162. Calzolari E, Bianchi F, Dolk H, Milan M. Omphalocele and gastroschisis in Europe: a survey of 3 million births 1980–1990. EUROCAT Working Group. *Am J Med Genet* 1995;58:187–194.

163. Tunell WP, Puffinbarger NK, Tuggle DW, Taylor DV, Mantor PC. Abdominal wall defects in infants. Survival and implications for adult life. *Ann Surg* 1995;221:525–528; discussion 528–530.

164. Chin T, Wei C. Prediction of outcome in omphalocele and gastroschisis by intraoperative measurement of intravesical pressure. *J Formos Med Assoc* 1994;93:691–693.

165. Salinas CF, Bartoshesky L, Othersen HB Jr, Leape L, Feingold M, Jorgenson RJ. Familial occurrence of gastroschisis. Four new cases and review of the literature. *Am J Dis Child* 1979;133:514–517.

166. Mahour GH, Weitzman JJ, Rosenkrantz JG. Omphalocele and gastroschisis. *Ann Surg* 1973;177:478–482.

167. Watkinson M, Dyas A. *Staphylococcus aureus* still colonizes the untreated neonatal umbilicus. *J Hosp Infect* 1992;21:131–136.

168. Harpin V, Rutter N. Percutaneous alcohol absorption and skin necrosis in a preterm infant. *Arch Dis Child* 1982;57:477–479.

169. Vivier PM, Lewander WJ, Martin HF, Linakis JG. Isopropyl alcohol intoxication in a neonate through chronic dermal exposure: a complication of a culturally-based umbilical care practice. *Pediatr Emerg Care* 1994;10:91–93.

170. Schick JB, Milstein JM. Burn hazard of isopropyl alcohol in the neonate. *Pediatrics* 1981;68:587–588.

171. Bennett J, Azhar N, Rahim F, et al. Further observations on ghee as a risk factor for neonatal tetanus. *Int J Epidemiol* 1995;24:643–647.

172. Bertone SA, Fisher MC, Mortensen JE. Quantitative skin cultures at potential catheter sites in neonates. *Infect Control Hosp Epidemiol* 1994;15:315–318.

173. Guvenc H, Guvenc M, Yenioglu H, Ayata A, Kocabay K, Bektas S. Neonatal omphalitis is still common in eastern Turkey. *Scand J Infect Dis* 1991;23:613–616.

174. Faridi MM, Rattan A, Ahmad SH. Omphalitis neonatorum. *J Ind Med Assoc* 1993;91:283–285.

175. Lally KP, Atkinson JB, Wooley MM, Mahour GH. Necrotizing fasciitis: a serious sequela of omphalitis in the newborn. *Ann Surg* 1984;199:101–103.

176. Monu JU, Okolo AA. Diffuse abdominal wall cellulitis in ascending omphalitis—a lethal association in neonatal necrotizing fasciitis. *J Natl Med Assoc* 1993;85:457–459.

177. Ryan CA, Fischer J, Gayle M, Wenman W. Surgical and postoperative management of two neonates with necrotizing fasciitis. *Can J Surg* 1993;36:337–341.

178. Samuel M, Freeman NV, Vaishnav A, Sajwany MJ, Nayar MP. Necrotizing fasciitis: a serious complication of omphalitis in neonates. *J Pediatr Surg* 1994;29:1414–1416.

179. Sawin RS, Schaller RT, Tapper D, Morgan A, Cahill J. Early recognition of neonatal abdominal wall necrotizing fasciitis. *Am J Surg* 1994;167:481–484.

180. Kosloske AM, Bartow SA. Debridement of periumbilical necrotizing fasciitis: importance of excision of the umbilical vessels and urachal remnant. *J Pediatr Surg* 1991;26:808–810.

181. Oudesluys-Murphy AM, Eilers GA, de Groot CJ. The time of separation of the umbilical cord. *Eur J Pediatr* 1987;146:387–389.

182. Wilson CB, Ochs HD, Almquist J, Dassel S, Mauseth R, Ochs UH. When is umbilical cord separation delayed? *J Pediatr* 1985;107:292–294.

183. Rais-Bahrami K, Schulte EB, Naqvi M. Postnatal timing of spontaneous umbilical cord separation. *Am J Perinatol* 1993;10:453–454.

184. Sarwono E, Disse WS, Ousdesluys-Murphy HM, Oosting H, De Groot CJ. Umbilical cord: factors which influence the separation time. *Paediatr Indones* 1991;31:179–184.

185. Novack AH, Bueller B, Ochs H. Umbilical cord separation in the normal newborn. *Am J Dis Child* 1988; 142:220–223.

186. Hayward AR, Harvey BA, Leonard J, Greenwood MC, Wood CB, Soothill JF. Delayed separation of the umbilical cord, widespread infections, and defective neutrophil mobility. *Lancet* 1979;1(8126):1099–1101.

187. Hoek T, Reifferscheid P, Hadam M, Gahr M. [LFA-1 defect: a rare granulocyte function disorders as a cause of therapy-resistant omphalitis in newborn infants]. *Monatsschr Kinderheilkd* 1991;139:418–420.

188. Chamberlain JM, Gorman RL, Young GM. Silver nitrate burns following treatment for umbilical granuloma [see comments]. *Pediatr Emerg Care* 1992;8:29–30.

189. Sinkin RA, Phillips BL, Adelman RD. Elevation in systemic blood pressure in the neonate during abdominal examination. *Pediatrics* 1985;76:970–972.

190. Reiff MI, Osborn LM. Clinical estimation of liver size in newborn infants. *Pediatrics* 1983;71:46–48.

191. Chen CM, Wang JJ. Clinical and sonographic assessment of liver size in normal Chinese neonates. *Acta Paediatr* 1993;82:345–347.

192. Ashkenazi S, Mimouni F, Merlob P, Litmanovitz I, Reisner SH. Size of liver edge in full-term, healthy infants. *Am J Dis Child* 1984;138:377–378.

193. Cortes-Gallo G, Mendez-Muniz MdC, Hernandez-Arriaga JL, Zamora-Orozco J. [The echographic dimensions of the liver in the term newborn and its relation to anthropometric variables]. *Bol Med Hosp Infant Mex* 1993;50:809–812.

194. Brion L, Avni FE. Clinical estimation of liver size in newborn infants [Letter]. *Pediatrics* 1985;75:127–128.

195. Urata K, Kawasaki S, Matsunami H, et al. Calculation of child and adult standard liver volume for liver transplantation. *Hepatology* 1995;21:1317–1321.

196. Mimouni F, Merlob P, Ashkenazi S, Litmanovitz I, Reisner SH. Palpable spleens in newborn term infants. *Clin Pediatr (Phila)* 1985;24:197–198.

197. Aoki S, Hata T, Kitao M. Ultrasonographic assessment of fetal and neonatal spleen. *Am J Perinatol* 1992; 9:361–367.

198. Klippenstein DL, Zerin JM, Hirschl RB, Donn SM. Splenic enlargement in neonates during ECMO. *Radiology* 1994;190:411–412.

199. Rosenberg HK, Markowitz RI, Kolberg H, Park C, Hubbard A, Bellah RD. Normal splenic size in infants and children: sonographic measurements. *AJR* 1991;157:119–121.

200. Scott JE, Hunter EW, Lee RE, Matthews JN. Ultrasound measurement of renal size in newborn infants. *Arch Dis Child* 1990;65(4 Spec No):361–364.
201. Chih TW, Teng RJ, Wang CS, Tsou Yau KI. Time of the first urine and the first stool in Chinese newborns. *Acta Paediatr Sin* 1991;32:17–23.
202. Verma A, Dhanireddy R. Time of first stool in extremely low birth weight (1000 grams) infants. *J Pediatr* 1993;122:626–629.
203. Jhaveri MK, Kumar SP. Passage of the first stool in very low birth weight infants. *Pediatrics* 1987;79:1005–1007.
204. Schwartz MA, Shaul DB. Abdominal masses in the newborn. *Pediatr Rev* 1989;11:172–179.
205. Hartman GE, Shochat SJ. Abdominal mass lesions in the newborn: diagnosis and treatment. *Clin Perinatol* 1989;16:123–135.
206. Belknap WM. Distended abdomen. In: Oski FA, DeAngelis CD, Feigin RD, McMillan JA, Warshaw JB, eds. *Principles and Practice of Pediatrics*. 2nd ed. Philadelphia: JB Lippincott; 1994:430–436.
207. Garcia VF, Randolph JG. Pyloric stenosis: diagnosis and management. *Pediatr Rev* 1990;11:292–296.
208. Tack ED, Perlman JM, Bower RJ, McAlister WH. Pyloric stenosis in the sick premature infant. Clinical and radiological findings. *Am J Dis Child* 1988;142:68–70.
209. Woolley MM, Felsher BF, Asch J, Carpio N, Isaacs H. Jaundice, hypertrophic pyloric stenosis, and hepatic glucuronyl transferase. *J Pediatr Surg* 1974;9:359–363.
210. Hernanz-Schulman M, Sells LL, Ambrosino MM, Heller RM, Stein SM, Neblett WW. Hypertrophic pyloric stenosis in the infant without a palpable olive: accuracy of sonographic diagnosis. *Radiology* 1994;193:771–776.
211. Forman HP, Leonidas JC, Kronfeld GD. A rational approach to the diagnosis of hypertrophic pyloric stenosis: do the results match the claims? *J Pediatr Surg* 1990;25:262–266.
212. Westra SJ, de Groot CJ, Smits NJ, Staalman CR. Hypertrophic pyloric stenosis: use of the pyloric volume measurement in early US diagnosis. *Radiology* 1989;172:615–619.
213. Breaux CW, Georgeson KE, Royal SA, Curnow AJ. Changing patterns in the diagnosis of hypertrophic pyloric stenosis. *Pediatrics* 1988;81:213–217.
214. Senquiz AL. Use of decubitus position for finding the "olive" of pyloric stenosis. *Pediatrics* 1991;87:266.
215. Buck JR, Weintraub WH, Coran AG, Wyman ML, Kuhns LR. Fiberoptic transillumination: a new tool for the pediatric surgeon. *J Pediatr Surg* 1977;12:451–463.
216. Buchheit JQ, Stewart DL. Clinical comparison of localized intestinal perforation and necrotizing enterocolitis in neonates. *Pediatrics* 1994;93:32–36.
217. Izraeli S, Freud E, Mor C, Litwin A, Zer M, Merlob P. Neonatal intestinal perforation due to congenital defects in the intestinal muscularis. *Eur J Pediatr* 1992;151:300–303.
218. Potter EL, Craig JM. *Pathology of the Fetus and the Infant*. 3rd ed. Vol. 1. Chicago: Year Book Medical; 1975.
219. Crelin ES. *Functional Anatomy of the Newborn*. New Haven, CT: Yale University Press; 1973.
220. Capraro VJ, Rodgers ED, Rodgers BD. The gyn exam for newborns, young children, adolescents. *Contemp Obstet Gynecol* 1982;20:43–57.
221. Sanfilippo J, Muram D, Lee PA, Dewhurst J, eds. *Pediatric and Adolescent Gynecology*. Philadelphia: WB Saunders; 1994.
222. Tran ATB, Arensman RB, Falterman KW. Diagnosis and management of hydrohematometrocolpos syndromes. *Am J Dis Child* 1987;141:632–634.
223. Mor N, Merlob P, Reisner SH. Types of hymen in the newborn infant. *Eur J Obstet Gynecol Reprod Biol* 1986;22:225–228.
224. Johnson A, Unger SW, Rodgers BM. Uterine prolapse in the neonate. *J Pediatr Surg* 1984;19:210–211.
225. Bayatpour M, McCann J, Harris T, Phelps H. Neonatal genital prolapse. *Pediatrics* 1992;90:465–466.
226. Jenny C, Kuhns MLD, Arakawa F. Hymens in newborn female infants. *Pediatrics* 1987;80:399–400.
227. Berenson A, Heger A, Andrews S. Appearance of the hymen in newborns. *Pediatrics* 1991;87:458–465.
228. Berenson AB. Appearance of the hymen at birth and one year of age: a longitudinal study. *Pediatrics* 1993;91:820.
229. Berenson AB. A longitudinal study of hymenal morphology in the first 3 years of life. *Pediatrics* 1995;95:490–496.
230. Kellogg ND, Parra JM. Linea vestibularis: a previously undescribed normal genital structure in female neonates. *Pediatrics* 1991;87:926–929.
231. Cook AS. Normal growth and development of the genitalia in infancy and childhood. In: Carpenter SE, Rock JA, eds. *Pediatric and Adolescent Gynecology*. New York: Raven; 1992:39–47.
232. Riley WJ, Rosenbloom AL. Clitoral size in infancy. *J Pediatr* 1980;1980:918–919.
233. Oberfield SE, Mondok A, Shahrivar F, Klein JF, Levine LS. Clitoral size in full-term infants. *Am J Perinatol* 1989;6:453–454.
234. Litwin A, Aitkin I, Merlob P. Clitoral length assessment in newborn infants of 30 to 41 weeks gestational age. *Eur J Obstet Gynecol Reprod Biol* 1991;38:209–212.
235. Sane K, Pescovitz OH. The clitoral index: a determination of clitoral size in normal girls and in girls with abnormal sexual development. *J Pediatr* 1992;120(2 Pt 1):264–266.
236. Griebel ML, Redman JF, Kemp SF, Elders MJ. Hypertrophy of clitoral hood: presenting sign of neurofibromatosis in female child. *Urology* 1991;37:337–339.
237. Ishizu K, Nakamura K, Baba Y, Takihara H, Sakatoku J, Tanaka K. [Clitoral enlargement caused by prepucial hemangioma: a case report]. *Hinyokika Kiyo* 1991;37:1563–1565.
238. Merlob P, Bahari C, Liban E, Reisner SH. Cysts of the female external genitalia in the newborn infant. *Am J Obstet Gynecol* 1978;132:607–610.
239. Callegari C, Everett S, Ross M, Brasel JA. Anogenital ratio: measure of fetal virilization in premature and full-term newborn infants. *J Pediatr* 1987;111:240–243.
240. Bellman A. Hypospadias and other urethral abnormalities. In: Kelalis PP, King LR, Belman AB, eds. *Clinical Pediatric Urology*. 3rd ed. Vol. 1. Philadelphia: WB Saunders; 1992:1467.

241. Ben-Ari J, Merlob P, Mimouni F, Reisner SH. Characteristics of the male genitalia in the newborn: penis. *J Urol* 1985;134:521–522.
242. Flatau E, Josefsberg Z, Reisner SH, Bialik O, Laron Z. Penile size in the newborn infant. *J Pediatr* 1975;87:663–664.
243. Feldman KW, Smith DW. Fetal phallic growth and penile standards for newborn male infants. *J Pediatr* 1975;86:395–398.
244. Aaronson IA. Micropenis: medical and surgical implications. *J Urol* 1994;152:4–14.
245. Lee PA, Mazur T, Danish R, et al. Micropenis. I. Criteria, etiologies and classification. *Johns Hopkins Med J* 1980;146:156–163.
246. Bourgeois MJ, Jones B, Waagner DC, Dunn D. Micropenis and congenital adrenal hypoplasia. *Am J Perinatol* 1989;6:69–71.
247. Maizels M, Zaontz M, Donovan J, Bushnick PN, Firlit CF. Surgical correction of the buried penis: description of a classification system and a technique to correct the disorder. *J Urol* 1986;136(1 Pt 2):268–271.
248. Bergeson PS, Hopkin RJ, Bailey RB, McGill LC, Piatt JP. The inconspicuous penis. *Pediatrics* 1993;92:794–799.
249. Ben-Ari J, Merlob P, Mimouni F, Rosen O, Reisner SH. The prevalence of high insertion of scrotum, hydrocele and mobile testis in the newborn infant (36–42 weeks gestation). *Eur J Pediatr* 1989;148:563–564.
250. Kallen B, Bertollini R, Castilla E, et al. A joint international study on the epidemiology of hypospadias. *Acta Paediatr Scand Suppl* 1986;324:1–52.
251. Kallen B, Winberg J. An epidemiological study of hypospadias in Sweden. *Acta Paediatr Scand Suppl* 1982;293:1–21.
252. Sweet RA, Schrott HG, Kurland R, Culp OS. Study of the incidence of hypospadias in Rochester, Minnesota, 1940–1970, and a case-control comparison of possible etiologic factors. *Mayo Clin Proc* 1974;49:52–58.
253. Barcat J. Current concepts of treatment. In: Horton CE, ed. *Plastic Reconstructive Surgery of the Genital Area.* Boston: Little, Brown; 1973:249.
254. Kallen B. Case control study of hypospadias, based on registry information. *Teratology* 1988;38:45–50.
255. Bauer SB, Retik AB, Colodny AH. Genetic aspects of hypospadias. *Urol Clin North Am* 1981;8:559–564.
256. Page LA. Inheritance of uncomplicated hypospadias. *Pediatrics* 1979;63:788–790.
257. Khuri FJ, Hardy BE, Churchill BM. Urologic anomalies associated with hypospadias. *Urol Clin North Am* 1981;8:565–571.
258. Shafir R, Hertz M, Boichis H, Tsur H, Aladjem M, Jonas P. Vesicoureteral reflux in boys with hypospadias. *Urology* 1982;20:29–32.
259. Zilka E, Laron Z. [The normal testicular volume in Israeli children and adolescents]. *Harefuah* 1969;77:511–513.
260. Cassoria FG, Golden SM, Johnsonbaugh RE, Heroman WM, Lariaux L, Sherins RJ. Testicular volume during early infancy. *J Pediatr* 1981;99:742–743.
261. Huff DS, Wu HY, Snyder HMd, Hadziselimovic F, Blythe B, Duckett JW. Evidence in favor of the mechanical (intrauterine torsion) theory over the endocrinopathy (cryptorchidism) theory in the pathogenesis of testicular agenesis. *J Urol* 1991;146(2 Pt 2)):630–631.
262. Cilento BG, Najjar SS, Atala A. Cryptorchidism and testicular torsion. *Pediatr Clin North Am* 1993;40:1133–1149.
263. Berkowitz GS, Lapinski RH, Dolgin SE, Gazella JG, Bodian CA, Holzman IA. Prevalence and natural history of cryptorchidism. *Pediatrics* 1993;92:44–49.
264. Hawtrey CE. Undescended testis and orchiopexy: recent observations. *Pediatr Rev* 1990;11:305–308.
265. Acquafredda A, Vassal J, Job JC. Rudimentary testes syndrome revisited. *Pediatrics* 1987;80:209–214.
266. Burge DM. Neonatal testicular torsion and infarction: aetiology and management. *Br J Urol* 1987;59:70–73.
267. Dewan PA, Walton JK. Spermatic cord torsion in the neonate. *Aust N Z J Surg* 1987;57:331–333.
268. Watson RA. Torsion of spermatic cord in neonate. *Urology* 1975;5:439–443.
269. Stone KT, Kass EJ, Cacciarelli AA, Gibson DP. Management of suspected antenatal torsion: what is the best strategy? *J Urol* 1995;153(3 Pt 1):782–784.
270. Kogan S. Cryptorchidism. In: Kelalis PP, King LR, Belman AB, eds. *Clinical Pediatric Urology.* 3rd ed. Vol. 1. Philadelphia: WB Saunders; 1992:1467.
271. Canavese F, Lalla R, Linari A, Cortese MG, Gennari F, Hadziselimovic F. Surgical treatment of cryptorchidism. *Eur J Pediatr* 1993;152(suppl 2):43–44.
272. Bica DT, Hadziselimovic F. Buserelin treatment of cryptorchidism: a randomized, double-blind, placebo-controlled study. *J Urol* 1992;148(2 Pt 2):617–621.
273. Huff DS, Hadziselimovic F, Snyder HMd, Blyth B, Duckett JW. Early postnatal testicular maldevelopment in cryptorchidism. *J Urol* 1991;146(2 Pt 2)):624–626.
274. Huff DS, Hadziselimovic F, Snyder HM, Duckett JW, Keating MA. Postnatal testicular maldevelopment in unilateral cryptorchidism. *J Urol* 1989;142(2 Pt 2):546–548; discussion 572.
275. Hadziselimovic F, Hecker E, Herzog B. The value of testicular biopsy in cryptorchidism. *Urol Res* 1984;12:171–174.
276. Frey HL, Rajfer J. Incidence of cryptorchidism. *Urol Clin North Am* 1982;9:327–329.
277. Morley R, Lucas A. Undescended testes in low birthweight infants. *Br Med J* 1987;295:753.
278. Hurwitz A, Yagel S, Abramov M, Adoni A. Prenatal ultrasonic detection of bilateral hydrocele. *Am J Perinatol* 1984;1:195.
279. Nagel P. Scrotal swelling as the presenting symptom of acute perforated appendicitis in an infant. *J Pediatr Surg* 1984;19:177–178.
280. Gunn LC, Ghionzoli OG, Gardner HG. Healed meconium peritonitis presenting as a reducible scrotal mass [Letter]. *J Pediatr* 1978;92:847.
281. Amoury RA, Barth RW, Hall RT, Rhodes PG, Holder TM, Ashcraft KW. Scrotal hemorrhage. Sign of intraperitoneal hemorrhage in the newborn. *South Med J* 1982;75:1471–1478.
282. Das S, Singer A. Controversies of perinatal torsion of the spermatic cord: a review, survey and recommendations. *J Urol* 1990;143:231–233.

283. Leach GE, Masih MK. Neonatal torsion of testicle. *Urology* 1980;16:604–605.
284. Timon Garcia A, Lopez Lopez JA, Blasco Beltran B, Ambroj Navarro C, Murillo Perez C, Lario Munoz A. [Prenatal torsion of the spermatic cord]. *Arch Esp Urol* 1995;48:85–87.
285. Tripp BM, Homsy YL. Prenatal diagnosis of bilateral neonatal torsion: a case report. *J Urol* 1995;153: 1990–1991.
286. Cartwright PC, Snow BW, Reid BS, Shultz PK. Color Doppler ultrasound in newborn testis torsion. *Urology* 1995;45:667–670.
287. Herman TE, Siegel MJ. Special imaging casebook. Neonatal spermatic cord torsion and testicular infarction. *J Perinatol* 1994;14:431–432.
288. Diamond FB, Shulman DI, Root AW. Scrotal hair in infancy. *J Pediatr* 1989;114:999–1001.
289. McGillivray BC. Genetic aspects of ambiguous genitalia. *Pediatr Clin North Am* 1992;39:307–317.
290. Migeon CJ, Berkovitz GD. Congenital defects of the external genitalia in the newborn and prepubertal child. In: Carpenter SE, Rock JA, eds. *Pediatric and Adolescent Gynecology.* New York: Raven; 1992:77.
291. Simpson JL. Disorders of abnormal sexual differentiation. In: Sanfilippo JS, Muram D, Lee PA, Dewhurst PJ, eds. *Pediatric and Adolescent Gynecology.* Philadelphia: WB Saunders; 1994:77–103.
292. Moshang T Jr, Thornton PS. Endocrine disorders. In: Avery GB, Fletcher MA, MacDonald MG, eds. *Neonatology: Pathophysiology and Management of the Newborn.* Philadelphia: JB Lippincott; 1994:764–791.
293. El Haddad M, Corkery JJ. The anus in the newborn. *Pediatrics* 1985;76:927–928.
294. Reisner SH, Sivan Y, Nitzan M, Merlob P. Determination of anterior displacement of the anus in newborn infants and children. *Pediatrics* 1984;73:216–217.
295. McGregor DB, Halverson K, McVay CB. The unilateral pediatric inguinal hernia: should the contralateral side be explored. *J Pediatr Surg* 1980;15:313–317.
296. Boocock GR, Todd PJ. Inguinal hernias are common in preterm infants. *Arch Dis Child* 1985;60:669–670.
297. Harper RG, Garcia A, Sia C. Inguinal hernia: a common problem of premature infants weighing 1,000 grams or less at birth. *Pediatrics* 1975;56:112–115.
298. Peevy KJ, Speed FA, Hoff CJ. Epidemiology of inguinal hernia in preterm neonates. *Pediatrics* 1986;77: 246–247.
299. Bilik R, Shandling B, Pope M, Thorner P, Weitzman S, Ein SH. Malignant benign neonatal sacrococcygeal teratoma. *J Pediatr Surg* 1993;28:1158–1160.
300. Boemers TM, van Gool JD, de Jong TP, Bax KM. Lower urinary tract dysfunction in children with benign sacrococcygeal teratoma. *J Urol* 1994;151:174–176.
301. Calenda E, Bachy B, Guyard MF. Sacrococcygeal teratoma and venous shunting through a tumor: biological evidence [Letter]. *Anesth Analg* 1992;74:165–166.
302. el-Qarmalawi MA, Saddik M, el Abdel Hadi F, Muwaffi R, Nageeb K. Diagnosis and management of fetal sacrococcygeal teratoma. *Int J Gynaecol Obstet* 1990;31:275–281.
303. Feldman M, Byrne P, Johnson MA, Fischer J, Lees G. Neonatal sacrococcygeal teratoma: multiimaging modality assessment. *J Pediatr Surg* 1990;25:675–678.
304. Havranek P, Rubenson A, Guth D, et al. Sacrococcygeal teratoma in Sweden: a 10-year national retrospective study. *J Pediatr Surg* 1992;27:1447–1450.
305. Havranek P, Hedlund H, Rubenson A, et al. Sacrococcygeal teratoma in Sweden between 1978 and 1989: long-term functional results. *J Pediatr Surg* 1992;27:916–918.
306. Kum CK, Wong YC, Prabhakaran K. Management of fetal sacroccocygeal teratoma. *Ann Acad Med Singapore* 1993;22:377–380.
307. Lahdenne P, Heikinheimo M, Jaaskelainen J, Merikanto J, Heikkila J, Siimes MA. Vertebral abnormalities associated with congenital sacrococcygeal teratomas. *J Pediatr Orthop* 1991;11:603–607.
308. Leon Sosa RR, Moore PJ. Sacrococcygeal teratomas in the fetus and newborn. *Int J Gynaecol Obstet* 1990; 32:61–66.
309. Lahdenne P, Heikinheimo M, Nikkanen V, Klemi P, Siimes MA, Rapola J. Neonatal benign sacrococcygeal teratoma may recur in adulthood and give rise to malignancy. *Cancer* 1993;72:3727–3731.
310. Malone PS, Spitz L, Kiely EM, Brereton RJ, Duffy PG, Ransley PG. The functional sequelae of sacrococcygeal teratoma. *J Pediatr Surg* 1990;25:679–680.
311. Milam DF, Cartwright PC, Snow BW. Urological manifestations of sacrococcygeal teratoma. *J Urol* 1993; 149:574–576.
312. Reinberg Y, Long R, Manivel JC, Resnick J, Simonton S, Gonzalez R. Urological aspects of sacrococcygeal teratoma in children. *J Urol* 1993;150:948–949.
313. Schropp KP, Lobe TE, Rao B, et al. Sacrococcygeal teratoma: the experience of four decades. *J Pediatr Surg* 1992;27:1075–1078; discussion 1078–1079.
314. Subbarao P, Bhatnagar V, Mitra DK. The association of sacrococcygeal teratoma with high anorectal and genital malformations. *Aust N Z J Surg* 1994;64:214–215.
315. Powell RW, Weber ED, Manci EA. Intradural extension of a sacrococcygeal teratoma. *J Pediatr Surg* 1993; 28:770–772.
316. Waibel F, Scherer G, Fraccaro M, et al. Absence of Y-specific DNA sequences in human 46,XX true hermaphrodites and in 45,X mixed gonadal dysgenesis. *Hum Genet* 1987;76:332–336.
317. Ramsay M, Bernstein R, Zwane E, Page DC, Jenkins T. XX true hermaphroditism in southern African blacks: an enigma of primary sexual differentiation. *Am J Hum Genet* 1988;43:4–13.
318. Duckett JW. Hypospadias. *Pediatr Rev* 1989;11:37–42.
319. Stringer M, Brereton R, Drake D, et al. Meconium ileus due to extensive intestinal aganglionosis. *J Pediatr Surg* 1994;29:501–503.
320. Gearhart JP. Bladder and urachal abnormalities: the exstrophy–epispadias complex. In: Kelalis PP, King LR, Belman AB, eds. *Clinical Pediatric Urology.* 3rd ed. Vol. 1. Philadelphia: WB Saunders' 1991:1467.
321. Willms JL, Schneiderman H, Algranati PS. *Physical Diagnosis. Bedside Evaluation of Diagnosis and Function.* 1st ed. Vol. 1. Baltimore: Williams & Wilkins; 1994.
322. Mikami R, Murao M, Cugell DW, et al. International Symposium on lung sounds. Synopsis of proceedings. *Chest* 1987;92:342–345.

323. Puhakka H, Kero P, Erkinjuntti M. Pediatric bronchoscopy during a 17-year period. *Int J Pediatr Otorhinolaryngol* 1987;13:171–181.

324. Hawkins DB, Clark RW. Flexible laryngoscopy in neonates, infants, and young children. *Ann Otol Rhinol Laryngol* 1987;96(1 Pt 1):81–85.

325. Zalzal GH, Anon JB, Cotton RT. Epiglottoplasty for the treatment of laryngomalacia. *Ann Otol Rhinol Laryngol* 1987;96(1 Pt 1):72–76.

326. Shohat M, Sivan Y, Taub E, Davidson S. Autosomal dominant congenital laryngomalacia. *Am J Med Genet* 1992;42:813–814.

327. Fah KK, Tan HK. An unusual cause of stridor in a neonate. *J Laryngol Otol* 1994;108:63–64.

328. Cunningham MJ, Eavey RD, Shannon DC. Familial vocal cord dysfunction. *Pediatrics* 1985;76:750–753.

329. Grundfast KM, Milmoe G. Congenital hereditary bilateral abductor vocal cord paralysis. *Ann Otol Rhinol Laryngol* 1982;91(6 Pt 1):564–566.

330. Grundfast KM, Harley E. Vocal cord paralysis. *Otolaryngol Clin North Am* 1989;22:569–597.

331. Nowlin JH, Zalzal GH. The stridorous infant. *Ear Nose Throat J* 1991;70:84–88.

332. Sherman JM, Lowitt S, Stephenson C, Ironson G. Factors influencing acquired subglottic stenosis in infants. *J Pediatr* 1986;109:322–327.

333. Laing IA, Cowan DL, Ballantine GM, Hume R. Prevention of subglottic stenosis in neonatal ventilation. *Int J Pediatr Otorhinolaryngol* 1986;11:61–66.

334. Morrish TN, Manning SC. Branchial anomaly in a newborn presenting as stridor. *Int J Pediatr Otorhinolaryngol* 1991;12:117–121.

335. Mitchell DB, Irwin BC, Bailey CM, Evans JN. Cysts of the infant larynx. *J Laryngol Otol* 1987;101:833–837.

336. Suhonen H, Kero PO, Puhakka H, Vilkki P. Saccular cyst of the larynx in infants. *Int J Pediatr Otorhinolaryngol* 1984;8:73–78.

337. Prasad S, McBride TP, Merida M, Katz NM. Double aortic arch. *Ann Otol Rhinol Laryngol* 1992;101:872–875.

338. Stark J, Roesler M, Chrispin A, de Leval M. The diagnosis of airway obstruction in children. *J Pediatr Surg* 1985;20:113–117.

339. Chan TS, Young LW. Radiological case of the month. Stridor due to double-aortic-arch anomaly. *Am J Dis Child* 1985;139:1047–1048.

340. Optican RJ, White KS, Effmann EL. Goitrous cretinism manifesting as newborn stridor: CT evaluation. *Am J Roentgenol* 1991;157:557–558.

341. Chan FL, Low LC, Yeung HW, Saing H. Case report: lingual thyroid, a cause of neonatal stridor. *Br J Radiol* 1993;66:462–464.

342. Jacobs RF, Yasuda K, Smith AL, Benjamin DR. Laryngeal candidiasis presenting as inspiratory stridor. *Pediatrics* 1982;69:234–236.

343. Nyquist A, Rotbart HA, Cotton M, et al. Acyclovir-resistant neonatal herpes simplex virus infection of the larynx. *J Pediatr* 1994;124:967–971.

344. Rosenfeld RM, Fletcher MA, Marban SL. Acute epiglottitis in a newborn infant. *Pediatr Infect Dis J* 1992;11:594–595.

345. Nielson DW, Heldt GP, Tooley WH. Stridor and gastroesophageal reflux in infants. *Pediatrics* 1990;85:1034–1039.

346. Orenstein SR, Orenstein DM, Whitington PF. Gastroesophageal reflus causing stridor. *Chest* 1983;84:301–302.

347. Cohen SR. Congenital glottic webs in children. A retrospective review of 51 patients. *Ann Otol Rhinol Laryngol Suppl* 1985;121:2–16.

348. Close LG, Rosenberg HS, Volgler C, Warshaw HE. Neonatal laryngeal fibromatosis. *Otolaryngol Head Neck Surg* 1981;89:992–997.

349. Williams WT, Cole RR. Lymphangioma presenting as congenital stridor. *Int J Pediatr Otorhinolaryngol* 1993;26:185–191.

350. Long SS. Pneumonia in young infants (birth through 3 months). In: Schidlow DV, Smith DS, eds. *A Practical Guide to Pediatric Respiratory Diseases.* Philadelphia: Hanley & Belfus; 1994:83–88.

Neuroskeletal Evaluation

10

The Extremities

Examination of the extremities is one of the easier sections of the neonatal physical assessment because of their accessibility compared with the internal organs, the overt presentation of major musculoskeletal anomalies, and the normal presence of more than one of everything for easy comparisons. Two potential difficulties in the process require comment. One difficulty emanates from attempting to apply traditional orthopedic terms that are laden with Latin and Greek. It is difficult to remember the correct terms when a need to apply them is relatively infrequent. Carefully describing a finding in relation to the anatomic position and using commonly understood terms eases this problem and allows communication or, at the least, finding the correct orthopedic term in a dictionary. A second challenge appears in interpreting the influence of gestational age, intrauterine position, and maternal hormones in shaping and deforming the extremities and affecting joint motility. It is easy to note a limb deficiency or duplication but more difficult to decide if a misshapen foot is simply deformed or malformed. Both having experience in examinations and allowing appropriate time to pass after birth for the gestational factors to diminish lessen this difficulty, but parents will force an educated opinion about the significance.

This regional examination overlaps the scrutiny of other regions but is intimately coupled to evaluation of neuromuscular function because most of an infant's motor activity involves moving the extremities. General observations about use and resting positions occur throughout each clinical assessment. Once it is determined that there are no congenital anomalies, an appropriate examination in the absence of specific symptoms would include merely inspecting for appropriate growth and function during infancy. An important exception to this is the need for repeated assessment of the hips until the end of infancy. A specific regional evaluation of the extremities ordinarily comes toward the end of the initial screening examination, when all four extremities are considered individually and in comparison. Indications for more detailed examination of the extremities are listed below.

Indications for detailed examination of extremities after cursory inspection:

1. Any visible abnormality in either form or use of the extremities and spine
2. After therapy with paralytic medications to assess for decreased range of motion (1)
3. Intrauterine history suggesting prolonged asphyxia or decreased fetal movement (2)
4. Swelling over a joint
5. Deep chemical or thermal injuries
6. Deep cellulitis or thrombophlebitis

7. Hematogenous infection with an organism that tends to spread to joints and bones (especially *Neisseria gonococcus, Staphylococcus aureus*)
8. Thromboembolic disease
9. Osteomyelitis
10. A positive family history for congenital bone or joint disease
11. Possible obstetric trauma
12. Presence of anomalies in other organ systems, particularly the cardiac and nervous systems

Simple inspection and palpation with comparisons are the major tools for the physical assessment of this region, but there are a few additional essential maneuvers that require practice for more skill in detecting subtle changes. Special techniques for assessing the hips and clavicles are discussed in separate sections in this chapter. In some instances, the landmarks used for measurements differ in newborn infants. These techniques are noted in the Appendix.

EMBRYOLOGY

There is such a strong association of certain types of limb defects with malformations in other organs that a full investigation for these association is warranted (e.g., radial or preaxial malformations) (3,4). Other defects are merely isolated or familial and carry no higher incidence of other malformations (e.g., little finger or postaxial duplication). Figure 1 depicts the development of the limbs, and Table 1 outlines the embryologic development of the extremities (5).

ANATOMY

The anatomic landmarks of the extremities are the bony prominences, including the acromion, anterior superior iliac spine, pubic symphysis, medial malleolus, axis of the limbs with the cranial or preaxial portion and the caudal or postaxial portion, joints, and

Table 1. *Embryologic development of the extremities*

Age (days)	Carnegie stage	Length (mm)[a]	Developmental characteristic
26–27	12	3–5	Upper limb buds appear.
28–30	13	4–6	Upper limb buds are flipperlike. Lower limb buds appear. Attenuated tail is present.
31–32	14	5–7	Upper limbs are paddle-shaped.
33–36	15	7–9	Hand plates formed; digital rays present. Lower limbs are paddle-shaped.
37–40	16	8–11	Foot plates formed.
41–43	17	11–14	Digital rays clearly visible in hand plates.
44–46	18	13–17	Digital rays clearly visible in foot plates.
47–48	19	16–18	Limbs extend ventrally. Trunk elongating and straightening.
49–51	20	18–22	Upper limbs longs and bent at elbows. Fingers distinct but webbed. Notches between the digital rays in the feet.
52–53	21	22–24	Hands and feet approach each other. Fingers are free and longer. Toes distinct but webbed. Stubby tail present.
54–55	22	23–28	Toes free and longer.
56	23	27–31	Tail has disappeared.

[a] The embryonic lengths indicate the usual but not full range of crown-rump length within a given stage.
Modified from Moore et al., ref. 5, with permission.

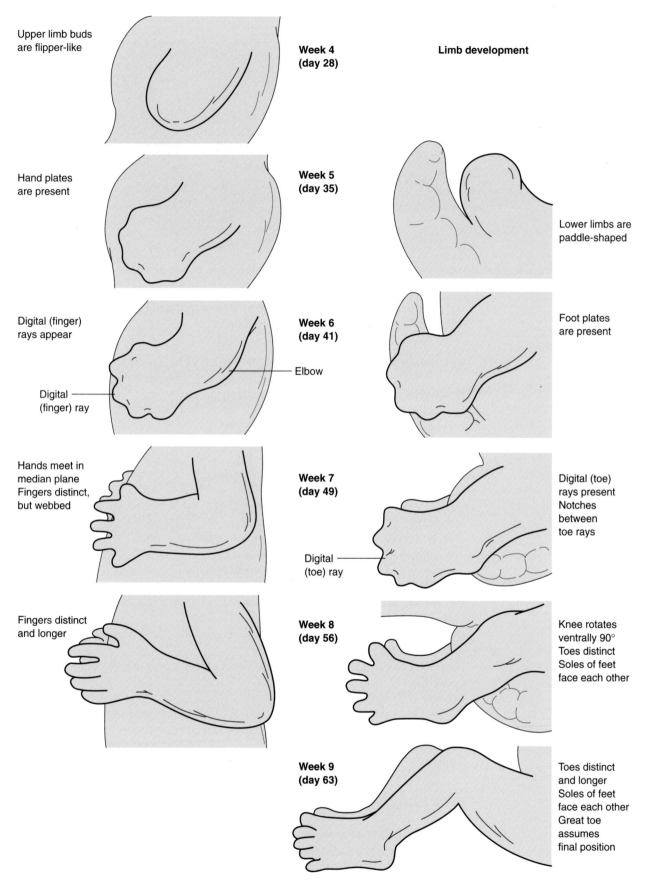

Figure 1. Development of the limbs. The upper limb buds are visible by days 26 to 27; the lower limb buds appear 2 days later. The stages for the limbs are similar except for the earlier process in the upper limbs.

Upper limb buds are flipper-like

Week 4 (day 28)

Limb development

Hand plates are present

Week 5 (day 35)

Lower limbs are paddle-shaped

Digital (finger) rays appear

Week 6 (day 41)

Foot plates are present

Digital (finger) ray

Elbow

Hands meet in median plane Fingers distinct, but webbed

Week 7 (day 49)

Digital (toe) rays present Notches between toe rays

Digital (toe) ray

Fingers distinct and longer

Week 8 (day 56)

Knee rotates ventrally 90° Toes distinct Soles of feet face each other

Week 9 (day 63)

Toes distinct and longer Soles of feet face each other Great toe assumes final position

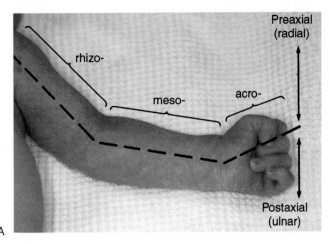
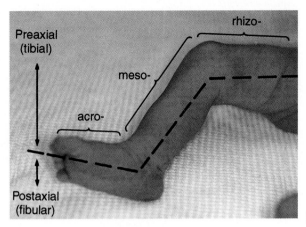

Figure 2. Anatomic landmarks of limb segments. **A:** Upper extremity. **B:** Lower extremity.

segments (Fig. 2). Areas on the limbs are also described according to region (e.g., deltoid, antecubital fossa, popliteal, axillary, or femoral).

TECHNIQUE OF EXAMINATION OF THE EXTREMITIES

Observe for spontaneous activity or in response to stimulation
Inspect the limbs for
    symmetry in lengths of arms and of legs
    symmetry in circumferences of arms and of legs
        symmetry of muscle mass
        evidence of muscular or vascular anomalies
    proportion of limb-to-trunk lengths
    presence of contractures or abnormal webbing
    symmetry and size of hands and feet
    proportion of each hand and foot to the rest of the extremity
    number, size, and symmetry of fingers and toes
    presence and appearance of fingernails and toenails
    distribution of the palmar and plantar creases
Measure any regions that appear disproportionate or asymmetric, using a specific anatomic
    landmark to define the site of measurement.
Determine range of motion across the joints in any areas that appear abnormal.
Feel and compare the pulses.
Palpate for tenderness, fluctuation, and temperature changes in areas of discoloration or
    swelling.
Palpate for hip stability.
Palpate for symmetry, tenderness, crepitation, or swelling along the clavicles.
If not already completed as part of the regional trunk examination, examine the spine for
    integrity, mobility, and the presence of any overlying cutaneous lesions or subcutaneous
    masses.

Upper Extremities

With the infant lying supine, assess the resting position of both upper extremities. Look for and compare spontaneous movement in all four extremities. If the infant does not have symmetry of position and movement in both upper and lower extremities, and the head is not in mid-line, gently center the head and verify that the previously extended limb flexes. If it does not, evaluate for paralysis, most commonly due to brachial plexus injury, or pseudoparalysis due to fracture or joint infection.

Inspect for symmetry of proportion in the arms, forearms, hands, and fingers. Esti-

mate the equality of length in the upper extremities by bringing the infant's wrists to-
gether. If the extremities are the same length and the back is straight with thoracic sym-
metry, the wrists will meet in the mid-line. If the point of approximation is not at the mid-
line, it deviates toward the side of the shorter extremity. Compare the size and shape of
the hands and the insertion of the thumb.

At term, the resting posture is one of flexion at the elbows with the hands loosely fisted. With increase in both chronologic age or prematurity, the flexion becomes less pronounced. When the resting position is with the head turned toward one side, the posture may be asymmetrical with the occipital side flexed and the mental (chin) side extended.

Determine if the length of the upper extremity is proportionate to the trunk by noting
where the hands reach on the lateral surface of the thigh. Keeping the infant's back
straight, bring both of the arms along the side of the trunk and note the point where the
wrist lies. If the two extremities are at different positions along the length of the trunk
and the spine is straight, flex each elbow to 90° and compare the height of the wrist. If
the wrists are at the same height, the discrepancy is in length of the forearm.

The arm span approximates the total length or height throughout most of life but is approximately 3 cm less in infancy, with the trunk proportionately longer than the extremities at birth. The arms should be long enough for the wrist to touch below the pelvic brim. With the hips flexed to 90° the fingertips should reach just to the back of the thighs. This length can be verified when checking range of motion in the elbows and fingers.

Due to their small size, it is easy to compare the circumferences of extremities across
their widest portion by encircling each with a thumb and forefinger while palpating the
muscle mass. If there is discrepancy between the sides, measure the circumference at the
same distance from a specific anatomical landmark. Should one side appear too large,
palpate for edema, induration, abnormal temperature, or tenderness suggesting fluid
stasis, hematoma, vascular malformations, thrills, or bony mass. If one area is too small,
palpate for lack of normal subcutaneous fat, muscle atrophy, or pulses. Inspect the over-
lying skin for evidence of vascular malformations, atrophy, ecchymoses, pallor, necro-
sis, or hamartoma. Measure any area that is asymmetrical or abnormal in length or cir-
cumference following the techniques recommended by Hall (6).

The muscles are not as defined as in older patients both because of immaturity and because of the overlying fat mass: atrophic muscles feel fibrous rather than doughy (their normal texture), and atrophic areas feel especially thin. Muscles that are clearly visible or easily defined by palpation may be hypertonic or contracted and fibrotic. Muscle hypertrophy will not be present at birth.

Edema is probably the most common reason for increase in size of an extremity. At birth, edema is often demonstrable in presenting limbs but its resolution is rapid. Its presence causes loss of normal skin creases and, eventually, a shininess to the skin with loss of anatomical landmarks and decreased range of motion in contiguous joints (Fig. 3). Pitting can be elicited in both lymphedema and edema, but lymphedema does not lead to loss of skin creases across joints as edema does. Unilateral vascular malformations can cause asymmetry at birth, although many conditions associated with later limb hypertrophy are not as notably asymmetrical in the newborn period.

Check range of motion in the shoulder, elbow, wrist, and interphalangeal joints by
passively moving each area and comparing the two extremities. Inspect the skin over the
joints for creases, redundancy, webbing, or dimpling. If there is asymmetry in range,
clear limitation in motion, or abnormalities in the overlying skin, measure the angles of
the joints in question (Figs. 4 and 5).

The range of motion for any joint is determined by structure and mobility of the joint itself, by muscle and tendon lengths across that joint, by muscle tone, and by interference from extra-articular soft tissue mass. In newborn infants the influence on range of motion by factors outside the joint is particularly strong such that gestational age, intrauterine position, body size, neurologic status, and state of relaxation may determine a comfortable passive range of motion as much as the joint structure itself. A term newborn has limitation of shoulder abduction, increased dorsiflexion and plantar flexion at the ankle, and flexion contractures at the elbow, knee, and hip (Table 2) (7–9). In the first few days after birth there is notable change in the range of motion as the effects of intrauterine constraint and maternal hormones abate. Our postnatal care patterns can influence range of motion, including how we swaddle or restrain the extremities. Even short periods of medically induced paralysis and disuse affect the demonstrable range of motion (1). For all joints except the hips, the range of normal reaches expected levels by 3 months of age. The hips take longer and may not reach adult ranges until the toddler has been walking for some time (7).

Fortunately, because it is possible to compare each joint with its contralateral counterpart, the infant serves as his own control. Importantly, many of the congenital conditions that have truly decreased range of motion have abnormalities of the overlying skin: absence of creases, unusual dimpling, or webbing (Fig. 6). Those with increased range may have more redundant skin. Most of the maneuvers needed to test range of motion are part of the neuromotor assessment and determination of gestational age, but if there are any notable

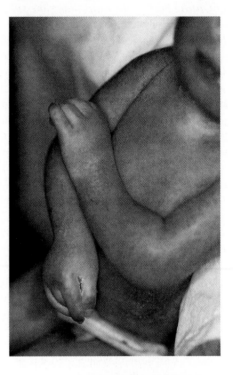

Figure 3. Decreased range of motion in hydropic infant with arthrogryposis. The swollen middle and ring fingers are fixed in flexion, and the thumb, index, and little fingers are fixed in extension. The skin creases over the joints are smoothed, indicating a lengthy period of absent mobility.

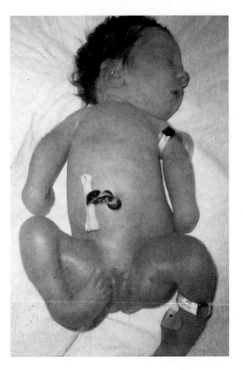

Figure 4. Congenital arthrogryposis with multiple joint involvement in a typical resting posture.

limb anomalies or abnormal movement patterns, specific evaluation of range of motion is indicated.

In most circumstances we are evaluating the passive range of motion as we extend, flex, and rotate the extremities. Because acquired decreased range of motion may be the primary presentation of joint pain or fractures, observations of active range of motion are important, although more challenging to elicit. For the most part, we use observations of unequal spontaneous motor activity to detect the pseudopareses of pain, but we can induce active movement in many circumstances by stimulating the skin reflexes over the area in question or by inducing movement against gravity. These reflexes and techniques are detailed in Chapter 11 Table 11.

Techniques for measuring ranges of motion as well as the definitions of the movements involved in the major joints as suggested by the American Academy of Orthopaedic Surgeons are depicted in the figures toward the end of this chapter (10).

Count the number of fingers on each hand. Assess and compare the shape and length of the fingers. Determine the course of the palmar creases and the presence or absence of creases across each of the digits. Inspect the nails for shape, width, and length of the fingernails. Note the presence of meconium staining and the color of the nail and its underlying tissue. Evaluate and compare the strength of the grasp and the resting position of the hand.

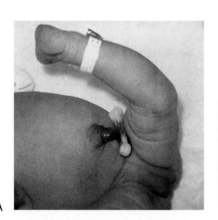 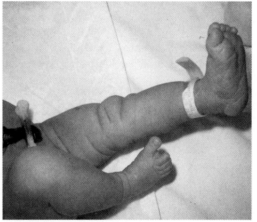

A   B

Figure 5. Genu recurvatum, the result of prolonged, forced hyperextension of the lower extremity. **A:** The curvature in the limb is marked, but the presence of popliteal creases indicates there has been flexion activity prenatally and suggests a better prognosis. **B:** The same limb appears normal when spontaneous activity allows the hip to be less flexed. No correction therapy was necessary.

Table 2. *Limitations and expected joint ranges of motion and torsion*

Joint	Motion	Newborn	3 mo	Adult
Spine		C-shaped	Cervical curve	—
Shoulder	Extension limitation	70–130°	Normal	177–191°
Elbow	Extension limitation	0–30°	Normal	−2 to 4°
Hips	Extension limitation	50–80°	45–70°	3–17°
	Internal rotation	40–80°	40–80°	41–53°
	External rotation	−30 to 0°	−20 to 0°	41–54°
	Anteversion	40°		15°
Knees	Extension limitation	0–35°	Normal	−1 to 4°
	Valgus	—	—	15°
	Varus	15°		—
	Tibial torsion	±5°	Normal	−20 to 10° lateral
Ankle	Dorsiflexion	40–80°	Normal	8–17°
	Plantar flexion	10–30°	Normal	50–62°

The ranges are for the terminal point of the range of motion, not for the full range of motion.

Modified from Dunne and Clarren, ref. 9, with permission.

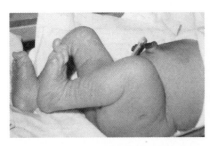
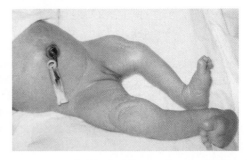

Figure 6. A: On first inspection this extremity appears unremarkable, but the presence of a dimple over the lateral thigh is a clue to an underlying abnormal articulation of long standing. **B:** Closer inspection and comparison of the limbs shown unequal leg lengths and shapes due to pseudoarthrosis of the left femur associated with a teratologic hip dislocation. Palpation of the thigh suggested a mobile fracture, but there was no accompanying pain, soft-tissue swelling, or discoloration.

Some instances of polydactyly have such normal-appearing digits that an extra one can be overlooked or hidden unless a count is routine. If there are extra digits, determine which digit is duplicated and if duplication is pre- or postaxial. Similarly, if there are too few digits, determine if the loss is longitudinal or transverse.

The length of the fingers and pattern of skin creases should be assessed by opening the hands. The fingers are not the same length, with the middle finger normally longer than the others. Similarly, the metacarpals vary in length, providing the curve in the distal margin of the palm. When the metacarpals are not varied in length, the hand has a straight distal margin and a single palmar crease, most commonly because of shortening of the middle metacarpal as seen in Down's syndrome.

A normal thumb reaches to a point close to mid-way along the proximal digit of the first finger. If not, the thumb may be hypoplastic if short or proximally inserted if of normal length. The distance from the tip of the index finger to the base of the thumb should be slightly more than one half the distance of the index finger to the carpal crease. If the thumb is proximally placed, the ratio will be greater than 0.58; if distal, it will be less than 0.43 (11). The Steinberg sign suggests Marfan's syndrome or excessive length if a thumb adducted across the palm extends beyond its ulnar margin. Because the palm is so flexible in most neonates, the hand must be held flat when assessing thumb length and insertion.

The fingernails are pliable and tear easily during the newborn period. There is a wide variability in size and shape that is primarily familial, but the nails should be somewhat uniform among the fingers. Small fingernails are more likely to indicate true hypoplasia than are small toenails (Fig. 7).

The resting position of the hand is a loose fist without significant overlap of the fingers. Infants who are in a quiet, awake state should actively open and close their hands, particu-

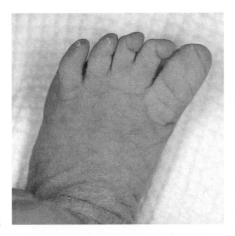
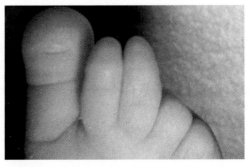

Figure 7. A: Nail hypoplasia and absent distant phalanx of the first three toes. The uniform pattern in both feet makes amputation from early chorionic villous sampling (47), amnionic bands, and vascular insufficiency unlikely. **B:** In contrast, the complete amputation without regrowth is characteristic of loss of the last two toes due to amnionic banding.

larly when they go through rooting movements. The thumb normally extends at the same time as the fingers and does not remain adducted across the palm. If fisting is normal and not accompanied by other abnormal posturing, the fingers and the thumb will extend when the back of the hand is stroked. As an isolated finding, absence of extension suggests radial nerve palsy (12,13). A resting position of thumb adduction is notable in X-linked hydrocephalus (14).

Lower Extremities

With the infant lying supine and the diapers removed or loosened, assess the lower extremities for their resting position and spontaneous movements. Inspect for symmetry and proportion of the thighs, legs, and feet. Holding one foot in each hand, extend the hips and knees with the medial malleoli together. Compare the position of the knees and the malleoli and the lengths of the lower extremities. If there is asymmetry in length, flex the hips to 90° and compare the height of the knees.

At birth there is a normal genu varum to about 10° (15). Coupled with common tibial bowing, there is often enough curve in the lower limbs that parents inquire about the unusual shape. In the absence of other pathology, they can be reassured that the legs will mold into a more normal shape in response to extrauterine forces. Some pathologic conditions directly relate to prolonged intrauterine compression so that hip dysplasia, genu recurvatum, metatarsus, and clubfoot all need to be considered when there is abnormal shape or mobility (16). If an infant was in breech position in utero for an extended period, the range of motion in the hips will be decreased so that extension is either quite decreased or is uncomfortable to the infant. The position of comfort for these infants may be quite unnatural (Fig. 6).

The upper to lower ratio at birth (1.7:1) is much higher than in adults (1:1), so comparison with standard curves based on age is important if there is a concern about disproportion (see Appendix figures 3–5, 8). Additionally, the landmarks used for determining the length of the lower extremities differ, so it is important to use the same techniques in comparing values.

If the knees are not at the same height with the hips flexed at 90° (Galeazzi sign), the most likely reason is a posterior dislocation of the hip on the shorter side. Other causes of unilateral femoral shortening include fractures and vascular insufficiency (Fig. 6). Abnormal lengthening of the femur due to hypertrophy is not as apparent at birth as in the later months of infancy but may occur in association with vascular malformations, with Klippel-Trenaunay-Weber and congenital cutis marmorata telangiectasia as examples.

Examine the plantar creases. Count the toes and examine the toenails. Determine range of motion for the ankle and forefoot. Grasp the foot proximal to the mid-tarsal joint and check for normal dorsiflexion and plantar flexion with the leg extended. If there is decreased dorsiflexion, flex the knee and retest. Improved dorsiflexion with knee shortening suggests a tightened Achilles tendon; no change suggests intrinsic joint inflexibility. Move the ankle and foot through the full range of rotation, supination, and pronation. Should there be a curve in the mid-foot, straighten the foot by gently applying pressure with one finger. Place the feet flat against the end of the bassinet or a vertical surface to simulate a standing position (Fig. 8).

As in the hands, the presence of creases correlates with fetal activity and compressions and the location reflects underlying anatomy. A prominent vertical crease develops when the foot is compressed on its long axis by prenatal position even in the absence of fetal movement. Horizontal creases across joints are more indicative of movement. Vertical creases also develop in association with a wide space between the great and second toes. The Goldstein toe sign of wide spacing is seen in some infants with Down's syndrome or hypothyroidism, but it is too prevalent in normal infants to be diagnostic.

Metatarsus abductus, or an incurving of the forefoot, is easily identified by the C curve of the lateral border of the foot. The creases on the sole of the foot are transverse, extending laterally from the apex of the concavity on the medial side of the foot. The space between the first and second toes may be increased. The deformity is most commonly associated with a fixed intrauterine position that is evident when the infant is encouraged to resume his intrauterine posture. There is an association with developmental hip dysplasia, so this should be carefully ruled out (15). Sometimes the deformation is marked and relatively rigid so that it is difficult to distinguish from talipes equinovarus (TEV). A flexible deformity can be corrected to a neutral position by placing the infant's feet against the bottom of the bassinet or applying gentle lateral pressure with one finger to the medial head of

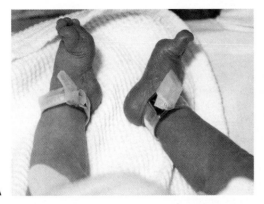
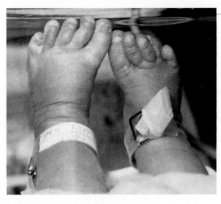

Figure 8. Positional deformation of feet. **A:** On cursory inspection, the deformation on the left seems to be the more significant. **B:** When the infant's feet are placed into a neutral position on the side of the bassinet, the left foot easily assumes a normal shape with straightening of both lateral margins. The right foot continues to have a metatarsus abductus with persistence of the medial and lateral curves, indicating a more significant deformation that requires passive stretching.

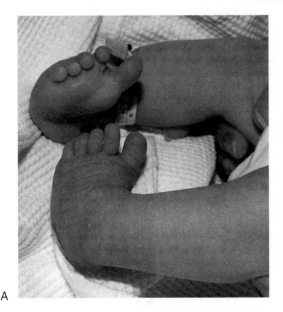
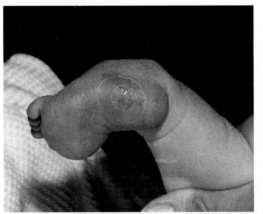
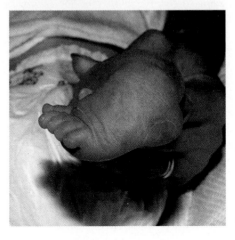

Figure 9. Bilateral TEV (clubfoot). Inspection from different angles as well as palpation and manipulation for range of motion are necessary to detail the characteristic findings and estimate the severity of the defect. **A:** The soles face medially in forefoot supination. **B:** Varus angulation of the forefoot with accentuated creases in the medial curve and posteriorly at the heel. **C:** Equinus posturing.

the first metatarsus. If correction to neutral is painful to the infant or causes the examiner's finger to blanch because of the amount of pressure required, the adductus may be rigid and indicate further evaluation for therapy (15) (Fig. 9).

Talipes equinovarus (15), or clubfoot, includes three specific deformities:

1. Adduction or varus angulation of the forefoot (Fig. 9B)
2. Varus angulation (inversion) at the ankle (the subtalar joint) so the sole of the foot points medially (Fig. 9A)
3. Equinus posturing with the toes down, the heel up, and the calcaneus difficult to feel (Fig. 9C)

The deformity develops either due to prolonged immobility from constraint or lack of neuromotor activity or due to abnormal joint formation early in gestation. TEV occurs in 1 to 2 per 1,000 deliveries, most often in otherwise normal infants. Fifty percent are bilateral and 70% are male. The recurrence risk is 2-5% unless it is associated with other syndromes. Maternal myotonia increases fetal risk for TEV (15).

Associations with TEV:

Conditions of decreased fetal movement either by constraint or by neuromuscular deficits:
 Spinal dysraphism, meningomyelocele
 Arthrogryposis
 Oligohydramnios
 Early amnion rupture sequence (amniotic band syndrome)
Primary malformation:
 Diastrophic dysplasia
 Larsen's syndrome
 Maternal aminopterin
 Maternal methotrexate in early gestation

Special Clinical Assessment: Examination of the Hips

Observations for diagnosing hip dysplasia:

Resting posture asymmetrical or in hyperflexion
Spontaneous movements decreased or unsmooth
Unequal leg length with one knee shorter than the other (Galeazzi sign)
Decreased range of motion in abduction
Inequality in extension (Thomas test)
Jerking thunk on relocation during abduction (Ortolani maneuver)
Shortening on dislocation during adduction (Barlow maneuver)
Excessive telescoping (Dupuytren's sign)

Observe how the infant is lying at supine rest and moving the lower extremities; look for equality in degree of abduction and extension during spontaneous activity. If the infant's lower extremities are extended and back is straight, hold the ankles and approximate the medial malleoli (Fig. 10). Compare the position of the knees and the length of the extremities. With the infant supine, flex the knees so the feet rest on the mattress and compare the height of the knees (Fig. 11). If the leg length or knee height differs (a positive Galeazzi sign), perform the Ortolani maneuver on the shorter extremity. If the sides are the same and both appear to have normal range of abduction, perform the Barlow maneuver before the Ortolani maneuver. If the infant is prone, compare the gluteal and popliteal skin creases with the hips both extended and flexed to 90°. An immobile, dislocated hip can also be the one to demostrate less extension.

Evaluate for flexion contracture with the Thomas test. Flex one hip to 90° to flatten the lumbosacral spine and stabilize the pelvis while extending the opposite. The angle that the extended thigh makes with the surface of the mattress is the degree of flexion contracture, normally 25° to 30° but as much as 45° in newborn infants. If there is inequality or an angle greater than 30°, the contracture may be in either the hip or the knee. The hip contracture normally found at birth relaxes over the first 2 to 3 months. If

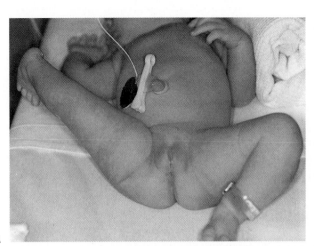
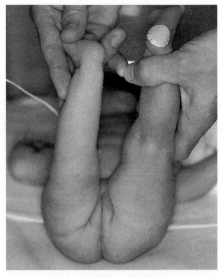

A   B

Figure 10. Signs of hip dysplasia. **A:** Twin with genu recurvatum who is most comfortable in her pre-natal position of a single breech. The extension of the right leg for a prolonged time is indicated by the absence of creases over the posterior popliteal angle (compare with Fig. 5A). Shortening of the quadri-ceps muscles prevented active or passive flexion of this knee until the muscles were gradually stretched. **B:** There is notable discrepancy in leg lengths due to posterior dislocation of the right hip. The Barlow and Ortolani maneuvers were both negative because the dislocated hip could not be relocated. Correc-tion was difficult. Infants presenting in a breech position with the hips flexed and legs extended are at highest risk for hip dysplasia (48).

there is asymmetrical extension, the more extended hip may be dislocated or unstable (17). An immobile, dislocated hip can also be the one to demonstrate less extension.

If the hips appear to be in place with equal knee height and equal angles of abduction, perform the Barlow dislocation maneuver on each side separately. The Barlow maneu-ver consists of applying a pressure along the axis of the femur and from medial to lateral at the head of the femur to push it posteriorly out of the socket (18) (Fig. 12). To accom-plish this, stand at the feet of the infant and examine one side of his pelvis while stabi-lizing the other. Position your hand with the infant's flexed knee in the space between your thumb and forefinger, your thumb as proximal on the medial side of the femur as possible and your other fingers on the lateral side (Fig. 13). Apply gentle but firm pres-sure posteriorly and laterally with your hand and thumb while adducting the hip toward and past the mid-line. If the hip is dislocated by this maneuver, the knees should now be at different heights (a positive Galeazzi sign).

If a hip appears to be out of the socket or after completing the Barlow dislocation ma-neuver, perform the Ortolani relocation maneuver (19) (Fig. 14). With your hand in the same position, and the long finger held on the greater trochanter, abduct the hip while applying a light medial and anterior pressure to lift the thigh toward the acetabulum. A

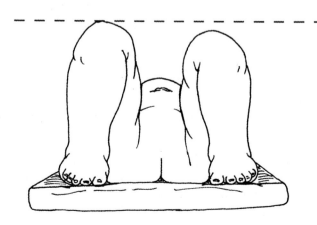

Figure 11. Positive Galeazzi sign of unequal knee height, demonstrating shortening of the left lower extremity due to posterior dislocation of the left hip.

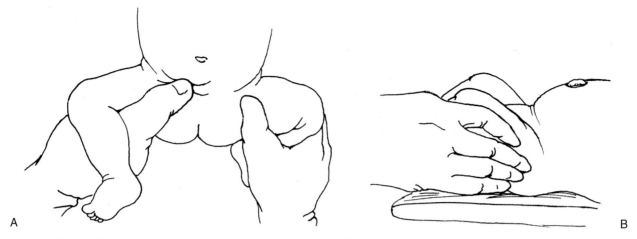

Figure 12. Hand position for examining the left hip. **A:** The right thumb is positioned proximally on the medial femur with the hand encircling the knee (important for the Barlow maneuver). The left hand stabilizes the pelvis. **B:** Position of the long fingers on the greater trochanter (important for the Ortolani maneuver).

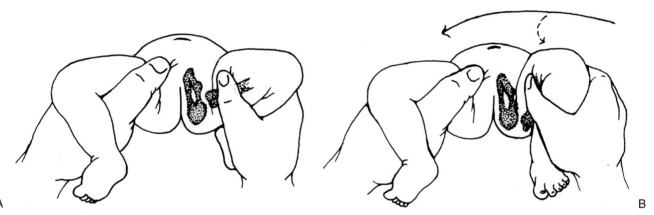

Figure 13. Barlow maneuver to dislocate an unstable left hip. **A:** With the hip initially abducted, the right hand is positioned to apply a soft pressure in the directions necessary to dislocate the femoral head posteriorly. **B:** As the leg is adducted to at least 20° past mid-line (*solid arrow*), the thumb applies a lateral pressure and the hand a posterior pressure to dislocate the hip (*interrupted arrow*). A positive test leads to knee height discrepancy.

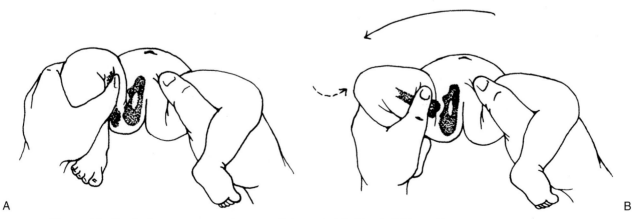

Figure 14. Ortolani maneuver to relocate a dislocated right hip. **A:** With the hip in neutral or partially adducted, the right hand is positioned with the long finger over the greater trochanter, the left hand stabilizing the pelvis. **B:** As the left hip is abducted (*solid arrow*), gentle medial pressure is applied to the greater trochanter to push the femoral head into the acetabulum (*interrupted arrow*). A positive test is felt as a clunk with a visible jerk as the femoral head moves into place.

positive Ortolani relocation sign is a thunking sensation felt as the hip slips into the socket. Assess joint laxity for excessive telescoping (Dupuytren's sign) by moving the femur up and down with the hip flexed. After completing the examination on one side, examine the other hip.

The Ortolani maneuver moves a dislocated hip into the socket while the Barlow maneuver will move a located but dislocatable hip out of the socket. The Ortolani maneuver will not be positive if the hip is not dislocated at that time or if it cannot be moved back into the socket. In the latter case, if there is unilateral involvement, unequal leg length, asymmetric skin folds, or incomplete abduction suggests the diagnosis. Hips that are dislocated will not spontaneously or freely abduct past about 50° unless they relocate during abduction. In the newborn period in some infants the hips may dislocate and relocate so freely that abduction is normal.

The sensation that makes the Ortolani maneuver positive is a thunk or jolt that occurs as the hip drops forward into the socket. It is very distinct from the cracking or clicking that occurs as a snap during joint movement. That cracking is just the same as cracking in knuckles and bears no clinical significance because it is present at some time in most infants. A true thunk is felt almost as much in the pit of the stomach as with the fingers and can sometimes be seen from a distance as a jolt.

Findings may be obfuscated if a fetal breech position was prolonged enough to limit range of motion in the knees and hips or if there are other anomalies present. In some instances, spontaneous movement by the infant is more effective in dislocating the hip than the Barlow maneuver and may be seen as a notable jerking of the lower extremity with flexion and extension as the femoral head goes in and out of the socket.

It is important to remember that both Barlow and Ortolani maneuvers will be negative if a hip is dislocated and cannot be relocated. In this instance leg length and range of motion may be the clinical indicators, but in some instances in which teratologic dislocations are suspected, imaging studies may be needed to make a diagnosis. It is not always possible to get a positive clinical examination with each assessment, even when the examiner is careful and experienced. If there is a strong historical indicator or a positive finding, further steps in evaluation are needed.

Hips may be dislocated, dislocatable, or subluxable. Dislocatable hips are those in place but completely dislocated upon the Barlow maneuver. Subluxation indicates that hips are in place but flexible enough to be partially displaced by the Barlow maneuver.

The hip joint is accessible for examination by ultrasound, and there is considerable literature on the use of ultrasound as both a screening and diagnostic tool for hip dysplasia. Whether its use as a screening tool is warranted and cost effective remains controversial, but the work done with ultrasonography at the least has helped to define the development of the hip in early infancy and to evaluate the efficacy of treatments (20–25). Diagnosis by ultrasound depends on the training and experience of the examiner, just as does the clinical detection, but it does not replace careful and repeated clinical evaluation with every opportunity during early infancy.

It is more accurate to call the dislocations and dysplasias of the hip occurring in the first half year of life developmental dislocation or dysplasia of the hip rather than congenital hip dysplasia. Previously when a hip dysplasia was first detected at several month of age, it was presumed to be a missed neonatal diagnosis. Now it is clear that there are several patterns of development and presentation, although dysplasia and dislocations are still missed clinically (21). Isolated hip dislocation that is clinically apparent in the neonatal period is more often unilateral on the left side with a higher risk in infants who are female (4:1), have a positive family history, or had a breech presentation (14:1) (9,26). Hip dislocations that present after the newborn period do not have the same left-sided predominance but have more bilateral occurrence and less female predominance (27).

Special Clinical Assessment: Examination of the Clavicles

With the infant lying supine, run your fingers along the margin of the clavicles and assess for swelling and tenderness. Compare both sides for uniformity along the mar-

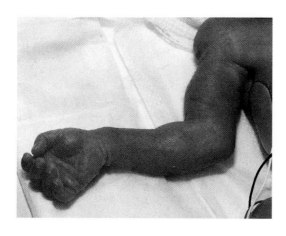

Figure 15. Fractured humerus in premature infant whose arm was around the neck of her twin at the time of delivery. There is discoloration and swelling, tenderness, pseudoparalysis, and irregularity in shape with shortening of the humerus. The arm healed quickly with normal shape, size, and function.

gins. Applying alternating pressure between the fingers, walk them along the clavicles to feel for a grating as the ends of the fracture site scrape across each other. It is helpful to flex or abduct the shoulder with the arm above the head while feeling over the bone to detect dislocation at a fracture line or to elicit pain on movement.

The examination of the clavicles is most efficiently done at the time of the neck examination but may be considered part of the regional examinations of the trunk or extremities as well.

The obstetrician often reports a cracking sensation or sound when a clavicle fractures at the time of delivery. The risk for fracture of the clavicle is higher in large infants delivered vaginally, particularly when there is shoulder dystocia and maternal history of high preg-

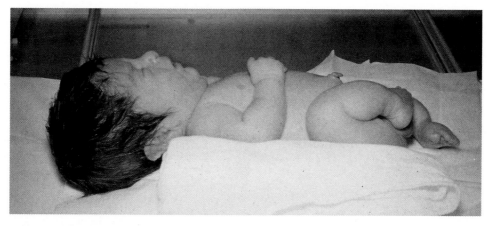

Figure 16. Osteogenesis imperfecta congenita (OI; type II) (49). The craniofacies are typical with shallow orbits, a small nose, and low nasal bridge, flat facial profile, and large fontanel. The extremities are short and the lower limbs remain in their fetal position because of severe deformation and multiple fractures. The sclera are deep blue in this form of OI (50). The defect is caused by heterozygous mutations of the COL1A1 and COL1A2 genes that encode the alpha 1(I) and alpha 2(I) chains of type I collagen, respectively. The severity of the clinical phenotype appears to be related to the type of mutation, its location in the alpha chain, the surrounding amino acid sequences, and the level of expression of the mutant allele. Most infants have their own de novo mutation, but the recurrence rate is about 7% from germline mosaicism in one parent (49).

nancy weight gain or obesity. Most fractured clavicles probably go undetected in the early neonatal period unless the obstetrician suggests the history because there are minimal symptoms and signs. The reported frequency of neonatally fractured clavicles ranges from less than 1% (28) to approximately 3% [2.9% (29) and 3.2% (30)]. Most fractures are not detected on initial examination and are more easily found at several days of age or when there is accompanying paresis (29). The clinical symptoms are subtle or absent because there appears to be little pain unless there is positional dislocation or swelling. One often overlooked sign is difficulty in feeding on the mother's breast opposite the side of the fracture (31). Callous formation at several weeks is not always detectable, but may be the presenting sign.

Fractures of other long bones, principally the humerus and femur, occur as birth injuries or in general conditions of exceptional bone fragility such as osteogenesis imperfecta or rickets associated with poor nutrition or disease (Figs. 15 and 16).

Special Clinical Assessment: Defining Direction and Range of Motion in Major Joints

The range of motion for key joints differs in neonates with notable limitations in the hips. Figures 17 through 30 depict the movements of the major joints involving more than flexion and extension.

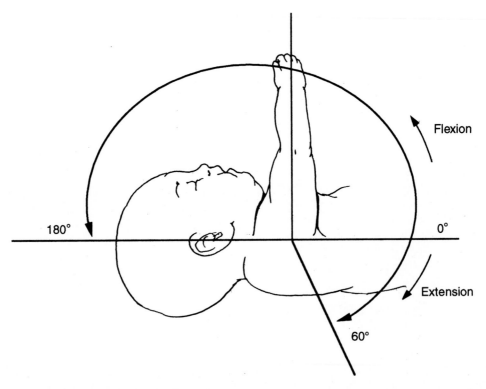

Figure 17. Flexion and extension of the shoulder. The zero starting position is with the arm at the side of the body. Elevation of the shoulder, flexion, or forward elevation is the maximum upward motion of the arm. This motion includes flexion of the humerus and elevation of the scapula. Slight external rotation and abduction are also required to reach maximal elevation. Extension of the shoulder, sometimes called posterior elevation, is motion in the opposite direction from forward elevation. Internal rotation is required for maximum extension.

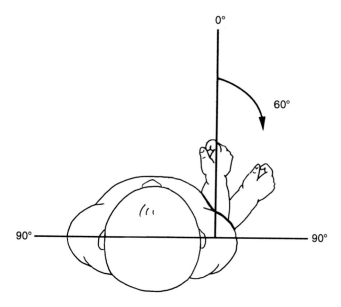

Figure 18. External rotation of the shoulder with the arm at the side (neutral position). The zero starting position is with the arm held comfortably against the thorax, the elbow flexed at 90°, and the forearm parallel to the sagittal plane of the body. The degree of external rotation is the maximum outward rotation of the arm from the sagittal plane. The trunk prevents accurate measurement of internal rotation in this position.

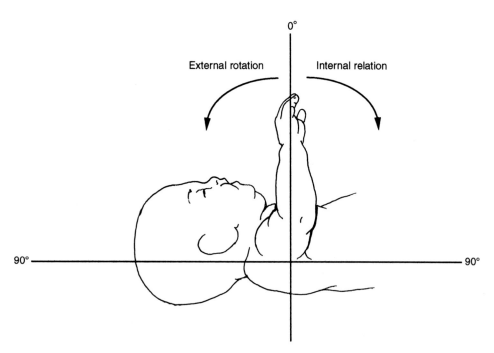

Figure 19. External/internal rotation of the shoulder with the arm in 90° of abduction. The zero starting position is with the arm abducted 90° and aligned with the plane of the scapula. The elbow is flexed 90°, and the forearm is perpendicular to the mattress. External rotation in abduction is the number of degrees the forearm moves away from the perpendicular toward the head. Internal rotation is the number of degrees the forearm moves away from perpendicular toward the feet. Adapted with permission (10).

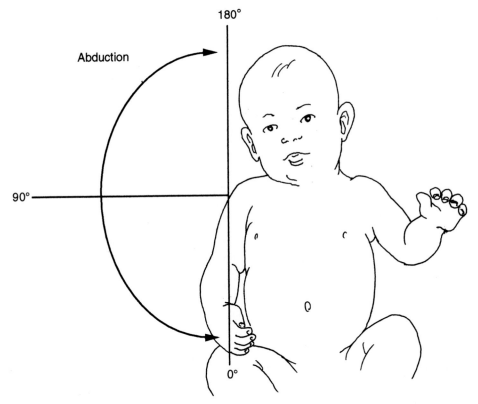

Figure 20. Neutral abduction of the shoulder. This is the upward motion of the arm in the coronal plane from the zero starting position.

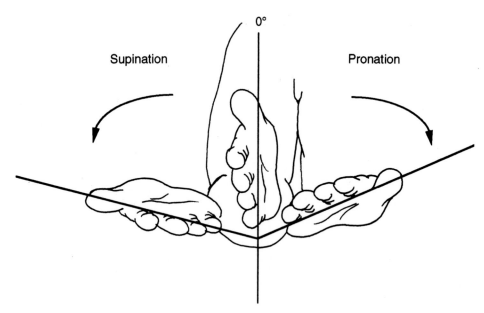

Figure 21. Forearm rotation, supination, and pronation.

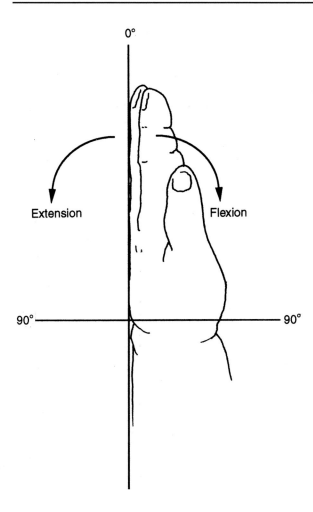

Figure 22. Flexion and extension of wrist. With the forearm in pronation, the zero starting position is with the ulnar border of the third metacarpal aligned with the axis of the distal forearm.

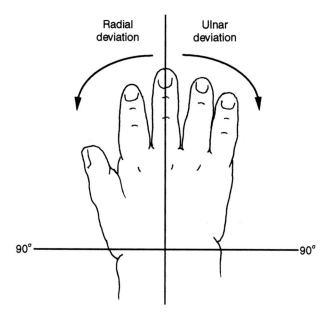

Figure 23. Radial and ulnar deviation. Zero starting position is with the forearm in pronation and the wrist in neutral position so the fingers are aligned with the axis of the forearm.

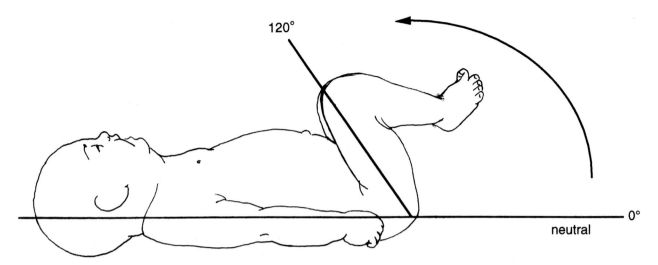

Figure 24. Flexion of hip. Maximum flexion is the point where the pelvis begins to rotate.

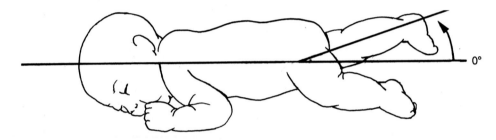

Figure 25. Extension of hip. Most neonates cannot reach a true zero starting position in prone to measure extension for at least several weeks because of limited joint extension but the angles of the two sides should be equal.

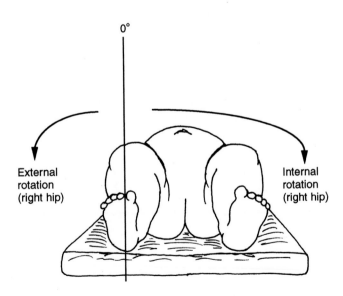

Figure 26. External/internal rotation of the hip. Rotation is measured by rotating the extended leg, thereby rotating the hip joint. Maximum external rotation is achieved when the pelvis starts to tilt, a movement that can be ascertained by keeping one hand on the pelvis.

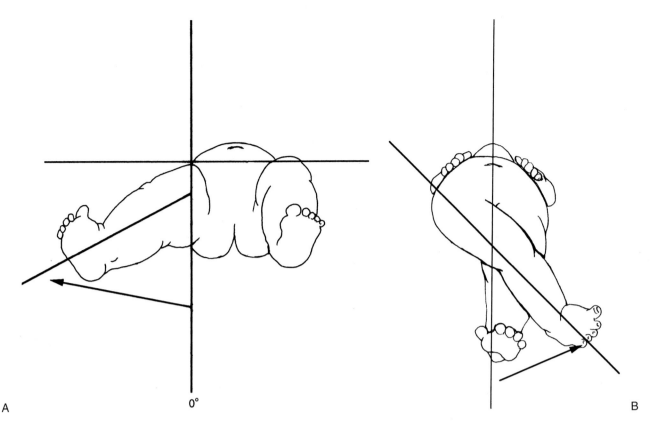

A   0°   B

Figure 27. A: Abduction of hip. Abduction is measured in degrees from the zero starting position. Maximum abduction is reached when the pelvis starts to tilt, a movement that can be detected by the examiner keeping his or her hand on the patient's pelvis when moving the leg. Adapted with permission (10). **B:** Adduction of hip. Because the limb at rest interferes with movement of the other across the midline, the extremity being measured can be lifted over the other. Alternatively, adduction can be assessed with the knee and hip flexed.

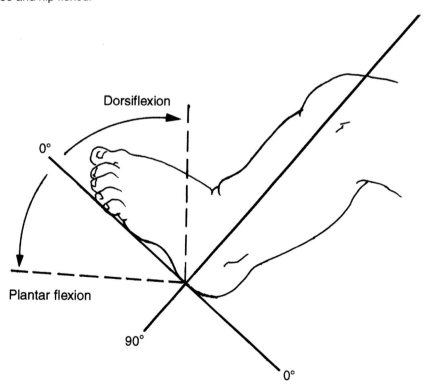

Figure 28. Dorsiflexion and plantar flexion of ankle. The zero starting position is with the knee flexed to relax the heel cord. The foot is perpendicular to the tibia. The lines subtending the angle to be measured are the long axis of the leg and the lateral side of the plantar surface of the foot. Note that when assessing flexion for gestational age and for motor tone, the leg should be fully extended so that both the gastrocnemius and soleus muscle tone is assessed. When assessing the joint itself for mobility, the knee is flexed to eliminate the affect of muscle tone.

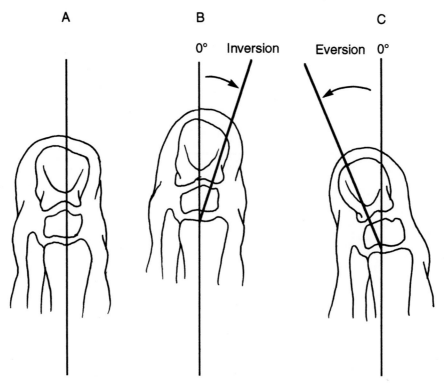

Figure 29. Zero starting position of right foot. **A:** The patient is lying prone with the knee flexed and the ankle in neutral dorsiflexion. **B:** Inversion of foot. The heel is moved medially, and the degree of inversion is measured from the zero starting position. **C:** Eversion of foot. The heel is moved outward and the degree of motion is measured from the zero starting position.

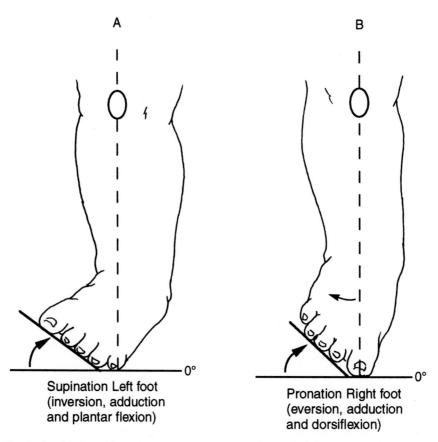

Supination Left foot
(inversion, adduction
and plantar flexion)

Pronation Right foot
(eversion, adduction
and dorsiflexion)

Figure 30. **A:** Supination of foot. Compound motion includes inversion, adduction, and plantar flexion. **B:** Pronation of foot. Compound movement includes eversion, abduction, and dorsiflexion.

CLINICAL EXAMPLES

A classification of malformations of the upper extremities has been proposed by Swanson and adopted by the American Society for Surgery and the Hand, the International Federation of Societies for Surgery of the Hand, and the International Society of Prosthetics and Orthotics (32). This classification based on developmental similarities replaces the more complicated systems that used only Latin and Greek terms or eponyms. Clinical examples are shown in the figures cited in the following outline.

I. Failure of formation of parts (arrest and develop)
   A. Transverse terminal deficiencies
   B. Longitudinal deficiencies
      1. Phocomelia: complete, proximal, distal (Fig. 31)
      2. Radial deficiencies (radial clubhand) (Fig. 32)
      3. Central deficiencies (cleft hand) (Figs. 33 and 34)
      4. Ulnar deficiencies (ulnar clubhand)
      5. Hypoplastic digits
II. Failure of differentiation (separation of parts)
   A. Synostoses: elbow, forearm, wrist, metacarpals, phalanges (Fig. 35)
   B. Radial head dislocation
   C. Syndactyly (Figs. 35 and 36)
   D. Soft tissue contracture
      1. Arthrogryposis (Fig. 4)
      2. Pterygium cubitale
      3. Trigger digit
      4. Camptodactyly
   E. Skeletal contracture
      1. Clinodactyly
      2. Delta phalanx
III. Duplication
   A. Duplicate thumb (preaxial polydactyly) (Fig. 37)
   B. Triphalangeal thumb
   C. Central polydactyly (polysyndactyly) (Figs. 38 and 39)
   D. Postaxial polydactyly (little finger polydactyly) (Figs. 40 and 41)
IV. Macrodactyly (overgrowth of all or portions of upper limb)
 V. Undergrowth (hypoplasia)
 VI. Congenital constriction band syndrome (Fig. 42)
VII. General skeletal abnormalities (Figs. 16 and 31)

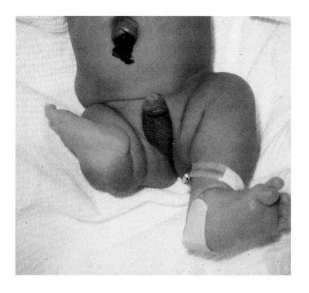

Figure 31. Caudal regression in diabetic embryopathy with bilateral proximal femoral focal deficiency and right tibial and fibular hypoplasia. Typically, in this clinical situation, the hip is held in flexion, abduction, and external rotation (15).

Most anomalies affecting the extremities are congenital reduction anomalies with deficiencies that are either transverse or longitudinal (15). The loss may be an entire limb (amelia), the distal portion, or intercalary with distal structures preserved and proximal ones lost. Partial loss of a limb is hemimelia. Preservation of the hands or feet with loss of the proximal and middle parts is phocomelia. Complete absence of the hand is acheiria, of the foot apodia, and of the finger adactylia. If a limb is short in the upper arm or thigh, it is called rhizomelic shortening; if in the forearm or calf, it is mesomelic; and if in the hand or foot, it is acromelic (Fig. 2). Because development of a distal segment depends in large measure on a normal proximal segment, complex involvement is usually categorized by the proximal abnormality.

Although the system proposed by Swanson is helpful, there are cases that do not clearly fall within these divisions. Anomalies of the lower extremities are not included in this classification, although some are comparable (33). Classification of limb anomalies is important for determining the probable causes, clinical associations, and potential for correction or amelioration. Any single cause may effect a wide range in severity of a malformation, likely reflecting variable timing. For example, in the caudal regression sequence, most often related to diabetic embryopathy, the lower extremity may be spared or severely affected as sirenomelia resembling a mermaid or as shown in Fig. 31. A classification of limb deficiencies based on morphologic differences suggested in the genetics literature is clinically useful and applies to both upper and lower extremities but this system also has overlap and some outliers (Table 3) (4).

Several large reviews of limb deficiency defects from population birth registries suggest the prevalence to be more than 1 in 1,000 births and higher when stillbirths are included

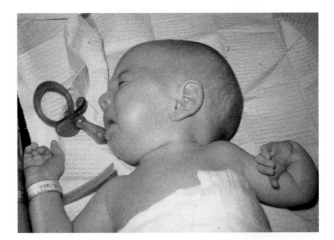

Figure 32. Radial hypoplasia in infant with VACTERL association. The forearm is markedly foreshortened, and the hand is radially deviated. In the presence of preaxial limb deficiencies the association with other malformations is so strong that complete evaluation is indicated.

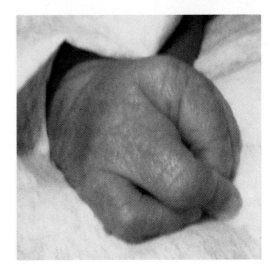

Figure 33. Cleft hand. Deficiency of the central digital rays results in a split hand or foot (lobster claw) also called ectrodactyly. The long finger with a part of the metacarpal is most often affected with other fingers showing camptodactyly, clinodactyly, oligodactyly, or syndactyly (51). When two or more limbs are involved, autosomal-dominant inheritance with variable penetrance is common. Frequently associated anomalies include cleft foot, cleft lip, cleft palate, imperforate anus, congenital heart disease, radial ulnar synostosis, and ectodermal dysplasia (35).

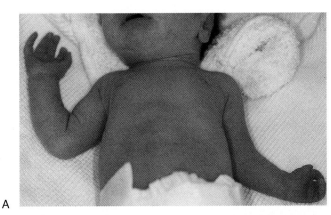
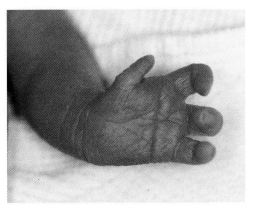

A

B

Figure 34. A: Abnormal resting posture of left-sided, radial hemimelia associated with arthrogryposis, short radius, hypoplastic thumb, and missing digit. There is shortening of the left forearm, mild radial deviation, and a small hand. The absence of creases in the antecubital fossa signal the lack of mobility at the elbow. **B:** Note the single transverse palmar crease and flexion contractures of the fingers. The thumbnail was rudimentary. An appropriate evaluation includes investigation of hematologic, gastrointestinal, and cardiac systems as well as bone films to determine the development of the radius and ulna and which digit is missing.

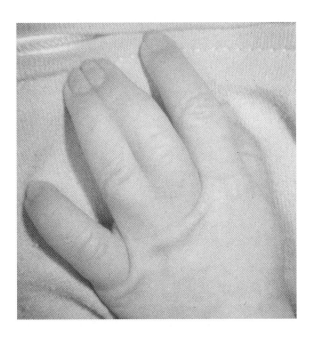

Figure 35. Syndactyly or simple synostosis of the middle and ring fingers. If only the soft tissue is involved, a synostosis is simple; if the bone is fused, the synostosis is complex. Radiographs are necessary to determine how complete fusion is.

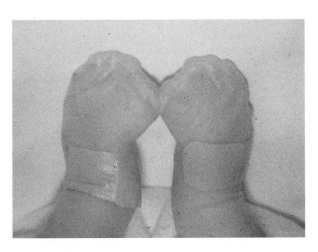

Figure 36. Severe complete, complex syndactyly in Apert's syndrome of craniosynostosis and syndactyly. The foot appears covered in a mitten of skin, so the fused toes are barely discernible.

(4,34). Deficiencies in upper extremities are far more common than in lower limbs and unilateral more than bilateral, although this latter variable is more affected by the type of deficiency (3,4,34). When a deficiency is preaxial, the association with malformations in other systems is far greater than in postaxial deficiencies. Radial defects in particular are strongly associated with other malformations, with reported involvement ranging up to 85% (3,4). Because one can assume an underreporting of subtle or undiagnosed internal malformations in birth registries, the clinical examination requires thorough evaluation of all systems in the presence of preaxial deficits.

Clinical Example: Preaxial Duplication

Figure 37 depicts duplication of the thumb (synonyms preaxial polydactyly, extra thumb). Duplications of the thumb may be classified by how far proximally the duplication occurs and by how complete the separation is (35):

Type I: duplication of the distal phalanx only
Type II: duplication at the proximal phalangeal level (Fig. 37)
Type III: duplication at the metacarpal level

Wood has proposed simplifying the classification of thumb anomalies to descriptions such as inadequate thumb, fingerlike thumb, contracted thumb, crooked thumb, extra thumb, and unusual thumb (36). Such simplification would make the Latin teachers groan but may be better for communication among the parent, the primary clinician, and the orthopedic surgeon.

Associations of anomalies of the thumb:

With hematologic problems as major association
    TAR syndrome (thrombocytopenia with absent radii)
    Aase syndrome (triphalangeal thumb and congenital anemia)
    Fanconi syndrome (radial hypoplasia, hyperpigmentation, and pancytopenia)
    Congenital hypoplastic anemia of Diamond-Blackfan

Table 3. *Morphologic classification of limb deficiency defects*

Type of deficiency	Description
Amelia	Complete absence of a limb
Rudimentary limb	Severe hypoplasia of all skeletal components of a limb
Terminal transverse	Absence or severe hypoplasia of distal segments of both axial sides of the limb with proximal structures essentially normal. Can be subdivided into aphalangia, adactyly, acheiria or apodia, and hemimelias.
Longitudinal preaxial	Absence or severe hypoplasia of preaxial structures. Can be subdivided into radial and tibial.
Longitudinal postaxial	Absence or severe hypoplasia of postaxial structures. Can be subdivided into ulnar and fibular.
Intercalary	Absence or severe hypoplasia of the proximal part of the limb with normal or near normal distal parts. Can be subdivided into deficiency of long bones, phocomelias and other, e.g., absent patellae.
Split hand/foot	Absence or severe hypoplasia of the central axis mainly involving the digits with normal or near normal lateral digits. Can be subdivided into typical or atypical "lobster claw" defect or fifth digit monodactyly.
Digital deficiencies	Asymmetric deficiencies of the digits usually associated with ring constrictions and/or syndactyly, often distal
Other	Limb deficiency defects not classifiable into the above categories
Mixed	Presence of limb deficiency defects of different morphologic types usually in different limbs.

Modified from Evans et al., ref. 4, with permission.

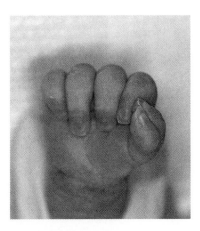

Figure 37. Duplication of the thumb, type II.

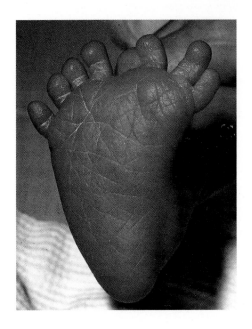

Figure 38. Preaxial polydactyly of toes. This form of polydactyly carries a much higher association with other anomalies compared with postaxial polydactyly.

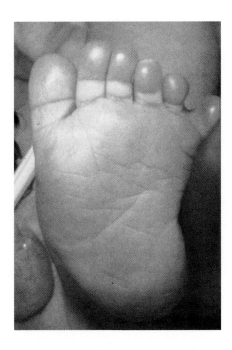

Figure 39. Metatarsus adductus with postaxial polydactyly.

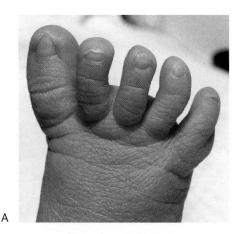
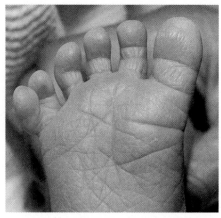

Figure 40. Postaxial polydactyly of toes. A cursory examination (**A**) without a toe count might not show the hidden extra digits (**B**).

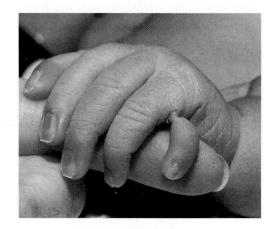

Figure 41. Postaxial extra digit (postminimus polydactyly) on left hand with a well-formed nail indicating the presence of underlying bone but with a thin attaching stalk. This type of polydactyly is familial (autosomal-dominant or dominant with variable penetrance) and most common in black infants. Little finger polydactyly is the most frequent type by at least 8 to 1 (35).

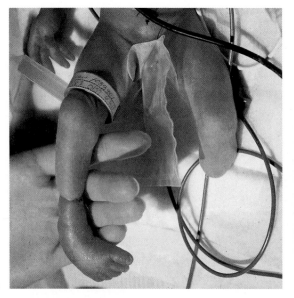
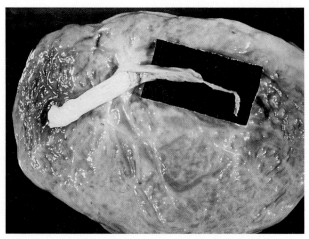

Figure 42. Amnionic band amputation. Such transverse amputations are characterized by nonuniformity between sides, with no attempt at regrowth more typical of vascular accidents.

Nonhematologic associations

Holt-Oram: skeletal defects of the upper extremities and congenital heart disease

VATER association: vertebral defects, anal atresia, tracheoesophageal fistula, radial dysplasia including thumb hypoplasia

Rubenstein-Taybi syndrome: short stature, downward-slanting palpebral fissures, broad thumbs and great toes, mental deficiency

Triphalangeal thumb: autosomal dominant or as part of the syndromes associated with preaxial abnormalities listed herein

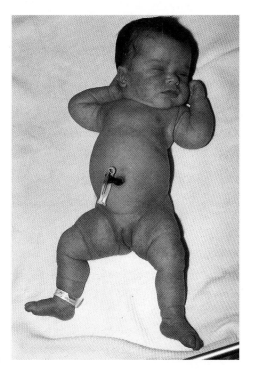
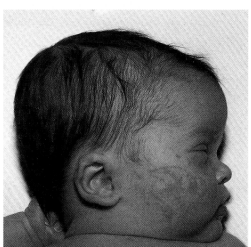
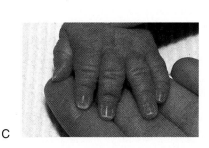
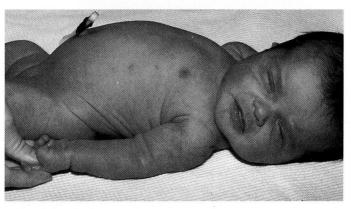

Figure 43. Achondroplasia. **A:** At first glance an affected newborn infant can appear normal, unless one looks more closely at the proportions of the body regions. The thorax is relatively small compared with the abdomen and head circumference. The upper to lower ratio was excessive, at greater than 1.7:1. **B:** Megalocephaly with mild mid-face hypoplasia, a low nasal bridge, and prominent forehead. Hydrocephalus secondary to a narrow foramen magnum is a consideration in achondroplasia. **C:** Trident hand. The middle fingers are the same length with short proximal and mid-phalanges. **D:** The humerus is short compared with the forearm. The point at which the hand reaches along the trunk is deceptively low because the infant's back is not straight.

Clinical Example: Abnormal Limb Length in Achondroplasia

The findings at birth are subtle because the proximal shortening typical in older patients is not as notable. This is the most common chondrodysplasia, with a frequency of approximately 1:26,000. This autosomal-dominant condition results after a mutation of the fibroblast growth factor receptor 3 (FGFR3). This receptor is expressed in cartilage and mediates the effect of fibroblast growth factors on chondrocytes (37,38) (Fig. 43).

Clinical Example: Abnormal Range of Motion in Arthrogryposis

When generalized, this condition is also called amyoplasia congenita or arthrogryposis multiplex congenita (AMC). The extremities are tubular and smooth, with an absence of flexion creases. The infants are born with rigid joints and adjacent muscle atrophy, the upper extremities have internally rotated shoulders, elbows locked in extension, and wrists in flexion. The lower extremities have dislocated hips, variable position of fixation in the knees, and clubfeet (Fig. 4) (39–43).

The condition occurs in approximately one per 3,000 births, with a variety of fetal neurologic or myopathic processes that lead to decreased fetal movement, muscle atrophy, and tight soft-tissue contractures around the affected joints. Most cases are neurogenic in origin (42,43). With prenatal diagnosis and elective termination, the incidence in live births is decreasing. Most cases are sporadic, but the findings can be associated with other conditions, including Potter syndrome, meningomyelocele, diastrophic dwarfism, and congenital muscular dystrophy. When affecting the hands and feet only, it may be an autosomal-dominant inherited condition as the distal arthrogryposis syndrome. An X-linked pattern is found is some types (44).

In the most common types of AMC there are often significant otolaryngologic findings with micrognathia, poor sucking, high arched palate, and an omega-shaped epiglottis. Airway compromise, achalasia, and aspiration pneumonitis are frequent complications as might be expected when there is a neurogenic etiology (45).

The prognosis depends primarily on the associated neuromuscular cause and with the local response depending on physical therapy, splinting, and orthopedic surgery (41).

GLOSSARY

The glossary includes general terms, as well as those describing movement and congenital limb absences (46).

Abduction   Movement away from mid-line of body in frontal plane; applied to hip, shoulder, fingers, thumb, and foot. The mid-line reference point is a central line in the body for proximal joints and the central part of a limb for distal joints (Figs. 20,27).

Acheiria   Absence of the hand (carpals, metacarpals, phalanges).

Adactylia   Absence of all five rays (metacarpals and phalanges).

Adactylia, partial   Absence of all or part of the first through fifth rays (phalanges and metacarpals).

Adduction   Movement toward the mid-line in frontal plane as opposed to abduction (see Abduction).

Amelia   Complete absence of a limb.

Amyoplasia congenita   Synonym *Arthrogryposis*. Disorder of fascia and muscle resulting in contracted joints during growth.

Amyotonia congenita   Muscle disorder of the newborn, usually fatal; characterized by muscle degeneration with failure of replacement (congenital hypotonia, Oppenheim's disease); several types include Werdnig-Hoffman disease (CNS origin), rod disease (microscopic rods forming within muscle cells), and central core disease, which is not fatal.

Ankylosis   Consolidation and abnormal immobility of a joint.

Anteversion   In reference to the neck of humerus or femur, is an anterior rotation.

Aphalangia, complete   Absence of one or more phalanges from all five digits.

Aphalangia, partial   Absence of the proximal or middle phalanx from one or more digits, one through five. A common deformity is a complete loss of the radius with the rest of the arm and hand being intact—intercalary complete paraxial hemimelia. Proximal focal femoral deficiency (PFFD) is an absence of a portion of the hip and/or proximal femur.

Apodia   Absence of the foot.

Apposition   Contact of two adjacent parts; bringing together as in a finger movement, the thumb to index finger.

Arthrochalasis   Abnormal relaxation or flaccidity of a joint.

Arthrodysplasia   Deformity of various joints; hereditary condition.

Arthrogryposis   Persistent flexure or contracture of a joint; usually related to a congenital neuromuscular disorder.

Avulsion   Tearing away of a part.

Camptodactyly   Bent finger; commonly referred to as a congenital flexion deformity of the proximal interphalangeal joint, usually of the little finger. It is associated with some syndromes involving multiple pterygia or trismus but is most often a minor variant that is inherited as an autosomal-dominant disorder.

Cartilage-hair hypoplasia   Rare dwarfism, similar to achondroplasia.

Circumduction   A maneuver or movement of a ball-and-socket joint in a circular motion; for example, the shoulder can circumduct 180° with six movements possible.

Clinodactyly   Angulation deformity of the finger, in either radial or ulnar deviation. Instead of the proximal and distal interphalangeal creases being parallel, they are trapezoidal, with the shorter dimension on the side toward which the digit is bent. The little finger is most commonly involved. Although associated with a variety of syndromes, it is a minor variant in most occurrences.

Clubfoot   Foot deformity resulting in the appearance of a golf club. The components include forefoot adduction with medial displacement of the talus, ankle equinus, and heel varus. The result is that the foot turns in with the heel pulled medially (Fig. 9).

Clubhand   (radial clubhand, talipomanus)   Position of the hand in strong flexion and radial deviation, caused by partial or incomplete absence of the radius and thumb.

Coxa brevia   Short hip with a small femoral head caused by premature closure of the epiphysis.

Coxa magna   Enlarged femoral head.

Coxa plana   Synonym *Legg-Perthes disease*. Flat femoral head (osteochondrosis) of the capitular epiphysis of the femur.

Coxa valga   Hip deformity in which the angle of the axis of the head and neck of the femur and the axis of its shaft (neck shaft angle) is increased.

Coxa vara   Reduced neck and shaft angle, usually caused by failure of normal bone growth; coxa adducta.

Delta phalanx   Deviation of the finger caused by a triangular, oval, or trapezoid bone with an abnormal epiphyseal plate. The abnormality is most often bilateral in the proximal phalanx of the thumb and little finger.

Deviation, radial   Deviation of the hand at the wrist such that the hand is directed radially; measured in degrees, from 0 with the hand in mid-line (Figs. 32,34).

Deviation, ulnar   Deviation of the hand at the wrist such that the hand is directed in an ulnar direction; measured in degrees, from 0 with the hand in mid-line.

Diastasis   May be one of two types: (1) a disjointing of two bones that are parallel to one another, for example, radius and ulna, tibia and fibula complex, or (2) the rupture of any "solid" joint, as in diastasis of the symphysis pubis. Such injuries tend to occur in association with other fractures and are then called fracture–diastases.

Diastrophic dwarfism   Autosomal-recessive dwarfism with flattening subluxation of various epiphyses.

Dislocation of the knee, congenital   A progressive anterior dislocation of the tibia caused by abnormal tissue remodeling. It is not equivalent to genu recurvatum.

Dislocation of the femoral head, anterior   Dislocation of the femoral head anteriorly.

Dislocation of the femoral head, posterior   One in which the femoral head slips posteriorly; more common than anterior dislocation.

Dorsiflexion   The toe-up motion of the ankle expressed in degrees, from the 0° position of the foot at rest on the ground in the standing position (Fig. 28).

Dysplasia of the hip, congenital   A failure of normal bony modeling of the hip socket (acetabulum) and/or ball (femoral head).

Ehlers-Danlos syndrome   Generalized joint capsular laxity occurring as a hereditary disease.

Eversion   When applied to the heel, describes the degree of motion of the heel pushed outward with the ankle in neutral position; when applied to the foot, describes the combined motions of dorsiflexion, pronation, and abduction (Fig. 29).

Extension   In the limbs, moving the extremity away from the body; in the spine, bending posteriorly (Figs. 17,25).

Familial periodic paralysis   Synonym *Myotonia intermittens.* Disorder of muscle metabolism in which periods of partial to nearly complete paralysis occur.

Flexion   To bend from the joint as in flexion movements of the spine at the waist (anterior or lateral) (Figs. 17,24).

Flexion, palmar   Bending the wrist with the palm up (Fig. 22).

Flexion, plantar   The toe-down motion of the foot at the ankle expressed in degrees, from the 0° position of the foot at rest on the ground in the standing position (Fig. 28).

Forefoot equinus   Plantar flexion of the forefoot on the hindfoot, producing a high arch foot with the apex of the deformity at the mid-tarsal joint.

Forefoot valgus   An everted structural position of the forefoot that causes abnormal pronation of the foot.

Forefoot varus   An inverted structural position of the forefoot that causes abnormal supination of the foot.

Fracture, depressed   Usually used to describe skull or particular surface fractures where the fragment is displaced below the overall level of the skull or articular surface.

Gastrocnemius equinus   An abnormal tightness of the Achilles tendon that restricts dorsiflexion of the foot in the ankle joint. This can be congenital or acquired.

Gaucher disease   (cerebroside reticulocytosis)   Bone disorder resulting from lipid storage disease that is due to the absence of glucocerebrosidase. Excessive production of histiocytes with interference of marrow function and destruction of bone occurs.

Genu recurvatum   Ability of the knee to bend backward; caused by trauma, prolonged intrauterine pressure, or general joint laxity (Fig. 10).

Genu valgum   Synonym *Knock-knee.* Deformity in which knees are close together, with ankle space increased. Even though valgum would indicate bending away from the midline, the valgum refers to the distal portion, which, when the knees are bowed in, forces the ankles away from the mid-line.

Genu varum   Deformity in which knees are bowed out and ankles are close in; may be associated with internal tibial torsion (ITT).

Hallux abductus   Great toe pointing toward second toe (transverse plane deformity).

Hallux adductus   Great toe pointing toward mid-line of body (transverse plane deformity). Hallux varus.

Hemimelia   Absence of the forearm and hand or leg and foot portion of a limb.

Hemimelia, complete paraxial   Lengthwise loss of one side or the other of the forearm and hand or leg and foot.

Hemimelia, incomplete paraxial   Similar to hemimelia, but a portion of affected bone remains, for example, complete absence of the ulna with a portion of the diameter of the radius intact.

Hemimelia, partial   Absence of part of the forearm or leg.

Hunter syndrome   Similar to Hurler syndrome, but less severely deforming; sex-linked inheritance; type II mucopolysaccharidosis.

Hurler syndrome   Severely deforming condition associated with blindness, mental retardation, and early death; type I mucopolysaccharidosis.

Infantile cortical hyperostosis   Painful hyperostosis with involvement of long bones and the mandible. This usually occurs in infants 5 months of age and younger and is associated with irritability, fever, and soft tissue.

Inversion   When applied to the heel, describes the degree of motion of the heel pushed inward with ankle in neutral position; when applied to the foot, describes the combined motions of plantar flexion, supination, and adduction (Fig. 29).

Kirner's deformity   Progressive, spontaneous incurving of the terminal phalanx of the fifth digit, not present in early infancy.

Limb absence, intercalary longitudinal   A congenital deficiency in the middle of a limb that leaves a longitudinal portion of the limb intact.

Limb absence, intercalary transverse   A congenital deficiency in the middle of a limb but that is a complete across the limb.

Limb absence, terminal longitudinal   A congenital deficiency at the end of a limb that leaves a longitudinal portion of the limb intact.

Limb absence, terminal transverse   A congenital deficiency at the end of a limb that is a complete across-the-limb loss.

Lobster-claw deformity   Absence of the central rays (metacarpals and fingers), resulting in a lobster-claw appearance (Fig. 33).

Luxatio coxae congenita   Congenital dislocation of the hip (CDH).

Macrodactyly   Overgrowth in size and diameter in one or more digits.

Madelung's deformity   Congenital or traumatic shortening of the radius with relative overgrowth of the distal ulna. Wrist is flexed and radially deviated.

Maroteaux-Lamy syndrome   Growth retardation, lumbar kyphosis, sternal protrusion; no mental retardation; type VI mucopolysaccharidosis.

Metatarsus abductus   Forefoot angles laterally from a midline axis.

Metatarsus adductocavus   Forefoot turned inward in association with a high arch, usually seen in clubfoot deformity that includes heel varus (talipes equinovarus).

Metatarsus adductus   Forefoot angles medially from a midline axis.

Metatarsus atavicus   Abnormal shortness of the first metatarsal bone so that it is the same length as the second metatarsus.

Metatarsus varus   Rotation of the forefoot (metatarsals) so that the plantar surface faces medially.

Morquio's syndrome   Dwarfing disease affecting mostly the spine and the hips; little or no mental retardation; type IV mucopolysaccharidosis, chondro-osteodystrophy.

Myasthenia gravis   Syndrome of attacks of muscle weakness that are episodic and reversible. Also called Erb-Goldflam disease.

Myatrophy   Muscle wasting.

Myoasthenia   Synonym *Amyosthenia.* Lack of muscle strength.

Myoclonus   Any disorder in which rapid rigidity and relaxation alternate; myoclonia.

Myoischemia   Local deficiency of blood supply in muscle.

Myolysis   Disintegration or degeneration of muscle tissue.

Myopalmus   Muscle twitching.

Myoparalysis   Synonym *Myoparesis.* Paralysis of muscle.

Myopathy   Any disease of the muscles.

Myotonia   Increased muscular irritability and contractibility with decreased power of relaxation; tension and tonic spasm of muscle.

Myotonia, congenital   Synonym *Thomsen's disease.* Disorder, found at birth, in which initiation and cessation of voluntary movement are delayed.

Niemann-Pick disease   Fatal fat storage disease marked by absence of sphingomyelinase affecting bone marrow in infancy.

Opposition   Applied mostly to the thumb but also to little finger; describes the motion required to bring about opposition, or the setting opposite, of the thumb against little finger (pulp surfaces). For the thumb, opposition is the combined action of abduction, rotation, and flexion (compare to apposition).

Osteogenesis imperfecta   Synonyms *Osteitis fragilitans, fragilitas ossium congenita, osteopsathyrosis idiopathica, brittle bones.* Condition in which bones are abnormally brittle and subject to fractures.

Osteomalacia   Rickets, a reduction of physical strength of bone caused by decreased mineralization of osteoid; may result from vitamin D, calcium, or phosphorus deficiency with or without renal disease. Osteomalacia in the child is associated with the growth deformities of rickets.

Osteomyelitis   Inflammation of bone marrow, cortex, tissue, and periosteum; can be caused by any organism, but usually bacteria.

Osteopathia striata   Synonym *Voorhoeve's disease*. Changes of bone giving distinct striped appearance on x-ray examinations; lesions characterized by multiple condensation of cancellous bone tissue, sometimes said to be in association with osteopetrosis.

Osteopenia   Any state in which bone mass is reduced below normal. This would include conditions of osteoporosis and osteomalacia.

Osteopetrosis   Synonyms *Albers-Schönberg disease, osteosclerosis, osteosclerosis fragilis*. Hereditary disease of bone, with areas of chalky condensed bone within bone.

Osteoporosis   Diminution of both the mineral and matrix components of bone such that the remaining bone is normal in composition but reduced in total bone mass. The secondary cause of osteoporosis is most commonly immobilization, such as casting. Primary osteoporosis is an age-related disorder.

Osteopsathyrosis   Osteogenesis imperfecta.

Phocomelia, complete   Presence of only a hand or foot.

Phocomelia, distal   Hand directly attached to upper arm; or foot directly attached to thigh.

Phocomelia, proximal   Presence of hand and forearm with absence of upper arm, or leg and foot with absence of thigh.

Poland syndrome   Absence of the pectoral head of the pectoralis major muscles associated with the deformities in the thumb ray or fingers. Simple absence of a portion of the pectoralis muscle is more common and functionally unimportant. The absence causes loss of an anterior axillary fold and cephalad positioning of the nipple.

Polydactyly   Congenital deformity, excess number of digits. It is most commonly postaxial, occurring on the ulnar side of the fifth digit (postminimus polydactyly). Tends to be hereditary (Figs. 37–41).

Polyostotic fibrous dysplasia   Synonym *Albright's syndrome*. Disease marked by fibrous tissue replacement of bone with resulting deformities and clinical appearance of café-au-lait skin pigmentation and precocious puberty.

Popliteal pterygium syndrome   Severe flexion of the knee and equinus deformity of the foot associated with the popliteal web extending from the ischium to the heel. Other concurrent deformities include toenail dysplasia and oral cavity abnormalities such as cleft palate or lip pits.

Postaxial   A position relating to embryologic development of the caudad portion of an extremity, thus including the third through fifth fingers; the ulnar side. On the lower extremity because of opposite rotation in human, the postaxial structures include the third through fifth toes; the fibular side.

Preaxial   A position relating to embryologic development of the cephalad portion of an extremity, thus including the thumb and index finger; the radial side. On the lower extremity because of opposite rotation in human, the preaxial structures include the great and first toes; the tibial side.

Pronation of foot   Complex motion of the foot that produces flattening of the arch. This motion is normal during gait: however, excessive pronation can lead to pathologic changes of the foot. The plantar surface turns down and out (Fig. 30B).

Pronation of hand   Palm-down position of hand with elbow at a 90° angle, brought about by the motion of the radius around the ulna (posterior rotation) (Fig. 21).

Retroversion   In reference to the neck of femur or humerus, a posterior rotation.

Rickets   Failure of disposition of bone salts within the organic matrix of cartilage and bone associated with stunting of growth and bone deformities.

Rocker-bottom flatfoot, congenital   Synonyms *Congenital vertical talus, congenital convex pes valgus*. Condition present at birth; abnormal equinus position of talus with valgus position of the heel, resulting in a foot that looks like a rocker and has a prominence below the medial ankle.

Rocker-bottom foot   Deformity of the foot such that the arch is disrupted and looks like a rocker bottom. This may be a complication of clubfoot treatment or myelomeningocele.

Rotation, external   In a frontal plane, away from mid-line (Figs. 18,19,26).

Rotation, internal   In a frontal plane, toward the mid-line (Figs. 18,19,26).

Sanfilippo syndrome   Mild skeletal deformity but more severe mental retardation than types I and II; type III mucopolysaccharidosis.

Scheie's syndrome No mental impairment but noted corneal clouding, aortic disease, and stiff joints; type V mucopolysaccharidosis.

Spondyloepiphyseal dysplasia Disorder of growth affecting both the spine and the ends of the long bones.

Subluxation Incomplete or partial dislocation in that one bone forming a joint is displaced only partially from its normal position; also a chronic tendency of a bone to become partially dislocated, in contrast to an outright dislocation, e.g., the shoulder, patella, and, in infants, hip.

Supernumerary digits Extra nubbins of fingers or thumb, usually possessing no function (Fig. 41).

Supination of foot Complex motion of the foot that produces an increase in the arch. The motion is normal during gait: however, excessive supination can lead to pathologic changes of the foot. The plantar surface turns inward (Fig. 30A).

Supination of hand Palm-up position of the hand with elbow flexed at a 90° angle, brought about by motion of the radius around the ulna (anterior rotation) (Fig. 21).

Symphalangism (multiple) Congenital fusion of multiple PIP joints or of a digit from end to end.

Symphalangism (true) Congenital fusion of a single PIP joint.

Syndactyly Fusion of two or more fingers in which there may be involvement of soft tissue only (simple) (Fig. 35) or that may include a fusion of bone or cartilage (complex) (Fig. 36). It is found most often between the second and third toes and the third and fourth fingers. It occurs as an isolated defect or as part of syndromes (deLange, Smith-Lemli-Optiz or Poland anomaly). Complete syndactyly occurs in Apert's syndrome (Fig. 36).

Talipes calcaneocavus High-arched foot with fixed dorsiflexion (pes cavus).

Talipes calcaneovalgus Abnormally dorsiflexed hindfoot with turning out of the heel.

Talipes calcaneovarus High arch associated with turning in of the foot.

Talipes calcaneus Synonym *Cavus foot.* Abnormally dorsiflexed hindfoot, with increased dorsiflexion of the calcaneus.

Talipes cavovalgus High arch and turning out of the heel.

Talipes cavovarus High arch associated with turning in of the foot.

Talipes equinovalgus Plantar flexion and turning out of the calcaneus.

Talipes equinovarus Turning of the heel inward with increased plantar flexion. More precisely, a clubfoot, often having the components of talipes equinovarus with metatarsus adductus. This condition can result from paralysis or from unknown causes (Fig. 9).

Talipes planovalgus Synonym *Pes planovalgus.* Depression of the longitudinal arch associated with heel valgus (pes planus).

Talipes planus Synonyms *Pes planus, flatfoot.* Depression of the longitudinal arch; no specified heel valgus is implied by this term. A flexible pes planus is flatfoot with general laxity but no other specific disease process (pes planus).

Valgus The distal part is away from the mid-line, e.g., genu valgus (knock-kneed).

Varus The distal part is toward the mid-line, e.g., genu varus (bowlegged).

References

1. Fanconi S, Ensner S, Knecht B. Effects of paralysis with pancuronium bromide on joint mobility in premature infants. *J Pediatr* 1995;127:134–136.
2. Molteni RA, del Rosario Ames M. Sclerema neonatorum and joint contractures at birth as a potential complication of chronic in utero hypoxia. *Am J Obstet Gynecol* 1986;155:380–381.
3. Froster UG, Baird PA. Upper limb deficiencies and associated malformations: a population-based study. *Am J Med Genet* 1992;44:767–81.
4. Evans JA, Vitez M, Czeizel A. Congenital abnormalities associated with limb deficiency defects: a population study based on cases from the Hungarian Congenital Malformation Registry (1975–1984). *Am J Med Genet* 1994;49:52–66.
5. Moore KL, Persaud TVN, Shiota K. *Color Atlas of Clinical Embryology.* 1st ed. Philadelphia: WB Saunders; 1994.
6. Hall JG, Froster-Iskenius UG, Allanson JE. *Handbook of Normal Physical Measurements.* Oxford: Oxford University Press; 1989.
7. Hoffer MM. Joint motion limitation in newborns. *Clin Orthop* 1980;148:94–96.
8. Forero N, Okamura LA, Larson MA. Normal ranges of hip motion in neonates. *J Pediatr Orthop* 1989; 9:391–395.

9. Dunne KB, Clarren SK. The origin of prenatal and postnatal deformities. *Pediatr Clin North Am* 1986;33: 1277–1297.

10. Greene WB, Heckman JD, eds. *The Clinical Measurement of Joint Motion.* 1st ed. Rosemont, IL: American Academy of Orthopaedic Surgeons; 1994.

11. Merlob P, Mimouni F, Rosen O, Reisner SH. Assessment of thumb placement. *Pediatrics* 1984;74:299–300.

12. Lenn NJ, Hamill JS. Congenital radial nerve pressure palsy. *Clin Pediatr* 1983;May:388–389.

13. Michelow BJ, Clarke HM, Curtis CG, Zuker RM, Seifu Y, Andrews DF. The natural history of obstetrical brachial plexus palsy. *Plast Reconstr Surg* 1994;93:675–681.

14. Halliday J, Chow C, Wallace D, Danks D. X linked hydrocephalus: a survey of a 20 year period in Victoria, Australia. *J Med Genet* 1986;23:23–31.

15. Mier RJ, Brower TD. *Pediatric Orthopedics. A Guide for the Primary Care Physician.* Vol. 1. New York: Plenum; 1994.

16. Carroll NC. Clubfoot. In: Morrissy RT, ed. *Lovell and Winter's Pediatric Orthopaedics.* 3rd ed. Vol. 2. Philadelphia: JB Lippincott; 1990:927.

17. Griffin PP. Orthopaedics. In: Avery GB, Fletcher MA, MacDonald MG, eds. *Neonatology: Pathophysiology and Management of the Newborn.* 4th ed. Philadelphia: JB Lippincott; 1994:1179–1194.

18. Barlow TG. Early diagnosis and treatment of congenital dislocation of the hip. *J Bone Joint Surg [Br]* 1962; 44:292–301.

19. Ortolani M. Un segno poco noto e sua importanza per la diagnosi precoce di prelussazione congenita dell'anca. *Pediatria* 1937;45:129–136.

20. Graf R. Hip sonography—how reliable? Sector scanning versus linear scanning? Dynamic versus static examination? *Clin Orthop* 1992;281:18–21.

21. Foster BK. Initial screening and diagnosis of and referral for developmental dysplasia of the hip. *Curr Opin Pediatr* 1995;7:80–82.

22. Davids JR, Benson LJ, Mubarak SJ, McNeil N. Ultrasonography and developmental dysplasia of the hip: a cost–benefit analysis of three delivery systems. *J Pediatr Orthop* 1995;15:325–329.

23. Andersson JE, Funnemark PO. Neonatal hip instability: screening with anterior–dynamic ultrasound method. *J Pediatr Orthop* 1995;15:322–324.

24. Sponseller PD. Screening and ultrasound for neonatal hip instability. *Curr Opin Pediatr* 1995;7:77–79.

25. Schuler P, Feltes E, Kienapfel H, Griss P. Ultrasound examination for the early determination of dysplasia and congenital dislocation of neonatal hips. *Clin Orthop* 1990;258:18–26.

26. Patterson CC, Kernohan WG, Mollan RA, Haugh PE, Trainor BP. High incidence of congenital dislocation of the hip in Northern Ireland. *Paediatr Perinatol Epidemiol* 1995;9:90–97.

27. Haasbeek JF, Wright JG, Hedden DM. Is there a difference between the epidemiologic characteristics of hip dislocation diagnosed early and late? *Can J Surg* 1995;38:437–438.

28. Farkas R, Levine S. X-ray incidence of fractured clavicle in vertex presentation. *Am J Obstet Gynecol* 1950; 59:204–206.

29. Joseph PR, Rosenfeld W. Clavicular fractures in neonates. *Am J Dis Child* 1990;144:165–167.

30. Walle T, Hartikainen-Sorri AL. Obstetric shoulder injury. Associated risk factors, prediction and prognosis. *Acta Obstet Gynecol Scand* 1993;72:450–454.

31. Waninger KN, Chung MK. A new clue to clavicular fracture in newborn infants? [Letter]. *J Pediatr* 1991;88: 657.

32. Swanson AB. A classification for congenital limb malformations. *J Hand Surg [Am]* 1976;1:8–22.

33. Froster UG, Baird PA. Congenital defects of lower limbs and associated malformations: a population based study. *Am J Med Genet* 1993;45:60–64.

34. Froster-Iskenius UG, Baird PA. Limb reduction defects in over one million consecutive livebirths. *Teratology* 1989;39:127–135.

35. Bayne LG, Costas BL. Malformations of the upper limb. In: Morrissy RT, ed. *Lovell and Winter's Pediatric Orthopaedics.* 3rd ed. Vol. 1. Philadelphia: JB Lippincott; 1990:563.

36. Wood VE. Congenital thumb deformities. *Clin Orthop* 1985;195:7–25.

37. Francomano CA. The genetic basis of dwarfism. *N Engl J Med* 1995;332:58–59.

38. Stoilov I, Kilpatrick MW, Tsipouras P. A common FGFR3 gene mutation is present in achondroplasia but not in hypochondroplasia. *Am J Hum Genet* 1995;55:127–133.

39. Hall JG. Arthrogryposis. *Am Fam Physician* 1989;39:113–119.

40. Sarwark JF, MacEwen GD, Scott CI Jr. Amyoplasia (a common form of arthrogryposis). *J Bone Joint Surg [Am]* 1990;72:465–469.

41. Shapiro F, Specht L. The diagnosis and orthopaedic treatment of childhood spinal muscular atrophy, peripheral neuropathy, Friedreich ataxia, and arthrogryposis. *J Bone Joint Surg [Am]* 1993;75:1699–1714.

42. Swinyard CA, Bleck EE. The etiology of arthrogryposis (multiple congenital contracture). *Clin Orthop* 1985; 194:15–29.

43. Vuopala K, Leisti J, Herva R. Lethal arthrogryposis in Finland—a clinico-pathological study of 83 cases during thirteen years. *Neuropediatrics* 1994;25:308–315.

44. Hennekam RC, Barth PG, Van Lookeren Campagne W, De Visser M, Dingemans KP. A family with severe X-linked arthrogryposis. *Eur J Pediatr* 1991;150:656–660.

45. Laureano AN, Rybak LP. Severe otolaryngologic manifestations of arthrogryposis multiplex congenita. *Ann Otol Rhinol Laryngol* 1990;99(Pt 1):94–97.

46. Blauvelt CT, Nelson FRT. *A Manual of Orthopaedic Terminology.* 4th ed. St Louis: CV Mosby; 1990.

47. Burton JK, Schulz CJ, Burd LI. Spectrum of limb disruption defects associated with chorionic villus sampling. *Pediatrics* 1993;91:997.

48. Suzuki S, Yamamuro T. Correlation of fetal posture and congenital dislocation of the hip. *Acta Orthop Scand* 1986;57:81–84.

49. Cole WG, Dalgleish R. Perinatal lethal osteogenesis imperfecta. *J Med Genet* 1995;32:284–289.

50. Chan C, Green W, de la Cruz Z. Ocular findings in osteogenesis imperfecta congenita. *Arch Ophthalmol* 1982;100:1459–1463.

51. Nutt JNd, Flatt AE. Congenital central hand deficit. *J Hand Surg [Am]* 1981;6:48–60.

11

Neuromotor Evaluation

The neurologic examination of the newborn infant is described in detail in several historically important publications (1–7). In each description there is a slightly different emphasis on which procedures are most informative. One common caveat is that a clinician must have experience to be able to tell if a particular finding in any infant is abnormal or if it is a normal deviation due to the infant's state, physical positioning, or gestational age, or to examiner technique. Some experts maintain that the experience recommended to make these distinctions involves observation under a tutor for months to years (2,3). Another recommendation to increase validity is to evaluate the same infant over several days. Most of these archetypal studies found that the most reliable examinations were performed after the first 2 days of life and on at least more than one occasion during the first month of age after term birth (3,5). Detailed and multiple observations are perhaps ideal but clearly unrealistic for most clinical situations.

For the practitioner it is important to have the examinations recommended by the clinical masters as resource guides, but it is impractical to use their entire examinations on every well infant or on any frail infants who might not tolerate the necessary handling. Instead, one selects the procedures that will give essential information and adds others as needed to supplement and confirm the findings.

Although there are volumes written in describing the examination on healthy term infants, there is often surprisingly little detail on how to get the same information when the subject is sick or coupled to restrictive equipment. Some procedures discussed in this chapter offer alternatives when the infant's condition and environment require.

The neonatal neurologic examination has several purposes:

1. Identify moderate to severe neurologic abnormalities.
2. Identify infants at risk for developmental difficulties to select for more specific follow-up or early intervention.
3. Indicate the severity and duration of an insult
   a. prognosis after asphyxia
   b. response of premature infants at 40 weeks corrected gestational age

Clearly, all infants do not require a lengthy neurologic examination as long as they demonstrate normal basic findings on each encounter. These basics include evidence of alertness, including visual interest and following response to sounds, normal tone and strength in the extremities and body, and normal control of the head and neck. Infants in intensive care require examinations in concert with their condition. Those admitted with either perinatal asphyxia or drug withdrawal need daily examinations but with different emphases. Premature infants should be examined at least weekly for assessment of their maturation. Any infant with a change in condition needs a neurologic evaluation as part of their work-up.

The detail of each examination is directed both by its purpose and the actual findings. For premature infants without specific neurologic insult, the examination emphasizes their level of maturation compared with that expected for their corrected gestational ages. When there has been neurologic insult, the examination emphasizes the findings expected with the affected areas; e.g., spinal cord or brachial plexus injuries compared with general hypoxic-ischemic encephalopathy. If the purpose is to assess narcotic withdrawal and treatment, the items emphasize the indicators of drug effect.

More recent authors have attempted to simplify the examination by shortening the original protocols and to apply a score (8–13). Abbreviating the process is reasonable as long as all aspects of neurologic function are covered because many of the observations included in the longer procedures are interesting reflexes and responses but are not necessarily pathognomonic. Selecting what are the most important features and leaving out others that are redundant, not helpful, or unnecessarily stressful has found popular favor in that it has shortened the examination and made it far more practical but not always better. By using stick figures to illustrate expected patterns on standardized forms, the various authors have helped make recording the findings more reproducible among observers (10,14,15). Unfortunately, by simplifying we have also probably lessened our system of observing or demonstrating to our trainees the nuances of possible responses that allow the very experienced observers to be the most accurate in the neurologic assessment. When there are subtle findings on any examination, it is appropriate to add more maneuvers to verify the observations so the clinician who has a variety of diagnostic tools and techniques in his armamentarium will be able to use them when required.

Assigning scores to the components of the examination scheme has attempted to serve two purposes: first, to separate normal from abnormal using a devised grading system instead of clinical impression, and second, to create a more precise quantification of findings in order to increase the interobserver reproducibility necessary for both clinical and research purposes. Scores are part of most of the formatted neurologic examinations, but the weighting or summing of the scores is sometimes based on the originator's opinion rather than on mathematical interrelationships or outcome (2,11,12,16). Even with detailed scoring systems, there is always an important category of suspect infants in whom the combination of findings is neither clearly normal nor abnormal. Although a definitive diagnosis should not be made when there is any question, those infants are still selected as requiring additional evaluations in follow-up testing just as are those infants with "abnormal" scores. For the most part, infants who are normal on a thorough neurologic examination remain normal, but many infants, particularly premature infants, who appear abnormal on a single examination, later become normal (13). Additionally, the reliability of the assessment depends both on the ability of the tester and the stage of development of the infant. The reliability increases with experience in the observer and with the age of the infant (17).

Not only is it necessary to understand what is normal in a generic sense for the term newborn but one must also understand what is the expected level of neurologic development for each gestational age and for each day after birth. The earlier writings make careful observation of the changes in the first weeks of life after term birth. More recent emphasis has shifted toward observing the neurologic maturation of premature infants, helped in part because of their prolonged hospital stays and in part because of the need to select which infants are at risk for poorer outcome and might benefit from earlier intervention. The emphasis of many examination systems in this country has been on predicting outcome after premature birth or perinatal episodes that carry an increased risk of neurodevelopmental deficit (5,6,11–13,18–23). With these attempts at prognostication has come not only a better understanding of the neurologic maturation of premature and term infants but a greater respect for the ability of the newborn infant to recover or, at the least, to keep his or her long-term outcome somewhat of a guarded secret.

PURPOSE OF NEONATAL NEUROLOGIC EXAMINATION

Assessing Behavior

Just as the neurologic examination in adults includes an assessment of mental status as a major component, so too should a similar description of the infant's personality or behavior be included in the neonatal examination. Neonates do have personalities, albeit not clearly defined by adult standards, but each baby shows differences and similarities in the ways he (or she) interacts with his environment. Because most of the items on the neurologic examination reflect either spinal or mid-brain responses, there should be some attempt to assess higher cortical functioning as part of a full evaluation. It is quite possible to get an impression of a "good brain" merely by observing how an infant controls his reactions or how aware of his environment he is. It is clearly reassuring to observe an infant instantly quieting down when he has found his own fingers or being able to adjust his emotions when presented with or removed from discomfort. Just as it takes parents time to get to know their baby, so too does it take experience for one to be comfortable in describing the various behavior patterns in neonates. It does not take a good physician long to realize that an observation by an experienced nurse of a change in the behavior of their patient is one of the most valuable diagnostic tools available in intensive care nurseries.

Brazelton et al. developed and continues to revise a standardized evaluation in the Neonatal Behavioral Assessment Scale (24,25). A full assessment takes at least 20 minutes with a cooperative infant in a controlled environment and is most informative if done on three separate days in the newborn period: on day 2 or 3, days 7 to 14, and at 1 month (26). Formal training and certification are suggested as necessary by the developers of this scale if results are to be used for research. Clearly, it is not clinically practical to apply this evaluation fully except in research situations or prolonged hospital stays, but knowledge of the various components helps anyone looking at babies understand and interpret their responses. The assessment has its greatest clinical application when it is performed in the presence of the parents because it helps them understand their own infant better and earlier (27–29). There has been no standardization of a shortened version of this evaluation, but, except for the items that require eliciting habituation responses, many of the same items can be observed as part of a regular physical examination. It is worthwhile to read the descriptions of how to elicit and interpret the responses to increase our understanding of the behavior capacity of neonates. These are detailed in the individual examination procedures below.

The term "neurobehavior" to title this aspect of physical examination is rather loose in that it implies a higher level, cortical reaction (behavior) when some of the responses are only lower level, more mid-brain reactions. The level of function of most of the reflex responses is relatively low even if not limited to the spinal cord and therefore may be seen in infants with severely limited cerebral capacity. It is by interpretation of the quality of response or of the pattern of extinction that one can try to estimate higher level cerebral capacity. One of the most striking examples of infants who appear remarkably normal at birth are those with hydranencephaly who have extremely limited or no cortical tissue and yet demonstrate a normal basic examination. It is only by failure to extinguish the primitive reflexes on repeated trial or to demonstrate expected behavior responses that such infants stand out as abnormal.

Other investigators have emphasized the differences in behavior due to prematurity (30–33). For the most part, the observations are made of the way the premature infant reacts to regular care activities as well as to elicited responses. The Assessment of Premature Infants' Behavior as developed by Als et al. is a detailed series of observations that, aside from research purposes, has a significant usefulness in demonstrating to caregivers how the environment is impacting on the infant patient (34). Understanding the expected behavior norms for the various gestational age groups is prerequisite to interpreting a neurologic examination because state and its regulation significantly affect the responses seen in virtually all neuromotor reflexes.

Infant State

The expected performance during an examination depends on what state the infant is in. Just as one would note the mental alertness of an older patient as part of an assessment, so too is it necessary to note what level of arousal or sleep the infant is in. There are three descriptions of state referenced most often by others in their examination schema (3,25,35). Each defines six states that are similar but not identical. For example, state 3 of Brazelton is essentially a transitional state between states 2 and 3 of Prechtl, but it is present often

Table 1. *Comparisons in descriptions of state: Prechtl versus Brazelton*

	Prechtl and Beintema (2, 3)	Brazelton (24, 25)
State 1	Eyes closed, regular respiration, no movements (may have spontaneous startles)	Deep sleep with regular breathing, eyes closed, no spontaneous activity, no eye movements (may have spontaneous startles or jerky movements at regular intervals; external stimuli produce startles with a delay; suppression of startles is rapid; change of state is less likely than from other states)
State 2	Eyes closed, irregular respiration, no gross movements (may have small, isolated movements of eyes, face, and hands with gross movements lasting several seconds as long as eyes are kept closed)	Light sleep with eyes closed; rapid eye movements; irregular respiration (low activity level, with random movements and startles or startle equivalents; movements are smoother and more monitored than in state 1; responds to stimuli with startle equivalents, often with a resulting change of state; sucking occurs intermittently; eyes may open briefly at intervals)
State 3	Eyes open, no gross movements (may have small, isolated movements of eyes, face, and hands)	Drowsy or semi-dozing; eyes open or closed, activity variable, movements usually smooth (If eyes are open, they are heavy lidded; if closed, eyelids flutter. Activity levels varies with startling from time to time. Infant is reactive to sensory stimuli but with delay and often followed by a state change. Movements are smooth. Infant may appear dazed and not interacting with examiner.)
State 4	Eyes open, gross movements, no crying (movements occur primarily in the extremities)	Alert, with bright look; minimal motor activity (Infant seems to focus attention on source of sensory stimulation; other stimuli may break through this attention but with some delay in response. There is a glazed look that is easily redirected to a more attentive state.)
State 5	Eyes open or closed, crying	Eyes open, considerable motor activity (Infant may show thrusting movements of the extremities and spontaneous startle. He reacts to stimuli with an increase in startle or motor activity but his overall general activity may obscure minor increases. He may have brief periods of fussiness.)
State 6	Other state: describe (e.g., coma)	Crying (This crying is intense and difficult to break through. The motor activity is high.)

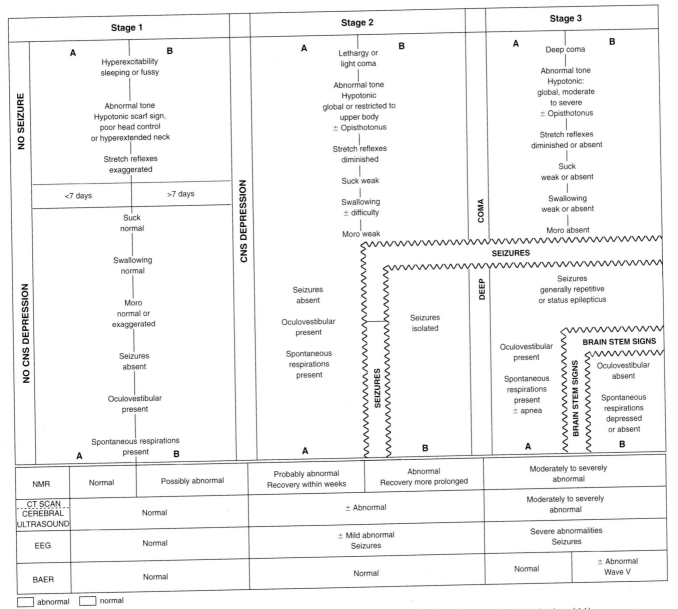

Figure 1. Clinical changes in hypoxic-ischemic encephalopathy. Reprinted with permission (41).

enough in both term and preterm infants to warrant separation when the state is particularly important in describing behavioral responses (Table 1). The behavior states described by Thoman are yet another variation, with 10 primary states (35). Combining the awake states and using computer analysis of infant movement patterns, he describes six derived states: quiet sleep, active sleep, active-quiet, transitional sleep, sleep-wake transition, and wakefulness (36,37). The Thoman descriptions are probably the least subjective because they are computer scored but they are not as clinically applicable for direct observation.

The formal descriptions of various infant states have somewhat different applications. The detailed computer analyses of Thoman allow comparisons of cycles of activity and behavior response in premature and term infants (35). The simpler ones of Prechtl and Beitema or of Brazelton, based on direct observation, promote better interpretation of infant response in reflex activity during a neurobehavior examination (2,25). Descriptions of infant state are part of evaluations for neonatal withdrawal from maternal drugs (38,39). They also serve in following infants treated with sedative or stimulant drugs. When the neurologic examination is assessing possible encephalopathy, other systems of classification assist in documenting status and estimating prognosis (7,40,41) (Fig. 1).

In general the ideal states for neurologic examination are the intermediate state levels where an infant is quiet but awake and alert. Noting the changes from one state to the next and the infant's ability to move between states is important as well for assessment of behavior.

THE GENERAL NEUROMOTOR EXAMINATION

Most of the neurologic examination is conducted by thoughtful observation during the rest of the regional assessments and synthesized as a system after adding any specific maneuvers that may be indicated. Except perhaps for the initial assessment just at birth, the first part of any evaluation should be a period of undisturbed observation of resting posture, spontaneous movements, and state: the state of the infant in a neurobehavior sense as well as the overall condition of the infant to determine what limitations may exist because of equipment, environment, gestational age, medical conditions, or malformations. Many of these observations can be made while approaching the infant's bedside.

All neurologic examinations include an assessment of the basic posture and movements of the infant both when he was undisturbed and when stimulated. How much any infant should be encouraged to respond to directed stimulation depends on how much information is needed to meet the clinical need and on how much the infant demonstrates through his or her own spontaneous activity.

Basic components of neonatal neurologic examination (7):

Level of alertness
Cranial nerves
Motor examination
    Tone and posture
    Motility and power
    Tendon reflexes and plantar responses
Primary neonatal reflexes
    Moro reflex
    Palmar grasp
    Asymmetrical tonic neck response
Sensory examination
    Vision
    Hearing

When a neurologic evaluation is not part of a general physical examination, then basic elements of a general assessment that screen for neurologic conditions are included. The head is assessed for size, shape, rate of growth, transillumination, size and character of the fontanelles, pattern of hair growth, and the presence of any extracerebral fluid collections such as caput succedaneum, cephalohematoma, or subgaleal hematoma. The skin is examined for café-au-lait spots, depigmented ash leaf spots, hemangiomas or vascular malformations, nevi, hairy tufts, dimples, or subcutaneous masses, particularly overlying the spinal cord and head, or areas of ecchymoses or petechiae. The extremities are inspected for range of motion and palpated for consistency of the muscles. Dysmorphic features are noted as is any evidence of seizures or apnea. Major organs are assessed for organomegaly. Historical facts about intrauterine activity and the perinatal course are noted.

Much of the traditional neurologic examination in older patients involves having the patient perform specific motor activities or sensory responses. When a patient is able to cooperate, the examiner simply asks him to follow directions or to report what he senses. Modified techniques are used when a patient is unable to cooperate. Just because a young infant cannot follow verbal directions does not mean he will be uncooperative and fail to communicate a response if appropriate techniques are used. Through careful observations of infants has come the recognition that even complex motor activities can be elicited to demonstrate the motor and sensory components of a detailed neurologic examination. There are many responses that are unique to young infants and enable us to get the active participation in an examination that provides meaningful information. Some of the reflexes and the brain levels involved are well detailed. Many others are yet to be defined but may play a role in some examinations. These reflexes are the primitive or primary reflexes and the skin reflexes. The primitive reflexes are present only in the early months of life. Some reappear in adults who have sustained severe cortical damage.

This chapter includes detailed descriptions of many reflexes and responses demonstrable in neonates in order to provide the reader with some historical observations as well as to allow comparison of techniques. There are usually several ways to induce an infant to demonstrate a specific response or a similar one that gives essentially the same information. Some are best chosen for an infant able to be held in suspension, but others are valid substitutes when the infant must be left examined with little or no contact or movement. Other reflexes and responses are included because they are unique to neonates even though we really do not know exactly what significance they carry.

Screening Examination

In the early newborn period after a term birth, a screening examination is sufficient unless there is a suggestion of increased risk based on either history or other physical findings. Examples of shortened and formatted examinations that are appropriate for screening infants of various gestational ages are reproduced at the end of this chapter (10,11) (see Figs. 31 and 32). The time saved in either of these formats comes primarily from eliminating the need for descriptive writing, but there is still benefit to including a descriptive synthesis in summary. The revised system proposed by Ellison puts more emphasis on infant interaction and awareness in response to the environment. It is important to remember that the best time to perform a neurologic evaluation is not in the first 24 to 48 hours of life because it is so difficult to elicit many of the reactions and responses necessary to indicate a normal examination. An examination at a 2-week evaluation is more informative.

Special Situations

Altered Mental Status

One of the important indications for a specific neurologic examination in newborn infants is an evaluation of possible encephalopathy from perinatal asphyxia. Neonates with decrease in level of alertness due to central nervous system insults should be evaluated for level of response with special attention to function of the cranial nerves and appearance of the fundus for optic disk hypoplasia-dysplasia or atrophy, retinal and vitreous hemorrhages, and chorioretinitis.

Sarnat and Sarnat described stages of hypoxic-ischemic encephalopathy as mild, moderate, and severe, based on clinical and electroencephalographic findings. Their classification was modified by Amiel-Tison (41) (Fig. 1). Volpe proposed a more simplified classi-

Table 2. *Levels of alertness in the neonatal period*

Level of alertness	Appearance of infant	Arousal response	Motor responses	
			Quantity	Quality
Normal	Awake	Normal	Normal	High level
Stupor				
Slight	Sleepy	Diminished (slight)	Diminished (slight)	High level
Moderate	Asleep	Diminished (moderate)	Diminished (moderate)	High level
Deep	Asleep	Absent	Diminished (marked)	High level
Coma	Asleep	Absent	Diminished (marked) or absent	Low level

Reprinted from Volpe, ref. 7, with permission

fication with only three general states or levels of alertness: normal, stupor, and coma (7) (Table 2). When encephalopathy is a consideration, assessment of these stages or levels of alertness should be repeated periodically. Whichever system for determining state or stages of coma is followed, one must verify that the infant is demonstrating a truly abnormal level of alertness for his or her condition and is not just deeply asleep or medically sedated.

Infant States in Drug Withdrawal

Another of the clinical situations when assessing infant state is important is in the evaluation and management of neonatal drug withdrawal. There are a number of assessment formats that include behavior state with other examination and physiologic parameters as measures of withdrawal (38,39,42) (Tables 3 and 4).

Spinal Cord Injury

When there is an obvious defect or a suspected injury in the spinal cord, basic observations to determine the level of injury include testing sensory response to touch or pinprick, observing the stream of urination, anal wink, and abnormal patterns of defecation. Constant dribbling or urinary retention with lower abdominal distention indicates neurogenic bladder. Obstipation or runny stools with a patulous anus may indicate poor neurologic function, but the timing and initiation of bowel patterns is so variable depending on gestational age and intake that this is a less reliable sign than in older infants (43–46). Apnea after spinal injury is suggested as carrying a particularly poor prognosis (47).

Table 3. *Neonatal drug withdrawal scoring system*

Signs	Score			
	0	1	2	3
Tremors (muscle activity of limbs)	Normal	Minimally increased when hungry or disturbed	Moderate or marked increase when undisturbed; subside when fed or held snugly	Marked increase or continuous even when undisturbed, going on to seizurelike movements
Irritability (excessive crying)	None	Slightly increased	Moderate to severe when disturbed or hungry	Marked even when undisturbed
Reflexes	Normal	Increased	Markedly increased	
Stools	Normal	Explosive, but normal frequency	Explosive, >8/day	
Muscle tone	Normal	Increased	Rigidity	
Skin abrasions	No	Redness of knees and elbows	Breaking of the skin	
Respiratory rate/min	<55	55–75	76–95	
Repetitive sneezing	No	Yes		
Repetitive yawning	No	Yes		
Vomiting	No	Yes		
Fever	No	Yes		

A score of >4 is consistent with neonatal withdrawal syndrome.
Reprinted from Lipsitz, ref. 38, with permission.

Table 4. *Neonatal abstinence syndrome assessment*

	Score
Central nervous system disturbances	
Excessive high pitched (or other) cry	2
Continuous high pitched (or other) cry	3
Sleeps <1 h after feeding	3
Sleeps <2 h after feeding	2
Sleeps <3 h after feeding	1
Hyperactive Moro reflex	2
Markedly hyperactive Moro reflex	3
Mild tremors disturbed	1
Moderate–severe tremors disturbed	2
Increased muscle tone	2
Excoriation (specify area)	1
Myoclonic jerks	3
Generalized convulsions	5
Metabolic/vasomotor/respiratory disturbances	
Sweating	1
Fever >37.2 but <38.2°C	1
Fever >38.4°C	2
Frequent yawning (<3–4 times/interval)	1
Mottling	1
Nasal stuffiness	1
Sneezing (>3–4 times/interval)	1
Nasal flaring	2
Respiratory rate >60/min	1
Respiratory rate >60/min with retractions	2
Gastrointestinal disturbances	
Excessive sucking	1
Poor feeding	2
Regurgitation	2
Projectile vomiting	3
Loose stools	2
Watery stools	3

Adapted from Rubaltelli and Granati, ref. 39, with permission.

Neurologic signs suggesting spinal cord injury in the newborn infant (7):

Motor: weakness, hypotonia, areflexia of extremities below the level of injury
Sensory: definable sensory level
Sphincter function: distended bladder and patulous anus (absent anal wink)
Other: Horner's syndrome, intact cranial nerves and normal level of alertness

Spinal Segment L1, L2: Cremaster Reflex (2). **Stroke the skin on the medial side of the thigh. If there is no response with stroking, use a superficial pin stick.**

A normal response is elevation of the testis on the stimulated side, most often on both sides with a contraction and blanching of the scrotal sac. The cremasteric response is at least partially present even in undescended testes. The presence of edema may decrease the visible response. Female infants may have a blanching of the skin over the vulva but not reliably.

Spinal Segment S4, S5: Anal Reflex (2). **Stroke the perianal skin and observe for contraction of the anal sphincter. If the response is not elicited by stroking, use a soft pin prick.**

The anal reflex should always be present in the first 10 days, although it is less brisk in marked prematurity.

Brachial Plexus Injury (48,49)

Brachial plexus injury is one of the most frequent abnormalities detected on the neonatal neurologic examination. Unilateral injury to the brachial plexus manifests as decreased

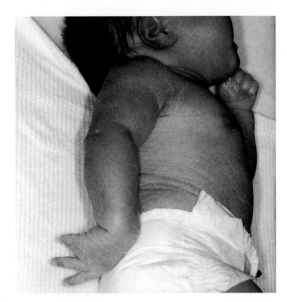

Figure 2. Hand and arm position in Erb's palsy involving C-5, 6, 7. See Table 5.

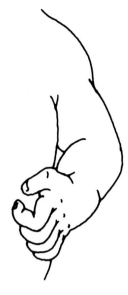

Figure 3. Hand and arm position in Klumpke's paresis involving C-8 and T-1. See Table 6.

Table 5. *Major pattern of weakness with Erb's (proximal) brachial plexus palsy*

Weak movement	Cord segment	Resulting position
Shoulder abduction	C-5	Adducted
Shoulder external rotation	C-5	Internally rotated
Elbow flexion	C-5,6	Extended
Supination	C-5,6	Pronated
Wrist extension	C-6,7	Flexed
Finger extension	C-6,7	Flexed
Diaphragmatic descent	C-4,5	Elevated

Reprinted from Volpe, ref. 7, with permission.

Table 6. *Major pattern of weakness with total brachial plexus palsy in addition to proximal weakness*

Weak movement	Cord segment	Resulting position
Wrist flexion	C-7,8; T-1	Extended
Finger flexion	C-7,8; T-1	Extended
Finger abduction	C-8; T-1	Neutral position
Finger abduction	C-8; T-1	Neutral position
Dilator of iris	T-1	Miosis
Full lid elevation	T-1	Ptosis

Reprinted from Volpe, ref. 7, with permission.

Table 7. *Reflex abnormalities in Erb's and total brachial plexus palsies*

Reflex	Cord segment	Response	
		Proximal palsy	Total palsy
Biceps	C-5,6	Absent	Absent
Moro			
Shoulder	C-5	Absent	Absent
Hand movement	C-8, T-1	Present	Absent
Palmar grasp	C-8, T-1	Present	Absent

Reprinted from Volpe, ref. 7, with permission.

movement and unequal resting posture in their upper limbs (Fig. 2). The reported incidence of this injury is from less than one to four per 1,000 births of term infants (48–51). The most frequently affected regions are C-5, C-6 almost twice as often as C-5, C-6, C-7 lesions. Involvement of the entire plexus is far less common. When it is the proximal upper extremity that is involved, the palsy is an Erb's palsy. When only the more distal extremity is affected (C-8, T-1), it is called a Klumpke's palsy (Fig. 3). Because injury limited only to the distal portion is extremely unusual at less than 1% of all brachial injuries, the term Klumpke's palsy is sometimes applied to total brachial plexus palsy (7,52).

The clinical presentation of Erb's is typically with an inability to abduct and externally rotate the shoulder, flex the elbow, and supinate the forearm. If C-7 is involved, the infant cannot extend his or her wrist and fingers, leading to the classical "waiter's tip" posture (Fig. 2). In a distal or Klumpke's palsy, the hand is more affected with complete loss of grasp. The clinical findings and the levels of involvement are detailed in Tables 5 through 7. Besides defining the level of motor involvement, one should also determine if there is sensory loss as well by examining the response to pain. Because brachial plexus injuries are associated with other traumatic lesions, the examination must include the other areas likely affected: the diaphragm, clavicle, humerus, shoulder, spinal cord, and facial nerve (49,53). Brachial plexus injuries are present from birth, although not always noted. When findings appear only later, postnatal trauma or a pseudoparesis due to septic arthritis or osteomyelitis are likely causes.

Development of Premature Infant

When a purpose for examination is to determine if neuromotor development is appropriate for the gestational and corrected chronologic ages, more detail is directed toward quality of the primitive reflexes and assessment of tone. Appropriate formats for following maturation include those suggested by Dubowitz or by Amiel-Tison that compare the infants over time with reflexes, tone, and postures expected with normal maturation (11,15). Follow-up studies have used a variety of formats, each of which again reflects the originator's preferences as to which items are the most informative. These assessments include the Neonatal Neurodevelopmental Examination (13), the Einstein Neonatal Neurobehavioral Assessment Scale (ENNAS), (54,55), the Neonatal Neurobehavioral Examination (NNE) (12), and the Neo Neuro & Up. For the clinician it is probably most important to pick one that he or she will use consistently and correctly to detect infants outside the ranges of normal. The Neo Neuro & Up is included at the end of this chapter.

SEQUENCE OF EXAMINATION

An important factor in accomplishing a neurologic evaluation on a newborn infant is being able to get essential information in a reasonable time frame without aggravating the infant to the point of losing all cooperation or unnecessarily stressing him or her. If the infant is mobile and unattached to equipment, the sequence is different than if one is encumbered by equipment or the fragility of illness or immaturity (Table 8). In reality, many of the steps of neuromotor function are interspersed with the examination of the head and neck (cranial nerves) and the extremities when a neurologic assessment is part of a full evaluation. When there are localized findings, the sequence and number of tests are adjusted to address patient tolerance and the information needed. Observations about levels of alertness, state, and behavior are made throughout the evaluation.

MUSCLE TONE

Assessment of muscle tone or tension is a major component of the neurologic examination (56). As applied to newborn and young infants, tone reflects both muscle tension and strength. Passive tone is assessed through an evaluation of how easily and fully muscle

Table 8. *Suggested sequence for basic neurologic examination according to infant status*

Mobile infant with normal tolerance	Immobile or fragile infant[b]
Observations of spontaneous activity and resting posture[a]	
Indicators of behavior and level of alertness[a]	
Root, suck, gag, facial activity[a]	
ATNR in supine	Observe for spontaneous presence
Palmar graps	
Square window	
Arm recoil	
Scarf sign	
Arm traction	
Pull to sit[a]	Delay
Neck flexors	Delay
Supported upright sitting	Delay
Neck extensors	Hypertonicity of neck extensors
Eye movements in rotation	Substitute dolls eye or caloric stimulation
Moro by body drop[a]	Substitute Moro by table bang
Body position in ventral suspension[a]	Delay in the presence of respiratory distress
Galant	Delay until infant can lie in prone
Slip through at shoulders	Delay until moble
Place and support[a]	Magnet
Stepping reflex	Crossed extensor, leg recoil, leg traction
Plantar grasp	
Babinski	
Ankle angle	
Ankle clonus	
Adductor angle	
Popliteal angle	
Heel to ear	
Tendon reflexes: patellar, adductors, brachioradialis, pectoralis	
Response to auditory stimulus[a]	Delay until in quieter environment
Pupillary response to light[a]	Delay until if less than 32 wk
Body position in prone	Delay until infant can lie in prone
Transillumination	

[a] Screening items for healthy infant; add other items as indicated by condition and findings.
[b] Except as noted for delay or sutstitution, use all items as tolerated.

groups stretch as various segments are moved and the infant lies passively. Tone should be described as normal, increased, or decreased for the axis or a particular segment. The tests that evaluate passive tone include the scarf, lateral rotation of the head, square window, adductor angles, heel to ear, popliteal angles, ankle dorsiflexion, and return to flexion after extension at the elbows or hips. For each of these maneuvers, an angle of response is estimated as the segment is slowly moved. In contrast to range of motion where specific angles are measured at the final endpoint, evaluation of tone does not require stretching to the greatest point for an estimate of range but rather to a point where resistance develops. Another evaluation of passive tone is the feeling of flappability, in which rapid shaking of the distal extremities triggers a compensatory breaking activity. This maneuver allows a comparison between extremities and, as a side effect, relaxes the distal muscles for more representative evaluation of passive tone or the deeps tendon reflexes (15).

Active tone is more an evaluation of muscle strength because it is an assessment of the infant's response to changes in position or to stimulation of skin reflexes. The infant initiates the movements spontaneously or the examiner can induce a fairly complicated series of movements. The tests and reflexes that assess active tone include the place, stepping, head movement and control, pull to sit, palmar grasp, crawling, arm release in prone, crossed extension, and magnet response.

Both active and passive tone change with gestational age. Passive tone develops first in the flexor muscles and progresses in a caudocephalic direction so that the legs assume a resting posture of flexion before the arms do (5). At less than 28 weeks there is little passive tone, so the extremities and trunk are relatively flaccid. At term, passive flexor tone is relatively increased. The pattern of development of passive tone is consistent enough to be of value in assessing gestational age, although intrauterine factors do affect the findings (see Chapter 3 Fig. 3). There is enough individual variability as well as error introduced by examiner technique and experience that the measures of maturity based on evaluation of passive tone are truly only estimates of gestational age with wide margins of error remaining (6,15). The pattern of tone and changes within an individual are more helpful than single examinations or comparisons among infants with differing environmental and medical histories. For instance, knowledge of a premature infant's tone on one day and finding a decrease in tone on the next can be a sign of the onset of a new medical condition or that the infant is not feeling well (56).

SPECIFIC EXAMINATION TECHNIQUES

Cranial Nerves

Cranial Nerve I: Olfaction

The sense of smell is rarely tested in newborn infants unless there is an apparent nasal anomaly or a specific indication to define function of all cranial nerves in a neurologically abnormal infant. Newborn infants have an ability not only to detect odors and respond to a strong enough stimulant, but they quickly learn fragrance discrimination (57,58). Within the first 48 hours after birth, infants are able to recognize odors associated with a pleasant response and to turn toward that odor while ignoring others (58). Early recognition of the odor of their own mother's breast milk is demonstrated with rooting toward the milk. Most infants of 32 weeks or more show a response to a strong odor, but at less than 32 weeks an absent response would not be abnormal (57).

Soak a cotton pledget in a strong odorant such as extracts of peppermint or cloves and bring it toward the nose from the side. Observe for sucking movements, grimace, or change in level of activity with arousal or quieting. If the infant is not capable of movement, observe for transient change in heart rate.

Cranial Nerve II: Vision

Optical Blink Reflex (Dazzle reflex): CN II and VII

The testing of an ability to see is essential for each newborn as it relays information about infant behavior as well as cranial nerve function. At term, awake, alert infants should be able to follow a high-contrast object horizontally from 30° to 60° (25), and most healthy 32-week infants fix at least briefly. Preterm infants may respond to varying intensity of visual input from as early as 26 weeks, but a lack of response to specific stimuli is not abnormal until much later (see Chapter 7, Table 6).

For general screening of alert, term infants, hold the infant en face so that you are in his (or her) line of vision with his eyes in a neutral position. If in the first week after birth, hold the infant no more than 1 to 1.5 feet from your face. If the infant fixes on your eyes, holding him still, move your face from side to side slowly, and watch for his gaze to follow yours. If there is no fixation, use a light source of increasing intensity until a blink reflex is elicited.

The infant needs to be in either light sleep or awake but not crying. In a room with the lights at a low ambient level, shine a bright light suddenly at the eyes.

Normal Optical Blink Reflex.   Quick closure of the eyes. There may be a slight dorsal flexion of the head as well.

This reaction will not occur until after there has been sufficient clearing of cloudiness of the cornea and vitreous after about 28 weeks gestational age. Its absence before 32 weeks is not abnormal, although it may be present much earlier. The response will diminish with repeated trials. Ambient light must be low enough and the light source sufficiently strong to allow a perceived contrast.

Abnormal Optical Blink Reflex.   No reaction because there is impaired perception of light. Consider obstruction to the light pathway (cataract) or cortical blindness.

Initiation of a mass reflex. If a general startle reaction occurs, there may be a state of hyper-
    irritability.
Absence in immaturity with cloudy vitreous.

Photic Sneeze Reflex

A bright light shown into the eyes causes reflex sneezing (59,60). This has been de-scribed as having a familial incidence with suggested autosomal-dominant transmission, but it is principally a reflex of interest in that it indicates visual perception of light. An ab-sence is not abnormal.

Cranial Nerve III: Pupils

The response of the pupils to light depends not only on an intact cranial nerve but also on clarity of the ocular medium allowing light to reach the optic nerve. Because of normal cloudiness in infants born at less than 32 weeks gestation, the pupillary reflex is not reli-ably present until after 35 weeks. The baseline pupil size varies with gestational age (see Chapter 7, Fig. 15).
   Hold your hands above the eyes to shield the environmental light, and encourage the infant to open his or her eyes spontaneously. Remove your hand and observe the reac-tion as the shadow is off the eye. If there is no reaction, use a stronger light source and bring it from the side to focus on a pupil; observe for constriction of both pupils. Avoid directly presenting a strong light and inducing the optic blink reflex.

   Major pupillary abnormalities and causes in the neonatal period* (7):

Bilateral increase in size
   Hypoxic-ischemic encephalopathy (reactive early, unreactive late)
   Intraventricular hemorrhage (unreactive)
   Local anesthetic intoxication (unreactive)
   Infantile botulism (unreactive)[†]
Bilateral decrease in size
   Hypoxic-ischemic encephalopathy (reactive)
Unilateral decrease in size
   Horner's syndrome (reactive)
Unilateral increase in size
   Convexity subdural hematoma, other unilateral mass (unreactive)
   Congenital third-nerve palsy ($\pm$ unreactive)
   Hypoxic-ischemic encephalopathy ($\pm$ unreactive)

---

*Most common reactivity to light is in parentheses.
[†]Usually mid-position and unreactive.

Cranial Nerves III, IV, and VI

Spontaneous extraocular movements are often not conjugate in the newborn period in both term and premature infants, but elicited movements show neuromotor function.

If an infant is alert and fixes and follows with his (or her) gaze, the horizontal eye movement can be tested by moving a high-contrast stimulus or diffuse light that is not too bright in a darkened room. If the infant can be moved, use the rotation test. If he cannot be moved except for his head, use a doll's eye maneuver or aural caloric stimulation. The eyes will deviate in the direction of the cooled ear.

Rotation Test (2) [Vestibular Reflex, Tonic Deviation of Head and Eyes and Nystagmus] (25)

The infant has to be awake and strong enough to have head control in a supported upright position. Hold the baby upright with your hands around the chest under the arms, facing you. Spin slowly to about 90° first in one direction and then in the other. On the first trial do not restrain the head. On a second trial, support the head with the hand so it cannot turn from neutral.

Normal Response to Rotation Test. With the head unrestrained, the head should turn toward the direction of the turn. With the head held, the eyes will turn toward the direction of the turn. At the cessation of the turning, the eyes return to mid-line. There may be brief saccadic movements of both eyes but no sustained nystagmus.

Abnormal Response to Rotation Test. Absent or inconsistent response in lesions that disturb vestibular response

Absence in one direction with a normal opposite response suggests abnormal cranial nerve (CN) VI and lateral deviation
Initiation of mass reflex
No return of eyes to mid-line after stopping turn
Sustained nystagmus

Doll's Eye Test (2,7)

Turn the head slowly to each side and observe the position of the eyes. Hold the head in each position for several seconds. The infant needs to be awake and not crying or with the eyes conjugate in the mid-line when the lids are held open.

As the head is turned, the eyes will not remain in mid-line. This response is normally present until visual fixation develops.

Cranial Nerve V: Facial Sensation and Sucking

Infants show a definite response to touching of the face through either stroking to induce rooting, or a painful stimulus to elicit a grimace. The motor portion of CN V controls the masseter and pterygoid muscles, involved in the jaw-closing phase of sucking.

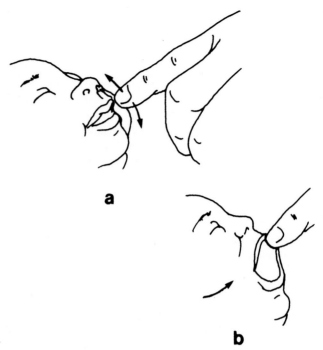

Figure 4. Rooting reflex.

Induce rooting by stroking adjacent to the side of the lips (Fig. 4). If there is no response, use a light pinprick to elicit a grimace. If there is no motor response, monitor the instantaneous heart rate for temporary changes. Use a gloved finger to encourage the infant to suck to assess the strength of jaw closure.

Corneal Reflex

Touch the cornea lightly with a sterile thread of cotton. If the eyes are not open at rest, bring the infant into a sitting position.

Normal Response.   Closure of the eyes as the object touches the cornea indicates an intact sensory function of CN V. Opening the eyes with position change demonstrates a vestibulo-palpebral reflex. This reflex differs from the corneal light reflex (CN II and VII).

Jaw Jerk Reflex or Masseter Reflex (2,7)

Sharply tap one forefinger against the other one resting on the chin well below the lips with the mouth slightly opened.

Normal Response.   Contraction of the masseter muscles elevates the chin. The response should be present in the first 2 weeks. It is easier to feel than to see the contraction and jaw movement.

Abnormal Response.   An absent or weak response after the first 2 days suggests a brain stem lesion or damage of CN V.

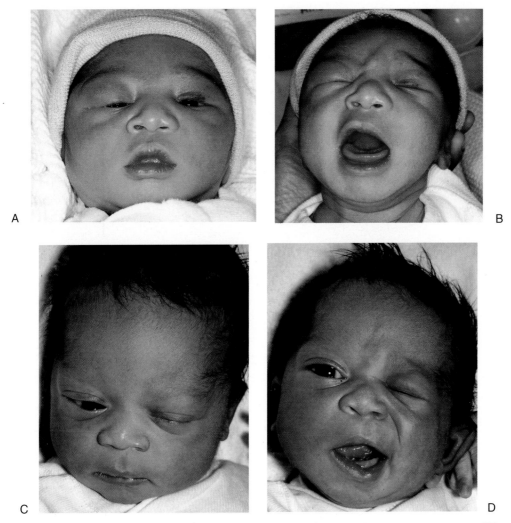

Figure 5. Left facial weakness at rest **(A)** and on stimulation **(B)**. Right facial weakness at rest **(C)** and on stimulation **(D)**.

Cranial Nerve VII: Facial Motility

Observations about changes in facial expression are made throughout the examination. It is easy to tell if an infant has a slack expression or normal changes that occur with yawning and crying (Fig. 5). Unequal opening of the mouth occurs with unilateral absence of the depressor anguli oris muscles, but in that situation the nasolabial folds and lid closure are unaffected (61). Failure to respond with a facial grimace to tactile stimulation may be due to failure through either the sensory portion of CN V or the motor portion of CN VII. The most frequent reason for facial weakness in the newborn period is compression of CN VII either from intrauterine position or forceps (62–64). When associated with forceps, there is almost always overlying dermal ecchymoses, abrasions, or induration. Most of these weaknesses are transient and last only a few hours. Absence of associated findings suggests more chronic compression or other causes of facial weakness as listed.

Observe the infant at rest for tightness of eye closure and fullness and equality of nasolabial folds. If there is no spontaneous facial movement, stimulate response to a painful stimulus to induce crying. Observe for equality in opening the mouth and closing the eyes.

Major causes of facial weakness in the neonatal period (7):

Cerebral
    Hypoxic-ischemic encephalopathy
    Cerebral contusion
Nuclear
    Möbius syndrome
    Hypoxic-ischemic encephalopathy
Nerve
    Traumatic neuropathy
    Posterior fossa hematoma
Neuromuscular Junction
    Myasthenia gravis
    Infantile botulism
Muscle
    Congenital myotonic dystrophy
    Congenital muscular dystrophy
    Facioscapulohumeral dystrophy
    Nemaline myopathy
    Myotubular myopathy
    Congenital fiber type disproportion
    Mitochondrial disorder-cytochrome *c* oxidase deficiency
    Hypoplasia of depressor anguli oris muscle

Lip Reflex (CN VII) (2)

Tap near the angle of the upper or lower lip sharply with a forefinger). Repeat on the opposite side. Crying or sucking interferes with the response.
This response decreases with repetitive stimulation and may not be present in a deep sleep state. A sustained contraction of the orbicularis oris muscle will cause a protrusion of the lips. Only a light touch is needed for a lightly sleeping baby.

Glabella Reflex (CN VII) (2)

Holding the head firmly, sharply tap on the forehead just above the nose and observe for tighter closure of the eyes and wrinkling of the brow.
Abnormal response includes asymmetry or an absent or exceptionally strong response with a sustained closure of more than 1 second or leading to a generalized startle response.

Cranial Nerve VIII: Hearing

Techniques for assessing hearing are discussed in more detail in Chapter 8. To have a valid assessment of hearing when using an external sound source, the environment must be quiet enough for sound discrimination and the infant in neither deep sleep nor an aroused state. The source of the sound must be kept out of the infant's view. Normal infants quickly habituate to repetitive sound sources, so a stimulus can be presented only once or twice. Suitable sound sources include a single tone bicycle horn, an automatic clapper toy, a bell, wrinkling of paper, or rattling of keys. If there is a definite response, then audition is present. A lack of response needs further assessment with a standardized environment and sound emitter. When motor responses are not evident or possible, evoked auditory brain stem responses determine the integrity and function of the nerve.
With the infant in a quiet awake or light sleep state and only a steady soft or absent background noise level, hold the sound source about one foot on either side of the infant. Observe for eye blinking, change in sucking rate, startle, or arousal response to the sound source. Repeat enough to determine reproducibility and habituation response. If

the infant is crying, approach the bedside without entering his field of vision, and speak softly. Observe for quieting activity. If the infant is either abnormally somnolent or in a deep sleep state and does not arouse to a loud sound source, test for evoked auditory potentials.

Acoustic Blink Reflex (Cochleopalpebral Reflex; CN VIII) (2,15,65)

The infant should be in a quiet state, either in light sleep or awake. Use a standardized noise source such as a strong bicycle horn or bell to elicit a loud noise.
The source of noise stimulation must be loud enough to be distinguishable from the environment but not damaging. The quieter the environment, the more likely there will be a response to the stimulation. A normal response is a strong blink that decreases after several trials. The initial response indicates an intact CN VIII. A decremental response indicates appropriate inhibition.

Abnormal Response. Persistence of response without any decrement of intensity or with initiation of a mass reflex. Absence of response after the first 2 days suggests impaired hearing response and indicates further evaluation.

Premature Infant Response. Immature infants are more likely to demonstrate a mass reflex reaction that can include complete shutting down of environmental interaction or difficulty in habituating with repeated trials.

Cranial Nerves V, VII, IX, X, XII (Sucking and Swallowing)

Sucking and swallowing is one of the most complex motor patterns a newborn has at birth. The muscles involved are relatively strong and well exercised by healthy fetuses in preparation for feeding after birth. If an infant is feeding extremely well, there is little need to test the function of these cranial nerves further, but without this history a quick assessment is indicated on the newborn examination.

Sucking and swallowing involves muscle groups that cause the jaw to close and open, the tongue to strip and to thrust, and, finally, swallowing with an interruption of breathing. For effective feeding, the infant must have good lip sealing around the nipple and rhythmic alteration of breathing and sucking. Coordination of sucking and breathing is learned after birth, and normal term infants can take several days before establishing a mature rhythm and pattern; premature infants take longer and do not reliably demonstrate a consistent pattern until after 34 to 35 weeks gestational age (66). Premature infants have less ability to coordinate the breathing and sucking and have weaker tongue propulsion (66). Neurologic evaluation of the suck must include a consideration of any degree of respiratory compromise that might interfere with a normal response.

The full response is tested by first stimulating rooting to get the infant to open his or her mouth spontaneously and turn toward the stroking finger and then allowing sucking for long enough to evaluate the strength of each of the steps involved. Abnormal responses include a tonic biting or a simple up and down motion of the jaw without use of the tongue to strip and propel the feed. The gag reflex (CN XII) may be tested by simply extending the finger further into the mouth or with a tongue blade when the palate is inspected.

Because premature infants occupy the greatest number of bed days in newborn intensive care nurseries, their problems with sucking and swallowing are those most frequently encountered in the neonatal period. Not only does their immaturity play a role in causing the problems, but also their higher incidence of chronic lung disease, high palates, and poor motor tone contribute. Other problems encountered are in infants with cleft palate, cleft lip, severe micrognathia syndromes, or tracheoesophageal fistula. Neurologic causes of sucking and swallowing are listed.

Major Causes of Impaired Sucking and Swallowing in the Neonatal Period (7):

Cerebral
    Encephalopathies with bilateral cerebral (pyramidal) involvement-diverse causes
    Extrapyramidal-adventitial movements
Nuclear
    Hypoxic-ischemic encephalopathy
    Möbius syndrome
    Werdnig-Hoffmann disease
    Arnold-Chiari malformation with myelomeningocele
Nerve
    Traumatic facial neuropathy
    Posterior fossa hematoma or tumor
    Bilateral laryngeal paralysis
    Familial dysautonomia (Riley-Day syndrome)
Neuromuscular junction
    Myasthenia gravis
    Infantile botulism
Muscle
    Congenital myotonic dystrophy
    Congenital muscular dystrophy
    Facioscapulohumeral dystrophy
    Nemaline myopathy
    Myotubular myopathy
    Congenital fiber type disproportion
    Mitochondrial myopathy-cytochrome *c* oxidase deficiency

Cranial Nerve XI: Sternocleidomastoid Function

Poor ability to flex and rotate the head in the early newborn period is difficult to detect unless head control is notably asymmetric. Rather than due to CN XI nerve dysfunction, abnormal function of the sternocleidomastoid (SCM) is more likely to be associated with congenital torticollis. This appears after the early newborn period in the second to fourth week, with fibrotic shortening of the SCM causing the head to be tilted so the chin points away from the affected side and the neck is laterally flexed toward the lesion (67).

Test for head control by providing good support to the infant's shoulders and bringing him (or her) into a sitting position. If the infant is able to fix and follow, he may turn

Table 9. *Infantile oral–motor reflexes*

Reflex	Description	Time of extinction
Rooting	Stroking around mouth elicits movement of head toward source of stimulus and latching onto nipple.	3–4 mo
Suck–swallow	Stroking anterior third of tongue or center of lips elicits suck/swallow movements.	6 mo (evolution to mature sucking)
Biting	Stroking gum elicits rhythmic vertical biting motion of the jaw.	6 mo
Gag	The stimulus to the posterior three fourths of the tongue of pharyngeal wall elicits constriction and elevation of the pharynx.	Sensitivity shifts to back one quarter of the tongue and the pharyngeal wall by adulthood
Babkin's	Stroking of the palm of the hand elicits mouth opening, eye closing, head moving forward and mid-line.	3–4 mo
Palmomental	Stroking of the palm of the hand elicits wrinkling of the mentalis muscle.	Can persist to adulthood

Reprinted from Walter, ref. 70, with permission.

his head toward a strong image. Inspect and palpate the length of the muscles on both sides for symmetry and definition of outline.

Cranial Nerve VII and IX: Taste

It is rarely necessary to evaluate the taste function in newborn infants, but they are capable of taste discrimination and demonstrating what they enjoy by facial expressions, rate of sucking, or changes in heart rate (68). Touching to the front and back of the tongue a small cotton tipped applicator dipped in any of a variety of safe but strong flavors can give quite obvious results.

Some of the reflexes combining cranial nerve interactions show a predictable pattern of maturation and extinction during early infancy, reflecting a change from brain stem function to voluntary control through encephalization (69). These reflexes are necessary for normal early feeding patterns, but their extinction signals more mature brain control. Extremely premature infants will not have well-developed oral motor reflexes at birth, precluding oral feeding. Exaggerated reflexes or failure to mature in an expected pattern suggests poor neurologic outcome (Table 9) (70).

Deep Tendon Reflexes

Test reflexes with infant in a relaxed supine position. If necessary, shake the extremity gently to encourage relaxation. Note the speed, strength, and amplitude of the response, the range of movement produced, and the duration of muscle contraction.
  Graded response:

0 = absent
± or Tr (trace) = very faint visible or palpable contraction but no movement
1+ = hypoactive
2+ = normal
3+ = hyperactive
4+ = hyperactive and reduplicated, inducing clonus or strong overflow, particularly to additional segments

A deep tendon reflex is dependent on

1. intact sensory or afferent nerve fibers,
2. functional synapses in the spinal cord,
3. intact motor or efferent nerve fibers,
4. functional neuromuscular junctions, and
5. competent muscle fibers.

The deep tendon reflexes are essentially the same as in older patients but their presence and the ease with which they can be elicited differ somewhat. Kuban et al. studied 10 classic deep tendon reflexes in premature infants born after more than 27 weeks of gestation (71). They found that they could elicit the pectoralis major readily in all infants regardless of maturity, and the Achilles, patellar, biceps, thigh adductors, and brachioradialis in at least 98% of babies born at more than 33 weeks of gestation. Infants born at less than 33 weeks of gestation had diminished rates for patellar and biceps reflexes and decreased intensity compared with older infants. They were least able to elicit the finger flexors, jaw, crossed adductors, and triceps reflexes. Factors that influence the response include infant state and medical treatment. The ideal state for testing DTRs is quiet and awake. In adults when an examiner needs to get the patient to relax, he can use Jendrassik's maneuver of reinforcement by asking the patient to look away and clench their hands or jaw. By creating a diversionary spinal arc at a level above the reflex being tested, cortical suppression of the reflex is blocked (72). Similar techniques of diversion and calming are important in infants not already in a quiet, awake state. Offering a pacifier or engaging the infant visually are helpful steps. Reflexes should not be attempted in a crying infant.

Treatment with theophylline tends to increase the Achilles response. The intensity of responses does not depend on whether or not an infant is ill but is less in infants born at less than 33 weeks of gestation (71,73) (Table 10).

Table 10. *Deep tendon reflexes*

Name of reflex	Normal response	Muscle	Nerve	Spinal level	Placement of examiner's finger or hammer strike and patient's extremity
Jaw	Elevation of the chin	Masseter	Trigeminal and facial	**Cr V**, VII	Place finger point over infant's chin with jaw slightly open
Deltoid	Elevation of arm	Deltoid	Axillary	**C5**, C6	On lateral aspect of humerus at junction of upper and middle thirds over insertion of deltoid Patient's shoulder slightly abducted
Pectoral	Adduction and slight internal rotation arm	Pectoralis major	Medial and lateral pectoral nerves	C5–**C6** clavicular head (medial)	Over front of the axilla with finger directed firmly across the muscle
	Clavicular fibers flex the arm			C7, **C8**, T1 sternocostal head (lateral)	Patient's shoulder slightly abducted.
Biceps	Flexion of forearm (sometimes some supination)	Biceps	Musculocutaneous	C5, **C6**	In the superomedial aspect of the antecubital fossa on the biceps tendon Patient's forearm semi-flexed and slightly pronated
Triceps	Extension of forearm	Triceps	Radial	C6, **C7, C8**	Over the triceps tendon above olecranon Alternatively, strike the muscle directly while partially flexing the forearm
Brachioradial	Flexion of forearm	Brachioradialis	Radial	C5, **C6**, C7	Strike directly over the distal third, lateral edge of the radius while slowly flexing and extending the arm in semipronation.
Finger flexors	Flexion of phalanges	Flexor digitorum superficialis and profundus	Median and medial part of the ulnar	**C8**, T1	Horizontally across the base of infant's fingers to elicit a partial grasp
Adductor and crossed adductor	Adduction of hip	Adductors	Obturator	L2, L3, L4	Index finger diagonally across the medial aspect above the knee with the little finger on the contralateral leg to maintain a 45° to 60° angle Thighs in slight abduction
Knee jerk	Extension of knee	Quadriceps femoris	Femoral	L2, **L3, L4**	Across patellar tendon just below knee in crease or just above patella on quadriceps tendon Hold knee and hip flexed at about 30°
Ankle jerk (Achilles reflex)	Plantar flexion of foot at ankle	Gastrocnemius and soleus	Tibial	L5, **S1**, S2	Horizontally across the plantar aspect of the infant's foot at insertion of Achilles tendon Foot is partially dorsiflexed, leg flexed

Reflexes listed are those likely present after 33 weeks' gestational age. Reflexes in **bold** indicate those most frequently tested, but Kuban et al. found pectoralis most reliably present regardless of gestational age. Spinal level in **bold** indicates primary supply.
Data from Kuban (71), and Slaby (73).

Skin Reflexes (74)

Stimulation of the skin induces a variety of regular and stereotyped motor responses of the limbs (74). The muscle groups involved are localized either under or at a distance from the specific skin site. In adults the superficial responses in the neurologic examination include the abdominal, gluteal, cremasteric, and plantar reflexes. There is a changing developmental pattern in these responses such that premature infants have the greatest number of responses and adults the least. Vlach has reported on the evolution of these skin reflexes. By stimulating the specific skin reflexes, an examiner can induce complex motor responses

Table 11. *Stimulation, innervation, and responses of the 28 skin reflexes*

Reflex (stimulation site)	Stimulation site nerve supply	Dermatome stimulated	Motor response[a]	Main myotome and muscles responding
Axillary (axillary fossa)	Lateral cutaneous branch of intercostal and medial cutaneous of arm	T2 + T3/4	3: full action of arm, slight head rotation, trunk incurvation, homolateral limb flexion	Pectoralis C5–T1, latissimus dorsi C6–8
		C8 + T1	2: moderate adduction	
			1: weak adduction (contraction)	
Cubital (cubital fossa)	Medial cutaneous of arm and forearm	C5 + T1	3: elbow flexion (>2 cm)	Biceps, brachialis C5 + C6, brachioradialis
			2: moderate flexion	
			1: slight contraction	
Digital (ulnar border of hand)	Volar branch of ulnar	C8	3: semi-extension 5th–2nd digits	Extensor(s) digitorum C6–8
			2: semi-extension 5th and 4th digits	
			1: slight extension 5th digit	
Finger extension (dorsal surface of fingers)	Radial, ulnar and median	C7, C8	3: semi-extension 5th–2nd digits (>150°)	Extensor(s) digitorum C6–8
		C7	2: semi-extension (70–90°)	
			1: slight extension	
Thumb adduction (palm of hand)	Volar branches of ulnar and median	C8	3: full adduction of thumb	Adductor pollicis C8, opponens pollicis C6–7
			2: moderate adduction	
		C7	1: weak adduction	
Hand-grasp (palm of hand)	Volar branches of median and ulnar	C7–8	3: strong flexion of fingers	Flexor(s) digitorum C7–T1
			2: weak flexion	
			1: slight movement	
Inguinal (Inguinal area)	Cutaneous branches of 12th intercostal and iliohypogastric	T12 + L1	3: strong hip joint flexion, slight knee and ankle flexion, slight trunk incurvation	Iliopsoas T11–L3, flexor(s) cruris L5–S2, anterior tibialis L4–5
			2: slight hip flexion	
			1: weak muscle contraction	
Abduction (lateral surface of thigh)	Lateral cutaneous of thigh	L4–5	3: thigh abduction (30°)	Gluteus medius L5–S1, tensor fascia lata L4–S1
			2: slight abduction	
			1: weak muscle contraction	
Anterior tibialis (anterior tibialis near ankle-dorsum)	Cutaneous branches of sural and fibula	L5	3: dorsal flexion of foot and toes, knee flexion	Anterior tibialis L4–5
			2: slight dorsal flexion	
			1: weak muscle contraction	
Foot (dorsal surface)	Fibula	L5	3: dorsal flexion of foot (90°)	Anterior tibialis L4–5
			2: slight dorsal flexion	
			1: weak muscle contraction	
Toe (dorsal surface of toes)	Fibula and profundus	L4–S1	3: dorsal flexion of toes, slight dorsal flexion of foot	Extensor(s) digitorum L5–S1
			2: slight dorsal flexion of toes	
			1: weak muscle contraction	
Plantar (plantar surface of foot, lateral border)	Plantar (lateral)	L5–S1	3: dorsal flexion and abduction of toes, dorsal flexion of foot, knee flexion	Extensor(s) and abductor(s) digitorum L4–S1
			2: slight dorsal flexion of toes	
			1: weak dorsal flexion	
Foot-grasp (distal sole of foot)	Plantar	L4–S1	3: strong flexion of toes, slight plantar flexion of foot	Toe flexors S1–2
			2: slight flexion of toes	
			1: slight movement of toes	
Abdominal (abdominal surface)	Cutaneous branches of intercostal	T7–12	3: strong muscle contraction and trunk incurvation, slight hip flexion	Obliqui T5–L1
			2: strong muscle contraction only	
			1: slight muscle contraction	
Lateral abdominal (lateral abdominal surface, axillary line)	Lateral cutaneous branches of intercostal	T7–12	3: trunk incurvation, slight hip flexion	Obliqui T5–L1
			2: slight incurvation	
			1: weak muscle movement	
Pubic (pubic area)	Iliohypogastric	T12 + L1	3: adduction and flexion of both hips	Adductors, iliopsoas L1–4
			2: slight adduction	
			1: weak adduction	
Crossed extension (sole of foot)	Plantar	L4–S1	3: flexion, extension and adduction of limb, big toe dorsiflexion	Flexors, extensors, adductors L1–S2
			2: flexion only (contralateral leg)	
			1: very slight flexion	
Magnet (sole of foot)	Plantar	L4–S1	3: strong extension of legs	Extensors L2–S2
			2: semi-extension	
			1: very slight extension	

continued

Table 11. *Continued.*

Reflex (stimulation site)	Stimulation site nerve supply	Dermatome stimulated	Motor response[a]	Main myotome and muscles responding
Placing (dorsal surface of foot)	Fibular	L5	3: placing and extensor thrust 2: placing only 1: very slight placing	Flexors, extensors L1–S1
Nuchal (dorsal surface of neck)	Dorsal branches of cervical	C3–4/5	3: neck extension, head elevation 2: slight neck extension 1: upper trapezius muscle contraction only	Trapezius (upper part) C2–5
Trapezius (over upper part of trapezius muscle)	Dorsal branch of supraclavicular	C4	3: shoulder elevation (>2 cm) 2: slight elevation 1: trapezius muscle contraction only	Trapezius C2–5
Scapular (over scapula)	Cutaneous branches of intercostal	T1–6	3: extension of shoulder and arm 2: slight extension (depression) of shoulder 1: very slight shoulder extension	Latissimus teres major C6–8
Interscapular (between scapula and vertebral column)	Cutaneous branches of thoracic	T1–7	3: trunk incurvation, head rotation, homolateral limb flexion 2: trunk incurvation, limb movements 1: weak incurvation or local contraction	Longissimus thoracis, iliocostal T2–L4/5
Lumbar (paravertebral lumbar)	Cutaneous branches of thoracic	T8–L1	3: trunk incurvation, leg movements 2: slight incurvation, leg movements 1: local muscle contraction	Obliqui T5–L1, quadratus T10–L2
Gluteal (over glutei)	Dorsal branches of lumbar and sacral	L5–S2	3: strong gluteal muscle contraction, rotation of leg 2: gluteal muscle contraction only 1: weak muscle contraction	Gluteus maximus, gluteus medius L4/5–S1/2
Sacral (sacrococcygeal area)	Sacral	S1–3	3: bilateral gluteal contraction, rotation of thighs 2: gluteal muscle contraction only 1: weak muscle contraction	Gluteus maximus, gluteus medius L4–S1/S2
Vertebral (over the spine)	Dorsal branches of thoracic and lumbar	C8–S1	3: elevation of pelvis, flexion of legs 2: slight elevation of pelvis 1: weak elevation of pelvis 1: weak muscle contraction only	Erectors of the trunk C3–L5
Popliteal (popliteal fossa)	Posterior cutaneous of thigh	S1–2	3: slight knee flexion 2: very slight flexion 1: muscle contractions only	Biceps, semitendinosus, semimembranosus L5–S2

[a] 3, strong; 2, medium; 1, weak, local contraction only.

that, to some extent, substitute for voluntary activity by the infant. These reflexes are used to execute many of the specific reactions that are detailed in the reflexes and responses comprising the neurologic examination. The reflexes, their innervation, and expected responses are detailed in Table 11.

Primitive Reflexes

The primitive reflexes (or primary reflexes) are stereotypic motor responses to various stimuli that develop before birth and disappear during early infancy in a predictable pattern. Caputo divides the primitive reflexes into three groupings depending on the age at which they appear and disappear (75). Primitive reflexes I are those that occur only during fetal development, so they are not present at term birth. These are not well defined but include a startlelike response that occurs in the first trimester only. Primitive reflexes II appear during late intrauterine development and disappear by at least 6 months of age. Primitive reflexes II include the Moro reflex, asymmetrical tonic neck reflex, tonic labyrinthine reflex (supine or prone), Galant reflex, positive support reflex, symmetrical tonic neck reflex, plantar grasp, placing reactions, upper extremity placing, stepping (walking) reflex, crossed extension reaction, and downward thrust. The late reflexes appear in early infancy when the second group are suppressed and include the postural reactions that appear just as voluntary motor functions such as turning from front to back and getting into a sitting position develop. These include two postural reactions: the Landau and the derotative righting response. Other postural reflexes that appear after 3 months and suppress by 10 months are protection, righting, and equilibrium reactions. These include the parachute, head righting in horizontal suspension, head righting in tilt from side to side, lateral extension of one arm toward the side of the fall, and upward counter movements of the arm and leg in forward and backward tilt from a sitting position. These reactions require a complex interplay of cerebral and cerebellocortical adjustments to multiple sensory inputs via proprioceptive, visual, and vestibular pathways. Detailed descriptions of each of these later reactions are provided in articles by Capute (9,76–78). These reactions that appear after the primitive reflexes wane are called by other investigators the "secondary responses" (1,79).

Individual investigators have their favorites among the primitive reflexes as being the most informative and indicative of neuromotor function and development. Delayed or asequential appearance of motor milestones is useful as an early, albeit not perfect, predictor of later motor dysfunction (13,75). In the neonatal period and in following infants who remain in intensive care for prolonged periods or require close sequential assessments because of developmental risk factors, these reflexes are part of a complete neurologic examination. Not only is the presence or absence of each reflex in relation to developmental age of importance, but also of value are the quality and habituation responses that should be present. For instance, infants in whom there is little or no functional cortical matter, such as in hydranencephaly, may have a technically normal initial primitive reflex response but then will fail to habituate and extinguish that response upon repeated stimulation. In contrast to the normally expected habituation and diminution of response, the reaction may increase with repetition and be one of the few abnormal signs in the neurologic examination (7). Therefore, it is important not only to know the timing of the development of these responses but also how to assess whether or not they are qualitatively normal. For practical purposes, using just a few reflexes is sufficient; Volpe suggests using the Moro reflex, palmar grasp, and tonic neck responses for all newborn examinations (7). When more detail is indicated or for more scrutiny in following neurodevelopment, more responses can be added to the examination. The techniques and expected responses for the earlier primitive reflexes are described.

INDICATORS OF BEHAVIOR

Evaluating behavior during an examination provides information about cerebral integrity that is indispensable in determining if neurologic function is normal or if an infant is in pain or otherwise ill. Caregivers are in the best positions to evaluate behavior of newborn infants on a continual basis, but some observations can be made during each physical assessment. Suggested observations of behavior include assessing irritability, cuddliness, self-quieting activity, orientation or decrement in response to visual and auditory signals, defensive reactions, demonstration of hunger, cycling of sleep/wake activity, responsiveness, and vocalizations. Brazelton has established a scoring system for observations of behavior that is helpful to understand some of the variability in possible responses (25). Als has added items that are more helpful in understanding the behaviors of premature infants (32).

Irritability (11,25)

Irritability is assessed in the infant's response by audible fussing or crying for at least 3 seconds to aversive stimuli such as uncovering, undressing, pull to sit, turn to prone or to supine, ventral suspension, the Moro reflex, walking, withdrawal, or the tonic neck reflex maneuvers. Observations include the presence of spontaneous fussiness as well as how many and how strong a stimulus must be to elicit a response.

A normal term infant should react after a noxious stimulation for several seconds but then, almost as soon as the stimulus is removed, begin to decrease the intensity and calm down. Relatively benign maneuvers should elicit no intense reaction. Maneuvers such as the Moro reflex are more noxious than undressing or pull to sit. Abnormal responses are those that are exaggerated compared with the type of stimulus, prolonged duration of reaction, or those absent despite a strong negative stimulus. Premature infants tend to show a less intense crying reaction to these noxious stimuli, particularly when much of their intensive care involves discomfort in pain or noise. Their reaction to an adverse stimulus may not be crying but rather decreases in oxygen saturation, apnea, or a mass reflex.

Cuddliness (25)

Cuddliness is a measure of an infant's response to being held while alert in both vertical and horizontal positions. The responses range from resistance to being held with pushing away, thrashing, or stiffening to nestling, turning the head toward the examiner, and molding to the examiner's body. Being limp should not be confused with cuddling.

Self-Quieting Activity (25)

When a baby is crying, he may make obvious efforts to quiet himself. The responses range from making no attempts without intervention from a caregiver to sustained self-quieting with no need for external intervention. Self-quieting activity includes rooting and finding an oral object, modulating the cry intensity, shifting position, or becoming visually attentive as examples.

Visual and Auditory Response Decrement (25)

With the infant in a quiet state after he or she has shown an aversive reaction to a bright light, the light is presented to the infant for 1 to 2 seconds and the response observed. The stimulus is repeated after 5 seconds up to 10 trials if there is no decrement in response. If there is a loss of response, it is repeated twice to verify. The response is evaluated for the infant's ability to control startles of the entire body and to delay and decrease localized startle response. Full decrement is when the infant shuts out any response to the light.

Similar decrement of response should be demonstrated with a disturbing auditory stimulus.

Visual and Auditory Orientation Responses (25)

If the infant is awake and alert, the infant is asked to fix on an object (red ball) that is moved horizontally. If there is horizontal movement of the head as well, the ball is moved vertically. The responses range from no response or brief fixation and interest to complex following. Similar response is demonstrable with a pleasant sound source. Absence of vertical head movement in the newborn period is not abnormal.

Defensive Reaction (25)

Following the technique of Brazelton, with the infant's head in the mid-line supine position, a cloth is placed over the infant's eyes and kept firmly in place by holding it close to the temporal regions but without occluding the airway. The cloth is held in place for up to

1 minute to observe the infant's best attempt to swipe at the cloth. If there is a swiping attempt, the hold on the cloth is released to see if he or she will remove it. Swiping directly and removing the cloth is the most mature response. Other responses include general quieting, twisting body action, head turning, or nondirected swipes. Pressure to the eyes by too tight a cloth should be avoided because of the risks of direct trauma to the eyes, bradycardia, and apnea. A poor response to the blindfold technique should not be followed by a tighter application of the cloth.

Dubowitz et al. described a technique for a similar maneuver by occluding the nose with either a cloth or hand, resulting in a variable response, as one can imagine. They expressed a hope that lack of response would predict a risk for later sudden infant death (11). This has not been confirmed.

GENERAL REFLEXES

Posture Supine and Prone (Resting Posture) (2,11)

Observation of resting posture is made on approach to the bedside and helps provide an immediate sense of the infant's health (Fig. 6). The resting posture is a sign of general tone and maturity, but it also reflects range of motion in the joints. At term the normal resting posture is symmetrical, with all limbs flexed and slightly abducted, but there is a wide variation depending on day of life, intrauterine position, and environment. For example, breech presentation generally is associated with more flexion at the hips, with limitation in extension. If a presentation was frank breech, the knees may be abnormally hyperextended with decreased tone in the legs and increased in the hips because of abnormal ranges of motion in the joints and shortening or stretching of the muscles rather than truly abnormal tone. After face presentation, the head may be retroflexed with the chin elevated, falsely suggesting opisthotonus or abnormal hypertonicity of the neck extensor muscles (see Chapter 6, Fig. 4).

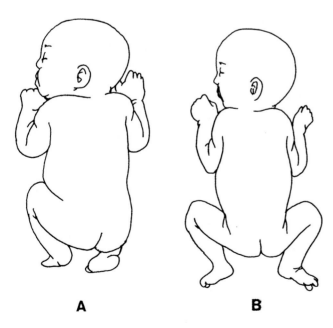

A   **B**

Figure 6. Resting positions in prone. The more mature a newborn infant, the more tightly flexed is the resting posture with more adduction of the shoulders and hips. **A:** Term resting posture. **B:** More premature resting posture.

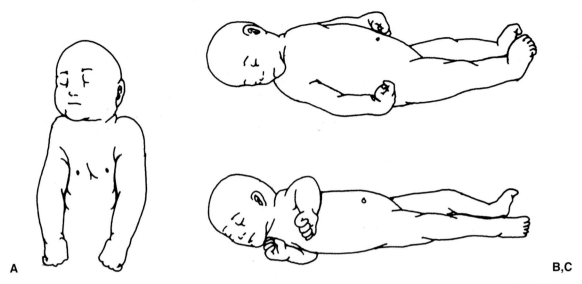

Figure 7. Abnormal posturing. **A:** Opisthotonic. The neck and arms are hyperextended. Legs and trunk may also be hyperextended. **B:** Decerebrate. The legs and arms are extended with the wrists flexed and hands fisted. **C:** Decorticate. The arms are flexed and legs extended.

Abnormal resting posture:

Limbs lying flat on the surface
Opisthotonic posture with the head retroflexed and the lower limbs extended (Fig. 7A)
Turning of the head consistently to one side with an asymmetrical posture
Exaggerated flexion of the extremities
Shoulder adducted and arms flexed such that the hands are held constantly in front of the mouth
Marked or consistent asymmetry in the posture of the limbs
Persistent spontaneous plantar grasp
Hands clenched tightly or persistently
Decorticate posture (Fig. 7C)
Decerebrate posture (Fig. 7B)

Spontaneous Motor Activity

Observe the infant before and after stimulation for the movements of all extremities (2,5,15,25). If the head is turned toward one side, an asymmetrical tonic neck reflex will affect the resting posture and, therefore, the pattern of spontaneous activity. If an ATNR is present, the head should be turned to mid-line. Evaluate for whether the movements are through a wide range or are limited, if they occur with the limbs in predominantly extension or flexion, and if there are alternating movements from side to side. They should be judged for speed of movement and intensity with activity graded as absent, weak, strong, or very strong with consideration of appropriateness to state and quality.

An expected pattern of activity in an awake infant is semi-purposeful stretching with alternation of flexion and extension. When an infant is asleep, there is little or no gross motor activity and his (or her) posture is relatively flexed. As a term infant becomes more used to living in his unconfined extrauterine space, his movements involve more extension and wider amplitude but should still remain equal from side to side.

The premature infant tends to lie more quietly even when awake but increases his activity with gestational age. In general, the healthier the premature infant, the greater the waking activity. In VLBW infants the movements of the arms or legs are a flinging out as the weight of the extremity seems to exceed the gross motor strength, so qualitatively there is a different pattern of activity. Because the period of time spent in the active awake condition increases both with gestational and chronologic age, activity should increase accordingly with time. Observation of spontaneous motor activity in an alert infant is especially telling about the overall well-being and remains one of the most important general observations for both regional and system assessments.

Abnormal patterns for spontaneous motor activity:

Repetitive, stereotypic movements such as bicycling or arm waving
Amount of activity inconsistent with level of alertness
Unequal activity among the extremities in the absence of restraints

Spontaneous Movements of the Head in the Prone Position (2)

The infant must be awake and active. Observe for lifting and turning of the head. If there is no spontaneous lift, firmly but gently stroke the back just off mid-line from the neck to the level of the scapula tip.

A normal response is lifting the head for a few seconds. In the first few days this response normally may be blunted. The ability to lift the head improves during the first month, so that by the end of the first month the infant should be lifting and turning the head regularly with more weight bearing on the elbows. Premature infants demonstrate an ability to lift their head in the prone position well before term. An abnormal response is either no attempt to lift or a sustained lift for longer than 10 seconds that accompanies other findings of opisthotonos.

Spontaneous Crawling or Bauer's Response (2)

With the infant awake and active in the prone position with the head in mid-line and the arms free from the body, watch for spontaneous crawling or alternating flexion of both lower extremities. If there is no spontaneous activity, press your thumb into the sole of a foot to induce a withdrawal or crawl. If there is asymmetry in the response, turn the head the other direction.

A normal response is a coordinated motion with vigorous activity; the infant lifts and turns his or her head. Normal infants may not demonstrate this reaction in the first few days of life. Premature infants will have a less fluid crawling action but become rather mobile with this activity well before they reach 40 weeks corrected gestational age.

Abnormal Spontaneous Crawling

Weak or absent response even with stimulation
Asymmetry even when the head is turned the opposite direction
Arching of the back with hyperextended neck and no relaxation
Stereotypic repetition in sleeping states
No attempt to free the face
Vigorous and repetitive movements enough to cause abrasion of knees

Athetoid Postures and Movements (2)

Some of the fingers are fully flexed with others extended, the elbow is flexed and the upper limb rotated, or the elbow is extended with the rotation at the wrist. The movements are slow changes. An expected pattern at term is occasional athetoid movements of the arms, forearms, hands, and fingers, especially in quiet awake or light sleep states. Athetoid postures in full-term infants occur throughout the neonatal period, but athetoid movements should not be continuous. More continuous athetoid movements are seen in premature infants. Athetoid movements are infrequent or absent in depressed infants. They may be exaggerated in asphyxiated infants or asymmetric in paresis.

Tremor (Jitteriness) (80–84)

Look for the incidence, frequency, and amplitude of movements in the extremities and jaw. (Frequency: Low is less than six times per second; high is more than six times per second. Amplitude: Low is less than about 3 cm; 3 cm or more is high.) A sustained low-frequency, high-amplitude tremor is equivalent to clonus.

High-frequency, low-amplitude tremor is normally present in term infants in the first few days of life, especially during or after crying, but is not normally present after the first 4 days. A benign tremor should extinguish when the infant begins sucking (84). Tremors of the chin are normal. Abnormal tremor continues even in the presence of sucking or other soothing activities in a noncrying baby. Brazelton suggests that aversive stimuli may set off a startle followed by tremulousness that subsides, but mildly aversive stimuli should not set off tremors (25). Tremulousness should not be consistent and repeated in all states. Normally more will be observed in the active, crying states.

Jitteriness is a frequently observed motor activity in newborn infants and one parents ask about, most often thinking it is shivering or nervousness. The prevalence and correlates of jitteriness were evaluated in a sample of 936 healthy full-term infants by Parker et al. (80). Jitteriness was seen in 44% of this sample: 23% were classified as mildly jittery, 8% as moderately jittery, and 13% as extremely jittery. Jitteriness was seen most commonly in infants who were sleepy or active and least commonly in infants who were quietly wakeful during the neonatal examination. Jittery infants were more likely to be difficult to console when crying and less visually alert than were nonjittery infants. Jitteriness was more likely in slightly smaller and shorter infants, in those more than 12 hours old, and in those not exposed to maternal general anesthesia. In an expanded sample of 1,054 healthy and sick full-term infants, jitteriness was observed more commonly in neonates who had been exposed prenatally to maternal marijuana use, but not to cocaine use (80). The magnitude of the drug effect was small.

In a study by Linder et al., the response of neonatal tremor to a suckling stimulation test was investigated in 102 healthy neonates born at term. In 84 the tremor resolved immediately; none had hypocalcemia, and only one had mild hypoglycemia. Eighteen in whom the tremor continued had either hypocalcemia or hypoglycemia. They considered the test was positive for excessive tremor if it stopped when sucking and returned when the supplied finger was taken out (84).

Moro Reflex (Fig. 8)

Method 1. Release after Traction Response (15)

With the infant supine, pull on both arms to raise the shoulders a few centimeters off the table. Release the arms to allow the infant to fall back to the table. There is no need to raise the infant more than enough to create a space between the neck and the table. Trials should be continued until there is extinction of response.

This technique means the infant's upper extremities are starting from a more extended posture than necessarily in the other techniques but allows a rapid combination of procedures when coupled with the evaluation of palmar grip and arm traction. If there is any question of abnormal response, these maneuvers might best be separated, but for most screening examinations, combining these reflexes is feasible and yields enough information.

Method 2. "Drop" of the Baby (2) (Fig. 8)

Suspend the baby by supporting the trunk with one hand and head with the other hand. Rapidly lower both hands 10 to 20 cm without flexing the neck. Remember not to tilt the baby during the "drop." Trials should be continued until there is extinction of response.

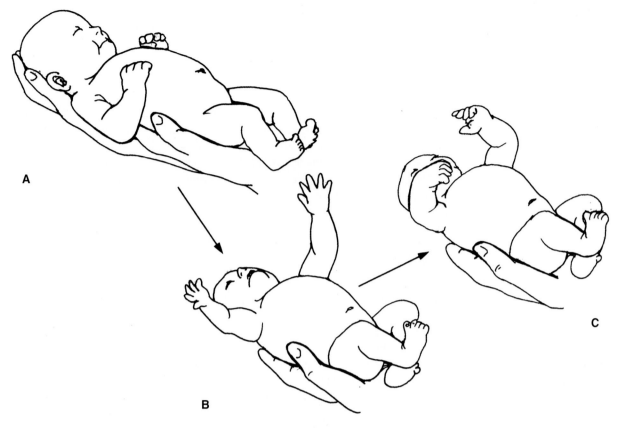

Figure 8. Moro reflex by body drop. **A:** Infant is supported with arms in comfortable resting position across the chest. **B:** Both hands are dropped without tilting the head. The first part of the response is extension at the elbows and abduction of the arms. Hands open fully. **C:** The second part of the response is adduction and flexion with curling of the fingers.

Method 3. Head Bang (85)

With infant lying supine in a symmetrically mid-line position, sharply slap the mattress with both hands, one on either side of the infant. Trials should be continued until there is extinction of response.

Eliciting a Moro reflex by striking the mattress is the only feasible technique for infants who are connected to major mechanical devices, in an incubator, or generally ill. Similarly, it is the method of choice for infants with possible spinal cord injuries. Other techniques, including pinching of the epigastrium, have been suggested (86,87). There is likely strong overlap in the elicited patterns of a Moro reflex and a startle reaction in these other techniques (88).

It is important to control the positions of the head and body during any method to ensure symmetry of response. An infant's extremities cannot be restrained in any way. Because of the noise from slapping the bed, a part of the response to the head bang technique may be a startle in reaction to the loud noise.

A normal response is symmetrical abduction of the arms and extension of the forearms followed by adduction and flexion of the forearms. The hands open completely. At the conclusion, the infant cries or grimaces. With repetition the full response should diminish in intensity and disappear as the infant habituates. In term infants the response should diminish after three tries. In premature infants more attempts may give a complete response, but it should extinguish by 10 attempts. Failure to extinguish or nonhabituation is an important indicator of lack of cortical inhibition and may be one of the major indicators of poor cerebral function above a brain stem level or of cortical irritability in the early newborn period (7). For example, infants with cortical irritability from drug withdrawal have exaggerated reactions and delayed habituation (89). Repeated attempts in normal infants leads to absence in the motor reflex in habituation but reactive anger.

Startle Reflex (88)

Throughout the course of the neurologic examination, evaluate for the number and intensity of startle responses, elicited both by noise or movement and spontaneously. If none are observed, with the infant in light sleep or quiet awake state, stimulate him with a sudden, loud noise or by tapping on the sternum.
Differing from the Moro reflex, this reaction involves flexion of the elbows while the hands remain closed, but there should be a total body reaction (3). When repeatedly presented with a stimulus to elicit a startle, a normal, mature response is to inhibit and react with less intensity until completely ignoring the stimulus or showing anger with intense crying. More immature infants may demonstrate a mass reflex.

Abnormal Startle Reflex

A markedly exaggerated or easily elicited response
Failure to habituate the response to repeated trials
Frequent spontaneous startles without any external stimulation
Initiation of mass response

Some observers consider the Moro reflex and startle to be the same response or at least that the Moro reflex is a form of startle response (88). The technique of stimulating the Moro reflex is understandably likely to stimulate a startle, but the complete sequence of movements that make up the Moro reflex are not normally seen with the frequency that less marked startles are.

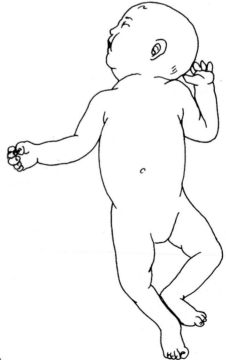

Figure 9. Complete asymmetric tonic neck reflex.

Asymmetrical Tonic Neck Reflex (2,10,15) (Fig. 9)

The infant should be in light sleep or awake but not crying. With the infant lying supine, the head mid-line, and the shoulders horizontal, the head is gently turned to the right until the jaw is over the right shoulder, held there for 15 seconds, and then released. Note the position of the extremities. Repeat by turning the head to the left.

The reflex can be seen in both prone and supine positions, but is most often tested in supine. Elicited response is a passive reflex; active reflex occurs spontaneously as the infant turns his or her own head.

A normal response is mental extension and occipital flexion. The arm and leg on the side toward which the face is turned will be extended. The extremities on the side opposite the face will be flexed. The response may be stronger in the lower extremities, especially in premature infants. After a few seconds the infant will either move out of this posture or lessen the degree of flexion and extension. Premature infants may normally lie at rest in this position in both supine and prone positions for indefinite periods. There are other combinations of responses normally seen.

Types of response in asymmetrical tonic neck reflex (ATNR) (90):

Complete: Both chin extremities extended and both occipital extremities flexed. Makes up
    approximately 50% of passive responses.
Leg ATNR: Chin lower extremity is extended, occipital lower extremity is flexed. Makes
    up approximately 25% of passive responses.
Arm ATNR: Chin upper extremity is extended, occipital upper extremity is flexed. Makes
    up approximately 4% of passive responses.
Unidirectional: Exclusively to right or left. Makes up approximately 15% of passive re-
    sponses.
44% of infants have spontaneous, complete ATNR.
Response time varies from 1 to 7 seconds, with resistance demonstrated by 15 seconds of
    holding the head in most.

Abnormal ATNR

Sustained or exaggerated response with failure to move out of the position while the head
    is held for 15 seconds or after the head is released. Obligatory means infant cannot break
    the reflex while the head is rotated.
Consistent failure to move an extremity.
Persistence of this response beyond 6 months of age (17,77).

Asymmetrical tonic neck reflex is an easily elicited reflex in the immediate newborn period and should not be considered pathologic in term infants unless it is obligatory and fails to subside. Although bidirectional responses are normally encountered, unidirectional responses are not uncommon. The majority of infants display the complete reflex, but the lower extremities are the most consistent participants (90). Because ATNR is so common in the newborn period, its impact needs to be considered before interpreting other tests of tone and position.

Some clinicians use the term "tonic neck reflex" for this reflex and designate it as asymmetrical when the response of the two sides is unequal and, therefore, considered abnormal (91). As originally described, the ATNR and the TNR are different reflexes as noted later in this chapter.

UPPER SEGMENTAL REFLEXES: PASSIVE TONE

Scarf Sign (15) (Fig. 10)

Hold the infant in a semi-reclining position by supporting the neck and head with one hand. Draw one hand and arm as far as possible across the chest toward the opposite

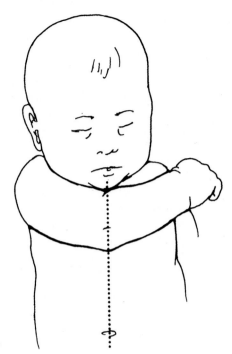

Figure 10. Scarf sign.

shoulder so the arm forms a "neck scarf." Determine the relationship of the elbow to the mid-line structures and evaluate the resistance to abduction of the shoulder. It is sometimes more informative to push the arm just above the elbow to avoid stimulating an arm traction response.

A normal response is symmetry between the sides and reaching the position expected for gestational age. The more premature the infant, and the lower the upper segmental tone, the farther the elbow passes mid-line. As extremely premature infants develop, they tend to have increased tone of the upper axial extensors, causing the scarf response to be more mature than expected. If an infant is obese, hydropic, or has a shortened humerus or fractured clavicle, the ability for the elbow to reach mid-line will be inhibited and not truly indicative of muscle tone.

Abnormal Scarf Sign

An abnormal response is either failure to reach the position expected for gestational age or an exaggerated response. Asymmetry suggests weakness in the side where the elbow reaches farthest. If there is unusual resistance unilaterally, it is more likely due to something other than neuromuscular tone, such as a fractured clavicle, for example, because high muscle tone is rarely unilateral at this age. Increased resistance bilaterally indicates increased tone in the shoulder girdle.

Recoil of the Forearm at the Elbow (3,6,15)

Optimum state for the baby is awake and active, lying supine with the head in a neutral position. Make sure there is nothing inhibiting free movement of the arms. Flex the infant's arms at the elbows for 5 seconds. Extend and then gently release them without causing a startle. Do not pull on the arms while extending the forearms.

A normal response is a brisk, symmetrical flexion at both elbows. This response is stronger in infants used to having their arms more flexed in utero, so is strongest in the term infant with less vigorous response in premature infants. Normal infants show a decremental response during early infancy, but a response should be present throughout the neonatal period. Premature infants who are at 40 weeks corrected gestational age will not demonstrate a pattern of recoil comparable with a term infant but are likely to have more ready recoil than they demonstrated at birth.

Abnormal Response in Recoil of Forearm

Absent, delayed, or weak recoil
Forceful flexion with stimulation of a mass reflex
Asymmetry that is consistent on several trials

Square Window (6,11,14,92) (Fig. 11)

With the elbows flexed, flex the wrist as far as possible and determine the minimum angle between the palm and the flexor surface of the forearm.

Dubowitz and Ballard use this item to assess gestational age, but Dubowitz does not include it in the formatted neurologic examination, relying more on tone in the lower segment (6,11,14,92).

A normal response is symmetry between the two sides with the angle somewhat dependent on intrauterine position as well as muscle tone. The angle decreases toward the latter weeks of gestation to the point of no space between the palm and forearm at term.

Abnormal Response in Square Window

An abnormal square window is asymmetry, or marked increase or decrease in resistance to movement beyond that expected for gestational age.

UPPER SEGMENTAL REFLEXES: ACTIVE TONE

Palmar Grasp (Upper Extremity Grasp, Tonic Reflex of the Finger Flexors, Hand Grasp) (2,10,15,25) (Fig. 12)

The infant should be in a quiet, awake state, and lying supine with the head in the midline and the arms semi-flexed. Without touching the dorsal surface of the hand, place your index finger across the palm and apply gentle pressure. Test both hands simultaneously. If the hand is too tightly clenched, stimulate opening by stroking along the ulnar

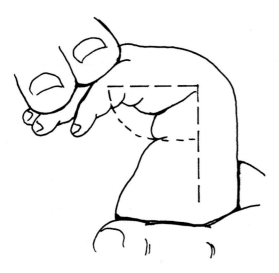

Figure 11. Square window.

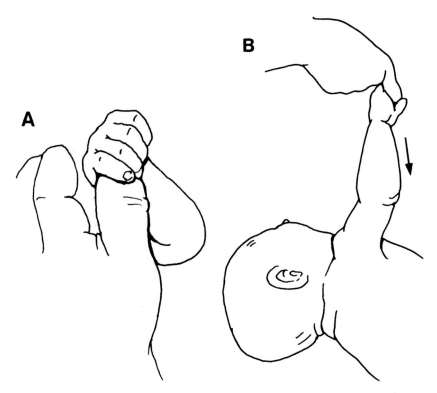

Figure 12. A: Finger grasp. **B:** The grasp can be so strong in even tiny infants that he can be lifted off the mattress.

surface of the hand and observe an unwrapping of the fingers. Similarly, firmly touching the dorsal surface of the hand may stimulate opening of the fingers.

All fingers should flex around the examiner's finger with a strong grasp that is sustained for several seconds and then relaxes. Allow the patient to suck on a nipple to facilitate a grasp if the initial response is poor. Before deciding there is asymmetry in strength, make certain the infant is perfectly symmetrical in position. There will be minimal response if the infant is either too deeply asleep or too irritable.

The strength and duration of the grasp is related to gestational age, although immature infants display remarkable strength in their grasp (Fig. 12B). The reflex is strongest at term, should weaken by age of 2 months, and disappear by 3 months.

Abnormal Response in Palmar Grasp

Any asymmetry in intensity between the two sides that may indicate a peripheral weakness
  due to Erb's or Klumpke's paresis (make sure head is in mid-line)
Persistence of the grip beyond a few seconds or so clenched that the fingers blanch
Bilateral weakness with a short attempt despite stimulation

Arm traction (Pull to Sit) (10,15) (Fig. 13)

After eliciting the palmar grasp, pull the infant up and forward to provoke flexion in the upper extremities and neck. If head lag is noted, test neck flexors in isolation. The infant should pull with his (or her) arms while keeping his head aligned with the axis of the trunk. The lower extremities flex for a few seconds. Premature infants will demonstrate less pulling and head control.

Some investigators consider arm traction and pull to sit to be the same maneuver (10). Others feel that the pull to sit is a later response when there is a volitional attempt to sit up as the arms are supported (15). There is a difference in the feeling of the two responses: the earlier response allows the examiner passively to lift the infant with his partially flexed extremities, and the later response includes volitional use of abdominal and neck muscles while the arms are actively pulling on the examiner's fingers. Whichever term is used in the neonatal period, the response involves noting head control in the neck flexors and active tone in the arm muscles.

Abnormal Response in Pull to Sit

Absent, weak, or asymmetric effort in the arms
Head lag without recovery at term

Arm Release in Prone Position

The infant, awake or in light sleep, is lying in prone with his (or her) head in mid-line and his arms extended next to his trunk so the palms face up (11). Make certain there is no restriction to movement for his upper extremities. Note the time it takes and how far

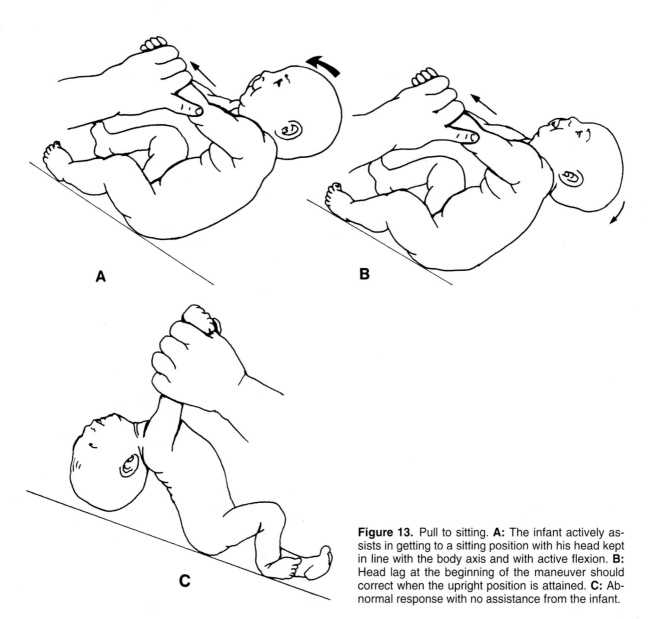

Figure 13. Pull to sitting. **A:** The infant actively assists in getting to a sitting position with his head kept in line with the body axis and with active flexion. **B:** Head lag at the beginning of the maneuver should correct when the upright position is attained. **C:** Abnormal response with no assistance from the infant.

the infant brings his arms forward. If a response is asymmetrical, particularly if the head has fallen to one side and stimulated an ATNR, turn the head to the opposite side.

This response is useful in sick infants who are prone but cannot be turned to evaluate arm recoil and strength. The presence of an intravenous line may inhibit movement.

At term a healthy infant will rapidly bring his hands near his face. This response is dependent on gestational maturity, although healthy preterm infants should be able to bring each arm to the same level.

Abnormal Response

No effort or inability to bring either wrist to the nipple level
Asymmetry of response may indicate a paresis in an upper segment

AXIAL REFLEXES

Active Tone

Evaluation of Neck Flexors (Raise to Sit Maneuver (10), Anterior Neck (15), Anterior Head Control) (Fig. 14A)

With the infant lying supine, grasp the shoulders and raise the infant into a sitting position at a gradual rate to allow time for the infant to flex the neck muscles and assist. Active contraction of the neck flexors brings the head forward before the trunk is fully upright. After the head is momentarily aligned with the slightly forward trunk, the chin should drop onto the chest.

If there is a normal response in neck flexion during traction of the arms or pull to sit, then it is not necessary to reassess them in a separate maneuver, but for purposes of assessing gestational age, or if there is a concern about the strength of these flexors, isolate the neck muscles by lifting at the shoulders.

Dubowitz suggests assessing anterior neck control by starting with the infants in a sitting position and allowing the head to fall back and then noting the degree of neck flexion within 30 seconds.

Any infant with a relatively large head may have difficulty lifting the head because of the weight but should demonstrate an attempt at neck flexion.

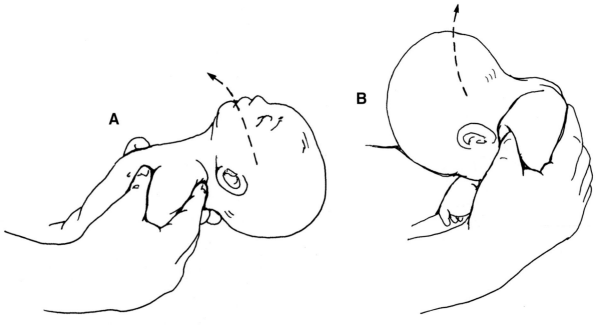

Figure 14. Neck control. **A:** Anterior neck muscles. **B:** Posterior neck muscles.

The tone of the neck flexors develops in a predictable enough pattern to be a reliable contributor to assessment of gestational age. There is little effort in raising the head before 34 weeks, when the control in the vertical position is poor. The term response is full flexion during the raising with the head maintained upright for more than a few seconds until the trunk is tilted further past vertical.

Abnormal Response

No or weak flexion attempt. This pattern indicates either specific flexor muscle weakness, general hypotonia, or central depression.

Head control "better" than expected for age. The head stays in an extended position and fails to fall toward the chest only when the trunk is tilted far forward. This pattern indicates abnormally increased tone of the extensor muscles.

Evaluation of Neck Extensors (Lowering from Sitting to Supine Position, Posterior Neck) (10,15) (Fig. 14B)

Support the infant at the shoulders, allowing him (or her) to lean forward in a sitting position so the head is flexed onto the chest. Wait at least 30 seconds to allow the infant to raise his head. Then move the infant backward to stimulate an active lifting of the head.

A term infant rocked around the vertical plane in sitting will alternately and symmetrically flex and extend his neck to attempt to keep his head upright. The neck extensors develop earlier in gestation than the flexors so some response in this maneuver should be evident by 32 weeks of gestation.

Abnormal Response

Poor or absent attempt

A response that is inappropriately brisk or strong for age, particularly if it represents imbalance between the extensors and flexors, most typically with an increase in tone of the extensor muscle groups and failure of the head to drop onto the chest

Held Sit (10)

Hold infant in an upright position using your hands to support the shoulders. Observe the length of time the head is held in an upright position. This may be done after raising the infant to an upright position in testing neck flexors. If there is a holding of the head for more than 10 seconds, determine the level of the lumbar vertebra from which the back bends.

An alert, term infant should hold his head upright for more than 10 seconds and may be facilitated with visual fixation at eye level. Premature infants with initial control will hold for a shorter period of time. The curve of the back should be rounded concave anterior. The stronger the back extensors, the lower the level of back curve. An abnormal response is failure to bring the head up or kept up for less than 3 seconds.

UPPER SEGMENTAL REFLEXES: PASSIVE TONE

Lateral Rotation of the Head (Fig. 15)

With the infant supine and lying symmetrically, turn the head toward each shoulder to determine the resistance of the contralateral muscles. Active rotation of the head can be elicited if the infant will follow a visual stimulus but is limited compared with passive rotation.

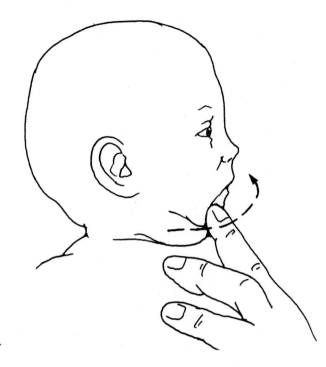

Figure 15. Head turning.

A normal response is equal range of rotation between the two sides. The range decreases with increasing gestational age.

Abnormal Response

Limitation that is asymmetrical due to shortening of the sternocleidomastoid muscle
Lack of limitation due to weakness of CN XII or low tone

Abnormal Hypertonia of Neck Extensors in the Supine Position (93)

With the infant resting supine, look for a visible space between the cervical spine and the table. The neck will be flexed with the muscles relaxed to leave little space between the cervical spine and the table. The finding does not change throughout gestation or postnatally.

A prominent occiput may complicate interpretation if the neck cannot then lie flat. Interpret the finding in light of other signs for muscle tension, such as change in tone with repeated ventral flexion of the head and head control in bringing it to the upright position.

Abnormal Response

Hypertonicity of the neck extensors prevents the infant from lying flat, leaving a visible space between the neck and the table. The resting position of the head will tend toward lateral rotation with posterior extension or nuchal opisthotonus.

Ventral Suspension (10,11) (Posture of the Head in Prone Suspension (3), Trunk Tone in Ventral Suspension) (Fig. 16)

Holding the infant by a hand under the chest, suspend him (or her) in a prone position and note the posture of the head, trunk, and limbs. Hold the head at a slightly higher level than the pelvis. The infant, who must be awake for this maneuver, should attempt to lift his head and flex his extremities. If there is no spontaneous lifting of the head, it may be stimulated by stroking firmly on the paraspinal muscles of the upper back. Prechtl noted the lifting of the head as the most significant component of this maneuver

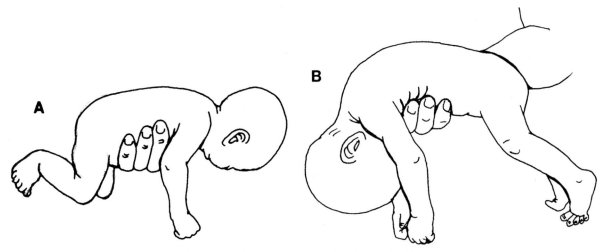

Figure 16. Ventral suspension. **A:** Good tone. **B:** Poor tone.

(3). If there is no attempt to extend the neck, stroke firmly up or down the spine to stimulate contraction of those muscles. (Perez and Vollmer reflexes are for up and down stroking on the spine, respectively.) Infants who are in respiratory distress may have little tolerance for this maneuver.

An expected response is general flexion of the extremities with extension of the trunk and head (Fig. 16A). With maturity there is a general increase in the strength of the limb flexion.

Abnormal Response in Ventral Suspension

No response to position change
Complete flaccidity (Fig. 16B)
Asymmetry of response with flaccidity on one side, in one extremity, or in the upper extremities but with a strong response in the lower extremities or vice versa.
A disproportionately good response in the neck and trunk extension, especially when accompanied by failure to head drop in forward sitting, suggesting abnormally increased extensor tone.

Perez Reflex (1)

With the infant in ventral suspension, apply pressure upward over the spine from the sacrum toward the head to induce flexion of the arms and legs with extension of the neck.
This reflex is useful if the position assumed in ventral suspension is complete relaxation. Note that the Perez reflex stimulates more response from the upper extremities with its upward stroke, whereas the Vollmer reflex stimulates more response from the lower trunk with its downward spinal stroking.

Abnormal Perez Response

Marked extension of the pelvis as well as the neck
Absent, weak, or asymmetrical response in failing to lift the head

Vollmer Reflex (94)

Holding the infant in ventral suspension, firmly stroke down the spine. The infant should not be crying. This response is similar to the Perez reflex but tends to stimulate more response in the lower trunk with flexion of the legs and extension of the lower back.

Abnormal Vollmen Response

Absent, weak, exaggerated, or asymmetrical response
Persistence of reflex beyond 3 months

Galant's Response (Incurvation of the Trunk) (2) (Fig. 17)

With the infant in the prone position either lying on the mattress or in suspension, rub lightly along either side of the spinal column from the shoulder toward the buttocks, first on one side and then the other.

A normal response is strong incurvation of the whole vertebral column with concavity on the stimulated side. Running the stimulation from the shoulders to the buttocks stimulates all the skin segments on the trunk.

Abnormal Galant's Response

Absent, asymmetric, or weak response to stimulation. There will be an absent response below the level of a transverse lesion of the spinal cord. Unilateral response may suggest a hemiparesis or sensory deficits along multiple dermatomes.
An exaggerated response to minimal stimulus with a rapid and sustained swing to the side.

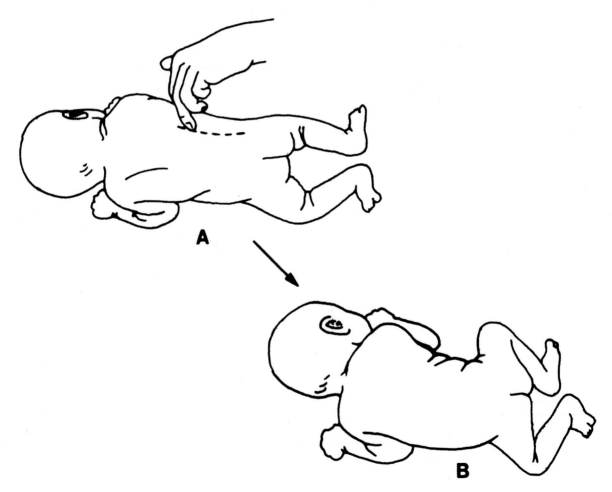

Figure 17. Trunk incurvation reflex. **A:** A stroke along the side of the spinal column. **B:** Reflex contraction of long muscles causing a C curve on the stimulated side.

LOWER SEGMENTAL REFLEXES: PASSIVE TONE

Heel to Ear Maneuver (15) (Fig. 18)

With the infant supine, hold the legs together and bring the feet toward the ears as closely as possible without lifting the pelvis off the table. Measure the angle made by the arc from the table to the infant's heels (15). Alternatively measure the angle made between the heel and the trunk (17).

If there is increased flexor tone, particularly in the first few days after birth, it will be impossible to extend the knees fully. If the knees cannot be extended because of anatomic restraint, measure the angle created by an imaginary line extended along the femoral axis and the pelvis at the intersection of the table. This maneuver presupposes absence of hip dislocations.

A normal response is equal angles on both sides and angles appropriate for age. By the technique of Amiel-Tison, the angle from the heels to the table decreases with advancing gestational age until 40 weeks corrected gestational age and then increases during the next 9 months after term. In other words, hip flexion decreases toward term and increases after birth.

Abnormal Response in Head to Ear Maneuver

Asymmetry
Increased angle for age suggests hypotonia
Decreased angle for age suggests hypertonia

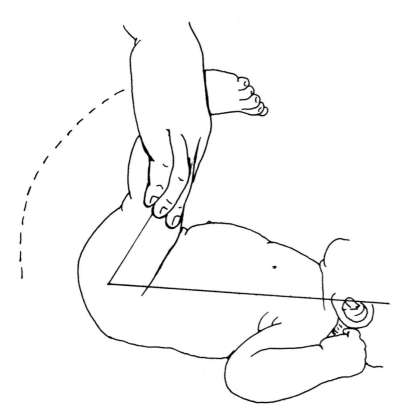

Figure 18. Heel to ear.

Popliteal Angle (Fig. 19)

With the infant lying supine, flex and abduct both hips and then extend the legs as far as possible by applying gentle pressure to the backs of the ankles. Measure the angle between the calf and thigh.

Some investigators do not first move the thighs away from the abdomen and assess these angles as part of the heel to ear maneuver (11). It is less stressful to ill babies, particularly those with abdominal distention, not to press the thighs against the abdomen but to follow the technique described by the French observers (15). Additionally, if both extremities are not tested simultaneously, it is more difficult to compare the angles and, hence, the symmetry.

A normal response is symmetrical angles that are dependent on gestational age and intrauterine position. The angle decreases progressively toward term and then increases in the 9 months after term. The angles normally held by a 32-week premature infant are in the same range as those for a 5-month-old infant. This angle is spurious in an infant who was in frank breech with extended legs. Similarly, the presence of a posterior hip dislocation prevents an initial positioning of hip abduction.

Abnormal Response

Asymmetry greater than 10° to 20° or outside the range expected for gestational age.

Adductor Angles (15) (Fig. 20)

The infant can be in any state as long as there is no active resistance during the maneuver. With the infant lying supine and the lower extremities fully extended, place the forefinger of each hand along the femoral axis and gently pull both legs apart as far as possible. Measure the angle formed by the legs. Note if there is any asymmetry in how far each leg can be abducted. The maneuver is abduction to measure the angle created by tone in the adductor muscles.

A normal angle at term is 40° to 80° and equal degree of abduction on both sides. The angle decreases with advancing gestational age to 40 weeks and increases over the first year. Abnormal hip development contributes to asymmetry in angles, and, conversely, abnormal adductor tone can lead to hip dysplasia.

It is convenient to check the femoral pulses during positioning for this maneuver.

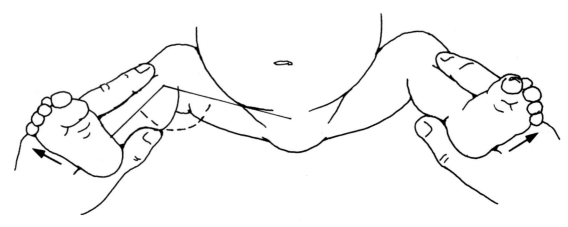

Figure 19. Popliteal angles.

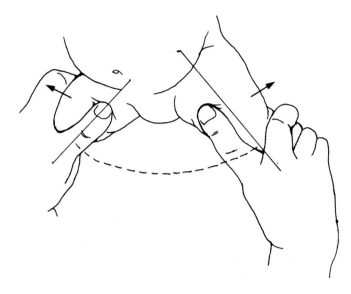

Figure 20. Adductor angles and tone.

Abnormal Response in Adductor Angles

Greater than 90° at term or asymmetrical.

Dorsiflexion Angle of the Foot (15) (Fig. 21)

Hold the leg extended and flex the foot toward the leg by applying pressure with the thumb to the plantar surface. Measure the angle formed by the dorsum of the foot and the anterior shin. With the leg fully extended, tone of both the soleus and gastrocnemius muscles is tested. If the knee is bent, only the soleus is tested. Testing tone in muscle groups across two joints is more informative, so it is better to test with the knee extended.

The French neurologists further divide this maneuver by first applying a slow, moderate pressure until the smallest possible angle is met (the "slow" angle) and then they apply a quick, sudden flexion (the "rapid" angle). Both angles should be equal with a difference of more than 10° indicating an abnormally exaggerated stretch reflex (15).

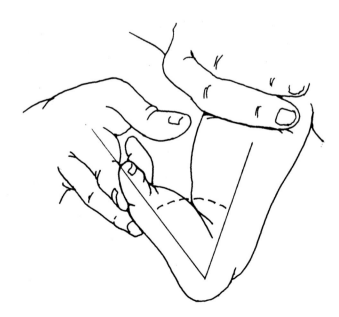

Figure 21. Dorsiflexion of the foot.

As the fetus becomes more compressed in utero, this angle decreases. Any factors that decrease uterine volume may decrease this angle beyond that expected for gestational age: e.g., oligohydramnios or twin gestation.

Leg Recoil (10,11)

With the infant lying supine and fully relaxed but awake, hold both ankles and fully flex the lower extremities for about 5 seconds. Next fully extend the extremities to the table, hold extended for 2 seconds, and then release. At term there should be an immediate, complete flexion at the hips and knees. The vigor of the response increases with gestational age.

Infants who have been in the breech position may normally resist extension of the hips but should still demonstrate symmetrical recoil from their point of maximum extension unless their legs have been in a hyperextended breech position.

Abnormal Response

Asymmetrical response at any gestational age
Decreased level of response in intensity or time to onset outside the range expected for gestational age

Leg Traction (11)

With the infant lying supine, grasp both legs near the ankles and pull up until the pelvis is off the table by 2 to 5 cm. Note the resistance of the legs to the pull and the popliteal angle. A normal response is flexion of both knees to an angle of less than 100° with strong resistance to pull.

This maneuver, always tested when changing diapers, is valuable for testing the strength of the lower extremity flexors, particularly when it is not feasible to change the infant's resting position.

Abnormal Response

An absent, weak, or asymmetrical response.

Flapping of Hand or Foots (15) (Fig. 22)

With the infant supine, grasp both upper or lower extremities simultaneously above the wrists or ankles and gently shake them while comparing the movements between the sides.

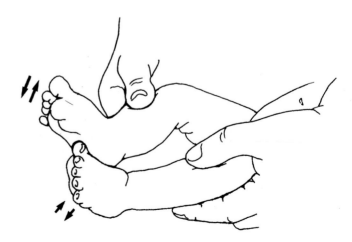

Figure 22. Flappability of the feet.

An increase in the flapping amplitude correlates with a decrease in tone. Although the amplitude may vary by gestational age, with more immature infants showing a wider range, the amplitude should be the same on both sides for any infant. When asymmetrical, it suggests paresis of the extremity with the higher amplitude. Flapping the extremities is helpful in relaxing the region before attempting tendon reflexes or general tone.

Abnormal Response

Asymmetry.

LOWER SEGMENTAL REFLEXES: ACTIVE TONE

Magnet Response (Heel Reflex) (2)

Method 1 (Fig. 23)

Position the infant supine with the lower extremities slightly flexed and symmetrical . The head should be mid-line. Apply light pressure to the soles of the feet.

Method 2

Percuss the heel away from the Achilles insertion and observe for extension of that limb (heel reflex).

A normal response is for the lower limbs to extend against the finger in a sustained response that gradually relaxes after a few seconds. This response is more difficult to elicit in the first days after birth while the infant's resting position shows a preference for marked

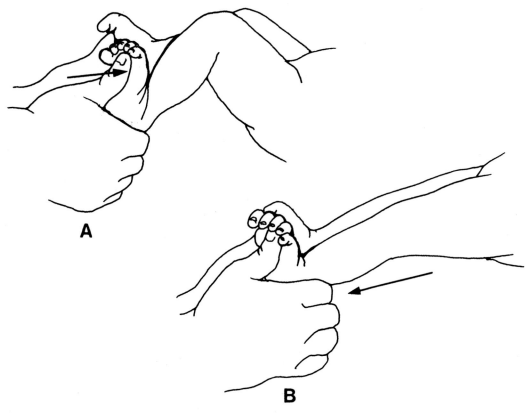

Figure 23. Magnet reflex testing strength of lower extremity. **A:** Pressure is applied to the plantar surface of each foot with the hips and knees slightly flexed. **B:** The infant responds with extension of the lower limbs.

hip flexion. The magnet response substitutes for a positive support response when an infant cannot be lifted because of illness or mechanical restraints.

Abnormal Response

Absent or asymmetrical response that may indicate a weakness in leg extensor muscles or decreased sensation to touch in lower spine defects
Prolonged sustained response with marked extension

Crossed Extension Reflex of Legs (1,15,75) (Fig. 24)

The infant is in a symmetrically mid-line, supine position, in light sleep or quiet awake. Hold one leg in extension and stroke the plantar surface of that foot. Repeat the trial on the opposite leg. The nonrestrained leg will demonstrate a three-stage response:
As described by Amiel-Tison these stages are (a) rapid withdrawal in flexion followed by extension, (b) fanning of the toes, and (c) adduction of the foot to bring it close to the stimulated foot (15).
As described by Illingworth these stages are (a) flexion of the nonstimulated leg, (b) adduction of the contralateral leg, and (c) extension of that leg (1).
The first two parts of the response should be present regardless of gestational age, but adduction of the foot will not be fully developed until 40 weeks, with a slight reaction at 36 weeks (15). Infants born at less than 30 to 32 weeks of gestation will have a more random, purposeless pattern of flexion and extension. This response should be disappearing by 1 month after 40 weeks gestational age.
This reflex is comparable with a stepping reaction but is applicable when the infant cannot be lifted. The response is defensive and should be quite vigorous to demonstrate normal lower extremity strength in flexion and extension muscle groups.

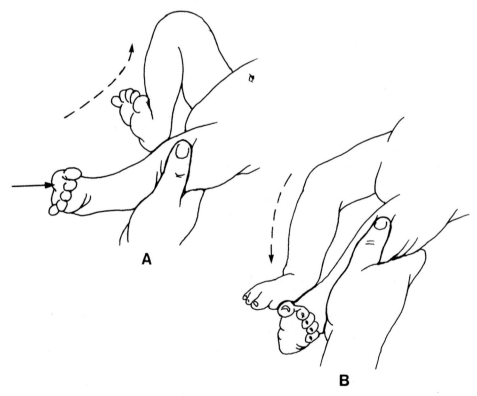

Figure 24. Crossed extensor reflex. **A:** A noxious stimulus is applied to the plantar surface of one foot, and holding that leg in extension causes initial flexion of the opposite foot. **B:** The free, unstimulated leg responds to push away the painful stimulus.

Abnormal Response

Asymmetrical, weak, or absent response
Persistence of full response after 44 weeks corrected gestational age

Placing Reaction (Fig. 25)

Hold the infant with both hands under the arms and around the chest. Support the back of the head with the thumbs and the jaw with the index fingers. Lightly touch the dorsum of the infant's feet to the side of the table or bassinet edge and lift him to draw the foot against the edge. The infant should flex the lower extremity enough to bring his foot up and place it on the surface.

Abnormal Response

Asymmetrical, absent, or weak response with poor movement of the lower extremity
Marked extension after initial stimulus

Supporting Reaction (Positive Support, Straightening of Lower Extremities and Trunk, Redressement du Tronc) (11,15,25,76)

Hold the infant around the chest in an upright position facing away from the examiner with the chin supported upright by the fingers. Allow the feet to touch the surface of the examining table. If necessary, stimulate the placing reaction first or bounce the infant lightly on his feet to look for extension of the lower extremity. Assess the support of body weight and the straightening of the trunk. Make certain that the head is in a neutral upright position.

The infant should straighten the lower extremities and trunk and somewhat support himself for a few seconds and should then relax by either taking a few walking steps or by flexing both hips. The knees may normally remain slightly flexed as long as there is some attempt at straightening the lower extremities and bearing weight.

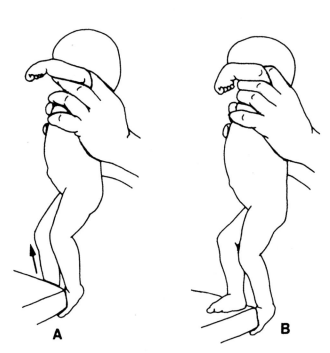

Figure 25. Placing response. **A:** The top of the foot is stimulated. **B:** The infant flexes his hip to place his foot on the surface and prepares to extend the leg and bear weight.

Before term, the duration of the positive support will be shorter but should still be symmetrical. By 5 months postterm, the infant will be unwilling to straighten unless the parents have frequently stimulated this position in their holding routines.

Abnormal Response

Trunk arching with hyperextension of legs, which indicates marked hypertonia of the posterior muscles
Complete absence of any extension of the hips and legs
Asymmetry

Stepping Movements (Automatic Walking) (5) (Fig. 26)

Hold the baby with both hands under the arms around the chest and the chin supported. Allow the feet to touch the examining table surface with the infant held leaning slightly forward. If necessary, shift the infant's weight from one side to the other to facilitate alternating weight bearing on the extremities. Extend the neck slightly if there is no initial response. There has to be a normal support reaction initially.

The infant should take at least three steps with clear flexion of the hips and knees on both sides. Infants who were in breech presentation may have difficulty attaining the full extension of their lower extremities necessary for this maneuver for the first few days.

This response increases after the first 2 to 3 days but generally lessens by the end of the first month after term. The full response can be elicited well past 1 month if the neck is extended. This response must disappear before voluntary walking can be acquired.

Abnormal Response

Absent, weak, or asymmetrical flexion
Hyperactive response with extreme extension or flexion response

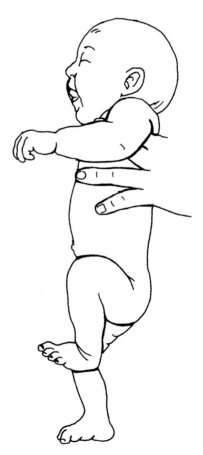

Figure 26. Stepping reflex. If infant has a positive support response, leaning him forward or from side to side stimulates an alternating stepping response.

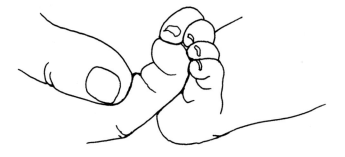

Figure 27. Plantar grasp.

Plantar Grasp (Lower Extremity Grasp, Grasp Reflex of the Foot) (1,2,10,15) (Fig. 27)

With the infant awake and supine, press your thumbs against the balls of the infant's feet close to the metacarpal-phalangeal joints. Do not touch the top of the foot. Take care not to elicit a Babinski response by applying a firm rather than tickling touch.

A normal response is a sustained grasp with plantar flexion of all toes that is symmetrical between the two feet and then gradually relaxes. The intensity of the grasp is minimally affected by gestational age. By 8 to 9 months, the response should disappear, usually as a predictable prelude to walking. In later months, a delay in disappearance of this response may indicate abnormally increased motor tone.

Abnormal Response

A weak or asymmetrical grasp that suggests lower spinal cord defects.
A grasp that does not relax suggests a generalized hyperirritable or hypertonic state.

OTHER LOWER SEGMENTAL REFLEXES

Babinski Reflex (Plantar Response) (2) (Fig. 28)

The legs should be semi-flexed. With a thumb nail, scratch the sole of the foot on the lateral side from the toes toward the heel. Be careful not to elicit a plantar grasp by stimulating the sole of the foot.

The first reaction of the great toe (normal flexion) is probably the most important component of the reflex because spreading of the toes is a far less consistent response. The response should be symmetrical for both feet with a dorsal flexion of the big toe and spreading of the smaller toes. There is no change in intensity during the neonatal period.

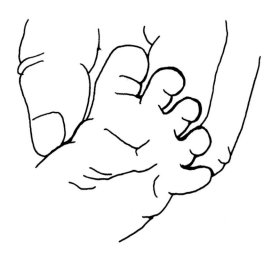

Figure 28. Babinski reflex.

Abnormal Response

Absent or weak response with minimal spread of toes
Asymmetrical response
Strong, obligatory response with no relaxation afterward
This response may be absent in severely depressed infants or in the presence of spinal cord
    injuries.

Ankle Clonus (10,11,15)

*With the infant supine and the head in the mid-line, flex the legs slightly. In an abrupt,
quick movement, press the thumb against the distal part of the sole to elicit a dorsiflexion of the foot. If there are beats elicited, repeat the maneuver and determine the average number of beats obtained. It is convenient to look for clonus after measuring the
Achilles angle, but for that test the knee is extended and for clonus the knee should be
flexed.*

Term infants should have fewer than five beats of extension with rapid decay in intensity. In preterm infants, there may be up to 10 beats.

Abnormal Response

Sustained beating
Asymmetry between the sides
Clonus elicited when testing for a deep tendon reflex.
Sustained response indicates lack of upper motor neuron inhibition.

MATURATION AND REFLEXES OF EARLY INFANCY

Many of the reflexes discussed in this chapter are useful in getting a newborn infant to
cooperate in moving specific muscle groups, but for some their presence also allows an estimation of gestational age. Reflexes unique to early infancy disappear before volitional
motor activity develops, and a delay in their disappearance signals delayed developmental
milestones. For example, the oral motor reflexes of automatic biting and sucking subside
before an infant can successfully chew solid foods. Other reflexes begin and then subside
in early infancy and reflect transitional changes from involuntary to volitional motor activity. Knowledge of the course and sequencing of these reflexes is essential to interpreting
the neurologic examination (Fig. 29).

The following reflexes are not expected in the neonatal period, although some infants
will demonstrate them. These reflexes may be part of a neurologic examination in patients
who remain in the hospital after the neonatal period or who require more careful examination as infants because of neonatal conditions.

Symmetrical Tonic Neck Reflex STNR (Cat Reflex) (1,9)

This response may be helpful to confirm other soft findings in infants well after the newborn period if it is pronounced and clearly abnormal. Its application should not be confused
with the ATNR.

Method 1

With the infant in prone suspension, raise and then lower the head (1).

Method 2

With the infant in a sitting position, extend the head (9).

With neck extension, there will be an increase in extensor tone of the arms and flexor tone of the legs with neck extension. With neck flexion, there is an opposite response with increase in flexor tone of the arms and extensor tone of the legs (1).

A symmetrical tonic neck reflex is present in fewer than 30% of the infants at any time with the maximum prevalence at 4 to 6 months of age using method 2 (78).

This response is incompatible with reciprocal crawl, so it must disappear if infants are to crawl normally. An exaggerated response is present if an infant can only extend his arms in kneeling when the head is raised and the legs are then fixed in flexion. As long as the head is raised, he cannot extend the legs (1).

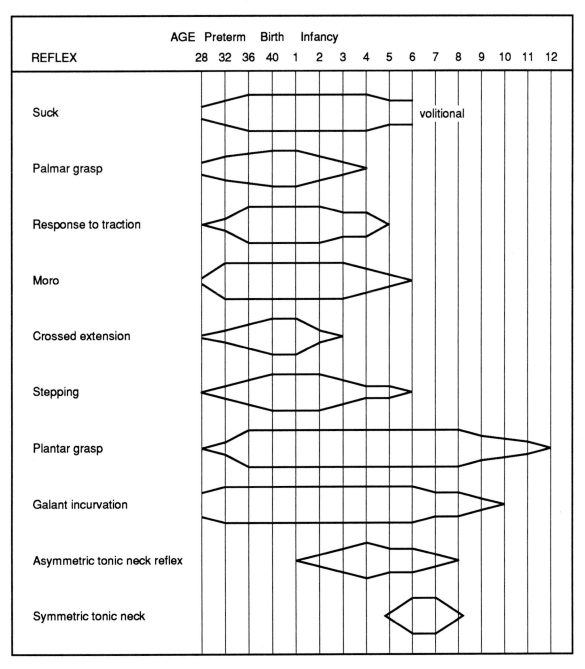

Figure 29. Maturation of infantile reflexes.

Tonic Labyrinthine Reflexes in Supine and Prone (1,9,76)

Supine: with the head mid-line, extend the head. Look for retraction of the shoulders with extension of the legs.

Prone: flex the head. Look for protraction of the shoulders with flexion of the legs (position needed to begin crawling).

A tonic labyrinthine response is seen in 80% of infants at 2 weeks of age, with a marked diminution by the age of 24 months (78). In normal infants at least 4 months of age, when the chin is raised with the infant in prone, there is a protective extension of the arms. If there is an abnormally strong tonic labyrinthine reflex, the infant draws the arms up in flexion and remains suspended by his or her head.

These reflexes interact closely with the tonic neck reflexes and so the pattern of manifestation will depend on whether the symmetrical tonic neck reflex predominates over the tonic labyrinthine reflex. As described by Illingworth, these reflexes are tested in a kneeling position after the neonatal period and have different responses than seen when the procedure is performed in the manner described by Capute (1,9,76).

Abnormal Response

An exaggerated increase in tone with marked resistance to passive movement. In older infants an abnormal response would be without a protective extension of the arms.

Landau Reflex (75,78,95)

Hold infant in ventral suspension. The head, spine, and legs will extend, forming an upward arc. Depress the head and observe for flexion of the hip, knees, and elbows or a reversal of the arc.

This reflex is sometimes confused in the literature with the Gallant, Perez, or Vollmer reflexes, but it normally appears at 2 to 3 months of age, with most infants 6 to 12 months of age having a normal reaction. After 12 months, the reaction is difficult to elicit (95). In a study by Capute the reflex was present in 44% of term birth infants at 2 months and in 95% at 4 months (78).

Abnormal Response

Absence of reflex after at least 4 months of age is seen in infants with motor weakness and cerebral palsy because the infant cannot lift the head in this position.

Derotative Righting Head on Body Reflex (75)

With the infant prone, turn the head 45° and observe for a series of derotative axial responses starting with the shoulders, followed by the body, hip, and lower extremities).

Neonatal response at term is a righting response from the head through the shoulders with a "loglike" roll of the lower extremities turning as a unit. This response becomes more mature as the flexor posture becomes more relaxed, allowing the hips to flex to assist in turning.

Abnormal Response

Persistence of a truncal roll without dissociation of the upper and lower movements beyond 3 to 4 months of age indicating hypertonia of the lower extremities.

Derotative Body (17,75) (Fig. 30)

With the infant supine, flex one leg and hip and roll toward the opposite side into prone. By 4 months, the turn of the hips should be followed by trunk rotation, and arm extension with completion of the turn.

Abnormal Response

Flexion of the arm, extension of the trunk and head, and failure to complete the turn.

Downward Thrust (75)

Hold the infant by the axilla and thrust the lower extremities toward the floor. When suspended, the infant flexes at the hips and knees. With the thrust, the infant fully extends his or her lower extremities. This reflex appears at 3 months of age.

Abnormal Response

The infant remains in a sitting in air position with failure to extend his lower extremities as long as infant is in hypotonic phase. If hypertonic, the legs may not flex at the hips when suspended.

Upper Extremity Placing (75)

Press and move the lateral surface of the forearm along the edge of the tabletop from the elbow to the wrist and dorsum of the hand. Upper extremity placing appears at 3 months of age. The infant responds with flexion, extension and placing of the hand on the tabletop.

Abnormal Response

Absent or asymmetrical response with extremity paresis.

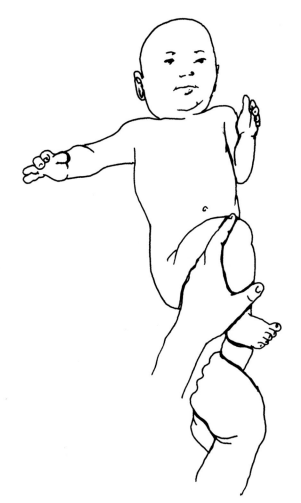

Figure 30. Derotative body reflex. As the examiner initiates a rolling over, the infant should extend the arm and adduct the shoulder to complete the turning motion. Lack of an assisting response is seen with low tone and immaturity. An abnormal response is for the arms to remain flexed or not to follow in rotation.

NEO NEURO & UP

Left margin labels: ASK CARETAKER · Corrected gestational age · Sex · Date of birth · Gestational age at birth · Name · Date

Item	Description						
1. CARETAKER MUST AWAKEN TO FEED		a) rarely	b) sometimes	c) often			
2. NUMBER OF FEEDINGS BETWEEN 6 PM - 6 AM		a) none	b) 1	c) 2	d) 3	e) 4 f) 5 g) 6 or more	
3. EASY OF CARING FOR		a) too easy	b) easy	c) not so easy	d) difficult		
4. HOW LONG CRIES BEFORE CONSOLED?		a) 1-3 min	b) 4-7 min	c) 8-12 min	d) 13-18min	e) 19-24 min f) 25 or more min	
5. POSTURE	Upper limbs / Lower limbs	a) extended / a) extended	b) semi-flexed or flexed / b) semi-flexed or flexed			c) strongly flexed / c) strongly flexed	
6. POSTURING		a) decorticate	b) decerebrate	c) opisthotonic	d) none of these		
7. HANDS OPEN/CLOSED		a) clenched	b) clenched with stress maneuver	c) closed	d) sometimes closed	e) open	
8. PALMAR GRASP		a) absent	b) weak flexion	c) medium flexion	d) strong flexion spread to	e) very strong lifts off bed	
9. PLANTAR GRASP		a) absent or weak	b) medium to strong	c) very strong			
10. ASYMMETRICAL TONIC NECK REFLEX		a) persistent or spontaneous	b) present, not persistent	c) absent			
11. SCARF SIGN		a) > 85°	b) 60° to 85°	c) 45° to 60°	d) 15° to 45°	e) 0° to 15°	
12. POPLITEAL ANGLE		a) >180°	b) 150° to 180°	c) 130° to 150°	d) 110° to 130°	e) 90° to 110° f) < 90°	
13. HEEL TO EAR		a) < 10°	b) 10° to 40°	c) 40° to 60°	d) 60° to 90°	e) 90° to 100° f) ≥ 100°	
14. KNEE REFLEX		a) absent	b) 1 + to 2 +	c) brisk	d) very brisk		
15. ANKLE CLONUS		a) > 2 beats	b) 1-2 beats	c) absent			
16. PULL TO SIT	Arm Flexion - angle at elbow	a) > 170°	b) 140° to 170°	c) 110° to 140°	d) 70° to 110° e) < 70°	
17.	Head Lag	a)	b)	c)	d)	e) f)	
18. HELD SIT		a) head stays forward or backward	b) head up < 3 sec	c) head up 3-10 sec	d) head up > 10 sec	e) bends from L3	
19. POSTERIOR NECK		a) no attempt to raise head	b) tries but cannot raise head	c) head upright by 30 sec, drops head	d) head upright by 30 sec, maintained	e) examiner cannot extend head	
20. ANTERIOR NECK		a) no attempt to raise head	b) tries but cannot raise head	c) head upright by 30 sec, drops head	d) head upright by 30 sec, maintained	e) examiner cannot flex head	
21. AUDITORY		a) no reaction or startle	b) brightens or stills	c) shifts eyes	d) shifts and turns	e) prolonged head turning	
22. VISUAL		a) no focus or following	b) focuses	c) follows 30° horizontally	d) follows 30°-60° horizontally	e) also follows vertically f) follows past midline g) follows full circle	
23. ALERT		a) 0-4 sec.	b) 5-10 sec	c) 11-30 sec	d) 31-60 sec	e) > 60 sec. f) regards hand or object in hand	
24. VENTRAL SUSPENSION		a)	b)	c)	d)		
25. ALL FOURS/PRONE		a) no head turning	b) turns head side to side	c) lifts head 45° drops	d) lifts head 45° holds	e) head up 90° drops f) head up 90° holds	
26. MORO		a) absent or minimal	b) partial	c) full	d) exaggerated - immediate brisk response		
27. SUCK		a) no attempt	b) weak	c) strong irregular	d) strong regular	e) jaw clenched	
28. TREMOR		a) all states	b) only in states 5, 6	c) also in state 4	d) only in sleep or after mono	e) none	
29. RESPONSIIVENESS		a) no smile	b) smiles to self	c) smiles responsively	d) gets excited anticipation of food	e) breathes heavily gets excited	
30. VOCALIZATION		a) none	b) small noises	c) talks back some way	d) chuckles	e) squeals, laughs outloud	
31. ATTENDS TO EXAMINER		a) no stimulus needed	b) with mild stimuli	c) moderate stimuli	d) really have to stimulate	e) does not attend	
32. ATTENDS DURING EXAM		a) does not attend	b) with stimulus only	c) some	d) recurrently	e) most of exam	

Figure 31. Neo Neuro & Up. Six areas are assessed: irritability/apathy as noted by caretaker, primitive reflexes, French angles, head control, neck and trunk tone, neurologic irritability/apathy, alertness, and responsiveness. This assessment is designed for neurologic evaluation of infants from 38 weeks' gestation to 16 weeks of age. The first four items are questions asked of the caretaker about the irritability/

Scoring-Use corrected gestational age   Factors

Assymmetry	38-39	0-4 weeks	4.1 - 8 weeks	8.1-12 weeks	12.1 - 16 weeks	1	2	3	4	5	6
				a = 5 b = 3 c = 1							
		d, e =5 c, f = 3 a, b, g = 1	c,d = 5 b, e = 3 a, f, g = 1	b, c = 5 a, d = 3 e, f ,g = 1							
			b = 5 c = 3 a, d = 1								
		a = 5 b = 3 c-f = 1		b, c = 5 a, d = 3 e, f = 1	c,d = 5 b, e = 3 a, f = 1						
R L d = levels ≥ 1	arms b = 5 c = 3 a,d=1		legs b = 5 c = 3 a,d = 1	Sum, divide by 2							
			d = 5 a, b, c = 1								
R L f = levels ≥ 2		c, d = 5 a, b, e, f = 1		d,e = 5 c = 3 a, b, f = 1	e = 5 d = 3 a, b, c, f = 1						
R L f = levels ≥ 2		b, c = 5 a, d = 3 e, f = 1		c, d = 5 b = 3 a, e, f = 1	b,c = 5 a,d = 3 e, f = 1						
R L d = levels ≥ 1		b = 5 a, c, d = 1									
R L d = levels ≥ 1		b, c = 5 a, d = 1			c = 5 b = 3 a,d = 1						
R L f = levels ≥2		d,e = 5 c = 3 a, b, f = 1			c, d = 5 b, e = 3 a, f = 1						
R L g = levels ≥ 2		d, e = 5 c, f = 3 a, b, g = 1			c, d = 5 b, e = 3 a, f, g = 1						
R L g = levels ≥ 2		d, e = 5 c, f = 3 a, b, g = 1			d = 5 c, e = 3 a, b, f, g = 1						
R L e = levels ≥ 2		b = 5 a, c = 3 d = 1									
R L d = levels ≥ 1		c = 5 b = 3 a, d = 1									
R L f = levels ≥2	b, c =5 a = 3 d, e, f = 1			c = 5 b = 3 a, d, e, f = 1							
	b, c =5 a, d-f = 1			c = 5 b, d = 3 a, e, f = 1	d = 5 c, e = 3 a, b, f = 1						
	b, c = 5 a, d, e = 1		c, d = 5 b, e, = 3 a = 1	d, e = 5 c = 3 a,b = 1	e =5 c, d = 3 a, b = 1						
		c = 5 b, d = 3 a, e = 1	c, d = 5 b = 3 a, e = 1	d = 5 c = 3 a,b = 1							
		c = 5 b, d = 3 a, e = 1	c, d = 5 b = 3 a, e = 1	d = 5 c = 3 a, b, e = 1							
* if assymmetry, consider hearing test		b-e = 5 c = 3 a = 1	c-e = 5 b = 3 a = 1	d, e = 5 c = 3 a, b = 1							*
	b-g = 5 a = 1	c-g = 5 b = 3 a = 1	d-g = 5 c = 3 a, b = 1	f, g = 5 d = 3 a - c = 1	g = 5 f = 3 a-e = 1						*
			b-f = 5 a = 1	c-f = 5 b = 3 a = 1 d-f = 5 c = 3 a, b = 1	f = 5 e = 3 a-d = 1						
		b, c = 5 a, d = 1		c,d = 5 b = 3 = 1	d = 5 c = 3 a, b = 1						
			a, b = 5	b, c = 5 a = 1	c-f = 5 b = 3 a = 1	d-f = 5 c = 3 a, b = 1					
R L e = levels ≥ 2		c = 5 b = 3 a, d, e = 1	b, c = 5 a = 3 d, e = 1	a, b = 5 c = 3 d, e = 1							
		d = 5 b,c = 3 a, e = 1			d = 5 c = 3 a, b, e = 1						
		d, e = 5 b, c = 3 a = 1	e = 5 c, d = 3 a, b = 1		e = 5 d = 3 a, b, c = 1						
	a,b = 5	b-e = 5 a = 1		c-e = 5 b = 3 a = 1	d, e = 5 c = 3 a, b = 1						
	a, b = 5	b-e = 5 a = 1		c-e = 5 b = 3 a = 1	d, e = 5 c = 3 a, b = 1						
	a-c = 5 d = 3 e = 1		a, b = 5 c = 3 d, e = 1		a = 5 b = 3 c-e = 1						
		b-e = 5 a = 1	c-e = 5 b = 3 a = 1	d, e = 5 c = 3 a, b = 1	e = 5 d = 3 a - c = 1						
					FACTOR SCORES						

Right side factor descriptions:

0-48 Hrs.
Severely abnormal = < 95
Moderately abnormal = 95 - 119
Mildly abnormal = 120 - 139
Normal = 140 up

48 Hrs. - 16 weeks
Severely abnormal = < 100
Moderately abnormal = 100 - 124
Mildly abnormal = 125 - 144
Normal = 145 up

* Abnormal auditory or visual requires hearing or vision testing. May be secondary to brain dysfunction

TOTAL SCORE

Figure 31. *(continued.)*
apathy of the infant. The last four items are observations by the examiner about the alertness of the infant (format and instructions kindly provided by Patrician Ellison. M.D., University of Colorado).

Figure 31. *(continued.)*

1. How often must the caretaker awaken the infant to feed?
2. How many feedings are given between 6 p.m. and 6 a.m.?
3. Describe how easy or difficult the infant is to care for.
4. How long does the infant cry before you can console him or her?
5. Posture: Observe both arms and legs of the infant lying quietly for strong flexion, semi-flexion, flexion, or extension.
6. Observe for decorticate (legs extended, arms flexed), decerebrate (legs and arms extended), or opisthotonic (neck hyperextended) postures.
7. Hands open or closed. Observe the hands for clenching (closed too tightly), clenched under stress (closed too tightly when crying or during the neurologic evaluation), closed, sometimes closed, or open positions.
8. Palmar grasp. Place your index finger in the palm of the infant's hands, approaching from the ulnar side and observe the flexion of the infant's fingers and arm.
9. Plantar grasp. Place your thumb on the ball of the foot and observe the flexion of the toes.
10. Asymmetrical tonic neck reflex. Use your hand to turn the infant's head from side to side with the infant supine. Observe for the fencing position: extension of the arm in front of the infant's face and flexion of the arm at the back of the head.
11. Scarf sign. Grasp the infant's upper arm near the elbow and move the arm across the chest until resistance is met. Measure the angle between a line dropped from the infant's armpit and the infant's upper arm.
12. Popliteal angle. Grasp the infant's lower leg near the knee and extend the leg until resistance is met. Measure the angle between the back of the upper leg and back of the lower leg with the back of the knee as the fulcrum.
13. Heel to ear. Keep the infant's buttocks on the table. Grasp the infant's upper leg and flex the legs at the hip until resistance is met. Measure the angle between the leg and the trunk.
14. Knee reflex. Relax the leg by some knee flexion, then tap below the patella and observe the quality of the reflex.
15. Ankle clonus. Grasp one foot and quickly flex it, counting any spontaneous beats.
16 and 17. Pull to sit. Grasp both wrists and pull the infant slowly to sitting position. Arm flexion and head lag are scored separately.
18. Held sit. Hold the infant in an upright position supporting each shoulder noting the amount of time the head remains upright. In an infant who has head control for over 10 seconds, support the infant on the trunk and observe the number of the lumbar vertebra from which the back is bent.
19. Posterior Neck. Support the infant at the shoulders, moving the trunk forward until head drops forward. Count the seconds until the infant returns head to upright position, noting also the ability to maintain the head upright.
20. Anterior neck. Support the infant at the shoulders, moving the trunk backward until the head drops back. Count the seconds until the infant returns head to upright position, noting also the ability to maintain the head upright.
21. Auditory. Ask the caretaker to call the infant's name from each side, holding the infant so the head can be easily turned. A rattle can be used instead at 6 to 10 inches from each ear.
22. Visual. Use a black-and-white bull's eye about 12 inches from the face first for horizontal tracking, next for vertical tracking, then for tracking well past the mid-line, and finally for following in a full circle.
23. Alert. The examiner uses voice or tongue clicking, holding the infant's face about 12 inches away from examiner's face, and notes that the infant is focusing and counts the seconds until the infant averts gaze.
24. Ventral suspension. The examiner supports the infant in the air under the abdomen, noting the infant's body position.
25. All fours/prone. Place the infant with the abdomen down on a firm surface, observe head and arm position.
26. Moro. Place one hand behind the infant's head, the other supporting the infant's back, then drop the infant 10 to 20 cm. Observe the hand and arm movements.
27. Suck. Wash your hands, place your finger in the infant's mouth with finger pad toward the palate, note sucking response. (Following universal precautions would mean using a gloved finger.)
28. Tremor. Note presence/absence of tremor and state of baby in which it occurs.
29. Responsiveness. The examiner talks to or clucks the tongue at the baby, trying to engage the baby and asks the caretaker about the infant's response to seeing a bottle or breast.
30. Vocalization. The examiner talks to or clucks the tongue at the infant and notes the infant's vocal response.
31. The examiner assesses the amount of stimulation needed to get the infant's attention.
32. The examiner assesses the infant's attention to the examiner throughout the evaluation.

GLOSSARY

Apathetic syndrome   Decreased responsiveness as defined by Prechtl (2,3). Infant displays a low intensity and high threshold for responses. Many responses absent; hypokinesis or decreased resistance to passive movements present. Infant is difficult to arouse.

Ataxia   Failure of muscle coordination. Motor ataxia indicates muscle incoordination; sensory ataxia indicates a loss of proprioception; truncal ataxia indicates a weakness of muscles of the trunk.

Athetosis   Slow writhing or wormlike repetitious movements of the distal portions of the extremities.

Chorea   Purposeless, nonrepetitive involuntary movements of the extremities and face, which interrupt a normal activity.

Double hemiparesis   Asymetrical spastic hemiparesis affecting the upper limbs more than the lower.

Hemiparesis   Weakness of the upper and lower extremities on the same side of the body, the arm usually being more affected than the leg.

Hemisyndrome   Asymmetry of response as defined by Prechtl (2,3). At least three items in an examination show an asymmetry in motility, motor system, posture, or responses.

Hyperexcitable syndrome Increased responsiveness to various stimuli as defined by Prechtl (2,3). Low-frequency, high-amplitude tremor, high or medium intensity of tendon reflexes, and Moro response with low threshold. There also may be hyperkinesis with increased resistance to passive movement, prolonged crying, and an instability of states.

Hypertonia of elevators palpebrae superiori   Upper part of the sclera and entire iris are visible but the globe is positioned normally. This gives a "bright eyed" appearance to an infant in its mildest form. This finding is rarely isolated and is seen with general hyperexcitability (15).

Monoparesis   Weakness of a single limb only.

Paraparesis   Weakness of the lower extremities only.

Paresis   Implies weakness rather than complete paralysis.

Plegia   Complete paralysis.

Sunset sign   Abnormal lowering of the globe in the orbit so that the lower lid covers more of the iris than usual and the sclera above the iris is visible. In newborn infants, particularly when they are drowsy, it is normal as long as it is not present at all times or in a fixed direction.

Tetraparesis   Synonym *Quadriparesis*. Weakness of all four limbs, which may or may not be symmetrical, the lower extremities usually being more affected than the upper. In the United States, the term "quadriparesis" is used, but it is a mixed word of Latin and Greek, compared with tetraparesis.

Tremor   Fine rhythmic involuntary movements with movement of agonist and antagonist muscles of equal amplitude. **Static tremor:** Present at rest. **Intention tremor:** Not present at rest but occurs when there is active movement. **Functional tremor:** Associated with anxiety or crying.

NEONATAL NEUROLOGICAL EXAMINATION (Dubowitz)

NAME	DATE OF EXAM	D.O.B./TIME	WEIGHT
HOSPITAL NO.	TIME	E.D.D.(L.N.M.P.)	LENGTH
	TIME AFTER FEEDING	E.D.D. (U-sound)	HEAD CIRC.
RACE	SEX	AGE	EXAMINER
GESTATIONAL AGE ASSESSMENT:	METHOD	SCORE	WEEKS

STATE | COMMENT | ASYMMETRY

CODE STATE AS FOLLOWS:
1 Deep sleep, no movement, regular breathing.
2 Light sleep, eyes shut, some movement.
3 Dozing, eyes opening and closing.
4 Awake, eyes open, minimal movement.
5 Wide awake, vigorous movement.
6 Crying.

HABITUATION (≤ state 3)

LIGHT
Repetitive flashlight stimuli (10) with 5 sec. gap.
Shutdown = 2 consecutive negative responses.

- No response.
- A. Blink response to first stimulus only. B. Tonic blink response. C. Variable response.
- A. Shutdown of movement but blink persists 2-5 stimuli. B. Complete shutdown 2-5 stimuli.
- A. Shutdown of movement but blink persists 6-10 stimuli. B. Complete shutdown 6-10 stimuli.
- A. Equal response to 10 stimuli. B. Infant comes to fully alert state. C. Startles + major responses throughout.

RATTLE
Repetitive stimuli (10) with 5 sec. gap.

- No response.
- A. Slight movement to first stimulus. B. Variable response.
- Startle or movement 2-5 stimuli, then shutdown.
- Startle or movement 6-10 stimuli, then shutdown.
- A. B. C. ─ Grading as above.

MOVEMENT & TONE
Undress infant.

POSTURE*
(At rest — predominant).

- (figures) (hips abducted). (hips adducted).
- Abnormal postures: A. Opisthotonus. B. Unusual leg extension. C. Asymm. tonic neck reflex.

ARM RECOIL
Infant supine. Take both hands, extend parallel to the body; hold approx. 2 secs. and release.

- No flexion within 5 secs.
- Partial flexion at elbow >100° within 4-5 secs.
- Arms flex at elbow to <100° within 2-3 secs.
- Sudden jerky flexion at elbow immediately after release to <60°.
- Difficult to extend; arm snaps back forcefully.

ARM TRACTION
Infant supine; head midline; grasp wrist, slowly pull arm to vertical. Angle of arm scored and resistance noted at moment infant is initially lifted off and watched until shoulder off mattress. Do other arm.

- Arm remains fully extended.
- Weak flexion maintained only momentarily.
- Arm flexed at elbow to 140° and maintained 5 secs.
- Arm flexed at approx. 100° and maintained.
- Strong flexion of arm <100° and maintained.

LEG RECOIL
First flex hips for 5 secs., then extend both legs of infant by traction on ankles; hold down on the bed for 2 secs. and release.

- No flexion within 5 secs.
- Incomplete flexion of hips within 5 secs.
- Complete flexion within 5 secs.
- Instantaneous complete flexion.
- Legs cannot be extended; snap back forcefully.

LEG TRACTION
Infant supine. Grasp leg near ankle and slowly pull toward vertical until buttocks 1-2" off. Note resistance at knee and score angle. Do other leg.

- No flexion.
- Partial flexion, rapidly lost.
- Knee flexion 140-160° and maintained.
- Knee flexion 100-140° and maintained.
- Strong resistance; flexion <100°.

POPLITEAL ANGLE
Infant supine. Approximate knee and thigh to abdomen; extend leg by gentle pressure with index finger behind ankle.

- 180-160°
- 150-140°
- 130-120°
- 110-90°
- <90°

HEAD CONTROL (post. neck m.)
Grasp infant by shoulders and raise to sitting position; allow head to fall forward; wait 30 secs.

- No attempt to raise head.
- Unsuccessful attempt to raise head upright.
- Head raised smoothly to upright in 30 secs. but not maintained.
- Head raised smoothly to upright in 30 secs. and maintained.
- Head cannot be flexed forward.

HEAD CONTROL (ant. neck m.)
Allow head to fall backward as you hold shoulders; wait 30 secs.

- Grading as above.
- Grading as above.
- Grading as above.
- Grading as above.

HEAD LAG*
Pull infant toward sitting posture by traction on both wrists. Also note arm flexion.

(figures)

VENTRAL SUSPENSION*
Hold infant in ventral suspension; observe curvature of back, flexion of limbs and relation of head to trunk.

(figures)

HEAD RAISING IN PRONE POSITION
Infant in prone position with head in midline.

- No response.
- Rolls head to one side.
- Weak effort to raise head and turns raised head to one side.
- Infant lifts head, nose and chin off.
- Strong prolonged head lifting.

ARM RELEASE IN PRONE POSITION
Head in midline, infant in prone position; arms extended alongside body with palms up.

- No effort.
- Some effort and wriggling.
- Flexion effort but neither wrist brought to nipple level.
- One or both wrists brought at least to nipple level without excessive body movement.
- Strong body movement with both wrists brought to face, or 'press-ups.'

SPONTANEOUS BODY MOVEMENT DURING EXAMINATION
Infant supine.
If no spont. movement try to induce by cutaneous stimulation.

- None or minimal. Induced.
- A. Sluggish. B. Random, incoordinated. C. Mainly stretching.
- Smooth movements alternating with random, stretching, athetoid or jerky.
- Smooth alternating movements of arms and legs with medium speed and intensity.
- Mainly: A. Jerky movement. B. Athetoid movement. C. Other abnormal movement.

TREMORS
Mark Fast (> 6/sec.) or Slow (< 6/sec.)

- No tremor.
- Tremors only in state 5-6.
- Tremors only in sleep or after Moro and startles.
- Some tremors in state 4.
- Tremulousness in all states.

STARTLES

- No startles.
- Startles to sudden noise, Moro, bang on table only.
- Occasional spontaneous startle.
- 2-5 spontaneous startles.
- 6+ spontaneous startles.

ABNORMAL MOVEMENT OR POSTURE

- No abnormal movement.
- A. Hands clenched but open intermittently. B. Hands do not open with Moro.
- A. Some mouthing movement. B. Intermittent adducted thumb.
- A. Persistently adducted thumb. B. Hands clenched all the time.
- A. Continuous mouthing movement. B. Convulsive movements.

*If asymmetrical or atypical, draw in on nearest figure.

						STATE	COMMENT	ASYMMETRY

REFLEXES

TENDON REFLEXES Biceps jerk. Knee jerk. Ankle jerk.	Absent.		Present.	Exaggerated.	Clonus.			
PALMAR GRASP Head in midline. Put index finger from ulnar side into hand and gently press palmar surface. Never touch dorsal side of hand.	Absent.	Short, weak flexion.	Medium strength and sustained flexion for several secs.	Strong flexion; contraction spreads to forearm.	Very strong grasp, infant easily lifts off bed.			
ROOTING Infant supine, head midline. Touch each corner of the mouth in turn (stroke laterally).	No response.	A. Partial weak head turn but no mouth opening. B. Mouth opening, no head turn.	Mouth opening on stimulated side with partial head turning.	Full head turning, with or without mouth opening.	Mouth opening with very jerky head turning.			
SUCKING Infant supine; place index finger (pad towards palate) in infant's mouth; judge power of sucking movement after 5 secs.	No attempt.	Weak sucking movement: A. Regular. B. Irregular.	Strong sucking movement, poor stripping: A. Regular. B. Irregular.	Strong regular sucking movement with continuing sequence of 5 movements. Good stripping.	Clenching but no regular sucking.			
WALKING (states 4,5) Hold infant upright, feet touching bed, neck held straight with fingers.	Absent.		Some effort but not continuous with both legs.	At least 2 steps with both legs.	A. Stork posture, no movement. B. Automatic walking.			
MORO One hand supports infant's head in midline, the other the back. Raise infant to 45° and when infant is relaxed let head fall through 10°. Note if jerky. Repeat 3 times.	No response, or opening of hands only.	Full abduction at the shoulder and extension of the arm.	Full abduction but only delayed or partial adduction.	Partial abduction at shoulder and extension of arms followed by smooth adduction. A. Abd>Add B. Abd=Add C. Abd<Add	A. No abduction or adduction; extension only. B. Marked adduction only.			

NEUROBEHAVIORAL ITEMS

EYE APPEARANCES	Sunset sign. Nerve palsy.	Transient nystagmus. Strabismus. Some roving eye movement.	Does not open eyes.	Normal conjugate eye movement.	A. Persistent nystagmus. B. Frequent roving movement. C. Frequent rapid blinks.			
AUDITORY ORIENTATION (states 3,4) To rattle. (Note presence of startle.)	A. No reaction. B. Auditory startle but no true orientation.	Brightens and stills; may turn toward stimuli with eyes closed.	Alerting and shifting of eyes; head may or may not turn to source.	Alerting; prolonged head turns to stimulus; search with eyes.	Turning and alerting to stimulus each time on both sides.			
VISUAL ORIENTATION (state 4) To red woolen ball.	Does not focus or follow stimulus.	Stills; focuses on stimulus; may follow 30° jerkily; does not find stimulus again spontaneously.	Follows 30-60° horizontally; may lose stimulus but finds it again. Brief vertical glance.	Follows with eyes and head horizontally and to some extent vertically, with frowning	Sustained fixation; follows vertically, horizontally, and in circle.			
ALERTNESS (state 4)	Inattentive; rarely or never responds to direct stimulation.	When alert, periods rather brief; rather variable response to orientation.	When alert, alertness moderately sustained; may use stimulus to come to alert state.	Sustained alertness; orientation frequent, reliable to visual but not auditory stimuli.	Continuous alertness, which does not seem to tire, to both auditory and visual stimuli.			
DEFENSIVE REACTION A cloth or hand is placed over the infant's face to partially occlude the nasal airway.	No response.	A. General quietening. B. Non-specific activity with long latency.	Rooting; lateral neck turning, possibly neck stretching.	Swipes with arm.	Swipes with arm with rather violent body movement.			
PEAK OF EXCITEMENT	Low level arousal to all stimuli, never > state 3.	Infant reaches state 4-5 briefly but predominantly in lower states.	Infant predominantly state 4 or 5, may reach state 6 after stimulation but returns spontaneously to lower state.	Infant reaches state 6 but can be consoled relatively easily.	A. Mainly state 6. Difficult to console, if at all. B. Mainly state 4-5 but if reaches state 6 cannot be consoled.			
IRRITABILITY (states 3, 4, 5) Aversive stimuli: Uncover Ventral susp. Undress Moro Pull to sit Walking reflex Prone	No irritable crying to any of the stimuli.	Cries to 1-2 stimuli.	Cries to 3-4 stimuli.	Cries to 5-6 stimuli.	Cries to all stimuli.			
CONSOLABILITY (state 6)	Never above state 5 during examination, therefore not needed.	Consoling not needed. Consoles spontaneously.	Consoled by talking, hand on belly or wrapping up.	Consoled by picking up and holding; may need finger in mouth.	Not consolable.			
CRY	No cry at all.	Only whimpering cry.	Cries to stimuli but normal pitch.	Lusty cry to offensive stimuli, normal pitch.	High-pitched cry, often continuous.			

NOTES Record any abnormal signs (e.g., facial palsy, contractures, etc.). Draw if possible.

Adapted with permission from Dubowitz L, Dubowitz V: *The Neurological Assessment of the Preterm and Full-term Newborn Infant*, Clinics in Developmental Medicine No. 79, London: William Heinemann Medical Books, Ltd. 1981. Copyright by Spastics International Medical Publications, 5A Netherhall Gardens, London NW3 5RN. Available in U.S. from J.B. Lippincott Company in Philadelphia 19105.

Figure 32. Dubowitz Neonatal Neuro Examination form.

References

1. Illingworth RS. *The Development of the Infant and Young Child.* 5th ed. Edinburgh, Scotland: Churchill Livingstone; 1974.
2. Prechtl H, Beintema D. *The Neurologic Examination of the Full-Term Newborn Infant.* London: SIMP Heinemann: 1964. [Clin Dev Med, Vol. 12.]
3. Prechtl H. *The Neurological Examination of the Full-Term Newborn Infant.* 2nd ed. Philadelphia: JB Lippincott; 1977. [Clin Dev Med, Vol. 63.]
4. André-Thomas, Chesni Y, Saint-Anne-Dargassies S. The neurological examination of the infant. Little Club *Clin Dev Med* 1960.
5. Saint-Anne Dargassies S. *Neurological Development in the Full-Term and Premature Neonate.* 1st ed. Amsterdam: Elsevier; 1977.
6. Amiel-Tison C. Neurological evaluation of the maturity of newborn infants. *Arch Dis Child* 1968;43:89–93.
7. Volpe JJ. Neurology of the Newborn. 3rd ed. Philadelphia: WB Saunders; 1995.
8. Tousen BCL, Bierman-Van Endenburg M, Jurgens-Van der Zee A. The neurological screening of fullterm newborn infants. *Dev Med Child Neurol* 1977;19:739.
9. Capute AJ, Palmer FB, Shapiro BK, Wachtel RC, Ross A, Accardo PJ. Primitive reflex profile: a quantitation of primitive reflexes in infancy. *Dev Med Child Neurol* 1984;26:375–383.
10. Ellison P. The infant neurological examination. *Adv Dev Behav Pediatr* 1990;9:75–138.
11. Dubowitz LMD, Dubowitz V. *The Neurologic Assessment of the Preterm and Full-Term Newborn Infant.* London: Spastics International Publications; 1981. [Clin Dev Med Vol. 79.]
12. Morgan AM, Koch V, Lee V, Aldag J. Neonatal neurobehavioral examination. A new instrument for quantitative analysis of neonatal neurological status. *Phys Ther* 1988;68:1352–1358.
13. Allen MC, Capute AJ. Neonatal neurodevelopmental examination as a predictor of neuromotor outcome in premature infants. *Pediatrics* 1989;83:498.
14. Dubowitz LM, Dubowitz V, Goldberg C. Clinical assessment of gestational age in the newborn infant. *J Pediatr* 1970;77:1–10.
15. Amiel-Tison C, Grenier A. *Neurological Assessment During the First Year of Life.* 1st ed. New York: Oxford University Press; 1986.
16. Sheridan-Pereira M, Ellison PH, Helgeson V. The construction of a scored neonatal neurological examination for assessment of neurological integrity in full-term neonates. *J Dev Behav Pediatr* 1991;12:25–30.
17. Ellison P. The neurologic examination of the newborn and infant. In: David RB, ed. *Pediatric Neurology for the Clinician.* Norwalk, CT: Appleton & Lange; 1992:19–64.
18. Allen MC, Capute AJ. The evolution of primitive reflexes in extremely premature infants. *Pediatr Res* 1986;20:1284–1289.
19. Cohen SE, Parmelee AH. Prediction of five-year Stanford-Binet scores in preterm infants. *Child Dev* 1983;54:1242–1253.
20. Howard J, Parmelee AH Jr, Kopp CB, Littman B. A neurologic comparison of pre-term and full-term infants at term conceptional age. *J Pediatr* 1976;88:995–1002.
21. Kopp CB, Sigman M, Parmelee AH, Jeffrey WE. Neurological organization and visual fixation in infants at 40 weeks conceptional age. *Dev Psychobiol* 1975;8:165–170.
22. Medoff-Cooper B, Delivoria-Papadopoulos M, Brooten D. Serial neurobehavioral assessments in preterm infants. *Nurs Res* 1991;40:94–97.
23. Parmelee AH Jr, Minkowski A, Saint-Anne Dargassies S, et al. Neurological evaluation of the premature infant. A follow-up study. *Biol Neonate* 1970;15:65–78.
24. Brazelton TB. *Neonatal Behavioral Assessment Scale.* 1st ed. Philadelphia: Spastics International Medical Publications with JB Lippincott; 1973. [Clin Dev Med, Vol. 50.]
25. Brazelton TB. *Neonatal Behavioral Assessment Scale.* 2nd ed. Philadelphia: JB Lippincott; 1984. [Clin Dev Med, Vol. 88.]
26. Brazelton TB. Behavioral competence. In: Avery GB, Fletcher MA, MacDonald MG, eds. *Neonatology: Pathophysiology and Management of the Newborn.* 4th ed. Philadelphia: JB Lippincott; 1994:289–300.
27. Widmayer SM, Filed TM. Effects of Brazelton demonstrations on early interactions of preterm infants and their teenage mothers. *Infant Behav Dev* 1980;3:79–89.
28. Myers BJ. Early intervention using Brazelton training with middle-class mothers and fathers of newborns. *Child Dev* 1982;53:462–471.
29. Worobey J, Belsky J. Employing the Brazelton scale to influence mothering: an experimental comparison of three strategies. *Dev Psychol* 1982;18:736–743.
30. Parmelee AH. Neurophysiological and behavioral organization of premature infants in the first months of life. *Biol Psychiatry* 1975;10:501–512.
31. Als H, Lester BM, Tronick EC, Brazelton TB. Towards a research instrument for the assessment of preterm infants' behavior (APIB). In: Fitzgerald HE, Lester BM, Yogman MW, eds. *Theory and Research in Behavioral Pediatrics.* Vol. I. New York: Plenum; 1982:35.
32. Als H, Lester BM, Tronick EC, Brazelton TB. Manual for the assessment of preterm infants' behavior (APIB). In: Fitzgerald HE, Lester BM, Yogman MW, eds. *Theory and Research in Behavioral Pediatrics.* Vol. 1. New York: Plenum; 1982:65.
33. Lester BM, Boukydis CF, MM, Censullo M, Zahr L, Brazelton TB. Behavioral and psychophysiologic assessment of the preterm infant. *Clin Perinatol* 1990;17:155–171.
34. Als H, Lawhon G, Brown E, et al. Individualized behavioral and environmental care for the very low birth weight preterm infant at high risk for bronchopulmonary dysplasia: neonatal intensive care unit and developmental outcome. *Pediatrics* 1986;78:1123–1132.
35. Thoman EB. Sleeping and waking states in infants: a functional perspective. *Neurosci Biobehav Rev* 1990;14:93–107.
36. Thoman EB, Glazier RC. Computer scoring of motility patterns for states of sleep and wakefulness: human infants. *Sleep* 1987;10:122–129.

37. Thoman EB, Davis DH, Denenberg VH. The sleeping and waking states of infants: correlations across time and person. *Physiol Behav* 1987;41:531–537.
38. Lipsitz PJ. A proposed narcotic withdrawal score for use with newborn infants. A pragmatic evaluation of its efficacy. *Clin Pediatr* (Phila) 1975;14:592–594.
39. Finnegan LP. Neonatal abstinence syndrome: assessment and pharmacotherapy. In: Rubaltelli FF, Granati B, eds. *Neonatal Therapy: An Update*. New York: Elsevier; 1986:122–146.
40. Sarnat HB, Sarnat MS. Neonatal encephalopathy following fetal distress. A clinical and electroencephalographic study. *Arch Neurol* 1976;33:696–705.
41. Amiel-Tison C, Ellison P. Birth asphyxia in the fullterm newborn: early assessment and outcome. *Dev Med Child Neurol* 1986;28:671–682.
42. Ostrea EM, Lucena JL, Silvestre MA. The infant of the drug-dependent mother. In: Avery GB, Fletcher MA, MacDonald MG, eds. *Neonatology: Pathophysiology and Management of the Newborn*. 4th ed. Philadelphia: JB Lippincott; 1994:1300–1333.
43. Jhaveri MK, Kumar SP. Passage of the first stool in very low birth weight infants. *Pediatrics* 1987; 79:1005–1007.
44. Verma A, Dhanireddy R. Time of first stool in extremely low birth weight (#1000 grams) infants. *J Pediatr* 1993;122:626–629.
45. Sherry SN, Kramer I. The time of passage of the first stool and first urine by the newborn infant. *J Pediatr* 1955;46:158–159.
46. Clark D. Times of the first void and stool in 500 newborns. *Pediatrics* 1977;60:457.
47. MacKinnon JA, Perlman M, Kerpalani H, Rehan V, Sauve R, Kovacs L. Spinal cord injury at birth: diagnostic and prognostic data in twenty-two patients. *J Pediatr* 1993;122:431–437.
48. Molnar GE. Brachial plexus injury in the newborn infant. *Pediatr Rev* 1984;6:110–115.
49. Walle T, Hartikainen-Sorri AL. Obstetric shoulder injury. Associated risk factors, prediction and prognosis. *Acta Obstet Gynecol Scand* 1993;72:450–454.
50. Baskett TF, Allen AC. Perinatal implications of shoulder dystocia. *Obstet Gynecol* 1995;86:14–17.
51. Jackson ST, Hoffer MM, Parrish N. Brachial-plexus palsy in the newborn. *J Bone Joint Surg [Am]* 1988;70:1217–1220.
52. al-Qattan MM, Clarke HM, Curtis CG. Klumpke's birth palsy. Does it really exist? *J Hand Surg [Br]* 1995;20:19–23.
53. Eng GD. Brachial plexus palsy in newborn infants. *Pediatrics* 1971;48:18–24.
54. Kurtzberg D, Vaughan HGJ, Daum C, Grellong BA, Albin S, LR. Neurobehavioral performance of low-birth-weight infants at 40 weeks conceptional age: comparison with normal fullterm infants. *Dev Med Child Neurol* 1979;21:590–607.
55. Majnemer A, Rosenblatt B, Riley PS. Influence of gestational age, birth weight, and asphyxia on neonatal neurobehavioral performance. *Pediatr Neurol* 1993;9:181–186.
56. Dubowitz V. Evaluation and differential diagnosis of the hypotonic infant. *Pediatr Rev* 1985;6:237–243.
57. Sarnat HB. Olfactory reflexes in the newborn infant. *J Pediatr* 1978;92:624–626.
58. Sullivan RM, Taborsky-Barba S, Mendoza R, et al. Olfactory classical conditioning in neonates. *Pediatrics* 1991;87:511–518.
59. Anderson RB, Rosenblith JF. Photic sneeze reflex in the human newborn. *Dev Psychobiol* 1968;1:65.
60. Peroutka SJ, Peroutka LA. Autosomal dominant transmission of the "photic sneeze reflex," *N Engl J Med* 1984:599–600.
61. Millen SJ, Baruah JK. Congenital hypoplasia of the depressor anguli oris muscle in the differential diagnosis of facial paralysis. *Laryngoscope* 1983;93:1168–1170.
62. Falco NA, Eriksson E. Facial nerve palsy in the newborn: incidence and outcome [see comments]. *Plast Reconstr Surg* 1990;85:1–4.
63. Saito H, Takeda T, Kishimoto S. Neonatal facial nerve defect. *Acta Otolaryngol Suppl (Stockh)* 1994;510:77–81.
64. Bergman I, May M, Wessel HB, Stool SE. Management of facial palsy caused by birth trauma. *Laryngoscope* 1986;96:381–384.
65. Allen MC, Capute AJ. Assessment of early auditory and visual abilities of extremely premature infants. *Dev Med Child Neurol* 1986;28:458–466.
66. Medoff-Cooper B, Verklan T, Carlson S. The development of sucking patterns and physiologic correlates in very-low-birth-weight infants. *Nurs Res* 1993;42:100–105.
67. Eng GD. Congenital torticollis. *Clin Proc Child Hosp Dist Columbia* 1968;24:75–81.
68. Crook CK, Lipsitt LP. Neonatal nutritive sucking: effects of taste stimulation upon sucking rhythm and heart rate. *Child Dev* 1976;47:518–522.
69. Stevenson RD, Allaire JH. The development of normal feeding and swallowing. *Pediatr Clin North Am* 1991;38:1439–1453.
70. Walter RS. Issues surrounding the development of feeding and swallowing. In: Tuchman DN, Walter RS, eds. *Disorders of Feeding and Swallowing in Infants and Children*. San Diego: Singular Publishing Group; 1994:27–35.
71. Kuban KC, Skouteli HN, Urion DK, Lawhon GA. Deep tendon reflexes in premature infants. *Pediatr Neurol* 1986;2:266–271.
72. Willms JL, Schneiderman H, Algranati PS. *Physical Diagnosis. Bedside Evaluation of Diagnosis and Function*. 1st ed. Vol. 1. Baltimore: Williams & Wilkins; 1994.
73. Slaby FJ, McCune SK, Summers RW. *Gross Anatomy in the Practice of Medicine*. 1st ed. Philadelphia: Lea & Febinger; 1994.
74. Vlach V. Evolution of skin reflexes in the first years of life. *Dev Med Child Neurol* 1989;31:196–205.
75. Capute AJ. Early neuromotor reflexes in infancy. *Pediatric Ann* 1986;15:217–226.
76. Capute AJ, Accardo PJ, Vining EPG, Rubenstein JE, Harryman S. *Primitive Reflex Profile*. Baltimore: University Park Press; 1978. [Monogr Dev Pediatr, Vol. I.]
77. Capute AJ, Shapiro BK, Accardo PJ, Wachtel RC, Ross A, Palmer FB. Motor functions: associated primitive reflex profiles. *Dev Med Child Neurol* 1982;24:662–669.

78. Capute AJ, Wachtel RC, Palmer FB, Shapiro BK, Accardo PJ. A prospective study of three postural reactions. *Dev Med Child Neurol* 1982;24:314–320.

79. Egan DF, Illingworth RS, MacKeith RC. Developmental screening 0–5 years. *Clin Dev Med* 1969;30:1–63.

80. Parker S, Zuckerman B, Bauchner H, Frank D, Vinci R, Cabral H. Jitteriness in full-term neonates: prevalence and correlates. *Pediatrics* 1990;85:17–23.

81. McGowan JD, Altman RE, Kanto WP Jr. Neonatal withdrawal symptoms after chronic maternal ingestion of caffeine. *South Med J* 1988;81:1092–1094.

82. D'Souza SW, Robertson IG, Donnai D, Mawer G. Fetal phenytoin exposure, hypoplastic nails, and jitteriness. *Arch Dis Child* 1991;66:320–324.

83. Wiswell TE, Cornish JD, Northam RA. Neonatal polycythemia: frequency of clinical manifestations and other associated findings. *Pediatrics* 1986;78:26–30.

84. Linder N, Moser AM, Asli I, Gale R, Livoff A, Tamir I. Suckling stimulation test for neonatal tremor. *Arch Dis Child* 1989;64:44–52.

85. Moro E. Das erste Tremenon. *Munch Med Wochenschr* 1918;65:1147.

86. Lesny I. A more sensitive way of eliciting the Moro response by pinching the epigastrium. *Dev Med Child Neurol* 1967;9:212–215.

87. Fredrickson WT, Brown JV. Gripping and moro responses: differences between small-for-gestational age and normal weight term newborns. *Early Hum Dev* 1980;4:69–77.

88. Bench J, Collyer Y, Langford C, Toms R. A comparison between the neonatal sound-evoked startle response and the head-drop (Moro) reflex. *Dev Med Child Neurol* 1972;14:308–317.

89. Chasnoff IJ, Burns WJ. The Moro reaction: a scoring system for neonatal narcotic withdrawal. *Dev Med Child Neurol* 1984;26:484–499.

90. Marinelli PV. The asymmetric tonic neck reflex. *Clin Pediatr* 1983;22:544–546.

91. Hoekelman RA. The physical examination in infants and children. In: Bates B, ed. *A Guide to Physical Examination and History Taking*. 5th ed. Philadelphia: JB Lippincott; 1991:561–635.

92. Ballard JL, Khoury JC, Wedig K, Wang L, Eilers-Walsman BL, Lipp R. New Ballard Score, expanded to include extremely premature infants. *J Pediatr* 1991;119:417–423.

93. Amiel-Tison C, Korobkin R, Esque-Vaucouloux MT. Neck extensor hypertonia: a clinical sign of insult to the central nervous system of the newborn. *Early Hum Dev* 1977;1:181–190.

94. Vollmer H. A new reflex in young infants. *Am J Dis Child* 1948;95:481.

95. Mitchell RG. The Landau reaction. *Dev Med Child Neurol* 1962;4:65.

APPENDIX

Appendix

GENERAL GROWTH MEASUREMENTS

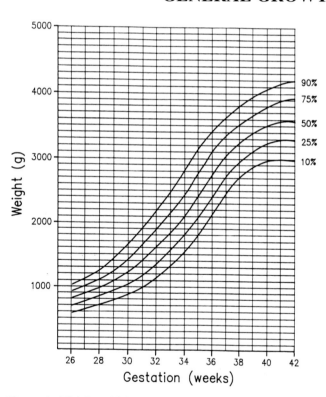

Figure 1. Weight at birth versus gestational age in female infants. Population is from singleton births, predominantly white, from middle socioeconomic class at low altitude. N = 13,564 females. The mean values for the lower gestational age infants is lower than those noted by Arbuckle (1), whereas the opposite is true for the older gestations. Reprinted with permission (2).

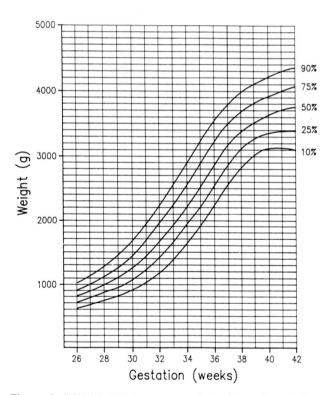

Figure 2. Weight at birth versus gestational age in male infants. Population is from singleton births, predominantly white, from middle socioeconomic class at low altitude. N = 14,399 males. The mean values for the lower gestational age infants is lower than those noted by Arbuckle (1), whereas the opposite is true for the older gestations. Reprinted with permission (2).

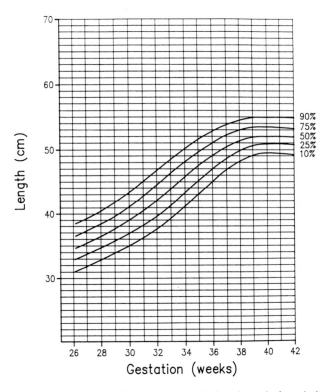

Figure 3. Length at birth versus gestational age in female infants. N = 13,544. Reprinted with permission (2).

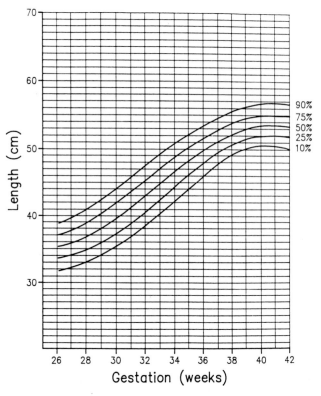

Figure 4. Length at birth versus gestational age in male infants. N = 14,609. Reprinted with permission (2).

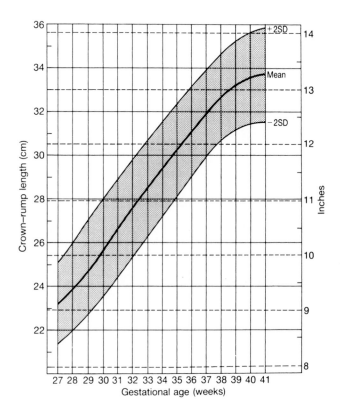

Figure 5. Crown–rump length at birth. Reprinted with permission (3). Data from Merlob et al. (4).

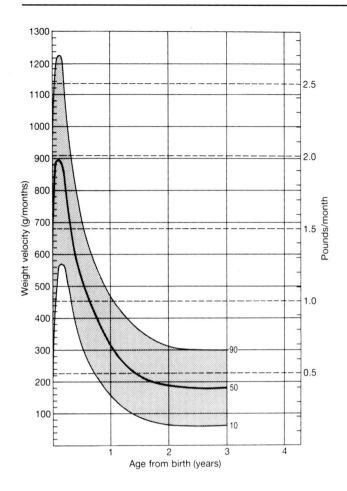

Figure 6. Weight velocity. Reprinted with permission (3).

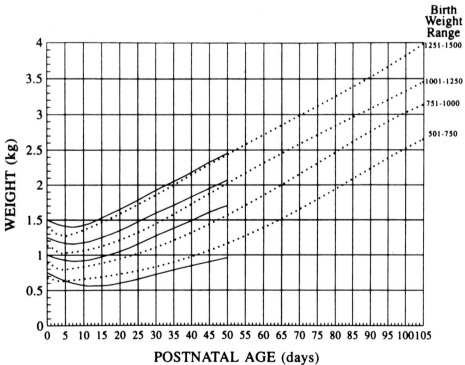

Figure 7. Average daily weight (grams) versus postnatal age (days) for infants with birth weight ranges of 501 to 750 g, 751 to 1,000 g, 1,001 to 1,250 g, and 1,251 to 1,500 g (dotted lines), plotted with the curves of Dancis (5), for infants with birth weights of 750 g, 1,000 g, 1,250 g, and 1,500 g (solid lines). Reprinted with permission (6).

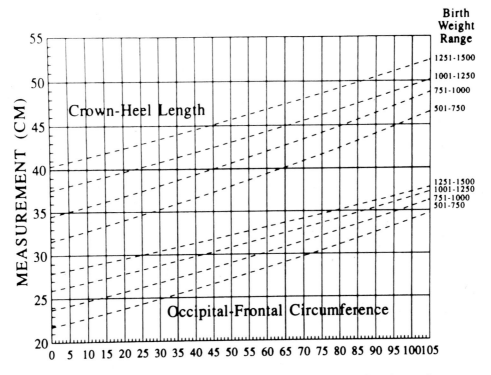

Figure 8. Average crown–heel length and occipital-frontal circumference (centimeters) versus postnatal age (days) for infants with birth weight ranges of 501 to 750 g, 751 to 1,000 g, 1,001 to 1,250 g, and 1,251 to 1,500 g. Reprinted with permission (6).

HEAD AND NECK REGION

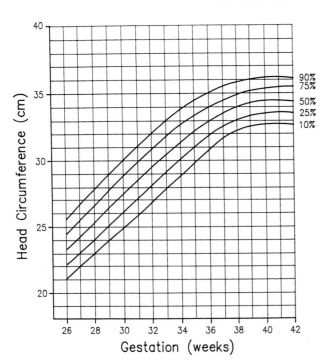

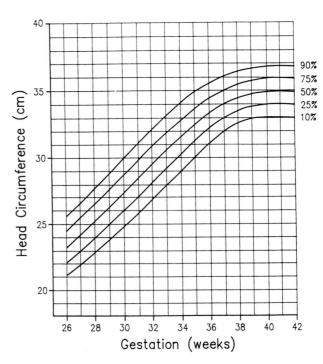

Figure 9. Head circumference at birth versus gestational age in female infants. N = 13,518. Reprinted with permission (2).

Figure 10. Head circumference at birth versus gestational age in male infants. N = 14,326. Reprinted with permission (2).

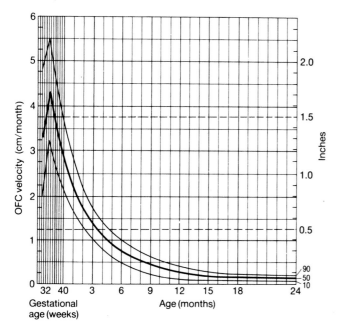

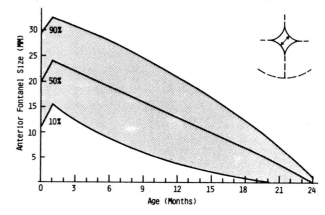

Figure 11. Velocity of growth in head circumference (OFC). Reprinted with permission (3). Data from Brandt (7).

Figure 12. Anterior fontanel size from term to 24 months of age for both sexes. Inset, technique of measurement of oblique diameter. Reprinted with permission (8).

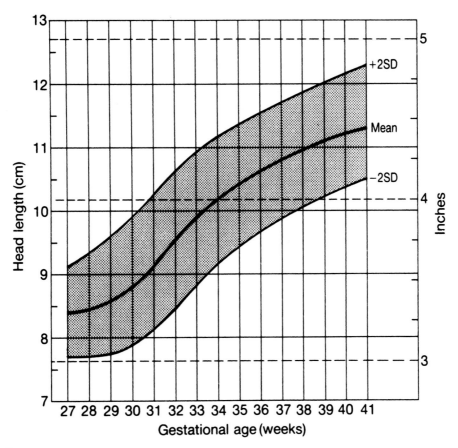

Figure 13. Head length at birth. Reprinted with permission (3). Data from Merlob et al. (9).

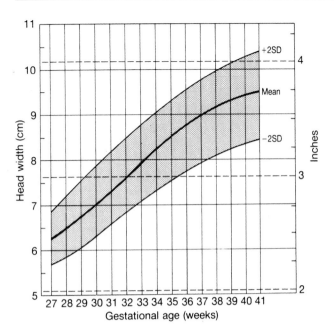

Figure 14. Head width at birth. Reprinted with permission (3). Data from Merlob et al. (9).

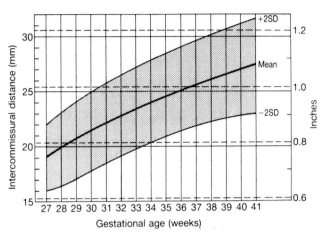

Figure 15. Intercommissural distance at birth. Reprinted with permission (3). Data from Merlob et al. (9).

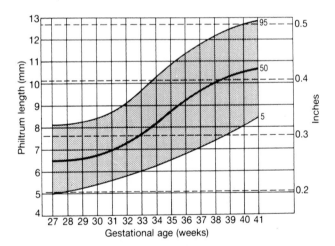

Figure 16. Philtrum length at birth. Reprinted with permission (3). Data from Merlob et al. (9).

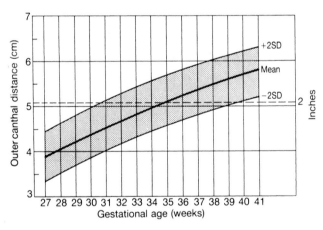

Figure 17. Outer canthal distance at birth. Reprinted with permission (3).

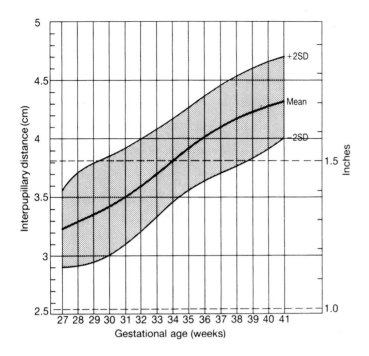

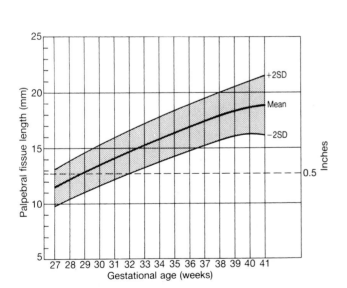

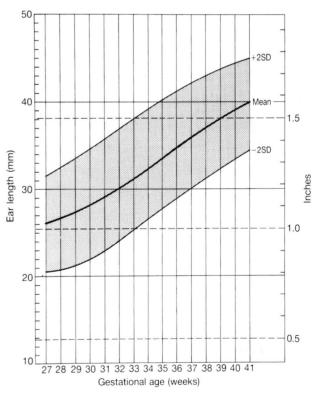

Figure 18. Interpupillary distance at birth. Reprinted with permission (3). Data from Merlob et al. (9).

Figure 19. Palpebral fissure length at birth. Reprinted with permission (3). Data from Merlob et al. (9).

Figure 20. Ear length at birth. Reprinted with permission (3). Data from Merlob et al. (9).

THE TRUNK REGION

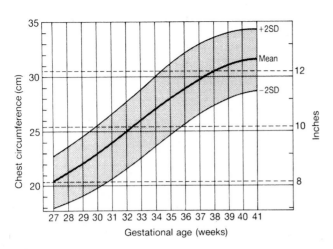

Figure 21. Chest circumference. Reprinted with permission (3). Data from Merlob et al. (9).

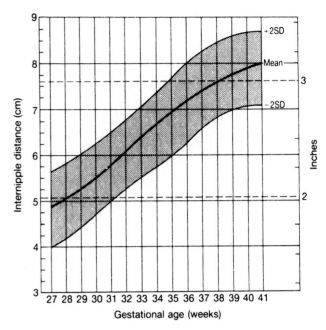

Figure 22. Internipple distance. Reprinted with permission (3). Data from Sivan et al. (10).

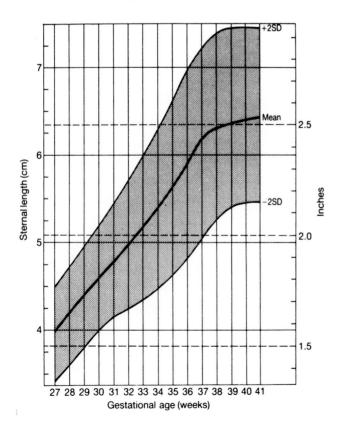

Figure 23. Sternal length of both sexes at birth. Reprinted with permission (3). Data from Sivan et al. (10).

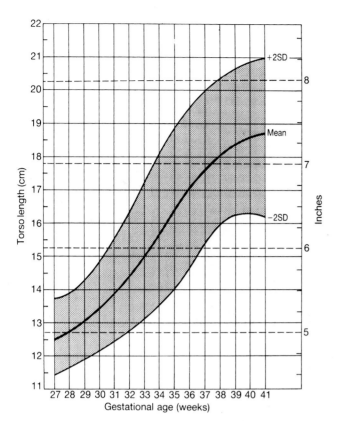

Figure 24. Torso length of both sexes at birth. Reprinted with permission (3). Data from Sivan et al. (10).

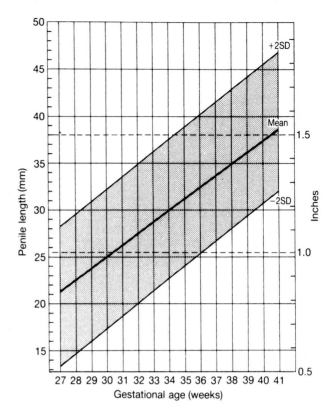

Figure 25. Penile length at birth. Reprinted with permission (3). Data from Feldman and Smith (11).

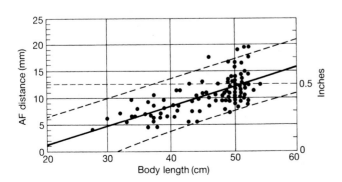

Figure 26. Distance (AF) from the anus to the posterior aspect of the introitus of the vagina (fourchette) in the female, or the end of scrotal skin in the male and the anterior border of the anal opening. A ratio of AF to anus–clitoris (AC) or fourchette–clitoris to AC has less variability. See glossary. Reprinted with permission (3). Data from Callegari et al. (12).

THE EXTREMITIES

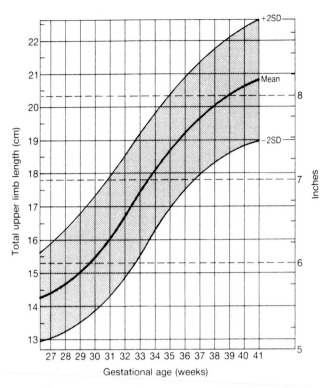

Figure 27. Total upper limb length at birth. Reprinted with permission (3). Data from Sivan et al. (13).

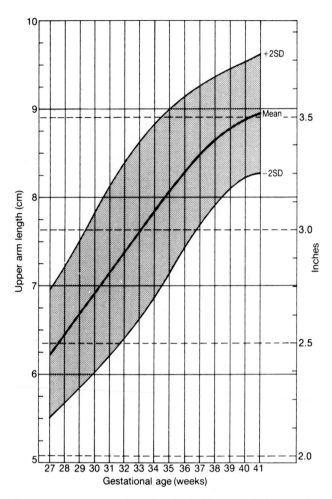

Figure 28. Upper arm length at birth. Reprinted with permission (3). Data from Sivan et al. (13).

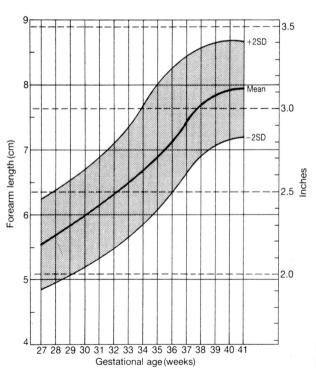

Figure 29. Forearm length at birth. Reprinted with permission (3). Data from Sivan et al. (13).

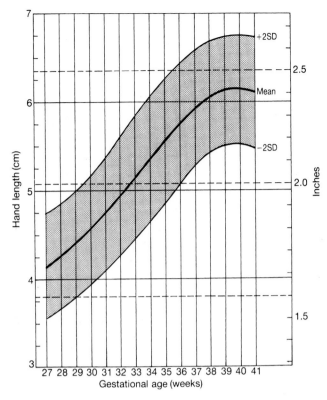

Figure 30. Hand length at birth. Reprinted with permission (3). Data from Sivan et al. (13).

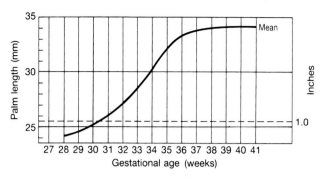

Figure 31. Palm length at birth. Reprinted with permission (3). Data from Sivan et al. (13).

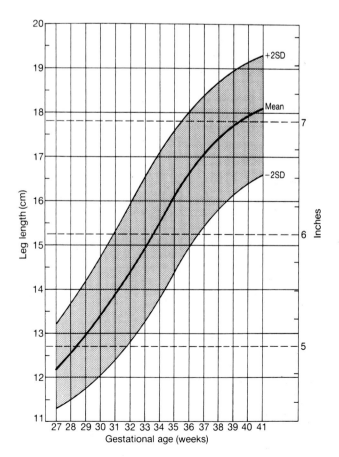

Figure 32. Leg length at birth. Reprinted with permission (3). Data from Merlob et al. (14).

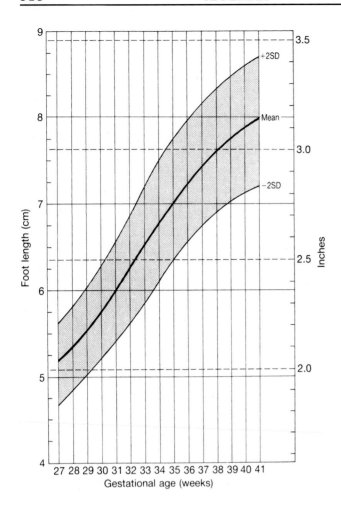

Figure 33. Foot length at birth. Reprinted with permission (3). Data from Merlob et al. (14).

PERIODS OF CRITICAL HUMAN DEVELOPMENT

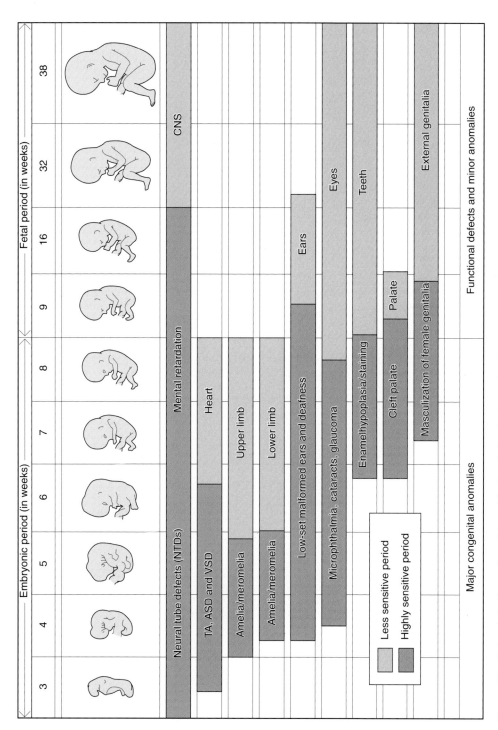

Figure 34. Schematic illustration of the critical periods of human development. Each part or organ of the embryo has a critical period when development may be disrupted, resulting in major congenital anomalies. Thereafter, environmental agents such as drugs and viruses may cause minor anomalies and functional disturbances. TA, truncus arteriosus; ASD, atrial septal defect; VSD, ventricular septal defect; NTDs, neural tube defects such as spina bifida. Adapted from (15).

BLOOD PRESSURE

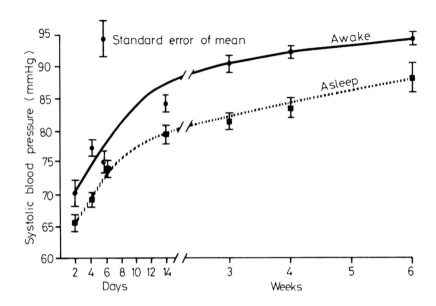

Figure 35. Increase in systolic blood pressure between ages 2 days and 6 weeks in infants awake and asleep. Values obtained by cuff measurements. Reprinted with permission (16).

Table 1. *Blood pressure values according to site and age*

Site and age (h)	Blood pressure (mm Hg)		
	Systolic	Diastolic	Mean
Right arm			
<36 (n = 140)	62.6 ± 6.9	38.9 ± 5.7	48.0 ± 6.2
>36 (n = 79)	68.4 ± 8.8[a]	43.5 ± 6.2[a]	53.0 ± 7.3
Total	64.7 ± 8.1	40.6 ± 6.2	49.8 ± 7.0
Calf			
<36 (n = 140)	61.9 ± 7.0	39.6 ± 5.3	47.6 ± 6.0
>36 (n = 79)	66.8 ± 10.1[a]	42.5 ± 7.3[a]	51.5 ± 9.0[a]
Total	63.6 ± 8.6	40.6 ± 6.3	49.0 ± 7.5

Values were obtained by cuff in 219 healthy term infants. Values are given as means ± SD.
[a] Significantly different from values in infants <36 h of age (p < 0.05).

Table 2. *Blood pressure ranges in different weight groups of a healthy population*

Birth weight (g)	n	Systolic (mm Hg)	Diastolic (mm Hg)
501–750	18	50–62	26–36
751–1,000	39	48–59	23–36
1,001–1,250	30	49–61	26–35
1,251–1,500	45	46–56	23–33
1,501–1,750	51	46–58	23–33
1,751–2,000	61	48–61	24–35

Values were obtained by cuff or umbilical arterial transducer in the first 3–6 h of life.
Reprinted from Hegyi T, Carbone MT, Anwar J, et al. Blood pressure ranges in premature infants. 1. The first hours of life. *J Pediatr* 1994;124:627–733.

Table 3. *Blood pressure ranges in different gestational age groups*

Gestational age (wk)	n	Systolic (mm Hg)	Diastolic (mm Hg)
<24	11	48–63	24–39
24–28	55	48–58	25–36
29–32	110	47–59	24–34
>32	68	48–60	24–34

Values were obtained by cuff or umbilical arterial transducer in the first 6 h of life.
Reprinted from Hegyi T, Carbone MT, Anwar J, et al. Blood pressure ranges in premature infants. 1. The first hours of life. *J Pediatr* 1994;124:627–733.

References

1. Arbuckle TE, Sherman GJ. An analysis of birth weight by gestational age in Canada. *Can Med Assoc J* 1989; 140:157–160,165.
2. Britton JR, Britton HL, Jennett R, Gaines J, Daily WJ. Weight, length, head and chest circumference at birth in Phoenix, Arizona. *J Reprod Med* 1993;38:215–222.
3. Hall JG, Froster-Iskenius UG, Allanson JE. *Handbook of Normal Physical Measurements.* Oxford, England: Oxford University Press; 1989.
4. Merlob P, Sivan Y, Reisner SH. Ratio of crown–rump distance to total length in preterm and term infants. *J Med Genet* 1986;23:338–340.
5. Dancis J, O'Connell JR, Holt LEJ. A grid for recording the weight of premature infants. *J Pediatr* 1948;33: 570–572.
6. Wright K, Dawson JP, Fallis D, Vogt E, Lorch V. New postnatal growth grids for very low birth weight infants. *Pediatrics* 1993;91:922.
7. Brandt I. Growth dynamics of low-birth-weight infants with emphasis on the prenatal period. In: eds. Falkner F, Tanner JM, eds. *Human Growth. A Comprehensive Treatise.* Vol. I. New York: Plenum; 1986:415–475.
8. Duc G, Largo RH. Anterior fontanel: size and closure in term and preterm infants. *Pediatrics* 1986;78: 904–908.
9. Merlob P, Sivan Y, Reisner SH. Anthropomorphic measurements of the newborn infant. *Birth Defects* 1984; 20:1–52.
10. Sivan Y, Merlob P, Reisner SH. Sternum length, torso length, and internipple distance in newborn infants. *Pediatrics* 1983;72:523–525.
11. Feldman KW, Smith DW. Fetal phallic growth and penile standards for newborn male infants. *J Pediatr* 1975; 86:395–398.
12. Callegari C, Everett S, Ross M, Brasel JA. Anogenital ratio: Measure of fetal virilization in premature and full-term newborn infants. *J Pediatr* 1987;111:240–243.
13. Sivan Y, Merlob P, Reisner SH. Upper limb standards in newborns. *Am J Dis Child* 1983;137:829–832.
14. Merlob P, Sivan Y, Reisner SH. Lower limb standard in newborns. *Am J Dis Child* 1984;138:140–142.
15. Moore KL, Persaud TVN, Shiota K. *Color Atlas of Clinical Embryology.* 1st ed. Philadelphia: WB Saunders; 1994.
16. Earley A, Fayers P, Ng S, Shinebourne EA, de Swiet M. Blood pressure in the first 6 weeks of life. *Arch Dis Child* 1980;55:755–757.

Subject Index